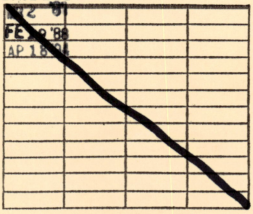

PRINCIPLES AND METHODS OF
ADAPTED PHYSICAL EDUCATION
AND RECREATION

PRINCIPLES AND METHODS OF
ADAPTED PHYSICAL EDUCATION AND RECREATION

DANIEL D. ARNHEIM, D.P.E., F.A.C.T.A.

Professor of Physical Education,
California State University at Long Beach,
Long Beach, California

DAVID AUXTER, Ed.D.

Professor of Developmental Physical Education,
Slippery Rock State College,
Slippery Rock, Pennsylvania

WALTER C. CROWE, Ed.D.

Professor of Physical Education,
California State University at Long Beach,
Long Beach, California

THIRD EDITION

with illustrations

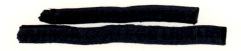

THE C. V. MOSBY COMPANY

Saint Louis   1977

THIRD EDITION

Previous editions copyrighted 1969, 1973

Printed in the United States of America

Distributed in Great Britain by Henry Kimpton, London

The C. V. Mosby Company
11830 Westline Industrial Drive, St. Louis, Missouri 63141

Library of Congress Cataloging in Publication Data

Arnheim, Daniel D
   Principles and methods of adapted physical education
and recreation.

   First-2d ed. published under title: Principles and
methods of adapted physical education
   Bibliography: p.
   Includes index.
   1.   Physical education for handicapped persons.
2.   Handicapped—Recreation.   3.   Physical education for
handicapped children.   4.   Handicapped children—Recreation.   I.   Auxter, David, joint author.   II   Crowe,
Walter C., joint author.   III.   Title.
GV445.A7 1977   613.7   76-46427
ISBN   0-8016-0320-X

CB/CB/B   9   8   7   6   5   4   3   2   1

To our families

PREFACE

The third edition has been extensively revised to reflect those changes in our society that 4 years ago, during our previous revision, were just emerging. In November 1975 President Gerald Ford signed into law P.L. 94-142, which defines the process by which education of the handicapped shall be conducted. This far-reaching legislation requires that, by 1978, school districts include in their programs individualized planning and due process guarantees for handicapped persons between 3 and 18 years of age. It is implied in this law that every teacher education agency should provide prospective teachers with experience in formulating individualized performance objectives based on assessment and in planning suitable programs that will enable handicapped persons to accomplish measurable objectives. The number of individuals requiring special services for various disabling conditions is expanding at an ever-increasing rate. There is today a pressing need for programs and specialists that will aid atypical individuals in developing to their full potentials. Physical education and recreation can play an integral role in this development.

In the early 1970's the Bureau of Education of the Handicapped, part of the United States Office of Education, listed physical education and recreation as a national educational priority for the handicapped. This emphasis at the federal level has stimulated innovation in physical education programming for the handicapped, as has the legislation included in P.L. 94-142. Educators are becoming more aware that each child can learn and develop at his own rate. Since each handicapped child is intrinsically different from other children, programming for the individual handicapped child based on his development and learning, in accord with his needs, should be emphasized.

This edition has retained descriptions of specific handicapping conditions and has included new sections on aphasia and autism in order to provide the physical educator with information about differing groups of children and acceptable generic programming for each group. However, the book also alerts the reader to educational processes that would tend to view children as children, irrespective of their handicaps. Therefore a new chapter on the developmental process has been added and the chapters on growth and development and perceptual-motor programs have been extensively revised and updated. New information has been included about somatotyping and about measuring nutritional status. Important relationships between assessment procedures, activity planning, and the use of performance objectives as they relate to programs for handicapped persons have been included. The concept of a systems approach (in which instructionally categorized objectives and diagnosis must be related before a specific need can be met in a specific child) is developed in Chapter 4 and in a new section on the profoundly mentally retarded. Over 100 new illustrations and numerous examples have been added throughout the book to clarify concepts presented.

This book is designed for the elementary and secondary school physical educator and the recreation specialist in adapted physical education. More specifically, it is intended as a text for colleges offering courses in adapted and corrective physical education and therapeutic recreation. The physical educator, recreational therapist, corrective therapist, school administrator, physician, school nurse, and physical therapist should all find the contents of this book pertinent to their particular fields.

Every effort has been made to show the reader both an academic and a practical approach to the field of adapted physical education. In all possible areas, theoretical material has been reinforced with information that is useful, practical, and feasible and that applies directly to the teaching situation.

The basic organization of this text is designed to lead the student from general to more specific concepts. There are four major divisions: the scope, key teaching and therapy skills, programming for specific problems, and organization and administration.

Part I provides the reader with an understanding of the diverse and complex nature of the atypical individual. In this section, we have focused attention on the way in which the handicapped are cared for in our society, the psychological implications of disability, the pertinent aspects of growth and development, and the perceptual implications for both typical and atypical individuals. A chapter on the developmental process directly relates these materials to meeting the individual needs of the handicapped person in our society.

Part II is designed to provide an in-depth discussion of the areas of therapeutic exercise, tension reduction, low vitality and physical fitness, and adaptive sports and games as they relate to all types of handicapped persons. Both individual and group approaches are presented to aid students in training and teachers in the field in preparing to readily apply these techniques and materials to their respective learning and teaching situations.

Part III supplies the reader specific information about the most prevalent types of disabilities found in the elementary school, high school, and college age groups and discusses the implications of these disabilities for the physical education program. Every attempt has been made to give timely and intensive coverage of these conditions and to discuss procedures for assessment and program planning.

Part IV includes information about the organization and administration of a district or school program, illustrates means of organizing adapted physical education classes for *instruction* in a variety of situations, and provides extensive coverage of facilities and equipment used in the adapted physical education and therapeutic recreation program.

Many hours and much hard work have gone into the creation of this edition. As is true of most productions of this type and magnitude, many individuals have assisted us. Therefore appreciation is accorded to those who have given their suggestions and comments on the first two editions, for their ideas have been incorporated into this edition. Special thanks are extended to Bob Fraleigh, Lyonel Avance, and Jim LaSasso for their excellent photographic contributions; Helene Arnheim and Carol Steffy for preparation of illustrations; and Helene Arnheim and Jessie Crowe for their help in typing and collating the final manuscript.

Daniel D. Arnheim

David Auxter

Walter C. Crowe

CONTENTS

ix

PART ONE

THE SCOPE

Part I is prepared for the reader as an introduction to the diverse and complex nature of disability and, more specifically, to the role of physical education for the handicapped. We have focused the reader's attention on how the handicapped child is cared for in our society, on the psychosocial implications of the handicapped child's disability, and on pertinent aspects of growth and development that affect the typical and atypical individual. In keeping with recent federal legislation and a trend of increased importance in several states, information is included on applying the developmental concept, performance objectives, and the systems approach.

1

SERVING THE DISABLED INDIVIDUAL

■ This is a time of great transition in the professional fields that deliver assistance to the mentally, physically, and emotionally inconvenienced. In our affluent society, no longer must the less endowed person be relegated to living outside the mainstream of life.

HISTORICAL IMPLICATIONS
Early history

In the highly developed countries of the world, the present level of concern for the well-being of the individual has evolved gradually over a period of many thousands of years. One of the characteristics of the typical early primitive cultures was their preoccupation with survival. Historians speculate that members of many early primitive societies who were unable to contribute to their own care were either put to death, allowed to succumb to a hostile environment, or forced to suffer a low social status. In some societies, persons displaying obvious behavioral deviations were considered—from a religious point of view—evil or, conversely, touched with divine powers.

These early inhabitants learned to fear the unknown and unexplained. Out of this anxious anticipation of danger or pain, they developed highly organized superstitions and religious expressions of the good and evil they saw in nature. The deviant individual, as the result, represented the unexplained and was often thought to be fraught with evil spirits.

Early sophisticated civilizations, such as China, Babylonia, and Egypt, depict in their writings the fear and superstition commonly associated with the atypical per-

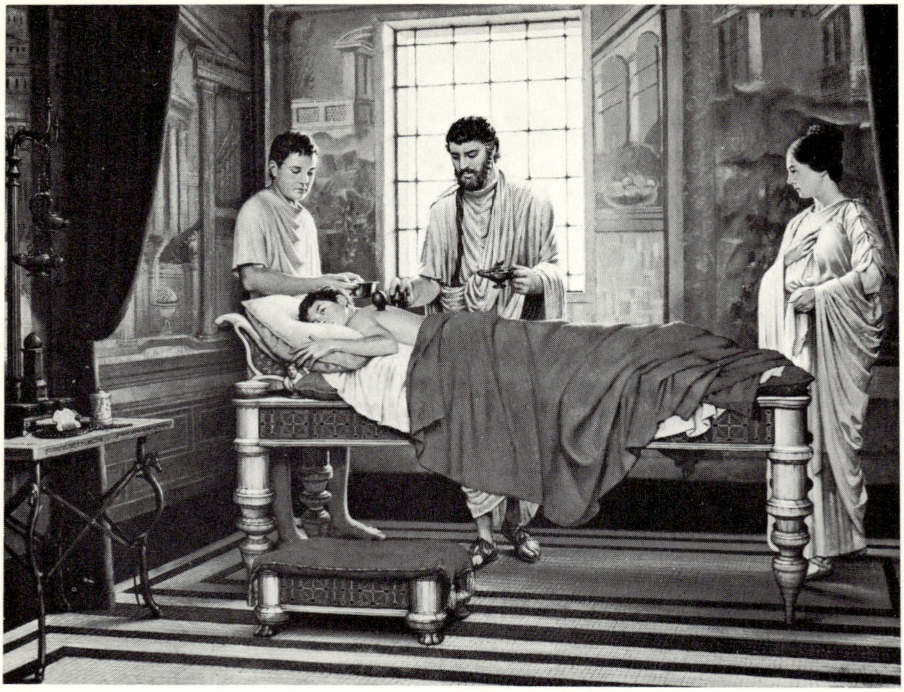

Fig. 1-1. Galen treating an ill child by cupping. (Courtesy Parke, Davis, & Co., Detroit.)

son. Even with the advent of modern science, the severely impaired or disabled were often regarded with disdain and suspicion, an attitude that is held by many persons in today's society.

The body perfection of the ancient Greeks and the rugged self-denial of the Spartans offered little, if any, place for the deformed or less endowed. Many deviant adults and children were made fools, jesters, and entertainers by the aristocrats of that period. Greek medicine, with the aid of Hippocrates (460-370 B.C.), made some inroads into changing man's reliance on supernaturalism by introjecting the logic of scientific reasoning. However, the chain of fear and superstition was not broken for long. After Greece's fall to the Roman Empire, its culture and scientific spirit degenerated. Even the brilliance of such persons as Claudius Galen (130-200 A.D.), a noted Greek physician, surgeon, and writer, could not impede the downward spiral (Fig. 1-1).

The medieval period brought with it self-denial for reasons of piety. As a result, the maimed, infirm, and mentally disturbed were often allowed to perish from a lack of care or become the recipients of cruel and inhuman treatment. Fear continued to cloud man's thoughts and found expression in the guise of religious doctrine. Any person different in behavior or appearance was thought to be a witch or possessed by the devil. Not until the late Renaissance period were man's primitive attitudes about the handicapped to be chipped away by scientific reason.

Humanitarianism and humanism

The Middle Ages gave way to the more positive period of the Renaissance, in which human dynamism again fulminated. Great social and cultural upheavals were about to take place. The seed of a social conscience had been planted. A genuine concern for the individual developed, giving the individual a dignity that was no longer sub-

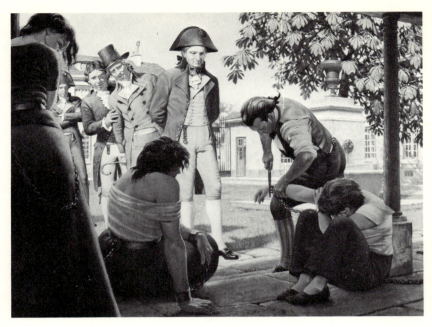

Fig. 1-2. Pinel unchains the insane. (Courtesy Parke, Davis, & Co., Detroit.)

merged in the extremes of asceticism. With a desire for social reform came a multitude of movements to improve man's life. Reforms dealing with peace, prison conditions, poverty, temperance, and insanity were organized and many social and moral problems were attacked in the first decade of the nineteenth century (Fig. 1-2). However, the main impetus for aiding the disabled did not occur until early in the twentieth century and as late as the early 1960's for the mentally retarded and the emotionally disturbed. The contributions of such figures as President Franklin D. Roosevelt, supporting the fight against crippling diseases such as poliomyelitis, and the Kennedy family, working to help the mentally retarded, can hardly be overlooked when discussing this country's humanitarian concerns.

In recent years, the philosophy of humanism, stemming primarily from humanitarian concerns as well as Gestalt psychology and existential philosophy, has emerged. In general, humanistic thought places the individual at the center of importance. Although cognitive and psychomotor factors are important in humanism, the affective domain takes precedence. Self-esteem, self-discovery, self-awareness, self-responsibility, self-evaluation, honesty in expressing feelings, and the courage to tempt failure stand out as highly important goals in the development of the individual.[8] Humanism is concerned with the individual's knowledge, understanding, and full, unconditional acceptance of the self, without which there cannot be acceptance by others.

Influences of war

Surges of social change often just precede or follow in the wake of great national upheaval. Such was the case with the United States just before and just after the Civil War. The national climate during the period that preceded the Civil War was gradually changing from the coldness of Puritanism to a greater warmth and a beginning acceptance of man's imperfection. A social awareness at this time indicated an interest in making the world a better place for all to live. However, social welfare institutions could not keep pace with the enigma created by the industrial revolution and the human exploitation that accompanied it. Not until public legislation, which occurred later, would many of these problems be resolved.

By the twentieth century, the public's interest in the physically handicapped had heightened to the extent that legislative action was taken to alleviate some of the financial burden on individuals in society. This stimulus for action came as a result of the great number of permanently injured industrial workers, the influenza pandemic, and the crippling infantile paralysis of 1916, plus the multitude of maimed World War I veterans who returned from fighting overseas.

World War I is marked as a period that greatly advanced medical and surgical techniques designed to help ameliorate many physically disabling conditions. Added to this, individuals were restored to usefulness by vocational and workshop programs. The interim between World War I and World War II marked a time in which state and federal legislation was enacted to promote vocational rehabilitation for both the civilian and the military disabled. The Smith-Sears Act of 1918 and the National Civilian Vocational Rehabilitation Act of 1920 were the forerunners of the Social Security Act of 1935 and the Vocational Rehabilitation Act of 1943, which provided the handicapped both physical and vocational rehabilitation.

With World War II came thousands of ill and incapacitated service personnel. Every conceivable means was employed to restore them to function as useful and productive members of society. Physical medicine became a new medical speciality. Many of the heretofore hospital services became autonomous ancillary medical fields. The paramedical specialties of physical therapy, occupational therapy, and corrective therapy considerably decreased the recovery time of many patients.

The present and future

How many handicapped persons currently reside in the United States? Until the 1970 census, this was a difficult question to answer. Reports indicate that there are over 11 million persons between the ages of 16 and 64 years who are not in institutions and are disabled and unable to work for 6 months or longer. In other words, 1 out of 11 Americans or 9% of its working force of 121 million were disabled by some chronically disabling condition. In general, the 1970 census revealed that those individuals who were handicapped and not in the mainstream of life earned less income, had less education, were employed less often, and represented more poverty than their working counterparts.[1, 12] In contrast to the proportion of handicapped persons of working age, there are estimated to be over 7.5 million handicapped children in America, representing 12% of the school-aged population.

Many disabling conditions are becoming extinct, while others are coming to the forefront. Poliomyelitis is almost a disease of the past and the destructive effects of German measles are being controlled, but as society imposes new and different demands on humans, other conditions emerge and become important. In recent years, more public and professional attention is being paid to the mentally retarded, learning disabled, and multiply handicapped child.

In the last few years, there has been a concerted effort made by those concerned with the handicapped to initiate *mainstreaming* of the handicapped wherever and whenever feasible. Mainstreaming, defined as the main impetus toward moving the inconvenienced into a fuller and more normalized life situation, has come primarily from the actions of parent groups throughout the country. By the exertion of political pressure on local and state boards of education and by other legal maneuvers, parents persuaded responsible leaders to provide more complete and comprehensive services for their disabled children.[1, 11]

Two recent court decisions have vastly affected mainstreaming of the handicapped child in school. The first decision, rendered in a suit by the Pennsylvania Association of Retarded Children (1971) in federal court, made it mandatory for a free public education to be given to all mentally retarded persons. A second court decision, *Mills v. the Board of Education of the District of Columbia* (1972), provided that all handicapped children in Pennsylvania, not just the mentally deficient, are to be given the right to an equal education. In summary, each school-aged child must be given ". . . a free and suitable publicly supported education regardless of the degree of the child's mental, physical or emotional disability or impairment. . . ."[1]

The Education Amendment of 1974, commonly known as P.L. 93-380, focuses on the placement for educational purposes of handicapped children in the least restrictive alternative environment. Implied in this law are means to ensure that these children will be educated with nonhandicapped children and that separate schooling of the handicapped will only occur when the nature of the disability is such that regular education cannot be effectively carried out.

P.L. 93-380 increases the heterogeneity of the classroom setting and thus places demands on the school and teacher that otherwise would not be present. This legislation requires individualization of the program for each learner. If the individual needs of all learners can be met, then the integration of the handicapped child into the mainstream of education becomes irrelevant. More current legislation, P.L. 94-142, ED, *Education for the Handicapped* (passed December 3, 1976), expressly states that the specially designed instruction must be conducted in physical education classes as well as in the academic classroom (Chapter 18).

Besides the obvious trend away from categorization, labeling, and separation of the inconvenienced from the mainstream of life, other trends in education are developing, for example, the large conventional clinical institution is giving way to more personal small group and home type settings. The halfway house as well as the sheltered workshop is increasingly being used to phase the handicapped into society.

Mainstreaming the atypical person into society ideally is a sound concept; however, it has many inherent problems. Not all handicapped individuals will profit from a totally mainstreamed existence and some may always require separate specialized care. Not every teacher is prepared or wants to be prepared to handle the handicapped. Finally, the American population in general must be educated to accept the "different" individual who was once kept apart from the mainstream of life.

One of the thrusts of this book will be to describe procedures for the assessment of each individual in order that plans for instructional intervention can be made and, where feasible, the individual can be mainstreamed.

Out of the concern of parents and small groups for the welfare of individuals grew many major organizations devoted to obtaining funds, establishing programs, and carrying on treatment and research activities. A sampling of some of these organizations follows:

1. Alexander Graham Bell Association for the Deaf, Inc.
   1537 30th St., NW.
   Washington, D.C., 20007
2. American Academy for Cerebral Palsy
   University Hospital School
   Iowa City, Iowa 52240
3. American Alliance for Health, Physical Education, and Recreation
   1201 16th St., NW
   Washington, D.C. 20036
4. American Association on Mental Deficiency
   5201 Connecticut Ave., NW
   Washington, D.C. 20016
5. American Cancer Society, Inc.
   219 East 42nd St.
   New York, N.Y. 10017
6. American Diabetes Association
   18 East 48th St.
   New York, N.Y. 10017

7. American Foundation for the Blind
   15 West 16th St.
   New York, N.Y. 10011
8. American Legion
   National Child Welfare Division
   P.O. Box 1055
   Indianapolis, Ind. 42206
9. American Medical Association
   535 North Dearborn St.
   Chicago, Ill. 60610
10. American Occupational Therapy Association, Inc.
    251 Park Ave., South
    New York, N.Y. 10010
11. American Physical Therapy Association
    1156 15th St., NW
    Washington, D.C. 20005
12. American Psychiatric Association
    1700 18th St., NW
    Washington, D.C. 20009
13. American Public Health Association, Inc.
    1015 18th St., NW
    Washington, D.C. 20036
14. Arthritis Foundation
    1212 Avenue of the Americas
    New York, N.Y. 10036
15. Association for the Aid of Crippled Children
    345 East 46th St.
    New York, N.Y. 10017
16. The Council for Exceptional Children
    1920 Association Dr.
    Reston, Va. 22091
17. Epilepsy Foundation of America
    111 West 57th St.
    New York, N.Y. 10019
18. Goodwill Industries of America, Inc.
    9200 Wisconsin Ave.
    Washington, D.C. 20014
19. ICD Rehabilitation and Research Center
    340 East 24th St.
    New York, N.Y. 10010
20. International Council for Exceptional Children
    1201 16th St., NW
    Washington, D.C. 20006
21. Joseph P. Kennedy, Jr. Foundation
    719 13th St., NW
    Washington, D.C. 20005
22. Muscular Dystrophy Association of America, Inc.
    1790 Broadway
    New York, N.Y. 10019
23. National Association for Mental Health
    10 Columbus Circle, Suite 1300
    New York, N.Y. 10019
24. National Association of the Deaf
    1575 Redwood Ave.
    Akron, Ohio 44301
25. National Association for Retarded Children (NARC)
    2709 Avenue E
    Arlington, Texas 76010
26. National Cystic Fibrosis Research Foundation
    521 5th Ave.
    New York, N.Y. 10017
27. National Easter Seal Society for Crippled Children and Adults
    2023 West Ogden Ave.
    Chicago, Ill. 60612
28. National Education Association
    1201 16th St., NW
    Washington, D.C. 20036
29. National Epilepsy League
    203 North Wabash Ave.
    Chicago, Ill. 60601
30. National Foundation for Asthmatic Children
    5601 West Trails End Rd.
    P.O. Box 5114
    Tuscon, Ariz. 85703
31. National Foundation for Neuromuscular Diseases
    250 West 57th St.
    New York, N.Y. 10019
32. National Foundation—March of Dimes
    1275 Momaroneck Ave.
    White Plains, N.Y. 10695
33. National Hemophilia Foundation
    25 West 39th St.
    New York, N.Y. 10018
34. National Kidney Disease Foundation
    342 Madison Ave.
    New York, N.Y. 10010
35. National Multiple Sclerosis Society
    257 Park Ave., South
    New York, N.Y. 10010
36. National Paraplegia Foundation
    333 North Michigan Ave.
    Chicago, Ill. 60601
37. National Rehabilitation Association
    1522 K Street, NW
    Washington, D.C. 20005
38. National Therapeutic Recreation Society
    1700 Pennsylvania Ave., NW
    Washington, D.C. 20006
39. National Tuberculosis Association
    1790 Broadway
    New York, N.Y. 10019
40. United Cerebral Palsy Association, Inc.
    66 East 34th St.
    New York, N.Y. 10016
41. United States Office of Education, Department of Health, Education, and Welfare
    7th and D Sts., SW
    Washington, D.C. 20202

CLINICAL SERVICES

Professional care of the temporarily or chronically inconvenienced is broadly based, encompassing the talents and dedication of many disciplines. All clinical services ideally join together, having as their primary goal the development of the physical, mental, social, cultural, and vocational potentialities of each disabled person they serve.

A number of disciplines are described herein to acquaint the reader with those hospital and institutional services particularly concerned with the handicapped. These services may be presented under three categories, namely, direct medical services, psychological services, and rehabilitative and habilitative services.

Direct medical services

In most clinical settings, there is direct medical service to the patient, including physicians' and nurses' care and support. Laboratory and x-ray services are extremely important adjuncts to the effective delivery of direct medical care to the patient.

All medical specialties lend their particular talents to the disabled, for example, a child with cerebral palsy might require the diagnostic or surgical ability of a neurologist, a muscle transplant by an orthopedic surgeon, and medical rehabilitation by the physiatrist. Behavioral problems would be seen by the psychiatrist or psychologist, whereas cases complicated by growth factors would require a consulting pediatrician.

Today's physicians, whatever their specialization, are beginning to see the value of taking the patient's care beyond the immediate pathological condition. In the rehabilitation or habilitation setting, physicians are concerned that their patients may live as fully as possible within the scope of specific handicaps and abilities. As members of intradisciplinary groups, physicians are usually charged with the responsibility of leadership and with final authority as to the care of the patient.

Psychological services

Almost always associated with any clinical setting concerned with the handicapped are the psychological services that deal with the client's emotional problems. The professional fields that usually come under this heading are psychiatry, psychology, clinical social work, and vocational counseling.

The psychiatrist is a physician who specializes in the study and treatment of mental illnesses. The psychiatrist focuses on the psychopathology that makes the individual unable to function effectively in society.

The psychologist, in contrast to the psychiatrist, is not a physician, but specializes in both normal and abnormal human behavior. Disciplines under the heading of psychology include clinical, educational, and counseling psychology. The clinical psychologist places the greatest emphasis on psychopathology, which stems from the disordered personality. In comparison, the educational and counseling psychologists place their emphasis on the normal personality. The educational psychologist is concerned with learning problems and maladaptation to the school setting, whereas the counseling psychologist deals primarily with normal personalities that exhibit problems.

As a specialist working with the handicapped, the psychologist must understand the many psychological problems that confront the patient and his family. A major handicap forces the individual to make many extreme personality adjustments. Faulty adjustments to these problems may result in psychopathological conditions requiring professional help. The rehabilitation psychologist serves to aid the patient by offering counseling on personal and occupational levels, making personality and vocational evaluations, and making referral to the psychiatrist in case of severe maladjustments.

The clinical social worker must have an understanding of the broad spectrum of intraprofessional specialties and how they affect each patient. The primary concern is with the personal effects of a disability, such as economics and the interpersonal relationship of family and friends. Often almost insurmountable problems involving social and environmental pressures are resolved by the professional and empathetic handling of the patient by the clinical social worker.

Vocational counseling in the total rehabilitation setting is one of the newest professions. The counselor is a specialist who has a broad knowledge of handicapping conditions, the rehabilitative process, and the needs of the disabled. An individual with a physical, mental, or emotional handicap is encouraged to achieve the maximum implementation of his capacities and abilities for employment. The fact must be emphasized that in our society, occupational independence is directly related to socioeconomic status and the individual's feelings of worth.

Rehabilitative and habilitative services

The term "rehabilitation" can generally be defined as the process of returning a disabled person to an effective level of physical, mental, and emotional health. On the other hand, the term "habilitation" refers to the process of assisting the disabled individual to live as effectively as his impairment will allow. There are many disciplines in the clinical setting (some of which have already been discussed) that are concerned with the ultimate functioning of the handicapped. Under this heading is a vast array of services for the disabled, depending on the type and scope of the clinical facility. Some of the more common professional practices are educational therapy, music therapy, orthotics and prosthetics, and the large number of therapies that concentrate on the movement of the patient.

Educational therapy

The educational therapist works primarily with the patient in the medium of communication skills. Through a variety of cognitive activities, the patient can attain self-expression, personal growth, and a sense of achievement. The patient in a hospital or institutional setting is provided with opportunities to take special classes to further his educational and vocational future. Recently, the educational therapist has gained importance, particularly in the area of learning disorders, acting within a psychoeducational setting. The educational therapist is usually an individual who has perhaps developed from a role in standard teaching to one in special education, for example, from remedial reading specialist to clinical educator.[9]

Music therapy

Because of its value as a recreational, creative, and therapeutic medium, music is becoming an increasingly important part of the treatment program in many hospitals and mental institutions. Music is known to produce varying degrees of physiological, psychological, and emotional responses in the human organism. Therefore its employment can serve as an important therapeutic adjunct to the total rehabilitation program. The music therapist can also encourage socialization of the patient through singing, dancing, and playing instruments.

Orthotics and prosthetics

When discussing the various kinds of professional assistance provided the physically impaired, it would be remiss to omit orthotics and prosthetics. Each has developed into a highly defined technology that aids the crippled patient in becoming more self-sufficient within the limitations of his particular disability. *Orthotics* offers the patient a number of possible benefits, namely, the prevention and correction of structural deformities, aid in supporting the body, and an adjunct to the control of involuntary movements. It provides the patient with a variety of self-help devices and splints made for his own requirements. *Prosthetics,* on the other hand, is the specialty of making and fitting artificial limbs and is becoming increasingly precise and sophisticated as new procedures and materials become available.[14]

Movement therapies

Of special interest to the physical educator are the many therapies found in institutions and hospitals that are based on movement behavior.

Physical therapy. Massage and heat have been used since the dawn of mankind for the amelioration of various illnesses. Physical therapy today is the process of treating physical impairments by the use of various physical modalities as prescribed by a qualified physician. The physical therapist utilizes a number of treatment devices to bring about a healing or rehabilitative response from the patient, namely, deep heat (diathermy, ultrasound), superficial heat (infrared heat, hydromassage, etc.), cryotherapy (cold therapy), electrical muscle stimulation, massage, mobilization techniques, manual muscle testing, and specific exercises for affected muscles and joints. Besides employing these modalities, the physical therapist may instruct the patient in the use of braces, wheelchairs, crutches, and prosthetic appliances and in activities of daily living.

Occupational therapy. Occupational therapy is a medically prescribed program that provides the patient with interesting activity that will develop varying degrees of physical strength, endurance, and, above all, hand dexterity. Through this medium, functional skills are learned that aid the patient's psychological outlook as well as help him to become self-sufficient and perhaps occupationally independent. The occupational therapists, in many institutions, train the patient in the use of special upper extremity self-help splints. They are also trained to assist patients requiring specific perceptual-motor activities. They may work in a mental hospital and engage the patient in body awareness and positive self-concept activities as well as other sensorimotor activities.

Currently, through the work of Ayres,[3]

occupational therapy has become increasingly interested in the broad field of learning disorders. Ayres has proposed a system of thought designed to assist the client in sensory integration. Through a variety of activities that stimulate vestibular functions, the patient develops the ability to effectively process information.

Recreational therapy. Therapeutic recreation, as recently defined by the National Therapeutic Recreation Society, is "a special service within the broad area of recreation services. It is a process which utilizes recreation services for purposive intervention in some physical, emotional, and/or social behavior to bring about a desired change in that behavior and to promote the growth and development of the individual."[13]

Recreational therapy gives to the rehabilitation armamentarium the aspect of enjoyable activities. Through recreational activities, the patient has the opportunity for emotional release while learning leisure-time activities. The therapist, through gross motor movements, uses the patient's physical capacities and those abilities that may give an impetus to restoring important physical or mental functions.

Dance therapy. In recent years, the use of dance as a therapeutic modality has been growing. It is found predominantly in mental hospitals, but it is beginning to be used as an adjunct to other therapy programs such as those for the mentally retarded, the emotionally disturbed, and the educationally handicapped who have minimal brain dysfunction. Through the medium of dance, the patient can find self-expression, nonverbal communication, and increased self-awareness and positive self-concepts. Body movement rhythmically initiated also provides a highly effective means of developing efficient motor patterns.[5]

Corrective therapy. The profession of corrective therapy emerged as a result of the needs created by World War II and the reconditioning programs instituted by Dr. Howard Rusk. *Corrective therapy is*

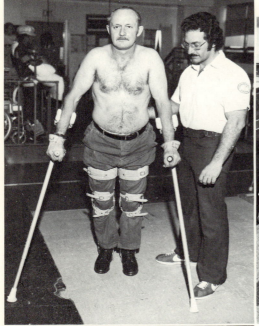

A

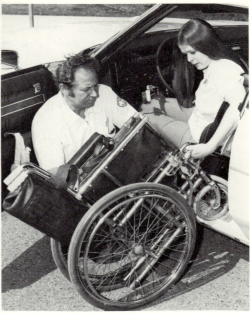

C

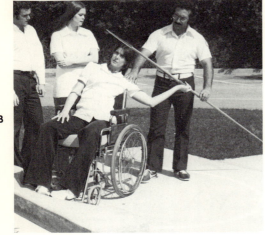

B

Fig. 1-3. Corrective therapy provides a wide variety of services in a clinical setting. **A,** Gait training. **B,** Wheelchair sports. **C,** Driver education and self-care activities. (Courtesy Long Beach Veterans' Administration Hospital, Long Beach, Calif.)

defined as the application of the principles, tools, techniques, and psychology of medically oriented physical education to assist the physician in the accomplishment of prescribed objectives.

Corrective therapy is contrasted to adapted physical education primarily in its delivery of services. Adapted physical education functions as an integral part of the various educational levels, including elementary, secondary, college, and university, whereas corrective therapy takes place within hospitals, clinics, and centers dedicated to physical, mental, and emotional restoration and/or habilitation.

The primary procedures employed by the corrective therapist are the following:
1. Offering conditioning and reconditioning exercises for the development of specific and/or general physical and mental requirements
2. Supplying socialization and resocialization activities for the mentally atypical, employing psychiatric objectives
3. Teaching fundamentals of transfer activities in daily living and the utilization of all types of orthotic and prosthetic devices, including the manually controlled motor vehicles

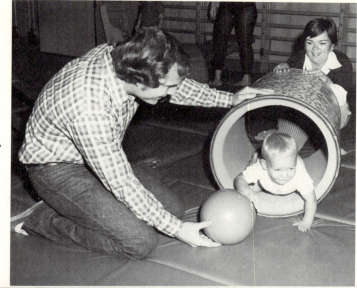

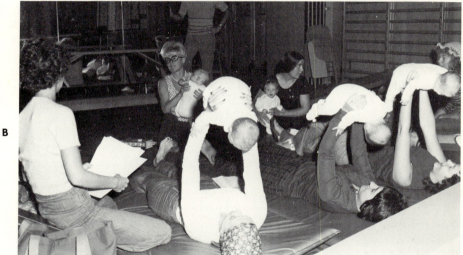

Fig. 1-4. Students learning to work in the area of motor therapy. **A,** Helping a child gain an awareness of spatial relationships. **B,** Infant stimulation through movement. (**B,** Courtesy, California State University, Audio-Visual Center, Long Beach, Calif.)

4. Instructing the individual in postural alignment and bodily movement through neuromuscular reeducation
5. Instructing the individual in developmental movement activities, employing basic motor-learning principles
6. Teaching adapted sports, games, and other activities

Motor therapy. As a result of the great interest in the perceptual-motor development and movement education that began in the early part of the 1960's and carried on to the 1970's, there has emerged a new field generally known as motor therapy. Although variously named sensorimotor therapy, perceptual-motor therapy, and psychomotor therapy, motor therapy is a burgeoning discipline dedicated to assisting the individual who, because of physical, mental, or emotional problems has difficulty in coordination. Through a planned program of intervention, a person's movement behavior is modified. "Motor Therapy provides a prescriptive program of selected developmental motor activities that are specifically designed to be employed for a particular movement ability level."[2] Motor therapy assists the individual in integrating specific tasks into efficient patterns of movement behavior that are essential to carrying out more complicated acts of coordination.

EDUCATIONAL SERVICES

The United States census of 1970 estimated that 30% of the population is under 21 years of age and that there are over 46 million persons between 5 and 17 years of age.

The National Health Survey determined that children under 15 years of age have approximately three bouts with acute illness annually. Respiratory conditions constituted about 55% of the reported conditions. Injuries from accidents also constitute a serious problem affecting one child in every three.[4, 7, 15] It has been estimated that almost one child in five, or 18% of the population under 17 years of age, has one or more chronic disorders. During one 2-year period, over 11 million children had one or more chronic conditions. Of those conditions reported, the most prevalent, which were hay fever, asthma, and other allergies (accounting for 32.8%) sinusitis, bronchitis, and other respiratory diseases (accounting for 15.1%), made up almost half of the chronic conditions of children under the age of 17.[7, 15] Paralysis, orthopedic disorders, hearing defects, speech defects, and heart disease also represented a considerable number of those conditions reported.

An ever increasing number of children with congenital malformations are surviving to a greater age each year. The conditions having the highest incidence are heart disorders, congenital dislocation of the hip, cleft palate and lip, spina bifida occulta, and meningocele.[7]

The number of individuals with multiple disabilities is also increasing.[17, 18] The reasons are many, but the primary ones seem to be the higher rate of survival among infants born prematurely and advanced techniques of medical science that are keeping children with one or more disabilities alive.

The exceptional child

It has been determined, from national public and private agencies and from state and local directors of special education programs, that over 12% of the school-aged population, which ranges from 6 to 19 years of age, is handicapped to the extent of needing special education assistance. This percentage represents 7,886,000 children (Table 1-1). From this total, 55% have been determined to be receiving some special education service. Of the 1,187,000 handicapped who are 0 to 5 years of age, only 22% are receiving special educational assistance (Fig. 1-5).

The term "exceptional child" in the educational environment may be defined as *a boy or girl who, because of some definite mental, physical, emotional, or behavioral deviation, may require a modification of school practices or an addition of some spe-*

Table 1-1. Percentages of handicapping conditions among school-aged children 6 to 19 years of age (1972 to 1973)

Handicapping condition	Percentage
Speech impaired	3.500
Mentally retarded	2.300
Learning disabled	3.000
Emotionally disturbed	2.000
Crippled and other health impared	0.500
Deaf	0.075
Hard-of-hearing	0.500
Visually handicapped	0.100
Deaf and blind and other multihandicapped	0.060
Total	12.035

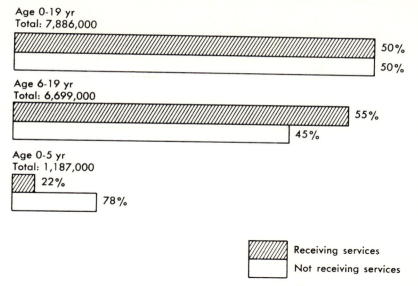

Fig. 1-5. Estimated number of handicapped children receiving and not receiving services grouped by age (1974 to 1975).

cial service in order to develop to his or her maximum potential.

Categories of children considered by the United States Congress to be eligible for special educational services under P.L. 89-313 and Title VI-A of the Elementary and Secondary Education Act are the mentally retarded, hard-of-hearing, deaf, speech impaired, visually handicapped, seriously emotionally disturbed, crippled, other health impaired or learning disabled children who may require educational services out of the ordinary. These conditions are specifically defined as follows:

Mentally retarded: Persons characterized by a level of mental development impaired to the extent that the individual is unable to benefit from the standard school program and requires special sevices. This includes such subcategories as slow learners, educable mentally retarded, and trainable mentally retarded.

Hard-of-hearing: Persons in whom the sense of hearing, although defective, is functional with or without a hearing aid. The hearing loss is generally of such a nature and severity as to require one or more special educational services.

Deaf: Persons in whom the sense of hearing is nonfunctional for the ordinary purposes of

life (inability to hear connected language with or without the use of amplification). This general group is made up of the congenitally deaf and the adventitiously deaf.

Speech impaired: Persons experiencing pronounced organic or functional speech disorders that cause interference in oral communication. This includes persons exhibiting language disorders resulting from such specific handicaps as stuttering, cleft plate, speech, or voice problems.

Visually handicapped: Persons who have such severe visual loss as to require special educational services. This includes subcategories such as blind, legally blind, partially sighted, and visually impaired.

Seriously emotionally disturbed: Persons having psychiatric disturbance without clearly defined physical cause of structural damage to the brain, which limits the ability of the individual to govern his own behavior. These are of such a nature and severity as to require one or more special services, particularly with reference to their education.

Crippled: Persons with orthopedic impairments that might restrict normal opportunity for education or self-support. This is generally considered to include individuals having congenital impairments, for example, clubfoot or absence of some body member, impairments caused by some disease, for example, poliomyelitis, bone tuberculosis, and encephalitis, neurological involvements that may result in conditions such as

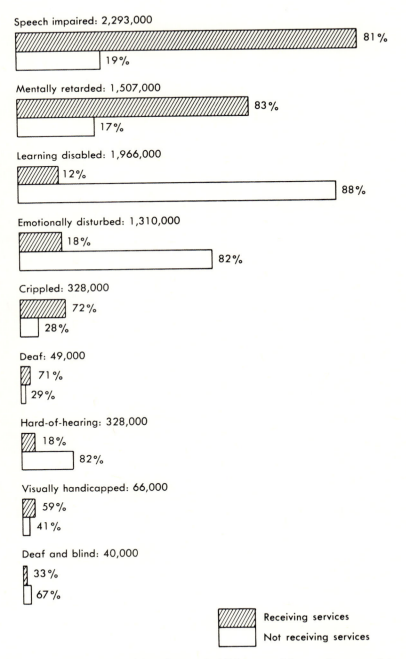

Fig. 1-6. Estimated number of handicapped children receiving and not receiving services grouped by type of handicap (1974 to 1975).

cerebral palsy, and impairments caused by accidents, for example, fractures or burns that cause contractures.

Other health impaired: Persons having health handicaps, not covered in other categories, of such a nature and severity as to require one or more special services, particularly with reference to their education. These could include asthma; rheumatic fever; conditions of less than the usual amount of strength, energy, or endurance; conditions resulting from chronic illness or environmental causes; epilepsy; diabetes; or cardiac disease.

Learning disabled: Persons with learning dysfunctions that prevent them from learning or functioning in a regular educational program. These individuals exhibit a disorder in one or more of the basic psychological processes involved in understanding or in using spoken or written language. These may be manifested in disorders of listening, thinking, talking, reading, writing, spelling, or arithmetic. They include conditions that have been referred to as perceptual handicaps, brain injury, minimal brain dysfunction, dyslexia, developmental aphasia, etc. They do not include learning problems that are a consequence primarily of visual, hearing, or motor handicaps; mental retardation; emotional disturbances; or environmental disadvantages.[4]

The scope of special education for the exceptional child is broad. Programs of instruction can be offered in a number of places, depending on the needs of the child, the staff, available facilities, and funds. State and local school district programs for the handicapped child vary considerably throughout the nation. Ideally, special education should be available in hospitals and special residential and day schools as well as in home instruction and special classes for the handicapped within the regular schools. It is necessary to remember, however, that the majority of handicapped students are attending regular schools.

The concern of all persons is that every individual should have the opportunity to reach full potential through a meaningful education.

ADAPTED AND THERAPEUTIC PHYSICAL EDUCATION

Physical activity as a remedial modality has been recognized since recorded history.

Early man became aware that movement of the body through massage, passive manipulation, and active exercise had an ameliorating effect on various physical and mental disorders. However, it was not until more recent times that concise systems of "medical gymnastics" were devised as a means to correct certain physical anomalies. One such system that was to become well known was created by Per Henrik Ling of the Royal Institute of Gymnastics, Stockholm, Sweden, in 1814. The Ling system, as it became known, consisted of specific formalized movements performed with the intent of developing or restoring the participant's health through proper body mechanics and posture. This system was brought to America in 1884 by Nissen and Posse. Requiring an exactness of movement, it soon won favor among American educators whose principal goals followed the European tradition of discipline and health through exercise. Harvard University became the first school in America to conduct a remedial physical education program. The school's program was designed by Dr. Dudley Sargent to help the students gain health through correct postural alignment and to prevent bodily deterioration from an increasingly sedentary life.

After World War I, physical education changed gradually from formality to play and sports activities. Even though many schools accepted the play concept, they still provided a special physical education class for students unable to take part in regular activities. At first, the primary concern of this special physical education class was to improve posture, but gradually the scope expanded to include a great variety of handicapping conditions.

Special physical education gradually expanded its offerings to incorporate sports, games, and rhythms adapted to the needs of the handicapped child. Through the efforts of such pioneers as George Stafford,[16] numerous physical education and recreational activities were found to benefit the total development of the exceptional person.

An identity crisis

Many names have been given to the specialized area of physical education that deals with the less endowed individual. These names have succeeded in causing confusion as to the real nature and the full scope of activities available to the handicapped through physical education. The paragraphs that follow contain numerous names attributed to physical education for the handicapped, along with descriptions of them.

Medical gymnastics: Term of European derivation commonly used before the turn of the century in America and still used in Canada and many other foreign countries; denotes a program of exercise given to remediate various pathological conditions.

Corrective, remedial, and *rehabilitative physical education:* Program titles implying that through exercise or specialized activity, disease conditions can be ameliorated.

Preventive physical education: Through a planned program of exercises and physical activities, various conditions can be prevented from occurring or, if present, can be prevented from resulting in deterioration.

Modified, restricted, or *limited physical education:* Alteration of the class in some way to meet the physical, mental, and social demands of its students.

Special physical education: Emphasis placed on the unique problems of individuals who are admitted to the class.

Orthopedic physical education: Applies to conditions primarily of the musculoskeletal system. Postural and body mechanics are of the utmost importance in this program. However, it is often used to encompass the majority of handicapping conditions.

Developmental physical education: Course title that is becoming more widely used, primarily to describe programs for the subfit individual, and has gained acceptance because of the positive connotation expressed by the title.

Perceptual-motor, sensorimotor therapy: Dedicated to aiding the child in the maximum development of his perceptual abilities. The specialist working with typical or atypical children attempts to establish a motor program in which the child accurately assesses the world through his senses and develops efficient movement.

As is readily apparent, the great number of names given to the area of adapted physical education only serve to emphasize the wide divergence of opinion as to what these classes really should mean to the student. Consequently, some course titles tend to stigmatize the student, limit scope, and, in essence, distort the real intention of the program.

Because of the great confusion as to the most descriptive title, a survey on recommended terminology was made by the Committee on Adapted Physical Education of the American Association of Health, Physical Education, and Recreation in 1947. This survey indicated that *adapted physical education* was the most appropriate title to describe the broad functions of the program. *It is defined as ". . . a diversified program of developmental activities, games, sports, rhythms, suited to the interest, capacities, and limitations of students with disabilities who may not safely or successfully engage in unrestricted participation in the vigorous activities of the general [physical] education program."*

It is generally agreed that adapted physical education classes should be provided for the severely disabled within each school. Also, classes should be provided for persons with moderate disabilities, postural deviations, obesity and for the subfit, all of whom cannot be adequately cared for in the regular physical education program. However, wherever possible, provisions within the regular physical education class should be made for students with minor afflictions. The adapted concept in which activities are individualized should be employed in all physical education, not only for special problems. A high quality regular physical education program utilizes the adapted concept by offering individualized instruction and opportunities for developing physical fitness, skill in sports activities, good body mechanics, rhythms, and relaxation techniques for all the students in the program.

Where are we going?

Adapted physical education has burgeoned in the past 10 years. An ever growing number of schools, hospitals, and institutions is utilizing the services of the adapted physical educator.

This current increase of interest in adapted physical education has been a result mainly of three factors: increased private and public funding, a broader scope of programming, and integration of disciplines. More money than ever before is being spent in research and program development in the area of special physical education. Universities and colleges are researching teaching methods and approaches in dealing with the exceptional child. School districts are innovating and putting into practice experimental plans for physically educating the handicapped child.

The scope of programming has broadened decidedly in the past 10 years. Whereas in the past, most adapted physical education took place at the elementary and secondary school levels, it is now conducted with the very young child, on every school level, and with citizens in retirement centers. Program coverage has expanded to involve almost all exceptional persons who can respond to physical education activities.

More and more frequently, the physical educator is coming together with the classroom teacher to talk about common problems. This getting together is particularly effective in the cases of the adapted physical educator and the special education classroom teacher. More than ever before, physical education is respected for the many positive effects it has on the exceptional child. No longer can disciplines dealing with aspects of the exceptional child work independently. The current trend is one of an interdisciplinary approach to the problems of children, with each expert joining his or her talents with those of others in the child's best interests.

Physical educators interested in the challenge of individuals with problems will find adapted physical education one of the most personally rewarding of all the many facets of physical education. Its future is bright.

REFERENCES

1. Abeson, A., editor: A continuing summary of pending and completed litigation regarding the education of handicapped children, Arlington, Va., 1973, The Council for Exceptional Children, State-Federal Information Clearinghouse for Exceptional Children.
2. Arnheim, D. D., and Sinclair, W. A.: The clumsy child: a program of motor therapy, St. Louis, 1975, The C. V. Mosby Co.
3. Ayres, A. J.: Sensory integration and learning disorders, Los Angeles, 1973, Western Psychological Services.
4. Better education for handicapped children, Annual report fiscal year 1969, Washington, D.C., 1970, U.S. Department of Health, Education, and Welfare.
5. Berstein, P. L.: Theory and methods in dance movement therapy, Dubuque, Iowa, 1971, Kendall/Hunt Publishing Co.
6. Denhoff, E.: Cerebral palsy: the preschool years, Springfield, Ill., 1967, Charles C Thomas, Publisher.
7. Health of children of school age, Washington, D.C., 1966, U.S. Department of Health, Education, and Welfare.
8. Hellison, D.: Humanistic physical education, Englewood Cliffs, N.J., 1973, Prentice-Hall, Inc.
9. Hellmuth, J., editor: Learning disorders. In Bryant, N. D.: Clinic inadequacies with learning disorders: the missing child educator, Seattle, 1966, Special Child Publications.
10. Mewett, F. M.: Mainstreaming the handicapped: concept and fact, third national conference on physical activity, Long Beach, Calif., 1974, Office of the Los Angeles County Superintendent of School, Division of Special Education.
11. Mann, P. H., editor: Mainstream special education, proceedings of the University of Miami conference on special education in the great cities, Bureau of the Handicapped, U.S.

Office of Education, U.S. Government Printing Office.

12. One in eleven handicapped adults in America: a survey on 1970 U.S. census data, Washington, D.C., 1970, U.S. Government Printing Office.
13. Program for handicapped: a clarification of terms, J. Health Phys. Ed. Rec. **42:**64, Sept., 1971.
14. Rusk, H.: Rehabilitation medicine, ed. 3, St. Louis, 1971, The C. V. Mosby Co.
15. Schiffer, C. G., and Hunt, E. O.: Illness among children, Washington, D.C., 1963, U.S. Department of Health, Education, and Welfare.
16. Stafford, G. T.: Sports for the handicapped, Englewood Cliffs, N.J., 1947, Prentice-Hall, Inc.
17. Service for handicapped youth: a program overview (R-12220-HEW), Washington, D.C., 1973, U.S. Department of Health, Education, and Welfare.
18. Wolf, J. M., editor: The multiply handicapped child, Springfield, Ill., 1969, Charles C Thomas, Publisher.

RECOMMENDED READINGS

Daniels, A. S., and Davies, E. A.: Adapted physical education, ed. 3, New York, 1975, Harper & Row, Publishers.

Kirk, S.: Educating exceptional children, Boston, 1962, Houghton-Mifflin Co.

Rusk, H. A.: Rehabilitation medicine, ed. 3, St. Louis, 1971, The C. V. Mosby Co.

Tilford, C. W., and Sawrey, J. M.: The exceptional individual, Englewood Cliffs, N.J., 1967, Prentice-Hall, Inc.

2

INDIVIDUAL DEVELOPMENT

■ This chapter is primarily concerned not with the entire field of growth and development but with highlighting some of the factors in personal development that are pertinent to the field of adapted physical education. Physical educators, particularly those teachers concerned with the exceptional individual, must have an understanding of the typical and atypical factors relevant to growth and development. Such knowledge provides the instructor with a sound rationale for following certain procedures and applying particular techniques.

Various meanings have been attached to the terms "growth," "development," and "maturation" by numerous authorities.

Therefore to provide the student with a common understanding, the following definitions are given. *Growth* refers to change in an individual's bodily structure and function. It implies a quantitative change in height, weight, and girth that can be assessed by the employment of some anthropometric techniques. *Development* is a general term indicating the process by which an individual attains maturity.[28] *Maturation* refers to the innate anatomical and physiological bodily changes that are predetermined by heredity.[8]

EARLY DEVELOPMENT

The typical unborn fetus is a unique entity undergoing a complex process of orderly cell division. This cell division develops into different types of tissue that ultimately develop into organs and organ systems that become a coordinated complex of physiological functions. Physical development and maturation usually follows a predictable pattern, occurring from the center of the body outward and from the head downward.

At first, the fetus within the mother displays movement that is random. Gradually, however, there occurs immature control of the head, then the arms, and, finally, the legs. The infant's movement control both before and after birth follows a similar pat-

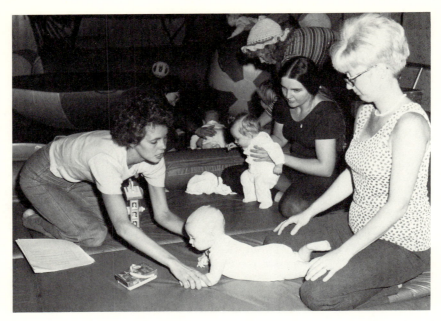

Fig. 2-1. An infant gaining head control. (Courtesy California State University, Audio Visual Center, Long Beach, Calif.)

tern of development.[14] Generally speaking, from gross undefined and uncoordinated behavior, the human infant gradually acquires complex behavior skills that continue throughout life.

The newborn is mainly dominated by primitive reflexes. Many of the reflexes seen in the infant directly after birth are designed to sustain life, for example, the rooting reflex, in which the infant's head turns when his cheek is tactually stimulated, is present in order that milk may be obtained from the breast. Other survival reflexes are breathing, yawning, coughing, sneezing, and sucking. The central nervous system matures slowly, starting with the spinal cord and ending with the higher brain centers. The infant's early development is controlled by the spinal cord. Each developmental milestone, for example, lifting the head, rolling over, and walking, is dependent on the maturation of the nervous system (Fig. 2-1). The primitive postural reflexes are designed so that eventually the individual will function effectively in the up-

right posture. From a completely grounded, helpless organism, the normal infant develops viable and efficient movement capabilities in the upright bipedal posture.[15, 16]

The infant seeks ultimate movement independence in order to move freely and explore the environment. In the beginning, the infant is almost completely dominated by the downward force of gravity; with increased strength and muscle control, he forces himself upward until he is balancing and propelling himself on two small feet. When in the upright posture, the child's hands are free to feel, to explore, and to learn from a variety of experiences that are limited only by the child's receptivity, the extent of his exploration, and the experiential richness of his environment. Full physical, mental, and emotional development can only occur when there is a constant variety of experiences provided by the environment.[32]

From relatively uncontrolled and purposeless movement behavior, the newborn prepares for the next big event by squirm-

Table 2-1. Early normal developmental characteristics: gross motor behavior

Age	Major events
4 weeks	Turns head to side. Holds hands in fist. Has sagging head. Shows tonic neck reflex. Displays crawling movement of legs.
8 weeks	Lifts head. Turns from side to back. Sits with support. Pushes self with arms and lifts chest.
12 weeks	Crawls prone. Holds head steady for 5 seconds. Raises chest. Holds hands mostly open.
16 weeks	Keeps head steady when sitting. Attempts to right self when tilted. Bears some weight on feet. Likes to sit.
20 weeks	Sits unsupported. Pulls self to sitting position. Supports weight on forearm and lifts head.
24 weeks	Lifts chest off floor. Bears some weight on feet. Controls head. Crawls backward. Reaches out with each hand. Stands by holding on. Rolls over from back to stomach.
28 weeks	Bounces self. Rocks on hands and knees. Supports weight on feet. Begins to crawl forward. Steps when supported under arms.
36 weeks	Crawls by moving hands and knees. Shows hand preference. Sits unsupported. Pulls self to standing position. Pulls self to sitting position.
40 weeks	Pulls self to feet. Stands by holding on. Creeps on hands and knees over obstacle 2 inches high. Stands unsupported for 1 minute.
48 weeks	Pulls self up to side of crib. Walks alone. Creeps by using hands and feet.
56 weeks	Walks short distances. Starts and stops. Walks backward. Throws objects. Stands up from lying on back.
62 weeks	Walks smoothly. Creeps upstairs. Stoops and stands up. Ascends stairs by walking.
18 months	Ascends stairs by marking time. Jumps in place. Walks sideways. Walks without falling. Runs awkwardly. Pulls toy.
24 months	Walks backward. Runs in preference to walking. Squats on floor. Descends ladder carefully by marking time. Jumps from 18-inch height with help. Throws object overhead.
27 months	Jumps off floor with both feet. Balances on one foot for 1 second. Ascends ladder carefully by marking time.
30 months	Walks straight line. Throws ball 4 feet or farther. Jumps from 18-inch height with one foot forward. Rides tricycle. Broad jumps 4 inches. Ascends ladder by marking time. Can walk on tiptoe.
36 months	Descends stairs by marking time. Jumps from 24-inch height with help. Jumps from 8-inch height with feet together. Hops on foot one or more times. Balances on one foot for 2 seconds. Kicks stationary ball. Climbs freely over furniture.
42 months	Hops 10 or more steps with both feet. Hops four or more steps on one foot. Throws 3-inch ball 6 feet. Walks heel to toe on a line for 10 feet. Balances on one foot for 5 seconds.
48 months	Ascends ladder by leading with alternate feet. Broad jumps 24 inches. Balances on one foot for 8 seconds. Hops on one foot. Catches object that has been thrown. Jumps in place with two feet. Jumps from 24-inch box with two feet.
52 months	Displays cross-pattern walking. Descends stairs by leading with alternate feet.
56 months	Descends ladder by leading with alternate feet. Hops seven or more steps on one foot. Throws 3-inch ball 10 feet.
5 years	Skips. Walks backward heel to toe. Walks like adult. Gallops. Throws 9-inch ball to feet. Hops 10 or more steps on one foot.

Table 2-2. Early normal developmental characteristics: social and adaptive behavior

Age	Major events
0	Responds to sounds. Responds to persons. Responds to brightly colored objects.
4 weeks	Shows awareness of persons. Searches for nipple. Regards persons' faces.
8 weeks	Smiles when talked to. Shows excitement when being approached by adult. Looks for source of sounds.
12 weeks	Likes to be around persons. Anticipates being fed. Tenses muscles when about to be lifted. Plays with own fingers.
16 weeks	Shows pleasure with certain toys. Laughs with persons. Plays with hands. Recognizes bottle. Brings objects to mouth. Is aware of self in mirror.
20 weeks	Plays peekaboo. Smiles at familiar person. Shows displeasure when toy is taken away. Inspects own hands.
24 weeks	Smiles at image in mirror. Wants to be talked to. May fear strange persons. Holds own bottle.
28 weeks	Makes noise to gain attention. Explores objects. Sucks food from spoon. Chews bananas and bread. Pats own image in mirror.
32 weeks	Plays pat-a-cake with help. Watches persons. Says "da da" and "ma ma." Uncovers toy.
36 weeks	Brings arms in front of face. Uses fingers to feed self from dish. Defends own possessions. Drinks from cup with some spill. Responds to questions.
40 weeks	Plays pat-a-cake. Likes to play. Looks at pictures in book. Responds to "no, no."
52 weeks	Puts everything into mouth. Uses fingers to feed self cracker. Chews in circular manner. Jabbers with expression. Imitates words. Plays nursery games.
64 weeks	Exhibits solitary play. Pulls socks off. Brings spoon to mouth. Drops things from crib and high chair to gain attention. Cooperates in dressing. Plays ball. Speaks two words.
16 months	Carries personal things. Dips spoon in dish. Indicates when diapers are wet. Unzips large zipper. Identifies common clothes.
18 months	Demonstrates side-by-side play. Is very possessive of own things. Helps feed self. Imitates scribbling. Follows simple directions.
21 months	Helps in washing self. Drinks from cup. Helps remove own clothes. Makes two-word sentences. Makes basic wants known. Identifies objects in picture.
24 months	Takes shoes off if laces are loosened. Feeds self with fingers. Holds and hugs doll. Pulls off own clothes.
27 months	Imitates other children's play. Eats with fork. Unbuttons large buttons. Indicates need to go to toilet.
30 months	Washes and dries hands. Dresses with help. Avoids specified dangers.
36 months	Takes turns. Feeds self with spoon and fork.
42 months	Puts on shoes. Functions independently in toileting. Plays with another child.
48 months	Plays highly structured games. May have imaginary playmate. Is very aggressive in play. Dresses self. Washes and dries hands. Cooperates in play.
5 years	Dresses without help. Plays in group of three.

ing, thrashing out, moving his head, rolling, and kicking. The ability to transport his body over a terrain evolves from the infant's early random movement and his rolling over, crawling, and creeping activities. Purposefully transporting the body forward stems from the infant's pushing with his legs at the same time that he is pulling and reaching with his arms. Although in the beginning, movements are highly unsophisticated, each new movement skill serves as a building block to a more complex skill. The concept that each new skill stems from and is built on a less complex skill can be applied to almost every learning situation that may be encountered by the child.

From the beginning locomotor skill of crawling, the infant gradually gains enough maturation and courage to raise himself to a four-point posture.[14] When the infant possesses the ability to effectively balance on hands and knees, the locomotor skill called creeping can be executed. Maturation and experience lead the child to pull himself from a four-point posture to the precarious two-point bipedal, or upright, position. The infant accomplishes something outstanding when he can bring himself to his knees and finally rise to balance unsteadily on the two small surfaces provided by the feet. Normally, it takes a development period of up to 14 months in order for the infant to achieve the upright position (Table 2-1).[17, 24, 26]

Besides transportation skills, effective object manipulation is highly important to the child's ultimate learning and physical development. Efficient object control stems from the child's ability to grasp and release an object at will. In the early days following birth, the infant reflexively grasps when pressure is applied to the palm of the hand. Gradually, the infant gains the ability to close and open the hand as desired. Purposeful manipulation in the beginning is performed by the child first with the palms of the hands and later with the fingers. Mature manipulation does not occur until about the sixteenth month of life, at which time the thumbs can be used in opposition (Table 2-2).[24]

All early behavior is dependent on the complex interweaving of visual, tactile, auditory, manipulative, and gross motor functions. It should also be noted that the senses of smell, taste, sight, hearing, and touch, taken together with the ability to move, provide the means by which the human organism learns about and makes adaptations to the environment. All senses act independently and in combination with one another to process and store information. A person who is deprived of adequate sensory experiences often has problems reaching full maturation and development that may carry throughout the individual's lifetime.

The proper coordination of the six pairs of eye muscles must take place before the child can adequately focus on objects. Inadequate coordination of both eyes may lead to problems in total body coordination as well as later difficulty in learning. The eyes are important to the child's normal development of body balance, postural awareness, spatial awareness, and self-image.

The sense of touch is the most mature sense that the infant has at birth. A variety of information about himself and surroundings comes to the infant through his tactile sense. The infant and the young child must have a rich backlog of touch experiences in order to develop maximally.

A variety of movement experiences is necessary to adequately stimulate the kinesthetic system. Body movement stimulates sensory organs that are located in the muscles, tendons, and joints as well as within the ear. A keen awareness of movement is necessary for the acquisition and maintenance of good posture, the ability to effectively deal with spatial relationships, and the ability to initiate synchronous motor patterns.[9]

Hearing and vocal language are synonymous to the human organism. The fetus begins to hear about 5 weeks after conception. After birth, the infant should be provided with a rich sound environment in order to acquire sound discrimination and sound identification for vocal communication (Table 2-3).

For the child's ultimate development, there must occur an effective processing of information through the senses. It is speculated that, from the time of conception, the human being is continually processing information and gaining a backlog of experience that will be used for future behavior.[3] It is imperative that the child be able to recognize, identify, and discriminate between different stimulants in order that behavior is accurate and effective according to individual requirements. Accurate perception and normal responses are necessary for normal behavior to take place.[5, 10, 17, 26]

Humans are by nature gregarious, needing stimulation from other persons to reach their full growth and development. From the first smile the child directs at a parent

Table 2-3. Early normal developmental characteristics: small muscle and visual-perceptual behavior

Age	Major events
4 weeks	Holds hands fisted. Attends to objects. Holds onto ring.
8 weeks	Swipes at objects. Begins to coordinate head and eyes.
12 weeks	Shows one- and two-arm control. Looks at interesting object and waves arms. Looks alternately at object and hands. Brings hands to front of body.
16 weeks	Holds hands mainly open. Brings hands to object. Reaches for objects. Picks up objects with palm.
24 weeks	Examines objects. Searches for hidden objects. Reaches for objects. Transfers objects from one hand to other. Visually tracks to midline. Lifts cup. Begins to rotate wrists horizontally.
28 weeks	Grabs objects with palms. Scoops raisins. Shows some hand preference.
32 weeks	Bangs objects on table. Tracks moving objects. Demonstrates rudimentary thumb opposition.
36 weeks	Rings a bell. Demonstrates pincer grasp. Takes objects out of container. Bangs objects together.
40 weeks	Releases objects awkwardly. Plays with fingers. Puts object into container. Holds own bottle. Attempts to hold three 1-inch cubes in one hand. Bangs two cubes together at midline of body.
48 weeks	Releases object easily. Chews and swallows. Makes marks with pencil.
64 weeks	Builds tower of two cubes. Puts raisins in box. Scribbles. Dumps raisins from container.
18 months	Picks up cereal with pincer grasp. Builds tower of four 1-inch cubes. Makes circular scribbles. Turns pages.
24 months	Builds tower of five 1-inch cubes. Turns pages of magazine one at a time. Unwraps paper covering from box.
27 months	Builds tower of eight 1-inch cubes. Turns doorknob. Unscrews lid of jar.
30 months	Holds pencil. Loosens shoelaces. Drinks from straw. Copies circle. Knows difference between vertical and horizontal lines.
36 months	Builds tower of 10 1-inch cubes. Holds pencil like adult. Draws vertical line. Strings four beads in 2 minutes. Cuts with scissors.
42 months	Traces diamond. Puts half-inch pegs into pegboard.
48 months	Draws man with three parts. Copies cross. Laces own shoes. Strings seven beads in 2 minutes. Buttons large button. Draws recognizable picture.
5 years	Copies square. Draws man with six parts. Knows difference between horizontal, vertical, and diagonal lines.

to his playing with other children, socialization is necessary for the development of an individual's self-concept and emotional stability. From the egocentricity of infancy, the side-by-side play of the toddler, and the cooperative play of the young child, there gradually emerges the ability to give and take graciously, to follow, to lead, to interact in many social situations, and, finally, to effectively compete in life under rigid rules of personal conduct (Table 2-4).[2]

PHYSICAL GROWTH

Physical growth is an extremely complex phenomenon that has a multitude of sensitive, interdependent variables. An individual's growth and development are affected mainly by heredity, prenatal factors, disease, and the environment.[21] The genetic plan of each cell provides the foundation for the potential size of an individual. However, ultimate growth can be adversely altered or exceed its natural potential through the influence of nutrition, exercise, and general health. To illustrate, the person who eats beyond his maintenance requirements will exceed the weight level that heredity has set or continued heavy weight lifting with low repetition, as conducted by many football players, will often produce a large bulky musculature, modifying considerably a person's natural inherited tendencies.

Many prenatal factors can adversely af-

Table 2-4. Early normal developmental characteristics: language and communication

Age*	Major events
0	Exhibits undifferentiated birth cry.
4 weeks	Watches person moving. Makes demand cry. Makes throaty cry.
8 weeks	Attends to person's voice. Shows discomfort. Gurgles. Coos.
12 weeks	Makes different sounds when touched or played with. Tenses when lifted. Shows vital or differentiated crying when cold, uncomfortable, or hungry.
16 weeks	Turns head to sound of voice. Recognizes mother. Laughs. Experiments with voice.
20 weeks	Turns to sounds. Shows displeasure. Responds to voices.
24 weeks	Responds to anger. Displays nonrhythmical crying. Babbles.
28 weeks	Squeals. Makes "M-m" sound. Smiles at mirror. Demands attention. Tries to imitate speech.
32 weeks	Combines babbling and gestures. Combines two syllables. Displays rhythmical babbling.
36 weeks	Cries to gain attention.
40 weeks	Understands "no." Waves bye-bye. Looks for hidden object. Imitates sounds. Says "da-da" and "ma-ma."
44 weeks	Shakes head "no." Says one word. Imitates new sounds. Listens to words. Anticipates playing pat-a-cake.
48 weeks	Knows own name. Indicates personal desires. Commands through gestures.
52 weeks	Knows names of objects. Shows likes and dislikes. Imitates words. Possesses three-word vocabulary. Anticipates being scolded. Responds to "Give it to me."
64 weeks	Points to things wanted. Shows variety of emotions. Possesses five-word vocabulary.
18 months	Knows three body parts. Imitates talking. Possesses 10-word vocabulary. Hums and sings to self. Uses words to indicate wants.
21 months	Tries to follow directions. Knows five body parts. Leads adult to object. Exhibits great curiosity. Connects three or four words. Possesses 20-word vocabulary.
24 months	Follows simple commands. Refers to self by name. Knows how some objects work. Names most objects played with. Imitates parents' speech. Expresses two- or three-word sentences.
27 months	Repeats two numbers. Knows three prepositions. Names most common objects in home. Uses plurals.
30 months	Identifies objects by use. Knows the number "one." Knows simple songs and rhymes.
36 months	Gives full name. Knows own sex. Identifies at least two objects from picture. Answers simple questions. Talks in simple sentences.
42 months	Counts to three. Follows simple verbal directions. Knows the concepts of longer and heavier. Can tell a story.
48 months	Uses conjunctions. Understands prepositions. Makes five- and six-word sentences. Names the colors "red," "blue," and "yellow." Possesses 800-word vocabulary. Gestures with entire body. Forms sentences.
5 years	Expresses mature articulation. Asks "Why?" Can define six words. Explains composition of materials.

*The ages at which the major events noted here occur are approximate.

fect the growing individual. Maternal conditions such as malnutrition, defective implantation, Rh incompatibilities, diabetes, or contraction of rubella or syphilis during the very early development of the unborn infant may alter the ultimate growth and development of the fetus, as may drug addiction or heavy cigarette smoking on the part of the mother.

Diseases of all types can result in significant hindrance of normal growth. Infec-

tions, for example, may prevent proper weight gain. A bedfast individual may fail to develop normally because of lack of exercise and fresh air. Motor development may also be impaired as the result of disease, compounded by inactivity and the lack of opportunity for proper skill development. Metabolic and endocrine gland disorders can directly and indirectly affect the growth process.

Increasingly, environmental factors are

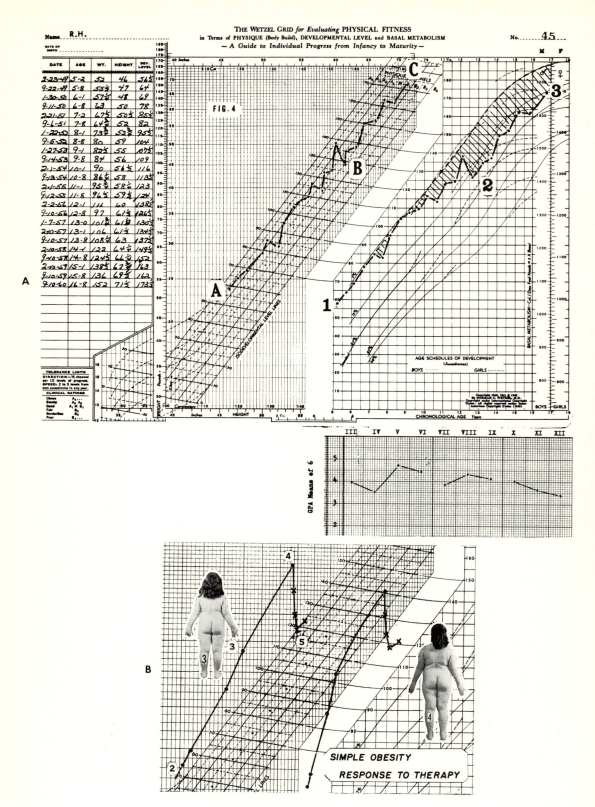

Fig. 2-2. For legend see opposite page.

identified as being the primary etiological factor in many growth and development problems. Poor living standards, together with inadequate health care and diet, constitute one of the major causes of mental retardation and deficient physical growth. Child neglect and lack of parental love also produce climates in which full maturation cannot be reached.

Accurate assessment of normal physical development is difficult because different parts of the body grow at different rates and at varied periods in life. Consequently, age and general height and weight charts serve only as estimates of a child's stage of development. A method that has proved of some benefit to the educator is the Wetzel grid. This type of system provides the teacher with a simple direct means for calculating a student's growth progress.

Conventionally, a child's physical growth has been compared with the corresponding *age means* of height or weight or as derived from samples (even as small as 100 or fewer subjects) and ethnic origin. Apart from comparing a child's own weight and height with the *mean* of a group to which he never belonged, judgment of growth in terms of weight or height is precarious at best, considering what is at stake and what the serious limitations of such procedures really are. The Wetzel grid,[29] on the other hand, avoids all such handicaps by providing, instead, a fixed parameter—

a universal and accurate standard for measuring and appraising the body *size* and *shape* (build) and the *direction* and *speed* of human physical development. These estimates are distribution free and independent of the original units of measurement as well as of ethnic and sample variability. The grid's applications to pediatrics, school health, and physical education have often been described (Fig. 2-2). Its principles, too, have been confirmed by worldwide data, including the very first observations of Quetelet in 1831. Yet the severest test of validity and reliability, of course, resides in the fact that the grid "predicts" the *preferred paths* of healthy development as observed in today's children.

Typical children display considerable variation in height and weight throughout their growing years. The rate of growth in height increases and decreases as the individual matures. With the exception of the adolescent growth spurt, at age 10 to 12 years for girls and age 12 to 14 years for boys, the rate of height increase decelerates at a continual rate. The most dramatic height increase occurs as the individual matures in the pubescent period of life. Weight, in contrast to the development of height, is less predictable, having a number of fluctuations in most individuals' lifetimes. Because of the wide divergence in factors affecting weight, it is difficult to

Fig. 2-2. A, Long-term (11-year) Wetzel grid record based on semiannual measurements of weight and height routinely made in the School Health Program, Shaker Heights, Ohio. *AB,* "Good growth" gradually but definitely changing to "early growth failure," with change in direction along *AB* and "slowdown" along *1-2*. These trends became even worse along *BC* and *2-3*. Note, too, the continuing drop-off in growth potential average (GPA). **B,** Characteristic direction and speed trends in childhood obesity clearly confirmed by the accompanying photos at points *3* and *4*, respectively. Section *4-5* shows the response (return to the Channel A_3A_4 boundary and to the "less advanced auxodrome expected from the first two observations"). (**A,** By permission of Newspaper Enterprise Association, Cleveland, Ohio, 1965, from special reprint of a paper by Hopwood, H. H., and Van Iden, S. S.: J. School Health **35:**337, 1965; **B,** From Wetzel, N. C.: Don't take growth for granted, Cleveland, Ohio, 1961, Newspaper Enterprise Association.)

predict. As an example, muscle growth increases from the 30% that is normal in childhood to almost 40% during adolescence. Commonly, children who mature early tend to be heavier than those that mature late. Similarly the longer period of growth of those maturing late results in proportionally longer legs when compared to the trunk. Abnormal weight gain and obesity during the pubescent period may cause both physical and personality development problems that can adversely affect individuals throughout their lives.

Structural changes

A number of methods are employed to assess the maturational state of an individual. Many utilize age, height, and weight, whereas others use anthropometric measurements such as skeletal breadth or body circumferences. However, the most accurate assessment is made by x-ray examination of dental and skeletal osseous development.

The most obvious methods of indicating skeletal maturity are through observing long bone growth and through x-ray study of carpal ossification. Anatomically, the long bone consists of a shaft known as the *diaphysis;* at each end of its shaft is the *metaphysis.* An epiphyseal cartilaginous plate, termed the *epiphysis,* separates the metaphysis from the end of the long bone. Growth of the long bones occurs by the laying down of osseous tissue at the metaphysis, which pushes the epiphyseal plate up, extending bone length. Gradually, during adolescence and early adulthood, through the influence of hormones, particularly thyroxin, the diaphysis and the epiphysis reach maturity by joining together in an ossified unit (Fig. 2-3).

The carpal index has proved to be one of the most valid and reliable growth measures. Through x-ray examination, the child's stage of development can be detected. Carpal bones do not begin to show ossification until 2 to 3 years of age and complete epiphyseal closure does not occur until late adolescence.

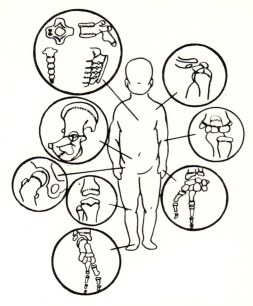

Fig. 2-3. Bones and their epiphyses. Carpal bones are often used as an index to determine the degree of ossification that has occurred at a particular age. Their development occurs between 2 and 18 years of age.

Before maturation, during the period when bones are predominantly cartilagious and have active epiphyseal growth centers, they are subject to stresses and trauma that may result in various structural deviations. This is a crucial period for injuries incurred by engaging in vigorous and traumatic sports activities. *Postural deviations occurring at this time may later develop into permanent structural changes, whereas diseases of the growth centers or of the epiphysis may result in disability and deformity.*

Postural adjustment

Good posture is that quality in which the body segments such as the head, trunk, pelvis, and lower limbs are in proper muscular and skeletal balance. Dynamically speaking, this means that the body is used in the most effective way with the least amount of strain placed on it supporting structures. Proper segmental alignment provides protection against acute injury or gradual deformity. The musculoskeletal system of the newborn child is extremely pliable and is subject to molding by the forces of gravity. Ossification and bone rigidity occur slowly with mineral salts, primarily calcium and phosphorus, replacing cartilaginous tissue. Muscle growth is associated with skeletal maturation. As the child uses his body, the musculoskeletal system is developed. Julius Wolff's law of functional adaptation, developed in 1876, clearly describes the influence of stress on the supporting structures of the body. It is stated as an *"early change in the form and the function of bones, or in their function alone, is followed by certain definite changes in their internal architecture, and equally definite changes in their external conformation, in accordance with mathematical laws."* This law indicates that the pull of gravity, coupled with muscle contraction, serves to inhibit or stimulate the growth rate of bones, depending on the degree and duration of the stress.

One of the greatest stresses placed on the musculoskeletal system is gravity. Ideally, the body should react against gravity by aligning its segments so that there is as little stress as possible. Constant faulty positioning of the young body can result in permanent structural deformities and asymmetry. Therefore the developmental process must be considered as playing an integral part in the posture of the child. The two most important changes that can be attributed to early posture are the development of the vertebral curvature and the transition of the center of gravity.

Because of the fetal position, in which the head and legs are placed in toward the trunk, the spine is forced into a single convex curve. In adjusting to the efforts at raising its head while in the supine position and, later, in attempting to crawl, the infant begins to develop the anterior cervical curve. Progressing through the stages of sitting, standing, and, eventually, walking, a compensatory anterior lumbar

curve develops in response to the gravitational force and the various musculoskeletal demands. However, it is not until late childhood that the mature vertebral curves occur. Adaptation of the spine to the stress of the upright posture is reflected in the increased size of the posterior aspect of the lumbar vertebrae and their thick intervertebral discs. The iliopsoas muscle serves to maintain the lumbar curve and the inclination of the pelvis and is one of the main stabilizers of the upright posture.

As the child develops posturally, there also occurs a lowering of the center of gravity, which gradually permits greater mobility in the upright position, freeing the upper extremities for fine motor activity. Lowering the center of gravity affords the child better balance and mobility.

Characteristically, the infant displays structural weaknesses until adjustment to the upright position has been accomplished. In preparation for locomotion, the child goes through various developmental periods such as sitting crawling, creeping, and standing, which prepare him for the next stage. In standing and walking during the early years, the infant often displays many normal postural characteristics that in later life may be deemed abnormal, for example, flat feet, knock-knees, pronated ankles (bearing weight on the inner side of the foot), and a pointing of the toes outward for a wider base of support. Many parents and educators become needlessly alarmed at the posture of small children when, in reality, it is normal for that particular maturational level. As the child develops strength and motor control, these postural adaptations usually give way to normal alignment. However, failure at adaptation may cause postural deviations that will eventually need to be corrected by professional help. Without proper balance, nutrition, sleep, relaxation, exercise, habit formation, and a general feeling of well-being, various postural asymmetries may occur to affect the individual adversely the rest of his life. The prevention of severe postural anomalies is of concern to all those who deal with children (Chapter 9).

Good postural adjustment, in reality, means good body mechanics and efficiency in the use of the body.[12] This is especially important to individuals requiring an increased conservation of energy, for example, those suffering from cardiorespiratory problems or chronic musculoskeletal disorders.

MORPHOLOGY AND SOMATOTYPING

Physical anthropologists as well as physical educators have long been interested in the relationship between human structure and the limitations it imposes on the movement of the body. Concern for body morphology dates back to early recorded history. In the last century, Kretschmer, a German psychiatrist, attempted to relate psychopathologies to specific morphological categories such as (1) the *pyknic* type, a person with a broad head, thick shoulders, large chest, short neck, and stocky body; (2) the *athletic* type, a person with well-defined musculature, long legs, and powerful trunk and arms; and (3) the *asthenic* type, a person with a thin, flat chest and poorly defined musculature. To this descriptive trichotomy, Kretschmer added a fourth dimension, which he called the *dysplastic*, or mixed, type.[35]

Emerging from the pioneering work of Kretschmer, William Sheldon and his collaborators produced an extensive system of classifying human morphology. This system, called somatotyping, is based on the body tissue that is derived from embryonic germ layers. These layers consist of the endoderm germ layer, which forms the primitive digestive and respiratory organs; the mesoderm germ layer, which develops into the musculoskeletal system and organs of circulation, reproduction, and excretion; and the ectoderm germ layer, which serves to create the nervous system and the sense organs. Sheldon characterized those individuals whose basic body morphology came predominantly from the endoderm germ layer as *endomorphs*—obese, having little muscle definition; small bones, large heads,

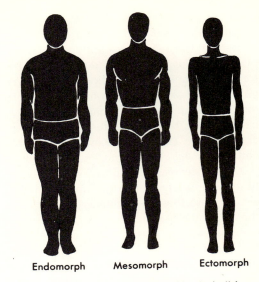

Endomorph Mesomorph Ectomorph

Fig. 2-4. A representation of body builds.

long trunks, short necks, short arms and legs tapered to the ends, little body hair, soft, smooth skin, and underdeveloped genitalia. In contrast to the endomorph, the *mesomorph* is described as having large bones, well-defined musculature, long neck, broad shoulders, slender waist, broad hips, long extremities, coarse skin, and well-developed genitalia. The third somatotype, the *ectomorph,* is linear in appearance, thin, and poorly muscled and has underdeveloped extremities and overdeveloped genitalia (Fig. 2-4).

Sheldon's original method considered an individual's body type as essentially unchangeable. Each of his somatotype components were evaluated on a seven-point scale. Many investigators have determined that Sheldon's initial findings are unsatisfactory and have proposed changes to overcome their inadequacies.[11, 14, 31, 34] Recently, a more valid and reliable method has been developed by Heath and Carter.[6, 7, 19] Their method of somatotyping uses the same descriptive categories as Sheldon but arrives at them by different means. The first component, endomorphy, is determined by taking skin fold measurements of the triceps, subscapular, and suprailiac regions. The

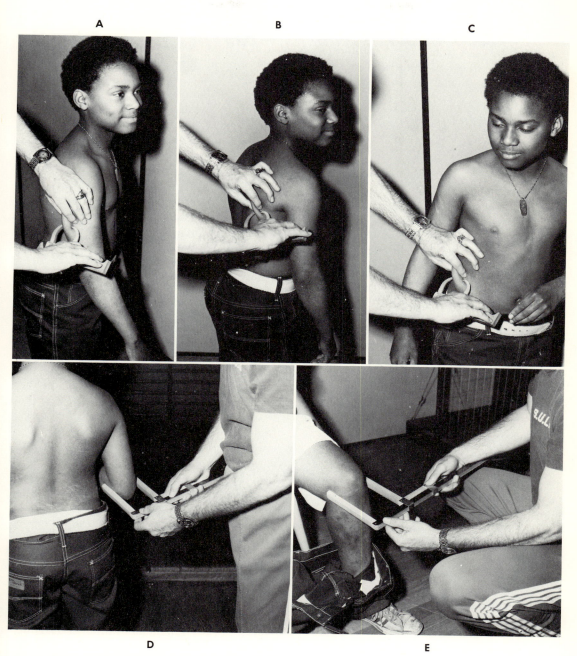

Fig. 2-5. Skin fold and biepicondylar diameter measurement. **A,** Tricep skin fold. **B,** Subscapular skin fold. **C,** Suprailiac skin fold. **D,** Humerus diameter. **E,** Femur diameter. (Courtesy California State University, Audio Visual Center, Long Beach, Calif.)

second component, mesomorphy, is arrived at by determining the subject's height; the biepicondylar diameters of the subject's humerus and femur; and the flexed muscle girths of the subject's biceps and calf, together with their skin fold corrections. (See Chapter 20 for techniques of girth measurement.) The third component, ectomorphy, expresses the linearity of the subject and is compiled by calculating as follows (Fig. 2-5):

$$\frac{Height}{\sqrt[3]{Weight}} = Linearity^*$$

Most studies in physical education and sports that deal with somatotyping have been mainly in the area of growth and athletic performance. In general, an individual who is less active than an athletic counterpart is usually more mesopenic or is lacking in mesomorphy and tends toward endomorphy.[6] Although genetics plays a major role in determining body build, factors such as exercise and nutrition can significantly alter somatotype ratings. Success in sport requires varying degrees of speed, strength, endurance, joint flexibility, and coordination. It has been determined that those individuals having a high mesomorphic and low endomorphic rating, in general, are better in their physical performance than those having a low mesomorphic and high endomorphic rating.

MOTOR BEHAVIOR

Whereas growth was earlier defined simply as the increase of body size, motor development is best characterized as the process by which a person, through maturation and experience, acquires management of his body. It is commonly accepted that as individuals grow, they become involved with integrating various segmental and random movements into complex patterns of motor behavior. From the very

*For further discussion of this calculation see Crowe, W. C., Arnheim, D. D., and Auxter, D.: Laboratory manual in adapted physical education and recreation, St. Louis, 1977, The C. V. Mosby Co.

beginning, the child is reacting to his environment with primitive reflexes that will gradually diminish as higher nervous system centers come into command.[16] The newborn attempts to orient himself in space and time and to adjust to the many physical forces imposed on him. He must learn to manipulate both his body and objects around him. The more specialized a cell, a tissue, or an organ system, the longer the period of maturation. This is particularly evident in nerve tissue. As myelinization of nerves occurs phylogenetically in the young organism, it is generally followed by an improvement of motor ability. At birth, the infant's lower brain centers are well developed as compared to his cerebral cortex. Reflexes such as sucking, swallowing, yawning, and sneezing are present at birth. However, reflexes such as grasping when the palm of the hand is touched, the "startle" (Moro) reflex, and the Babinski reflex (extension of the great toe and flexion of the other toes in response to stroking the plantar aspect of the foot) disappear as development progresses.

Fiorentino[16] divides normal reflexive development into the following three levels: the *apedal*, or spinal and/or brain stem, level with motor response of supine and/or prone lying; the *quadropedal*, or midbrain, level with a postural response of crawling and sitting; and the *bipedal*, or cortical, level with allowance for the action of standing and/or walking. If the normal sequential development of reflex maturation is disrupted because of neurological dysfunction, there often occurs delayed sensorimotor integration, for example, children who are diagnosed as having cerebral palsy may retain many reflexes that would normally have been replaced by the inhibiting functions of a higher neurological level.

The normal infant has rudimentary control of his head and neck in the first 4 to 6 months; then, during the seventh month, he begins to roll over from his stomach to his back. Sitting up, moving on all fours, and creeping occur in the first 7 months. With skeletal and neuromuscular maturity, the child progresses from crawling and creeping to the upright posture and then, between the ninth and eighteenth months, to taking independent steps.

In the early stages of walking, the young child toes out to provide a wider base of support. As strength is increased, the foot begins to realign to a straighter position. By the age of 3 or 4 years, most children have acquired a mature walking habit. A wide number of variations to the original walking pattern occur in the next 2 to 3 years, each requiring successively greater skill, for example, standing on one foot, running, climbing up and down stairs, jumping and hopping, riding a tricycle and a scooter, skipping and galloping, jumping over something, and kicking an object. All these skills can be executed by the normal youngster by the age of 5 or 6 years.

Man's upright position frees his hands for fine coordinated activity. The use of the hands in prehension stems from the early grasping reflex. Purposeful manipulation by the hands can take place only when the thumb develops opposition, the eyes are able to fix on a single object, and the coordination between hands and eyes matures. Shirley[36] described the maturational sequence of hand development as (1) reaching and missing an object; (2) reaching and touching an object; (3) reaching, grasping, and holding an object; and (4) reaching, grasping, and manipulating an object (Chapter 4).

The rudimentary patterns of throwing, catching, and striking objects can be seen in early childhood, but a number of years is required before these become competent skills. However, proficiency in these movements is seen in typical children between the ages of 6 and 7 years. A lack of proficiency in these basic motor skills may eventually cause difficulty in engaging in play activities.

Sex difference in movement behavior is apparent early in life. From an early age, boys can be noted to perform better than girls in most types of motor activities, which is more indicative of cultural influences than differences in physical potential. This difference gradually becomes greater during adolescence. Because of the dramatic changes in bodily proportions and functions, the pubescent boy develops increased strength, leverage, and stamina, which aid in all motor skills. Girls also go through marked physiological changes, which result in broad hips, narrow shoulders, and a low center of gravity, all of which tend to cause a failure in improvement in motor skills. Many of the differences between adolescent girls and boys in performance have been attributed to body structure; however, social aspects are the most important. In the last few years, girls' participation in vigorous physical activity has increased considerably. Since this increased interest, physical activity for girls has become more socially acceptable. In addition, there are fewer indications of sexual differences in physical performance than once were thought to exist.

As the typical child grows and matures, his motor abilities develop in an orderly and continuous manner from the simple to the more complex. In this way, the human organism is able to make adaptations to its particular developmental and experiential levels. Consequently, the major problem for the teacher, in relation to the developing child, is to help him engage in activities that are appropriate for his particular developmental level. Oxendine[30] describes readiness for motor activities as dependent on maturation, physical development, and specific prerequisities of learning. Although teachers are not able to alter a child's readiness for a maturational level, they can still provide appropriate readiness activities. Children who, as a result of some physical, mental, or environmental factor, fail to develop motor skills appropriate for their maturational level must be considered motorically retarded.

Children who become ill or who receive inadequate nutrition become less active in order to conserve their energies. Evidence indicates that prolonged inactivity and lack of movement experiences results in physical deterioration and motor retardation in the young. Besides affecting musculoskeletal functions, neural stimulation is also diminished. Hebb[20] indicated that inadequate physical and mental stimulation of humans and animals results in a break down of their total behavior. Whether or not the child is typical or atypical (normal or handicapped), motor development is a factor of maturation and involves the individual's ability to organize his behavior in varying situations. Although a physical or mental disability may create distinct retardation of motor responses, every opportunity for a great diversity of movement experiences must be afforded the child. Only by being able to make a wide variety of movement responses can the growing child face the numerous challenges that are placed before him by his internal bodily functions and the external demands of the environment. Each challenge, when surmounted, provides the child with a backlog of useful tools for overcoming additional and more complex problems in the future. Competency in physical play is of the greatest importance for a child's self-esteem and positive self-concept. Children, especially boys, who have poor motor ability find themselves left out of peer activities. Involuntary exclusion from play, whatever the reason, may cause the child to have feelings of devaluation.

Throughout the country, a number of special programs have been established to aid the motor retardate as well as the normal child in the area of sensorimotor activities. The concept of *movement education,* which originated in Europe, has important implications for the motor development of the child. This approach has grown out of the ever increasing concern over the restrictiveness of the child's environment, which disallows free, uninhibited play. Years ago, a child could climb trees, run, jump, and play at will, whereas now, in most cases, city life makes this impossible. Through movement education, the child can become mentally, emotionally, and physically involved in moving, exploring, and solving problems with his body. Each child moves individually in discovering his own personal environment. Having no predetermined standards, the child participates at his own rate of speed and within his own physical and mental capabilities.

With the growing awareness of the developmental needs of handicapped children has come the realization that motor proficiency tests are neither adequately evaluating the problem nor providing sufficient information for program planning. It is becoming more apparent that information regarding child growth and development should be applied in planning and administering physical education programs. Disregarding growth patterns leads to wasted efforts in teaching; a child cannot be taught activities he is not ready for and efforts to teach him these may result in his becoming frustrated and using awkward movements to compensate for his inability to function at a desired level.

There can be physical growth without corresponding motor learning. Such "learning is achieved through experience and experimentation with movements and patterns of movements." Physical education planned on the basis of sensorimotor experiences would be highly structured, developmental in nature, and seeking improvement in other areas through motor training.

Basic motor skill development

Whoever coined the term "first things first" said a great deal in a few words. Basic skill development is of paramount importance to the development of the specific and more complex skills and therefore should not be overlooked in physical education programs. Among the gross motor movements listed as basic skills are the following:

1. *Balancing:* Innervation of one side of the body against the other to maintain

body equilibrium against the forces of gravity

2. *Bending:* Flexion, extension, abduction, adduction, circumduction, rotation, eversion, inversion, and utilization of all the dimensions of movement of each joint of the body.

3. *Bouncing:* Short bipedal jumps involving a series of small jumps

4. *Carrying:* Exploration of lifting weights relative to base of support and experimentation with muscle groups most capable of coping with objects carried by the body

5. *Catching:* Executing the complicated match between hand and eye in an attempt to control an external moving object

6. *Climbing:* Using arms and legs to raise the body against the gravitational force

7. *Crawling:* Developmental pattern involving alternate use of opposite hand and leg to move in a prone position

8. *Creeping:* Pattern of locomotion in which the individual propels himself on hands and knees

9. *Crouching:* Flexion of ankles, knees, hips, and trunk

10. *Dodging:* Ability to stop and change direction relative to visual or auditory cue

11. *Dribbling:* Matching hand and eye, while moving the entire body, in order to control a ball bouncing on the floor

12. *Falling:* Acceptance of force as a result of gravitational pull

13. *Galloping:* Running with a leap interpolated after every other stride

14. *Hanging:* Resistance of weight against gravitational pull with arms or legs fixed and supported by an object

15. *Hitting:* Swift contact by hand with an external object (implement not used)

16. *Holding:* Exerting enough upward force against an object to balance gravity's pull so that the object has no vertical motion

17. *Hopping:* Propulsive force exerted by one foot, followed by landing on same foot

18. *Jumping:* Propulsive force exerted by one or two feet, but both feet contact the ground simultaneously

19. *Kicking:* Matching foot and eye so that leg and foot may exert force to propel an object

20. *Landing:* Acceptance of loss of kinetic energy when contacting a surface

21. *Leaping:* Propulsive force made by one foot with the landing made on the other

22. *Lifting:* Overcoming the gravitational force of an object by employing external resistance of muscles of the body

23. *Passing:* Propulsive force given to an object held in hands (many times a graded response)

24. *Pivoting:* Transference of weight to one foot with angular velocity applied so as to move body around a fixed point

25. *Pulling:* Overcoming a resistance so that the object will move toward the body

26. *Punching:* Hitting with no preliminary movement

27. *Pushing:* Overcoming a resistance in a direction away from the body

28. *Reaching:* Movement of arms away from the medial aspect of the body and over head

29. *Rising:* Raising the center of gravity

30. *Rocking:* Rhythmic transfer of center of gravity

31. *Rolling:* Throwing underhand so an object travels along a horizontal surface or turning body on floor

32. *Running:* Locomotion in which a flight phase is generated (from continuous movement)

33. *Skipping:* Continuous movement in which a hop is followed by a leap

34. *Starting:* Overcoming inertia of the body at rest by a muscular contraction

35. *Stooping:* Hip, knee, and ankle flexion that lowers the center of gravity over the base

36. *Stopping:* Overcoming the inertia of the body while it is in motion to bring it to a rest

37. *Stretching:* Movement at a joint that takes the limb as far as it can go
38. *Striking:* Using an implement to hit an object
39. *Swinging:* To-and-fro movement with the body suspended from a fixed object (body parts and object can also swing)
40. *Tagging:* Reaching, touching, and running activities
41. *Throwing:* Imparting force to an object held in the hand and releasing it to give it desired direction
42. *Tossing:* Short throw with graded impetus
43. *Touching:* Tactile stimulation to hand rendering it possible to discriminate the texture, size, and shape of an object
44. *Trotting:* Slow run in which there is a flight phase
45. *Tumbling:* Continuous transfer of weight from one part of the body to the other in a smooth fashion
46. *Twisting:* Rotation of a body part with or without accompanied movement
47. *Vaulting:* Transfer of weight and center of gravity from feet to hands to feet in a continuous direction
48. *Walking:* Continuous locomotor movement with the body in an upright posture involving a swing phase, contact, double support, and propulsion sequence that gives the body a linear direction

PSYCHOSOCIAL IMPLICATIONS

To understand the atypical individual adequately, the physical educator must become sensitive to the innumerable psychological and sociological factors that interact within each person. To explain human behavior fully as it relates to exceptionality would be an extremely difficult task. Therefore this section is intended to survey some of the more relevant psychosocial areas that relate to the handicapped person.

The terms "impairment," "disability," and "handicapped" often denote a negative state, one in which the recipient is less capable than his typical peer. For the sake of clarification, *impairment* is defined as a defect or deviation; *disability* will be considered a physical, mental, and/or emotional deviation that can be described clinically; and *handicap* will refer to the barriers that a disability imposes between the person and his optimal functional status. Broadly speaking, a handicap could be any encumbrance or disadvantage that makes personal goals more difficult to attain than if the disability were not present. If this concept is accepted, it can be speculated that the majority of persons are handicapped in some manner. It should be apparent to all that whether one wears glasses, is a member of an ethnic minority, or is unable to continue his job because of paralysis, *an individual's psychological reaction to a disability is personal, unique, and relative to the social milieu in which he finds himself.* In other words, an individual with a particular disability must not be expected to act in a prescribed manner nor must handicapped persons in general be expected to cope differently with life's problems than the nonhandicapped population.[4]

One must recognize that the child who is handicapped by a disability must adjust not only to his own limitations but also to the demands of society. Because of the numerous adjustments required of the severely disabled, psychological problems may be more frequent and serious than with individuals who are not handicaped.[11] However, there is no guarantee that because an individual is mentally, physically, or emotionally disabled, he will react differently than a person who does not have such a disability.

Individual adaptation

Man's adaptation and adjustment to the stresses of life are dependent on individual personality. Allport[1] broadly defined personality as *"what a man really is."* More descriptively, personality is *"the dynamic organization within the individual of those psychophysical systems that determine his unique adjustments to his environment."* This definition implies that personality is ever changing and consists of a balance between the mind and the body. The total human organism is in a constant state of flux. To acquire a healthy or positive adjustment to life, an individual must constantly be able to interact with his environment. The well-adjusted person is realistic in the requirements he places on himself and on his environment.

Adaptation by the individual begins at conception and continues throughout life. In the primary years, life's problems are resolved through the method of trial and error. As successes and failures are gradually incurred, the individual builds a backlog of ways of handling his various psychosocial problems. The exceptional individual may be denied many of life's experiences. Placed frequently in new psychological situations, the handicapped may find coping with their disabilities difficult and may resort to numerous adjustment mechanisms to alleviate the psychological pain. However, whether this adjustment is healthy or unhealthy is primarily dependent on how the individual has met the primary psychological growth stages, which include (1) *dependence and deprivation,* (2) *autonomy and discipline,* (3) *sexual development,* and (4) *management of aggression.*[38]

The first 6 months of a child's life represent a time of complete dependence, in which his primary concern is satiation of his immediate biological needs. Unsuccessful efforts to fulfill personal needs may result in a denial of the reality of the world. This early period helps to establish foundations for later behavior and determines whether the individual learns to trust or mistrust his immediate surroundings. If personal requirements are satisfied without undue duress, there is a good chance the individual will develop self-confidence and a positive self-concept, whereas a constant struggle to satisfy basic needs may lead to personal discontent and an environmental mistrust. Janov[22] describes the primary needs of the infant as being "fed, kept warm and dry, . . . held and caressed, and . . . stimulated."

As the child emerges from the helpless period, he gradually seeks independence. Increasingly, the child strives to control his immediate surroundings. As successful authority is gained over the environment, self-confidence is also gained. However, a constant thwarting of desired independence, as experienced by many disabled children, may eventually lead to discouragement and feelings of devaluation. With the second and third years of life, the individual stores a milieu of experiences as he explores the new vistas of movement and speech. This also becomes a time for learning discipline. Through the imposition of guidelines and rules, the child learns to control his actions. Complete freedom of expression produces within the individual an egocentricity that is unruly, whereas a lack of adequate freedom produces fears and a rigidity of personality. Therefore the right amount of discipline and freedom becomes a subtle matter of creating or establishing a firm, but loving and accepting, environment.

Sexual development is of primary importance to the total personality of an individual. Most authorities concur that sexual needs are apparent from earliest childhood. Feelings of affection, jealousies, and desires for bodily contact and caresses are basic to personality development. It is not until puberty, coupled with its obvious physiological changes, that the powerful sexual motive often presents overt problems of adjustment. Changes of body structure and the development of secondary sex characteristics, together with a newly acquired sex drive, serve to create unique conflicts for the individual. The individual views himself and others in a new perspective. Peer acceptance becomes uppermost in the thoughts and actions of the adolescent. The turmoil of adolescence becomes an extremely crucial period for the handicapped person, when he must face the added burden of his impairment and perhaps the depressing realization that love of the opposite sex, courtship, and marriage may be difficult or impossible for him.

The maturing individual must also cope

with aggression, a general term referring to the emotion of anger or hostility that stems from frustration. The seeds of aggression and its attending anxiety are sown early in a child's life when his attempts at environmental control are thwarted. Psychologists have described three basic ways that persons manage their anger or aggression: (1) *directing anger toward the environment,* (2) *directing anger toward the person,* and (3) *coping with anger in socially acceptable ways.* Depending on individual personality and circumstances, the venting of anger can be rational or irrational, overt or covert. Misplaced hostility acted out on society may become expressed in violence, prejudice, or bigotry. Also, a fear of the consequence of acting out anger may become inverted to a feeling of self-hate that may be manifested, in its most severe state, in self-annihilation. A healthy ability to cope with anger requires an understanding of its cause, an acceptance of its presence, and the ability to direct it into acceptable channels of expression. Anger is one of the most difficult emotions to manage because of its numerous social implications. As a result, the handicapped person could feel threatened by acting out normal anger because of his extreme dependency on others or, on the other hand, he may strike out in retaliation against a world that has caused him much pain and unhappiness. Aggression for the handicapped child may also take the form of tantrums as a means of gaining attention or of controlling the environment.

Social development follows closely the other factors of personal development already mentioned. Man is a "social being," with much of his success based on how well he gets along with others. Basically, the involvement of the individual in group situations emerges slowly from the complete egocentricity of the body to the gregariousness of the teenager.

The family

The family has a great influence on the total life-style of the disabled child.

Children who have severe or prolonged disabilities often are delayed in normal growth and development. Their life experiences are limited, with childhood extending far beyond the normal period. Long suffering often results in a preoccupation with the self and an emotional dependency on parents. Through the family and parental influences, personality strengths and weaknesses are forged to form adaptive mechanisms against the psychosocial stresses of life. The child has a tendency to view his disability in the same manner as his parents. If they regard him unrealistically, then the child fails to understand his limitations. Kessler[23] described the most common parental attitudes as oversolicitude, rejection, pushing the child to succeed beyond his abilities, and inconsistency in behavior toward the child. "The impact of an abnormal child on the family defies generalizations. Each child and each family presents an individual set of problems, requiring individual solutions. Any meaningful assessment of the impact of an abnormal child on the family requires an understanding of the family members as people —how they feel, how they live, their hopes and aspirations, their fears, their [religious] beliefs, their cultural, social, educational, and economic background."[23] Ideally, genuine love, warmth, and acceptance of their handicapped child on the part of the parents are the most important factors for the development of a well-adjusted personality.

Of great importance to the parents of a disabled child are the problems of overprotection, dependence, and independence. As is true with every child, the disabled child needs to develop independence wherever possible. Overprotection or extended help, especially when the child is very capable, confines and narrows his growth possibilities. The feeling of dependency can be both a frightening and a depressing experience.[4]

Many stresses and strains can be experienced in a family with a disabled child. The husband and wife may feel guilt and remorse for having this child. Anger and frustration may be displaced and vented on the child or siblings. Brothers and sisters may feel deprived of the attention of the parents, sensing that they are relegated to second place in the hearts and minds of the parents. Kohut stated:

It is not surprising, then, that well children become bitter and vent their anger on the abnormal child. In some instances, children act out the underlying hostility and anger felt by parents. . . . Older children are sometimes ashamed of an abnormal brother or sister. . . . Also, some will wonder if the disability is inherited and how this will affect their chances for marriage.[25]

No matter what the disability, the handicapped child must have responsibilities within the scope of his particular capabilities and must be depended on to carry them out. Praise and acknowledgment must follow each new accomplishment; however, caution must be taken that a parent does not become oversolicitous and overindulgent. A child who becomes too much the center of attention, or egocentric, fails to experience the pleasure that comes from sharing with others.

The school

Because of the limited opportunities for experiencing social situations, the disabled child may find school difficult. Cruickshank[11] indicated that the handicapped child very often finds difficulty in verbalizing or communicating his frustration, self-consciousness, and disappointment. The child often hesitates in new social situations, wondering whether he will be accepted, pitied, patronized, praised, rejected, or ignored. Therefore feelings of inferiority may crop up when the child attempts new things or suddenly finds himself in a competitive situation with normal children. It is extremely important that the exceptional child be accepted by his peers. Although family acceptance is vital for healthy psychological adjustment, a positive self-concept is largely attributable to the attitudes of peers and how they relate to the exceptional child. Although children are readily accepted by their peers in

elementary schools, they may become the recipients of malicious tricks. Derogatory names can be humiliating and devastating to the wholesome self-concept of the handicapped child. A concerted effort must be made by schools and teachers to help normal children understand and accept their atypical schoolmates.

The National Easter Seal Society for Crippled Children and Adults offers the following list of suggestions to aid the relationship between nondisabled and disabled persons*:

1. First of all remember that the person with a handicap is a person. He is like anyone else, except for the special limitations of his handicap.
2. A disability need not be ignored or denied between friends. But until your relationship is that, show friendly interest in him as a person.
3. Be yourself when you meet him.
4. Talk about the same things as you would with anyone else.
5. Help him only when he requests it. When a handicapped person falls, he may wish to get up by himself, just as many blind persons prefer to get along without assistance. So offer help but wait for his request before giving it.
6. Be patient. Let the handicapped person set his own pace in walking or talking.
7. Don't be afraid to laugh with him.
8. Don't stop and stare when you see a handicapped person you do not know. He deserves the same courtesy any person should receive.
9. Don't be overprotective or oversolicitous. Don't shower the handicapped person with kindness.
10. Don't ask embarrassing questions. If the handicapped person wants to tell you about his disability, he will bring up the subject himself.
11. Don't offer pity or charity. The handicapped person wants to be treated as an equal. He wants a chance to prove himself.
12. Don't separate a disabled person from his wheelchair or crutches unless he asks it. He may want them within reach.
13. When dining with a handicapped person, don't offer help in cutting his food. He will ask you or the waiter if he needs it.

---

*From When you meet a handicapped person. By permission of the National Easter Seal Society for Crippled Children and Adults, Chicago.

14. Don't make up your mind ahead of time about the handicapped person. You may be surprised at how wrong you are in judging his interests and abilities.
15. Enjoy your friendship with the handicapped person. His philosophy and good humor will give you inspiration.

Self-esteem

How the handicapped child views himself as a person is extremely important to his total psychosocial adjustment. The child constructs a sense of uniqueness and exclusiveness from the responses he elicits from other persons. If, for the most part, others' reactions are affirming, then a positive self-perception is acquired. If, however, a negative response is elicited, a variety of defense mechanisms may be used unconsciously by the disabled person to protect himself against the threat to self-esteem and the feelings of pain and anxiety.

The sense of personal worth or self-esteem is attained by the individual from his earliest strivings for autonomy and independence. A feeling of competence comes from accomplishing intended goals. However, when failure becomes the person's predominant experience, he develops a low self-evaluation. How the individual values himself is predominantly determined by society. Acquisition of feelings of personal worth begins with the family, expands to the playground and the school, and, subsequently, encompasses an individual's total experience.

The child's early group acceptance and self-esteem stem almost solely from his appearance and ability to engage actively in play. A child who deviates considerably in looks and actions often finds group membership denied him. Without active participation within the group, the child with a handicap may find personal adjustment difficult. Because opportunities for peer approval and recognition may be lacking, the courage to face many of life's problems fails to develop.

The atypical child soon becomes aware that others consider him different, treat him differently, and hold different expectations of him. He soon realizes that society places a high premium on an attractive appearance and a normal body. Cruickshank[11] described the disabled as being in an extremely untenable position in society. The disabled are denied the satisfaction of being disabled; to be accepted by society, they must continually strive to overcome their handicaps, often with minimal success. Such social pressures may cause psychological problems of adjustment and adaptation. Experiencing prejudice, discrimination, and lack of status, the child perceives himself a less worthy and capable individual. To the disabled, society may serve only to produce emotional distress, conflict, and development of a defense system.

Physique is one of the most important factors in the total development of personality. It is primarily through exploring and discovering the functions of the body that a child conceptualizes himself as a distinct person. Body image has been described as the way in which one pictures his body or, in other words, it is a system of ideas and feelings that the individual has about his physical structure. Wittreich and Grace[39] incorporated the concept of body image into expectation of present and future behavior by stating that "in every percept, or in every act, the individual is making some prediction as to what his body can do."

A physically or mentally less endowed child may be denied the many experiences that can be derived from movement. Lacking a positive body image, the child may consider himself a marginal person, rejected from the mainstream of life.

The well-adjusted person uses defense mechanisms moderately without jeopardizing his personal identity or a positive self-concept. A sense of being a distinct person in society requires an understanding and acceptance of the self with its strengths and its weaknesses. The various qualities of a person, his physical makeup, temperament, mental abilities, and special abilities, are reflected in his behavior, affecting his outlook on life and his unique perception of himself.

Reaction to sudden physical loss

The individual who suddenly receives a severe physical disability must face many crucial psychosocial adjustments. Because the body becomes an integral part of a person's total personality, any alteration in its function or appearance constitutes a threat to the total organism. A number of typical reactions have been observed to occur in patients who have experienced a physical loss.[18, 37] In general, they can be listed as (1) denial, (2) mourning and depression, (3) overt anger, and (4) return to a premorbid personality.

Denial is a common early reaction to a physical disability—the individual is unable to face reality. Denying the existence of the condition or the disability protects the individual against the pain of loss of self-esteem. *Mourning* and *depression* are common reactions for those individuals who have just experienced a physical loss. It can be compared to the bereavement and grief over a recently deceased loved one. The affected person believes he has now been denied the accomplishment of important goals. Wright[40] suggested that mourning becomes resolved when a realization is made that there are worse conditions or when one becomes weary of mourning and reestablishes positive values. *Overt anger,* or aggression and hostility, has been described by Rusk[33] as the third in the triad of basic emotions, with anxiety being first and depression second. A common early reaction of the disabled person is striking out in anger against a fate that was unkind. An outward expression of anger is much preferred to that of repressed anger because it can be dealt with accordingly. Anger that is not acted out finds devious means of expression. The energies of anger can be rechanneled by the physical educator to socially acceptable activities, sports, or other recreative pursuits. The *premorbid state* may be reached when a person who has incurred a physical loss has overcome his initial suffering, has accepted the fact of his loss, and has overcome his period of grief.

The ultimate adjustment to a recent handicapping condition is dependent on the individual's mental health at the time the condition occurs. Ideally, the person with a handicap should not only fully acknowledge his limitations but, above all, be realistically aware of his personal attributes and capabilities. In doing so, he shows the ability to adapt to new situations and to grow to become a more positively functioning person. The experienced teacher or therapist in a well-planned program of adapted physical education can do much to help the handicapped individual adjust satisfactorily to his own limitations and to his environment.

A developmental point of view seems most essential to program planning for disabled children. It takes as its point of departure the child's basic nature and needs. It acknowledges the racial implications that determine sequences and the distinctive growth patterns of each individual child. Because of the great variability in the motor skills of the generic handicapped population, this philosophy seems particularly applicable. A perceptiveness of growth appears most indispensable for accurate guidance in establishing programs in physical education and recreation. It demands that the teacher be alert to the growth needs of the child and be able to answer the following questions: "How does the child grow?" "How does he learn?" and "How does he advance from stage to stage as he matures?" These three questions are really one: "How can the tremendous heterogeneity in needs among the handicapped population be met?"

Programs should intervene, assist, direct, postpone, encourage, and discourage many turns of development. They should create the most favorable conditions for self-regulation and self-adjustment.

It is necessary to remember that growth is a unified process and that the forces affecting one phase of development make an imprint on others as well. There is no step in the growth process that can be bypassed without consequence to subsequent development.

It becomes apparent that there should be a reduction in the tendency to adhere to chronological and mental age norms and scales. Rather the child should be viewed in terms of maturity. The disabled child's behavior at the moment is a result of a composite of factors that cannot be defined adequately by chronological or mental age alone. The label "handicapped" tells little about the needs, characteristics, motor abilities, and limitations of the child. A diagnosis should be made of each child regarding motor and physical characteristics and subsequent plans should be implemented to meet the defined needs.

REFERENCES

1. Allport, G. W.: Personality: a psychological interpretation, New York, 1937, Holt, Rinehart & Winston, Inc.
2. Ansubel, D. P.: Theory and problems of adolescent development, New York, 1954, Grune & Stratton, Inc.
3. Arnheim, D. D., and Sinclair, W. A.: The clumsy child: a program of motor therapy, St. Louis, 1975, The C. V. Mosby Co.
4. Baldwin, C. P., and Baldwin, A. L.: Personality and social development of handicapped children. In Psychology of the handicapped child, Washington, D.C., 1974, U.S. Department of Health, Education, and Welfare.
5. Bayley, N.: Manual for the Bayley Scales of Infant Development, New York, 1969, The Psychological Corporation.
6. Carter, J. E. L.: The somatotype of athletes —a review, Hum. Biol. 42:536-569, 1970.
7. Carter, J. E. L., and Heath, B. A.: Somatotype methodology and kinesiological research, Kinesiology Rev., 1971. (Reprint.)
8. Cratty, B. J.: Movement behavior and motor learning, Philadelphia, 1967, Lea & Febiger.
9. Cratty, B. J.: Perceptual and motor development in infants and children, London, 1970, Macmillan and Co., Ltd.
10. Cratty, B. J.: Perceptual-motor behavior and educational processes, Springfield, Ill., 1969, Charles C Thomas, Publisher.
11. Cruickshank, W., editor: Psychology of exceptional children and youth, Englewood Cliffs, N.J., 1966, Prentice-Hall, Inc.
12. Cureton, T. K., Jr.: Physical fitness appraisal and guidance, St. Louis, 1947, The C. V. Mosby Co.
13. Damon, A.: Adult weight gain, accuracy of stated weight and their implications for constitutional anthropology, Am. J. Phys. Anthropol. 23:307-311, 1965.
14. Espenschade, A. S., and Eckert, H. M.: Motor development, Columbus, Ohio, 1967, Charles E. Merrill Publishing Co.
15. Fiorentino, M. R.: Normal and abnormal development, Springfield, Ill., 1972, Charles C Thomas, Publisher.
16. Fiorentino, M. R.: Reflex testing methods for evaluating C.N.S. development, Springfield, Ill., 1963, Charles C Thomas, Publisher.
17. Frankenberg, W. K., and Dodds, J. B.: The Denver Developmental Screening Test, J. Pediatr. 71:181-191, 1967.
18. Garrett, J. F., editor: Psychological aspects of physical disability, Washington, D.C., 1962, U.S. Department of Health, Education, and Welfare.
19. Heath, B. H., and Carter, J. E.: A modified somatotype method, Am. J. Phys. Anthropol. 27:57-74, 1967.
20. Hebb, D. O.: The mammal and his environment, Am. J. Psychiatry 3:826-871, 1955.
21. Hughes, J. G.: Synopsis of pediatrics, ed. 4, St. Louis, 1975, The C. V. Mosby Co.
22. Janov, A.: The primal scream, New York, 1970, Dell Publishing Co., Inc.
23. Kessler, J. W.: The impact of disability on the child, J. Am. Phys. Ther. Assoc. 46:153-159, 1966.
24. Knobloch, H., and Pasamanick, B.: Gesell and Amatruda's developmental diagnosis, 1974, Harper & Row, Publishers.
25. Kohut, S. A.: The abnormal child: his impact on the family, J. Am. Phys. Ther. Assoc. 46:160-167, 1966.
26. Koontz, C. W.: Koontz Child Developmental Programs training activities for the first 48 months, Los Angeles, 1974, Western Psychological Services.
27. LeWinn, E. B.: Human neurological organization, Springfield, Ill., 1969, Charles C Thomas, Publisher.
28. Logan, G. A.: Adaptations of muscular activity, Belmont, Calif., 1964, Wadsworth Publishing Co., Inc.
29. Montoye, H. I., editor: An introduction to measurement in physical education, Indianapolis, 1970, Phi Epsilon Kappa Fraternity.
30. Oxendine, J. B.: Psychology of motor learning, New York, 1968, Appleton-Century-Crofts.
31. Parnell, R. W.: Somatotyping by physical anthropometry, Am. J. Phys. Anthropol. 12:209-239, 1954.

32. Roach, E. G., and Kephart, N. C.: The Purdue perceptual-motor survey, Columbus, Ohio, 1966, Charles E. Merrill Publishing Co.
33. Rusk, H. A.: Rehabilitation medicine, ed. 3, St. Louis, 1971, The C. V. Mosby Co.
34. Sheldon, W. H.: The varieties of human physique, New York, 1940, Harper & Row, Publishers.
35. Sheldon, W. H., Hartl, E. M., and McDermott, E.: Varieties of delinquent youth, New York, 1949, Harper & Row, Publishers.
36. Shirley, M. M.: The first two years; a study of twenty-five babies, Minneapolis, 1931, University of Minnesota Press.
37. Strickler, M., and LaSor, B.: The concept of loss in crisis intervention, J. Ment. Hygiene **54:**301-305, 1970.
38. White, R. W.: The abnormal personality, New York, 1964, The Ronald Press Co.
39. Wittreich, W. J., and Grace, M.: Body image development, unpublished progress report to the Office of Naval Research, 1955.
40. Wright, B. A.: Physical disability—a psychological approach, New York, 1960, Harper & Row, Publishers.

RECOMMENDED READINGS

Baldwin, A. L.: Theories of child development, New York, 1967, John Wiley & Sons, Inc.

Barker, R. G.: Adjustment to physical handicap and illness: a survey of the social psychology of physique and disability, New York, 1953, Social Science Research Council.

Bayley, N.: The development of motor activities during the first three years, Soc. Res. Child Dev. Monogr. 1:1-26, 1935.

Cruickshank, W. M., editor: Psychology of exceptional children and youth, Englewood Cliffs, N.J., 1966, Prentice-Hall, Inc.

Fisher, S., and Cleveland, S. E.: Body image and personality, ed. 2, New York, 1968, Dover Publication, Inc.

Garrett, J. F., and Levine, E. S.: Psychological practices with the physically disabled, New York, 1962, Columbia University Press.

Ginott, H. G.: Between parent and child, New York, 1965, Macmillan Publishing Co., Inc.

Kephart, N. C.: The slow learner in the classroom, Columbus, Ohio, 1964, Charles E. Merrill Publishing Co.

Telford, C. W., and Sawrey, J. M.: The exceptional individual, Englewood Cliffs, N.J., 1967, Prentice-Hall, Inc.

Wright, B. A.: Physical disability: a psychological approach, New York, 1960, Harper & Row, Publishers.

3

FACTORS IN PERCEPTUAL-MOTOR DEVELOPMENT

■ Perception is the integer between a child and his environment. Thus it enables him to interpret objects and events and assists in the acquisition of learning.

There is a growing awareness in the field of physical education that the factors that differentiate poor and proficient performance in motor skills are related to perceptual characteristics. Therefore the perceptual development of children cannot be overlooked. Worthy of emphasis is that perception can be developed. Therefore programs that are task oriented and sequentially constructed to develop these essential perceptual characteristics of the learner are of paramount importance not only to adapted physical education but also to the total physical education program.[12, 13]

It is generally accepted that normal perception is essential for the acquisition of higher order motor skills as well as to the development of cognitive skills. A child must accurately interpret symbols that form words before meanings can be attached to these words. There is evidence that fulfillment of sensorimotor prerequisites may assist in the development of higher cognitive abilities.[3, 8, 10, 11]

Reading is one of man's highest cognitive abilities, requiring many integrative perceptual functions; consequently, children prior to the age of 5 years usually cannot read with fluency. With regard to children who function at preschool levels, perceptual-motor training programs are essential to total development, particularly the development of those individuals having impaired perception (Fig. 3-1).

PERCEPTUAL-MOTOR DEVELOPMENT AND THE DISABLED

There is a need for perceptual training programs for disabled children. Besides cognition, normal development of the senses of vision and audition have been purported to be a prerequisite to the development of a sound motor base. Through appropriate use of kinesthetic information, together with movement experiences that are paired with audition and vision, normal perception is made possible. It then follows that children who are physically, mentally, or emotionally impaired may be limited in their perceptual ability and may require some form of perceptual training intervention. It is also accepted that children who are mentally retarded possess deficiencies in the ability to appropriately utilize sensory information and past experience to solve efficiently current problems. The basic interrelated components that are involved in the perceptual process need assessment and treatment in the case of each individual learner, whether he is handicapped or not. It has been indicated that 20% of a normative population may need training to appropriately use perceptual information that poses a problem to efficient learning. Therefore perceptual development appears to be a global trait that is specifically relevant to the total development of the majority of handicapped children and generally relevant to all children (Fig. 3-2).

Handicapped children, more often than not, are limited in their ability to physically explore the environment, thus experiencing deficiencies in the development of perception. Furthermore, depending on the nature of the handicap, adaptation that will compensate for the lack of perception in the handicapped child may be needed. The following are examples of such adaptation:

1. Blind children must perceive spatial objects through audition or touch.

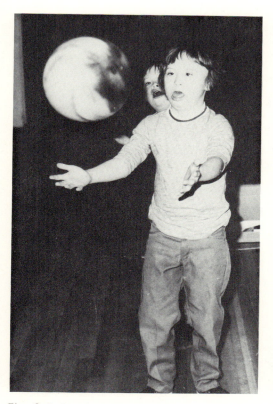

Fig. 3-1. Handicapped children who function at preschool cognitive and motor levels learn to focus attention on a ball and track with their eyes.

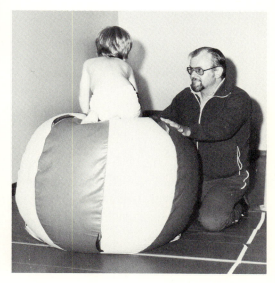

Fig. 3-2. Learning to statically balance on an unstable base of support. (Courtesy California State University, Audio Visual Center, Long Beach, Calif.)

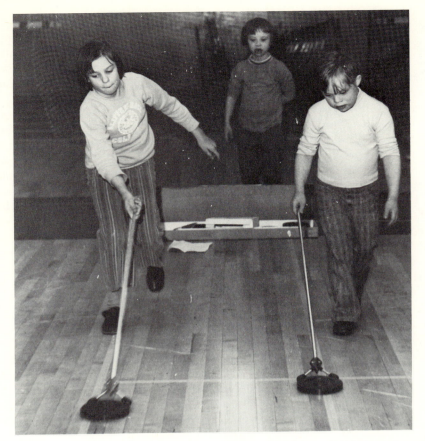

Fig. 3-3. Handicapped children move their bodies and shuffleboard disks in space as their eyes inspect.

2. The blind read through touch and can be instructed in physical activity through manual kinesthetic guidance or audition.
3. Deaf children must develop refined perceptual skills in vision to read lips for instructional purposes.
4. Physically handicapped children may have had limited motor experience and therefore not have developed a kinesthetic awareness of movement capability; thus adaptation may be needed (Fig. 3-3).
5. Minimally brain-injured children or slow learners often are deficient in the total process of perception.

Lack of consideration by the physical educator for the perceptual capability of the handicapped child and its impact on his total development severely limits the possibility for positive change.

Perceptual development

Children need primary perceptual-motor experiences to master higher order perceptual-motor skills. It is essential that the requirements of any prescribed task selected by the instructor for the learner be in accord with the learner's current abilities; otherwise, the perceptual process functions less than optimally.

It is accepted that early perceptual learnings are provided through differential movement experiences.[2, 9, 10, 14] Early in development, a child moves his body randomly and thus gains strength and mobility. As the child's body moves from object to object, the pairing of the eye functioning with the muscular energy expended in movement among objects tends to structure objects visually in space from the self. For instance, if a child sees a table that is 15 feet from him, the visual placement of the table in space from the child has been developed through a visual-motor match. This match involves an experiential history of comparing muscular energy through movement of the body to the table with ocular motor adjustments of the eye in which the child perceives the table as large when he is close and small when he is far away. As the child moves toward the table, he perceives it as becoming larger and larger; the distance that the table is from the child can only be accurately measured in space through a comparison of the muscular energy expenditures produced by the body as he moves toward the table and the relationship to changing visual imagery as interpreted by the eye. Thus the confirmation of objects in space, as interpreted by the eye, are the result of movement experiences paired with visual experiences. Kephart[11] has indicated that motor movements accompany the development of vision and of location of visual and auditory objects in space.

Perceptual development is cumulative, in that the utilization of each new additional experience provides opportunities for the person to seek out greater differential experiences. The extension of motor capability through engagement in new experience expands perceptual-motor capability almost to geometric proportions. On the other hand, stereotyped motor activity may contribute to a lag in perceptual development because of the lack of new developmental experience. *Furthermore, handicapped children who lag in early motor development may be afflicted with maldevelopment in the social and emotional spheres.*[15] It has been hypothesized that these aspects of development are interrelated and that deficiency in one area of development (motor) may adversely affect other aspects of development such as the social and/or emotional factors. Society has expectations for a child at each level of development. Therefore if the individual is unable to fulfill the expectation at a certain age, particularly in the areas of self-help skills, psychosocial stresses may arise. Furthermore, if a child is incapable of accurately perceiving environmental reality, then his adaptability to his environment is adversely affected.

EDUCATIONAL APPROACHES

There are several systems of perceptual-motor training. Among them are those proposed by Frostig,[7] Dunsing and Kephart,[5] and Ayres.[2] The Frostig approach is primarily concerned with visual perceptual skills as they relate to reading and the purpose of the training is to achieve skills related to these particular ends. Frostig also incorporates gross motor behavior in her program of educational remediation.[6] Kephart poses training based on a theory of perceptual-motor development in which the child's orientation to his environment is emphasized. Kephart's concern is with learning problems in which the perceptual process is incomplete. Therefore in training the child, he frequently returns to basic motor patterns and motor experiences that enable one to attain adequate relationships of one's body to the environment in a spatial-temporal context. Ayres,[2] on the other hand, proposes a neurophysiologically based program intended to assist the child with a learning disorder in developing normal sensory integration through techniques that stimulate the tactile, vestibular, and proprioceptive systems (Fig. 3-4).

THE PERCEPTUAL PROCESS

Perception has been defined as the meaning that is attached to objects and events that occur in the environment. Therefore accuracy in the interpretation of what is perceived by an individual will be directly related to the quality of a motor response. For instance, if a handicapped child is in-

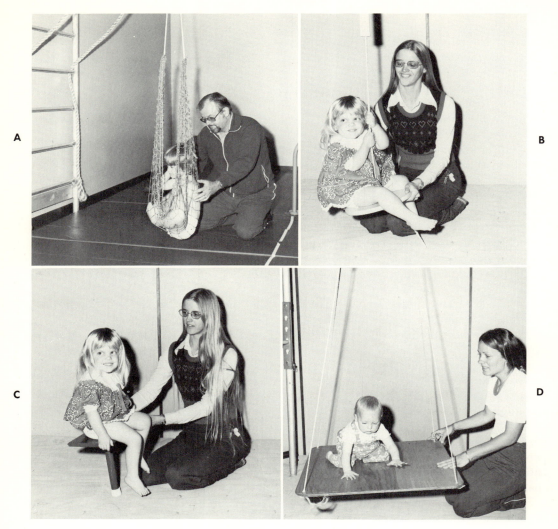

Fig. 3-4. Assisting sensory integration through vestibular stimulation. **A,** Swinging and twisting in a net. **B,** Bouncing and turning on a swing. **C,** Balancing on a "T" stool. **D,** Maintaining balance on a platform swing. (Courtesy California State University, Audio Visual Center, Long Beach, Calif.)

volved in basketball and cannot accurately interpret his distance from a basket, the chances for successful shooting are reduced because of his inability to perceive the proper distance. A successful basketball player must be able to determine how much force is required to direct the ball to the basket. If this distance cannot be interpreted accurately, then task success will be impaired. Another example might be when

a golfer attempts to putt a ball in a hole. If he cannot perceive the appropriate force to be applied to the ball through the club head, the possibility of task success may be reduced. If a disabled softball player cannot perceive the speed of a thrown ball and determine where it is spatially in relationship to the bat as it approaches the plate, there is a possibility of error when the bat contacts the ball. Every instance in

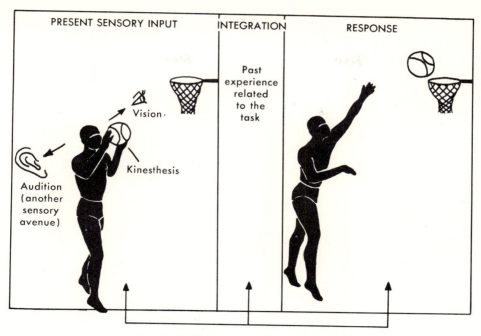

PRESENT SENSORY INPUT   INTEGRATION   RESPONSE

Vision·

Past
experience
related
to the
task

Kinesthesis

Audition
(another
sensory
avenue)

Fig. 3-5. Model of perceptual process.

sports involves the interpretation of stimuli to which a response is to be made. Impairment in perception will detract from the pupil's ability to perform motor tasks in a great many spheres of physical activity (Fig. 3-5).

Perceptual development involves hypothesized opportunities in activity to interpret visual objects, auditory symbols, and kinesthetic events so that an individual may behaviorally adapt to the response that is desired. In essence, perceptual development involves adequate storage of past experience for the interpretation and solution of future problems. In its simplest form, the perceptual process involves interpreting current stimuli associated within a specific content integrated with past experience from which a response is made. Information is provided regarding the appropriateness of the response and is then fed back to the organism for storage. Thus prior experience is utilized to assist in solving current motor problems. A perceptual training program seeks varied but similar experience

for the learner for the purpose of building a background of differential experiences so that he may solve other similar problems in the future. One should note that *redundant repetitious activities that lie inside the behavioral repertoire of the learner do not contribute to perceptual development.* For example, if a child can walk a 4-inch beam efficiently, there is little perceptual development value in performing the activity again, for he is not struggling to extend his behavioral repertoire. However, if a child were to walk a 4-inch balance beam and were required to struggle with his balancing mechanism to stay on the beam or were to fall off (and be provided with the knowledge that he fell off), then the assumption could be made that this particular experience was outside his current behavioral repertoire. Information probably would be provided of the consequences of not properly equating innervation of one side of the body to the other as he moved down the balance beam. Such an experience would be in accord with the

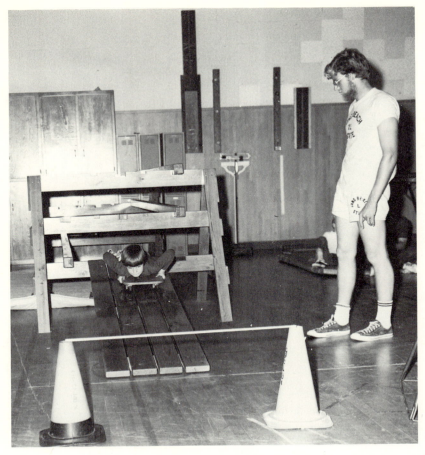

Fig. 3-6. Gaining perceptual-motor experiences. (Courtesy California State University, Audio Visual Center, Long Beach, Calif.)

development of perception that involves the balancing mechanism.

Perceptual development involves a greater variety of different instructional strategies than does the acquisition of specific motor skills. The selection of such strategies should be precise. With the selection of the precise activity, a new experience should be provided for the learner. Therefore *similar but not identical elements must be part of the composition of tasks in the perceptual-motor training program* (Fig. 3-6). The concern of perceptual development is to provide a broad base of varied motor experience for solutions to skillful performance in more specific complex skills.

Analysis of skill proficiency

Four component parts of the perceptual process must be operative before the performer can achieve desired task mastery. An example of the skill of shooting a basketball will be used as the task. The four component parts are as follows:

1. The learner must be able to perceive or conceptualize the desired response.
   EXAMPLE: The ball must pass through the basket.
2. The learner must make a response relevant to current sensory input as it relates to his past experience.
   EXAMPLE: He must be aware of his distance from the basket and remember

the amount of force he gave to the ball from similar distances from the basket in the past.

3. The learner must be aware of consequences of the response made in comparison to the desired response.

    EXAMPLE: Did the ball go into the basket? If not, why?

4. The learner must store the information for subsequent use to perform better next time. Appropriate storage of new experience with its functional utilization at a subsequent time is the essential element of the perceptual process.

    EXAMPLE: He must remember the outcomes of the shot and the conditions under which they occur so that performance can be corrected next time.

Such a model provides a basis for the analysis of deficiency in task performance of a learner who possesses a disabling condition. For instance, if the defined task for a performer, impaired or normal, is to hit a softball and he cannot hit the ball, the question that must be asked in light of the model of the perceptual process is "why?" There may be several reasons why he fails to achieve mastery of the tasks. They may be as follows:

1. *Inability to interpret current stimulation:* The performer may fail to interpret the speed, direction, or position of the ball in the spatial area where the ball is to be hit.

2. *Inappropriate past experience:* The performer may not have prior experience for space-time predictions as to when the ball will meet the bat to hit it properly.

3. *Lack of physical prerequisites to make the response:* The performer may not be strong enough or coordinated enough to move the bat with sufficient speed to hit the ball.

4. *Inability to interpret the desired response through inappropriate utilization of feedback:* The performer may inappropriately interpret information concerning the performed act as compared to the desired response because of inappropriate feedback or he may not re-

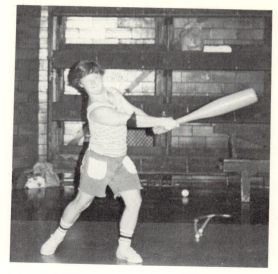

Fig. 3-7. A plastic bat, which provides a wider hitting surface, enables the learner to successfully respond to an adapted softball activity.

member the conditions of prior performances. Improvement may be impaired for incorrect alterations of the swing cannot be made when similar conditions occur. Stated another way, the performer is likely to make the same mistake twice and thus prevent storage of differential information because of inadequate retention of feedback.

5. *Any combination* of the reasons mentioned above may be a deterrent in learning (Fig. 3-7).

Utilization of a perceptual process model

The application of the model of the perceptual process enables an instructor to precisely identify target deficiencies of a handicapped learner. For instance, in the case of the learner trying to hit the softball, there are several reasons why the learner may fail. Application of such a model would explore the following possibilities:

1. It may be that the visual mechanism is at such a level of development that the ocular motor muscles cannot track the ball with the ability needed to

master the task. If this is the case, prerequisites for achieving task success have not been developed within the framework of the learner. Therefore developmental programs are needed to establish better functioning of the oculomotor mechanism before the ball can be hit with the desired proficiency. In some instances, the refractory portion of the eye may be unable to perform the physiological functions of the eye for task success. Thus prior practice experiences to move the eye with expediency have not been developed to the point of consistent task mastery. Therefore sequential tasks that lead to the development of the ocular motor ability of the eye as it relates to the skill are in order.

EXAMPLE: Use a larger ball and throw it slowly so that the eye can track the object.

2. If the child is incapable of moving the bat fast enough because of his lack of strength development, he may need to fulfill this prerequisite for task mastery. In this particular instance, a strength development program might be needed to provide the pupil with needed prerequisites for obtaining task mastery.

EXAMPLE: Throw the ball from a greater distance or use a heavier ball. In addition, the child may perform special developmental exercises.

3. Inappropriate functioning of the feedback mechanism may be a deterrent to learning. It may be that the pupil is unable to accurately interpret and rectify errors that have occurred at a prior time or, because of prior task failure earlier in similar learning situations, tends to repress prior information that may assist in task mastery.

EXAMPLE: Arranging successful experience with stronger feedback for hitting the ball may be added to the process. This may better activate use of the feedback mechanism. Hitting a ball suspended on a string may be effective.

4. The child may be unable to relate the

consequence of the motor act to the conditions under which the motor act took place.

EXAMPLE: Let us use the case of the child hitting the ball. In this particular instance, feedback is expressed by the distance and direction the ball travels as a result of its being hit by the child. Therefore the adaptation to facilitate feedback for this specific task is the introduction of a large light ball. With relatively little force applied, the ball travels a considerable distance. The projection of the ball provides feedback that is paired by the child to

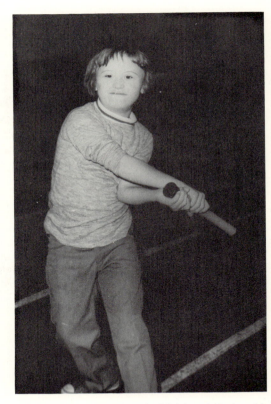

Fig. 3-8. A handicapped child has failed to hit the ball. He (1) could make the response, that is, swing the bat, (2) did not interpret the ball in time and space, (3) may not have had appropriate and adequate prior practice or experience, and (4) may not utilize or determine alternatives to failures.

the motor response and the conditions under which the ball was projected. Therefore the size of the ball enables the child to be repetitively successful and provides positive feedback regarding distance that the ball travels as a result of his efforts. The input conditions, hitting response, and its consequence may be retained better because of the provision of strong positive feedback.

The interpretation of information may be made sequentially more difficult by a reduction in size of the ball or heavier bats could be gradually introduced into the activity. Eventually, the child might be able to hit a ball using a bat that approximates one used in a conventional softball game (Fig. 3-8).

Generalizing perceptual-motor experience

With few exceptions, perceptual-motor training programs indicate that training activities are specific to the skill that has been practiced. There is a need to explore a generalized activity experience that might be transferred to perceptual-motor skills other than those that have been practiced. Therefore the nature of the perceptual-motor experience consists of searching for a reservoir of motor experience that, hopefully, will provide the ability for learning a broad group of skills with greater facility.

ASSESSMENT AND ACTIVITIES FOR SPECIFIC PERCEPTUAL DEFICITS

Specific components of perceptual-motor structure have been hypothesized by Dunsing and Kephart.[5] Such a classification system of perceptual components enables the identification of specific target traits to be developed within the framework of the visuomotor structure. Thus once the specific subdomains are identified, activities that develop these specific domains may be paired with measured needs for treatment of handicapped children. Furthermore, through the generation of a profile of ability and disability on specific perceptual characteristics, it is then possible to select appropriate activities to enhance the visual-perceptual subdomains of a specific child.

There are several types of perceptual-motor assessments that yield different kinds of data. Two types of data result from tasks that are observed for qualitative performance. Observational assessment involves a study of the patterns of movement, from which an inference is made with respect to a perceptual-motor deficit. On the other hand, behavioral performance usually results in a quantifiable score to compare pupil skills with chronological age performance. Whatever form testing takes, it is essential that activities that constitute the program be directly related to assessment and that the ability level of the specific child be reached when prescriptive activity is implemented (Chapter 4).

Types of perceptual inputs during physical activity

There are essentially three types of sensory input utilized in physical activity: vision, kinesthesis, and audition. All senses are used to some degree in the performance of motor activity; however, in a given task, one form of input may predominate over the others or a task may rely on two of the sensory inputs more than on others.

Vision. Vision refers to sensation interpreted by the eye and to the meaning that is attached to the interpretation of the event. Visual skill is particularly important in those activities involving projectiles (Fig. 3-9).

Kinesthesis. Kinesthesis is the awareness of the position, direction, and extent of movement of the limbs and the whole body. Also, closely associated with kinesthesis is the vestibular mechanism. This mechanism is found in the inner ear and informs the body of its rate of movement and its position in space. It is particularly important in successful participation in activities that involve changes in body position such as performing stunts as well as refined skills requiring precise movement and accuracy.

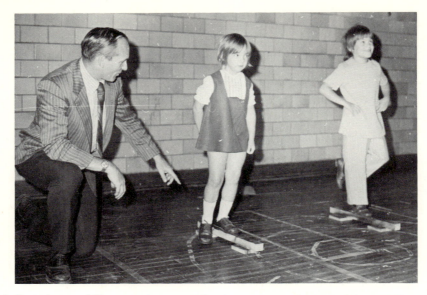

Fig. 3-9. Balance ability may be generalized into many physical activities. The girl on the right has generalized it, so her vision is off the task. The girl on the left searches for visual cues in the environment to maintain balance.

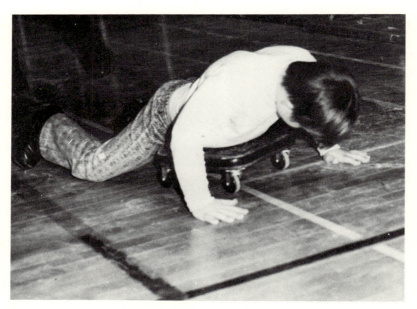

Fig. 3-10. A handicapped child moving a scooter at different rates. Moving the scooter with the body placed in different positions develops kinesthetic awareness of the body parts involved in the motor task.

The utilization and development of this sense in handicapped children is essential for gaining motor control (Fig. 3-10).

Audition. Audition refers to the reception of sound by the ear and its interpretation by the auditory center in the brain. Many activities in the adapted physical education curricula rely on audition; those groups of activities that are particularly concerned with auditory perceptual ability are rhythms.

• • •

Specific activities in the physical education curriculum may be associated with the reception of information through specific sensory avenues. The knowledge of the nature of sensory inputs in activity is important because it assists the teacher in sequential selection of activity and facilitates more accurate pairing between difficulty of the task and ability level of the child. Following are examples of pairing sensory avenues of reception to motor tasks:

1. *Development of kinesthetic awareness* is obtained through participation in motor experience. Programs of this nature would include activities that involve gross motor movement such as beam walking and movement exploration activities.

2. *Visual development* in physical education may occur through developmental programs that involve the ocular management of objects in space, which includes both their reception and projection. Examples of such activities are ball activities in which the eye tracks the object in coordination with the hands in the act of throwing or catching.

3. *Auditory perception development* can be effected by rhythm programs. In such programs, auditory inputs are paired with motor movements.

4. *Perceptual development programs* can be made more complex by requiring more elaborate integration of sensory input with motor output. The following are examples of visual-kinesthetic movements:

    a. Such activities might involve qualitative movements in catching or hitting projectiles, which require kinesthetic perception for proper application of force and appropriate positioning of limbs. Activity becomes more complex when the eye must track objects that involve distance-time ratios.

    b. Auditory-kinesthetic movements occur in the more elaborate dances and floor exercise routines (gymnastics).

    c. Rhythmical gymnastics may involve throwing and catching balls to music and engaging the body in qualitative movement; thus there is expression of the integration of all senses.

Regardless of the nature of the act performed, it is important to be aware of the complexities of perpetual inputs and the responses expected to be made so that the degree of task difficulty can be matched with the level of the handicapped child's ability. Appropriate selection of activity is essential to perceptual development for it is the instrument that enables progression for each child (Fig. 3-10).

HIERARCHY OF PERCEPTUAL DEVELOPMENT

Getman[10] and Dunsing and Kephart[5] have provided information that suggests a hierarchy of motor behaviors that serve as prerequisite functions for the acquisition of higher order visual perceptual abilities. This is of great significance to the physical educator, since application of a prerequisite structure makes possible the specific positioning of an individual on that structure; thus it enables selection of appropriate activities for a specific child.

A normal child is born with innate responses, which appear to be the initial base from which motor responses will develop. Established innate responses are interwoven with the first random movement and later with the basic locomotor patterns such as crawling, creeping, walking, hopping, skipping, and jumping, which all humans acquire to develop visual-motor potential.

Locomotor systems

It is through the development of the loco-motor system that the child gains the capability to explore first himself and later himself as he relates to the environment. Through locomotion, the concept of distance of objects from the self in space is formulated by moving the body from object to object. This helps the individual to gain experience in calculating differences in size by moving toward and away from specific objects. The locomotor system thus serves as the integrating factor between the development of the eye and objects in the environment. However, when the child initially tends to the *skill itself* and fails to interpret the complex arrangement of environmental objects, visual development progresses at a slower rate. If this is the case, the child cannot effectively use information provided to the eye regarding his movements to and from objects. Therefore for vision to develop further, the eye needs to be freed from the locomotor skills themselves. It is necessary for these loco-motor patterns to be built in as subroutines where little or no attention is on the loco-motor skill itself, but primary attention is on the environment, for example, disabled children often focus their attention on the placement of their feet as they walk. Vision thus is being directed to execution of the walking skill. There is impairment in the use of vision to orient the body to the environment as the child moves among objects. The integration of the visual mechanism with the locomotor skill of walking increases the possibility that combined hand and eye activity will take place while the child is in locomotion (Fig. 3-11).

Specific motor systems

Locomotor systems also serve as subroutines that enable the development of hand-eye, hand-foot, hand-hand, eye-foot, and foot-foot relationships (Fig. 3-12). We must assume that when a child reaches the stage of development in which his feet and hands function independently of vision, locomotion functions at a subroutine level,

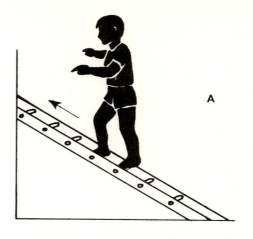

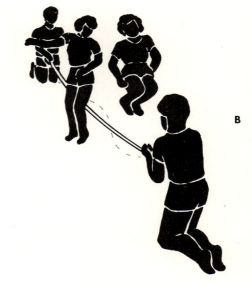

Fig. 3-11. A, Foot-eye coordination and antero-posterior balance. **B,** Rhythm and locomotion. The rope is moved back and forth so that the child must raise both his feet at the same time and transfer his weight.

thus enabling vision to be directed toward specific tasks involving greater refinement of the hand and the eye in three-dimensional space (Fig. 3-13). Ball activities involving hand manipulation or kicking activities involving the eye and the foot all contain this particular dimension of the perceptual motor structure. It is during this period that the hand and the eye become paired. Actual information from the hand provides the eye with data in order that the visual mechanism can be developed with refinement and can accurately structure objects in space. Authorities have hypothesized that 20% of vision consists of focusing light onto the retina and 80% consists of development of interpretation. Vision refers to both sensation interpreted by the eye and the meaning attached to it. When hand and eye and foot and eye are coordinated

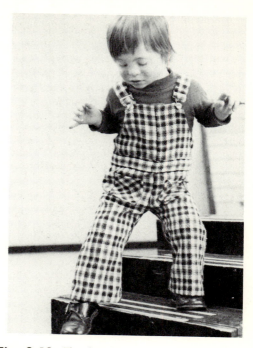

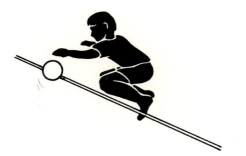

Fig. 3-12. Locomotor and hand-eye coordination. This task involves jumping back and forth across a line while bouncing a ball.

Fig. 3-13. The handicapped child learning to walk down stairs.

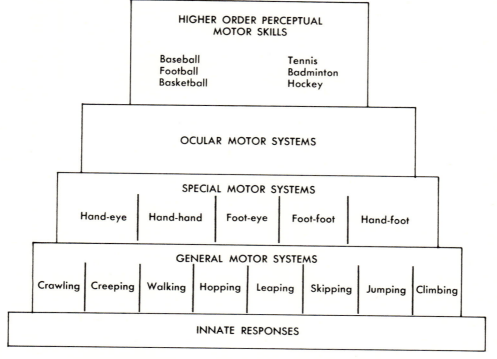

Fig. 3-14. The hierarchical sequence for visuomotor development.

with locomotor patterns functioning at subroutine levels, the prerequisites are fulfilled for the next level of development to take place (Fig. 3-14).

Oculomotor development

After perceptual information is provided to the brain via hand and foot experience, there eventually develops an autonomous capability to interpret and track visual stimuli without the aid of kinesthetic movements for spatial identification. This has been labeled the "ocular motor level of development."[10] An example of a pupil functioning at this level in sport skills involves projectiles that make it necessary for the eye and brain to track objects and interpret speed, direction, and spatial positioning appropriately. Although there are other progressive steps that lead to more elaborate perceptual structures,[10] oculomotor development is perhaps the highest level

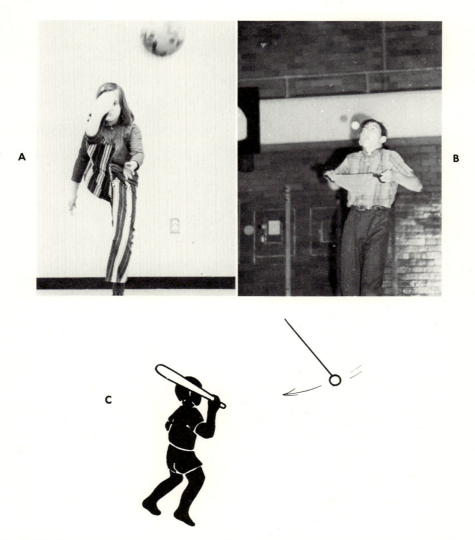

Fig. 3-15. Gaining oculomotor control. **A,** Oculomotor control is needed to accurately kick a ball. **B,** Engaging in ocular tracking task to catch a ball in a net. **C,** The child strikes a ball as many times as possible with a bat as it swings toward him.

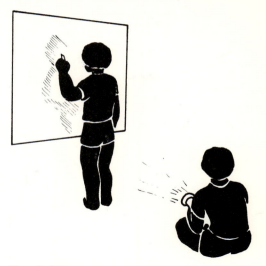

Fig. 3-17. Producing a movable image with a flashlight.

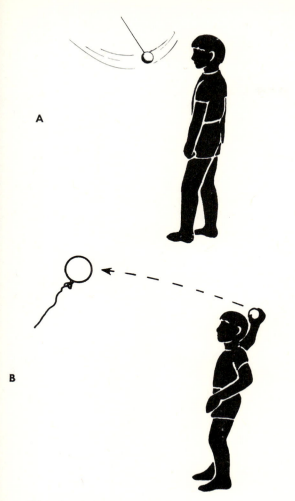

Fig. 3-16. Ocular tracking and distance duration. **A,** Tracking a moving ball. **B,** Throwing a sponge rubber ball at a descending balloon.

of functioning applicable to activities found in physical education (Fig. 3-15).

It is essential that the physical educator be aware of the hierarchical levels of visual-motor development for the implementation of a perceptual-motor training program. Curricula that take into account the development of visual-motor perception can be constructed. Once the hierarchical structure of visual development is established as a frame of reference, programs may be conducted, handicapped children measured for appropriate placement on the hierarchy,

and activities selected in accord with the needs of specific pupils (Fig. 3-16).

Body image

Body image is the perception of the relationship of body parts to external objects and the position of the body to gravitational forces. With the progressive acquisition of motor ability and movement experience as a result of vestibular and kinesthetic exploration, there is a concomitant development of spatial knowledge. This contributes to an awareness of the body and the development of body image. The growth and development of body image gives a person a perceptual set or a stable platform for the reception of vision from the outside world. Sensations received by the nervous system are based on this perceptual set. Consequently, this results in a need to test body image experiences to see which parts will fit into the perceptual whole or a particular time frame. Authorities believe that the developmental aspects of body image involving the integration of body parts with sensation mature near the age of 7 years in a normal child. Handicapped children often lag in body image development.[9]

To project visual perceptions outside the

body, the development of body image is a prerequisite. Impaired body image may produce impaired visual perception and a lack of awareness of one's bodily functions and capability impairs optimal use of the visual sense (Fig. 3-17).

Kephart[11] and Barsch[3] have hypothesized components of the body image that develop through qualitative movement. These hypothesized constructs are as follows:

1. *Kinesthetic motor awareness:* Awareness of what the motor capabilities are and the ability to assess and interpret motor responses
2. *Laterality:* Internal awareness of two sides of the body
3. *Verticality:* Awareness of the vertical alignment of the segments of the body
4. *Directionality:* Ability to relate objects and space in relationship to the body (space-time-body relationships)

Kinesthetic motor awareness. Kinesthetic motor awareness has been purported to be an important component of the development of body image. According to Dunsing and Kephart,[5] movement input is stored by the systematic gathering of initial information that is a result of movement exploration. This storage provides feedback data that are associated with movement output. The term given to this process is "motor awareness." Thus motor awareness enables the body to predict and interpret motor data and motor capability based on past experience.

Kinesthetic motor awareness is important in the development of visual perception because it is the central avenue through which motor movements are interpreted and paired with visual estimates in space. Stated another way, it provides the wherewithal for accurate assessment of energy expenditure over time to predict distance by the visual mechanism. Kinesthetic motor awareness is essential in accurately establishing visual objects in relationship to oneself in space (Fig. 3-18).

Kinesthetic motor awareness is also essential for successful execution of higher order complex skills that require the appli-

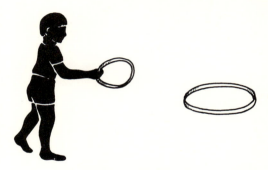

Fig. 3-18. Developing kinesthetic motor awareness and oculomotor tracking by throwing a ring through the hoop.

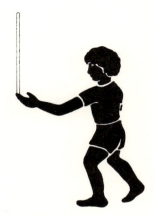

Fig. 3-19. Gaining kinesthetic motor awareness and the ability to conduct oculomotor tracking by balancing a wand on the index finger while running as far as possible.

cation of qualitative force, for instance, refined kinesthetic motor awareness must be present when a performer is putting a golf ball, bunting a baseball, shooting a basketball, or executing a dropshot in tennis or badminton. If motor awareness is inaccurate in terms of the precise amount of force that is to be applied in various game activities requiring striking, mastery may not be accomplished (Fig. 3-19).

Verticality. Another proposed construct that is part of the perceptual-motor structure is verticality. It has been hypothesized that this construct aids erection of the body on the vertical axis and thus contributes to

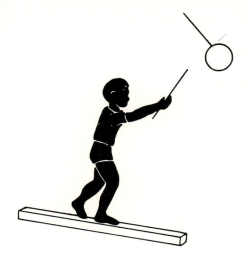

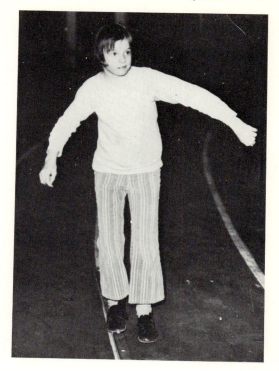

Fig. 3-20. Engaging in oculomotor tracking and laterality by standing with one foot ahead of the other on the balance beam. A ball is swung so that the child must track laterally with his eyes. He tracks the ball with the point of the wand as it moves back and forth.

Fig. 3-21. A child attempts to walk a balance beam to develop laterality. It is developed through the innervation of one side against the other to maintain body equilibrium through the lateral plane.

vision in regard to accurate assessment of objects along vertical axes.[3] Vision is therefore used to accurately interpret objects on a vertical continuum. Impairment of this factor may cause a batter to hit over or under a projectile (Fig. 3-20).

Laterality. Laterality is an important developmental construct in the cognitive development of children. Barsch[3] indicated that laterality is related to the structuring of symbols and objects in space on a lateral coordinate. It appears to be an internal awareness of the rightness and leftness of the body. This construct is purported to be developed through participation in lateral tasks of balance (Fig. 3-21).

Directionality. Although spatial-temporal relationships are inseparable, for the purpose of this presentation, five components relevant to an individual's perception of space-time are investigated. The constructs of the organization of space and time[5] are the following:

1. Distance duration
2. Time
3. Space
4. Synchrony
5. Rhythm

Distance duration. Distance duration is concerned with the movement of objects or the body through space in a given period of time. This may result from the movement of a projectile or of one's own body to and from objects as the projectile covers a specified distance in a specified time. Perceptual judgments of persons and objects that are moving in relationship to distance and time are essential in task mastery in almost every game activity in the physical education curriculum (Fig. 3-22), for example, if a *football passer* is to throw to a receiver, he must be able to predict with precision the length of time it will take the ball to reach a specified spot so that the receiver will not have to retard progress for reception. It means that the passer must accurately perceive the speed of the receiver in relationship to the length of time the ball will

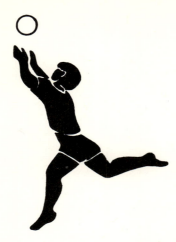

Fig. 3-22. Gaining the ability to judge distance duration and oculomotor tracking by throwing a ball into the air and running to catch it.

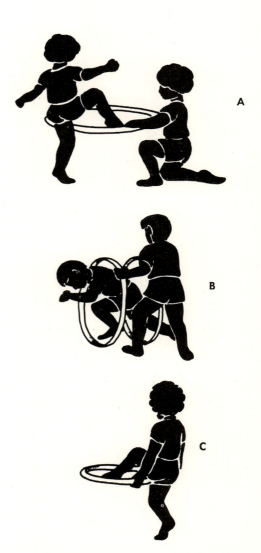

be in flight. Any deficiency in distance-duration perception will hinder task mastery. Also, a diver or a gymnast must perceive specific points in time at which a tucking or twisting action is to be executed. With practice, the distance-duration component within a specific task may become a subroutine. A baseball hitter must be able to predict the speed of the ball as it travels over a distance and derive some assessment as to the precise time it might arrive at the most advantageous spot for him to hit the ball with his bat. In addition, the baseball batter must have some knowledge as to how fast his bat can be swung to contact the ball at the optimal spot. Therefore without perception of the distance-duration construct, it is difficult to perform complex tasks that call for time-space interpretations of objects outside oneself. Acquisition of this characteristic is particularly essential in the projectile sports.

Time. Although time and space are inseparable, some motor activities are more highly loaded with the prediction of an event at a specific time relative to its position in space. An example of an activity that would be highly oriented to time would be rhythmical activities. An auditory

Fig. 3-23. Learning spatial relationships. **A,** With a hoop held level so that it is off the ground, the child steps over the front edge of the hoop and pulls it over his head without touching his body. **B,** With two hoops held apart and vertical to the ground, the child crawls through the hoops without touching them. **C,** With the hoop held in front of the belt area, the child swings it like a jump rope and jumps through it each time it comes around.

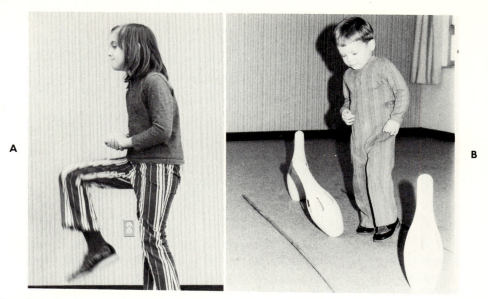

Fig. 3-24. Synchrony in rhythm. **A,** Marching and clapping hands at the same time. **B,** Weaving in and out of the bowling pins is difficult without synchrony of movement.

stimulus is provided by music or a beat and the body must project movements on a precise time interval. Spatial consideration may thus be considered a subsidiary to time. If it is not possible to predict time data between beats with the body, then motoric performance will not coincide with the rhythmical auditory beats.

Visual time is another component part of the total time structure that must be interpreted by sensory organs. Visual time is concerned with the inspection of objects and then with the prediction of where an object will be at a specific moment. In physical activity, this is essential because a response must be made at specific time intervals for successful participation in many tasks. Thus motor activity provides the opportunity for structuring the general developmental components of visual and auditory time. If a pupil cannot interpret perceptual time intervals visually, kinesthetically, and auditorially, difficulty may be encountered in higher order perceptual-motor tasks.

Space. Space is another essential percep-

tual component that must be interpreted by the visual mechanism. Children who have problems relating the body kinesthetically in space and time to visual objects will not perform well in a task requiring these spatial relations (Fig. 3-23). An example of inappropriate perception of space would be a hitter who swings at an object too soon; since he has not accurately interpreted the object in space in relationship to the hitting implement, he may fail to hit properly. While learning to play, many elementary school baseball outfielders will stand still long after the ball has been hit and will not make the catch. Inability to interpret the ball in space is reflected by movement toward the ball only a short time before the ball is to fall to the ground. Children who perform in this manner may be improperly relating the ball in space to themselves (Fig. 3-24).

Synchrony. Synchrony is a component of the time-space structure. This construct is concerned with the transformation of one motor act to another in a time block for the purpose of proficiency of muscular control designed for a specific purpose. It is prevalent in many gross motor acts and also refined motor tasks. Examples of motor tasks that involve synchrony are as follows:

1. Starting and stopping a gross motor pattern.
2. Running a zigzag line or moving between objects and changing direction.
3. A springboard dive such as a forward somersault half twist. The somersault is one discrete action from which direction and body position must be transformed to the half twist. Many gymnastic tasks include this perceptual-motor component. Synchrony is also prevalent on fine motor levels such as prehensive skills in which directional control must be made by muscles to manipulate objects.

Rhythm. Synchrony is the disruption of rhythmical activity or movements of equal blocks of time and their transformation into other movements. Rhythm involves similar repetitive cyclic motor acts performed in approximately the same time blocks.[3] The dance is an obvious example of rhythm in that beats represent equal time intervals between sounds, requiring the learner to pair similar body movement with repeated auditory beats over intervals of time. Such tasks as walking and swimming are also rhythmical in that repeated movement cycles must occur within a sequence of equal time blocks.

Although synchrony and rhythm appear to be antithetical in nature, both are essential in the development of a broad base of activities that enable the learner to adapt efficiently to his environment (Fig. 3-24).

• • •

In summary, the development of perceptual ability is of critical importance to handicapped children for it is closely associated with skill learning. If environmental cues cannot be accurately interpreted, the production of desirable motor response will be less efficient. Inasmuch as most handicapped children have some perceptual deficit and perception can be developed, it is the responsibility of physical educators to include perceptual-motor development opportunities in their curriculum.

REFERENCES

1. Arnheim, D. D., and Sinclair, W. A.: The clumsy child: a program of motor therapy, St. Louis, 1975, The C. V. Mosby Co.
2. Ayres, A. J.: Sensory integration and learning disorders, Los Angeles, 1973, Western Psychological Services.
3. Barsch, R. H.: Achieving perceptual-motor efficiency approach to learning, Seattle, 1967, Special Child Publications.
4. Cratty, B. J.: Perceptual and motor development in infants and children; New York, 1970, Macmillan Publishing Co., Inc.
5. Dunsing, J., and Kephart, N. C.: Motor generalizations in space and time. In Hellmuth, J., editor: Learning disorders, Seattle, 1965, Special Child Publications.
6. Frostig, M.: Movement education: theory and practice, Chicago, 1970, Follett Publishing Co.
7. Frostig, M., and Horne, D.: The Frostig program for the development of visual perception, Chicago, 1964, Follett Publishing Co.
8. Gearheart, B. R.: Learning disabilities—educational strategies, St. Louis, 1973, The C. V. Mosby Co.
9. Gesell, A., and Amatruda, C. S.: Developmental diagnosis, ed. 3, New York, 1975, Harper & Row, Publishers.
10. Getman, G. N.: Visuomotor complex in the acquisition of learning skills, Seattle, 1965, Special Child Publications.
11. Kephart, N. C.: Motor aids to perceptual training, Columbus, Ohio, 1968, Charles E. Merrill Publishing Co.
12. Kiphard, E. J., and Leger, A.: Basic psychomotor education, Flottman, Gutersloh, 1975, West Germany.
13. Muller, H., et al., editors: Motor behavior of preschool children, Schorndorf, Germany, 1975, Hofmann.
14. Piaget, J.: The psychology of intelligence, Totowa, N.J., 1967, Littlefield, Adams & Co.
15. Wundelich, R. C.: Learning disorders, Phys. Ther. **47:**700-708, 1969.

RECOMMENDED READINGS

Ball, T. S., Itard, S., and Kephart, N. C.: Sensory education—a learning interpretation, Columbus, Ohio, 1971, Charles E. Merrill Publishing Co.
Falik, L. H.: The effects of special perceptual-motor training in kindergarten on second grade reading, J. Learning Disabilities **2:**325-329, 1969.
Frostig, M.: Visual perception, integrative func-

tions, and academic learning, J. Learning Disabilities **5**:1-15, 1972.

Gearheart, B. R.: Learning disabilities—educational strategies, St. Louis, 1973, The C. V. Mosby Co.

Hammill, D. D., and Bartel, N. R.: Teaching children with learning and behavior problems, Boston, 1975, Allyn & Bacon, Inc.

Hammill, D. D., Goodman, L., and Wiederholt, J. L.: Visual-motor processes: what success have we had in training them? The Reading Teacher **27**:469-478, 1974.

Kirk, S. A., and Kirk, W. P.: Psycholinguistic learning disabilities: diagnosis and remediation, Urbana, Ill., 1972, University of Illinois Press.

Larsen, S., and Hammill, D. D.: The relationship of selected visual-perceptual skills to academic abilities, J. Educ., 1975.

Lerner, J. W.: Children with learning disabilities, Boston, 1971, Houghton Mifflin Co.

Mann, L.: Perceptual training: misdirections and redirections, Am. J. Orthopsychiatry **40**:30-38, 1970.

Myklebust, H. R., editor: Progress in learning disabilities, New York, 1971, Grune & Stratton, Inc.

Turner, R. U., and Fisher, D.: The effects of a perceptual-motor training program upon the readiness and perceptual development of culturally disadvantaged children, ERIC ED 041 633, Washington, D.C., 1970, U.S. Government Printing Office.

Waugh, K. W., and Bush, W. J.: Diagnosing learning disorders, Columbus, Ohio, 1971, Charles E. Merrill Publishing Co.

4

APPLICATION OF THE DEVELOPMENTAL CONCEPT

■ Education is a lifelong process that relates to overall human development. We grow and develop physically, mentally, socially, and emotionally along rather predictable paths. Allowing for individual differences, a teacher can thus use behavior as an observable indication of development. Such information can be used in a viable process for delivering educational benefits to handicapped children. The application of the developmental concept to instruction implies that benefits to be delivered to handicapped children should be specified in terms of behavioral characteristics in order to determine where a student *is* within a hierarchical sequence of objectives, where he *should be* at present, and where he *might be* at a specified point in time as a result of some instructional intervention. (This approach to instruction is the basis of legislation and court decisions of the 1970's.)

LEGISLATION

The philosophy that education is for individual development and is a right of every child is implicit in the historic 1972 consent decree of the United States District Court for the Eastern District of Pennsylvania in the case of *PARC etc.* vs. *Commonwealth of Pennsylvania et al.*, Civil Action No. 71-42. Whereas this court action was directed at the inclusion of all children in the educational process, other judicial rulings as well as legislation in many states require the mainstream education of handicapped children.

More recent legislation, "Education for the Handicapped" (P.L. 94-142, Nov. 29, 1975), has as its main theme individualized instruction and due process guarantees. This legislation is of paramount significance to the physical education profession inasmuch as physical education is specified in the instructional process. The law* reads as follows:

(16) The term "special education" means specially designed instruction, at no cost to parents or guardians, to meet the unique needs of a handicapped child, including classroom instruction, instruction in physical education, home instruction, and instruction in hospitals and institutions.

(19) The term "individualized education program" means a written statement for each handicapped child developed in any meeting by a representative of the local educational agency or an intermediate educational unit who shall be qualified to provide or supervise the provision of, specially "designed" instruction to meet the unique needs of handicapped children, the teacher, the parents or guardian of such a child, and, whenever appropriate, such child, which statement shall include (A) a statement of the present levels of educational performance of such child, (B) a statement of annual goals, including short-term instructional objectives, (C) a statement of the specific educational services to be provided to such child, and the extent to which such child will be able to participate in regular educational programs, (D) the projected date for initiation and anticipated duration of such services, and appropriate objective criteria and evaluation procedures and schedules for determining, on at least an annual basis, whether instructional objectives are being achieved.

Although all components of the individualized education program are impor-

*From Education for all handicapped act of 1975, P.L. 94-142, December 2, 1975, Washington, D.C., Weekly Compilation of Presidential Documents, Vol. 11, No. 49.

tant and interdependent, those aspects that will receive most discussion in this chapter are *present levels of educational performance*, which are extended by the acquisition of the *short-term instructional objective*, which thus ignites the developmental process. The definitions of these two essential terms are as follows: *Present level of educational performance* means the present level from which short-term instructional objectives are formulated. *Short-term instructional objective* means an activity performed by the pupil, described in specific, objective, and measurable terms, that is an intermediate step and extends present levels of educational performance toward "annual goals."[11] Thus regulations are explicit in the relationship between measurable activities and are implicit in that the focus of the instructional process is on the development of the child.

MAINSTREAMING

The concept of mainstreaming is predicated on the application of the developmental concept, which implies that each individual is unique with respect to specific abilities. Since the abilities of each individual are at different developmental levels, the developmental concept cannot be applied unless there is individualization of instruction. If individualization of instruction is practiced, there is less need for homogeneous grouping, allowing handicapped children to be educated in the mainstream of education. A more recent legislative statute, P.L. 412-664, provides support for this concept.

Modern educational technology has made the implementation of the developmental process feasible by applying the concept of behavioral objectives. These objectives are organized into prerequisite order in the form of programmed instruction, which leads the learner to mastery of preconceived goals. Thus the application of the developmental process involves the establishment of a sequence of hierarchical behavioral objectives. Current legislation is quite clear that there must be a direct relationship between assessment and programming and that there must be precise monitoring of all behaviors as an individual progresses through these sequences en route to mastery of specific tasks.

DEVELOPMENTAL CONCEPT OF EDUCATION
Hierarchy and developmental tasks

Hierarchies facilitate the ordering of instructional activities for the purpose of development. A hierarchy is a continuum of ordered events in which a task of a lower order and of lesser difficulty is prerequisite to acquisition of a task of greater difficulty. It thus can serve as a measure of student development and answers three vital educationally relevant questions: (1) *What is the student's present level of educational performance on the hierarchy?* (2) *What short-term instructional objectives should be provided to extend present levels of educational performance or development?* (3) *How much development has already occurred?* Task analysis therefore is a valuable tool for the development of instructional hierarchies.

The application of the developmental concept to education was an attempt by the United States Office of Education to promote the accountability of the measured educational progress of each child. It has as its central concern the development of instructional procedures that involve the following factors:

1. *Curricula* that provide learning experiences that state educational progress in terms of developmental concept and from which diagnosis of the unique needs of children is possible
2. *Trained teachers* to implement the curricula
3. *Evaluation procedures* that are addressed to individual teacher competency, curricula quality, and pupil competency

Individualizing instruction

Procedures employed in applying developmental concepts to individualized instruction vary greatly from traditional instruction designed to teach groups. Table 4-1 compares the essential differences between these two teaching approaches.

Programmed instruction

Modern trends call for the individualization of instruction, particularly with those children who function at preschool levels; however, as the typical child begins formal education during his fifth year of life, he usually has developed the capability to begin to direct some of his own learning. With the acquisition of the skills to be self-directing and self-evaluating, the student is freed from dependency on the teacher. The

Table 4-1. Traditional versus developmental systems approach to instruction

Traditional approach	Developmental systems approach
Teachers design curricula according to their experiences in areas of intended interest.	There must be measurable predetermined objectives to be taught by teachers.
Teachers develop their own curricula within framework of guidelines. Assessment instruments are at discretion of teachers.	There must be programmed materials or behavioral inventories that indicate what child can and cannot do prior to program implementation.
Teachers' skills are a composite of their particular learning experience.	There must be specifically trained teacher competencies that will enable reproducibility of curricula to yield predictably similar learning results.
Lesson plans tend to be general and follow guidelines.	Lessons of teachers must be so specific that they are reproducible by another person.

possibilities for unlimited instructional input and feedback become a reality. It is at this point in development that self-instructional and self-evaluative learning materials in the form of programmed instruction should be introduced into the educational schema. One major goal of an individualized instructional system is to develop a communication system between the student and teacher by which they can become as independent of one another as possible. The teacher's ultimate primary role is one of guiding and managing instruction according to the student's individual needs and learning characteristics. This approach enables the teacher to cope with heterogeneous groups of children and to accommodate large numbers in the same class without sacrificing instructional efficiency. In order to implement such a program, however, three major factors must be taken into consideration: (1) programming must be constructed on the basis of scientific principles,[2, 3, 6] (2) learners must be trained in specific behaviors,[7] and (3) learning principles must be applied through the use of programmed curricula.

The most expeditious way to manage an average-sized class in a public school, using the individualized developmental approach, is through the use of behavioral objectives that shift learning conditions to create developmental task sequences. Behavioral objectives take the form of self-instructional and self-evaluative programs that are appropriate for typical children and for atypical children functioning at a relatively high level. However, for the child who cannot self-instruct and self-evaluate, task analysis and pattern analysis will facilitate his development. The child functioning at a low level and the child who strives to reach upper limits of development for competitive purposes will need special types of programming and thus specific attention by instructors when the teacher-student ratio is low. A list of characteristics for such a program has been suggested by Lindvall and Bolvin.[5]

1. Definition of the objectives the students

are expected to achieve must be clear and specific.
2. Objectives must be stated in behavioral terms.
3. Objectives must lead to behaviors that are carefully analyzed and sequenced in a hierarchical order so that each behavior builds on the objectives immediately preceeding and is prerequisite to those that follow.
4. Instructional content of a program must consist of a sequence of learning tasks through which a student can proceed with little outside help and must provide a series of small increments in learning that enable the student to proceed from a condition of lack of command of behavior to a condition of command of behavior.
5. A program must permit the student to begin at his present ability level and allow him to move upward from that point.
6. A program must allow each student to proceed independently of other students and learn at a rate best suited to his own abilities and interests.
7. A program must require active involvement and response on the part of the student at each step along the learning sequence.
8. A program must provide immediate feedback to the student concerning the adequacy of his performance.
9. A program must be subjected to continuous study by those responsible for it and should be regularly modified in the light of available evidence concerning the student's performance.
10. A program must accommodate the ability range of many students, thus enabling continuous progress.

Developmental diagnosis of children

The systems approach to education requires that the instructor formulate general objectives for his students and assess each learner to determine the degree to which he has achieved these general objectives. *The overall goal of such an instructional*

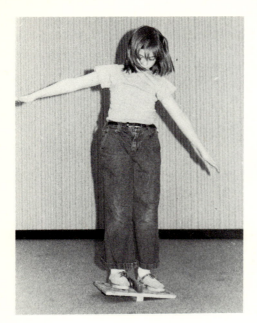

Fig. 4-1. Equipment that relates to a program. Balance sticks are different widths. The board can turn to the other side for a more difficult task; the eyes can be used in a different way; constraints can be placed on movement of the arms. To form either a less or more difficult sequence, activities can be constructed so that one is a required prerequisite to another.

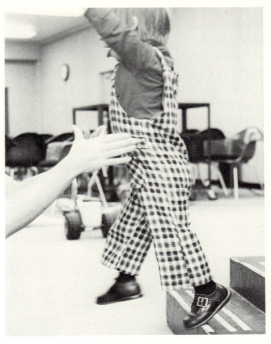

Fig. 4-2. A handicapped child who cannot jump and land on two feet. The behavioral objective is to land on two feet.

procedure is to enable measured learning of each child, handicapped or not, along developmental continua. In the following sections of this chapter are discussed diagnostic techniques that enable programmed curricula to be linked directly with diagnostic information in order to produce measured educational progress of children (Fig. 4-1). Some of these diagnostic techniques are as follows:

1. Diagnosis of motor development tasks as measured against *normative developmental scales* with suggested techniques for subsequent programming based on task analysis and knowledge of the *principles of development*
2. Diagnostic information obtained through task analysis of *skills from behavioral inventories*
3. Diagnostic information obtained through the placement of the individual in *hierarchical learning curricula* that take the *form of programmed instruction*
4. *Pattern analysis of skills*

INSTRUCTIONAL OBJECTIVES

The behavioral objective is a specific predetermined learning experience on which subsequent development is built. Instructional objectives take several forms; it is the purpose of this discussion to establish objectives in relationship to the total instruction process.

Objectives occur at different levels of curricular development and must be appropriate for the ability levels of a specifically diagnosed individual (Fig. 4-2). They require an assessment of the learner in relationship to what he can and cannot do within a specific activity domain (present level of educational performance). In the event that mastery of a specific behavior is not possible by a learner, the question is asked, "What prerequisites are needed for this individual to achieve mastery of this task?" This question, once answered, is restated until the current ability level of the student is determined and the appropriate instructional objective is derived. A sequence of prerequisite activities thus provides a chain of instructional events that lead the learner from lower to higher levels of mastery within the instructional content. The utilization of this instructional process requires that detailed records be kept on each learner in order to understand where he is in his learning activity sequence. The mastery of one objective is the prerequisite that gives rise to a more complex objective, making development progressive (Chapter 18).*

The behavioral objective must incorporate four concepts: (1) it must possess an action, (2) it must establish conditions under which actions occur, (3) it must establish a criterion for mastery of a specific task, and (4) it must lie outside the child's present level of educational performance.

The action concept

The action aspect of the behavioral objective indicates what the learner will do in the execution of the task. It is important that the action take a verb form. (For the purpose of this discussion, it will be assumed that affective and cognitive aspects are essential prerequisites for efficient behavioral performance in programs of motor development of students and psychomotor performance of teachers. Thus the focus of the discussion will emphasize performance aspects of teaching and the development of motor activity in the student.)

---

*See also assignments 29 and 30 in Crowe, W. C., Arnheim, D. D., and Auxter, D.: Laboratory manual in adapted physical education and recreation, St. Louis, 1977, The C. V. Mosby Co.

Establishing action conditions

It is necessary to specify the conditions under which the performance of the instructional objective is to occur. This is particularly necessary when programming instruction to preserve developmental sequences that lead to target objectives. The specification of the movement to be demonstrated is most important in preserving the hierarchical elements of a programmed activity. The boxed material on p. 74 gives an example of conditions from which a behavioral objective can be developed.

The violation of any of the conditions that make up a behavioral objective render it inappropriate and a deterrent to measured development. If the conditions are not specified, there can be little agreement as to the capability level of a student and thus as to the appropriate selection of a developmental activity. It should be noted that specified conditions facilitate achievement of target objectives and prevent circumvention of a task by the performer (Fig. 4-3).

Criterion for mastery of a specific task

The criterion for mastery of a specific task indicates when students have mastered assigned tasks. It serves notice that one prerequisite has been mastered, allowing for progress toward a more difficult task and thus increasing the efficiency of performance. Criteria for task mastery can take several different forms, as may be seen in the following examples:

1. Number of repetitions (10 repetitions)
2. Number of repetitions over time (20 repetitions in 15 seconds)
3. Distance traveled (8 feet on a balance beam without falling off)
4. Distance traveled over time (200 yards in 25 seconds)
5. Number of successive trials without a miss (four times in a row)
6. Specified number of successful responses in a block of trials (three of five)
7. Mastery of all the stated conditions of the task

GENERAL OBJECTIVE: Develop the elbow extensors and arm flexors with "push-up" activity.

Specification of conditions	Rationale
1. Straighten back and hips to 180 degrees.	Bending either part of body reduces length of resistance arm and decreases degree of difficulty of task.
2. Place hands shoulder width apart on floor.	Spreading hands wider than shoulder increases difficulty of task.
3. Tuck chin against sternum.	Raising head while performing tends to bend the back and shorten resistance arm.
4. Touch forehead to floor.	Touching forehead indicates starting and ending position of push-up.
5. Straighten arms to 180 degrees.	Straightening arms indicates degree of movement of arms (will count as one repetition).
6. Support weight on hyperextended toes, which rest on floor.	Supporting weight indicates the point of the fulcrum to control length of resistance arm.

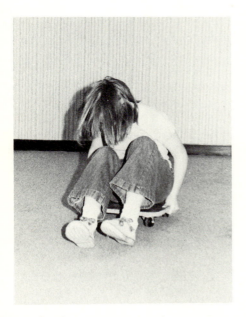

Fig. 4-3. The measurement of this task is the distance that the scooter can be moved over a given period of time.

8. Number of degrees of movement (flexibility in degrees of movement in starting and terminal positions)

There are other forms of measurement for the criterion of mastery. The intent of the criterion of mastery is to objectively communicate to all parties concerned when the task has been mastered. This is important to the learner for the following reasons: (1) it is immediately reinforcing, (2) it provides an immediate target of performance mastery, and (3) it acts as an indicator of readiness to be assigned more advanced tasks (Fig. 4-4).

It should be noted that objectives are not valid unless they are directed at the acquisition of behaviors that lie outside the current repertoire of an individual's capability. The intent of the instructional process is to add new behaviors; therefore a prerequisite for stating a behavioral objective is to assess each learner on a continuum of activities to determine what he can and cannot do. Hierarchies are important for the construction of appropriate behavioral objectives. Once a behavior on a hierarchy can be mastered by an individual, all behaviors falling below it are not worthy of being considered behavioral

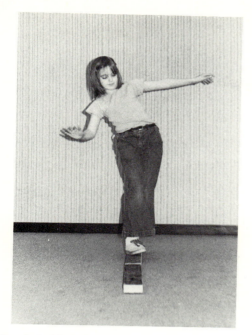

Fig. 4-4. The criterion for mastery in this task is walking 8 feet, the length of the 4-inch wide balance beam.

Table 4-2. Acceptable and unacceptable objectives

Action	Condition	Criterion
Acceptable objectives		
Run	1 mile	In 5 minutes 30 seconds
Walk	A 4-inch balance beam, heel to toe, eyes closed, and hands on hips	For 8 feet
Swim	Using the American crawl in a 25-yard pool for 50 yards	In 35 seconds
Unacceptable objectives		
Run		As fast as you can
Walk	On a balance beam	Without falling off
Swim		To the end of the pool

objectives for that person (thereby reducing the amount of initial testing). Therefore the hierarchically structured learning curriculum must be considered a very efficient instructional instrument in managing accountable educational data.

Acceptable and unacceptable behavioral objectives

There are three central features essential to fulfilling the developmental systems model of instruction through behavioral objectives: (1) there must be justification that the objectives are relevant to the learner, (2) objectives must possess the capability of being reproduced when implemented by independent instructors, and (3) there must be an agreement as to what is to be taught and when it is to be mastered by the student.

The unacceptable behavioral objectives presented in Table 4-2 are discussed in more detail in the following outline:

1. Run as fast as you can.

CONDITIONS: The condition of distance or other environmental arrangements such as hurdles and nature of the course are not specified.

CRITERION: An objective distance over measured time is not in the objective. The perception "as fast as you can" is subjective. A player or student may think that he is running as fast as he can. The coach or teacher may evaluate the performance differently.

2. Walk on a balance beam without falling off.

CONDITIONS: The width of the balance beam makes the task more or less difficult. It is not specified. The position of the arms and utilization of the visual mechanism are other conditions that affect performance.

CRITERION: The distance to be traveled and distance over time are not specified.

3. Swim to the end of the pool.

CONDITIONS: The type of stroke is not specified.

CRITERION: Swimming pools are different

lengths. The behavior in the performer's pool cannot be generalized to another pool.

Effective utilization of instructional objectives

There has been considerable controversy concerning the functional use of the behavioral objective in instruction. Concerns that have been indicated by critics include (1) behavioral objectives are difficult to manage, (2) they take too much time, (3) they require too much testing, (4) more important aspects of instruction are not stressed and cannot be measured, and (5) they impersonalize instruction. Many of these concerns are well founded; however, with the effective management of programmed instruction and the proper utilization of behavioral objectives, an accounting of measured learning and a systematic revision of the instructional processes can be achieved.

Task analysis

There are several procedures for the analysis of abilities that are the basis for the behavioral objective of a specific learner. Some of these procedures involve (1) analysis of higher order skills or abilities that require open-ended development for leisure activity or vocational pursuits, (2) analysis of a skill or task to serve as a prerequisite for engaging in a more complex task, (3) acquisition of a behavior within the pattern of a skill, and (4) analysis of behaviors through inventory of subtasks to determine needed prerequisite behaviors. Whatever the procedure, the behavioral objective is usually the result of an analysis of higher order tasks that lead to a given task. It then becomes necessary to perform task analysis to determine the prerequisite behaviors that lead to the attainment of higher order objectives (Figs. 4-5 and 4-6).

Examples of task analysis to formulate behavioral objectives (terminal objectives)

EXAMPLE A

I. Correct reversals of a child in visualiz-

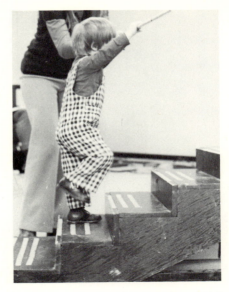

Fig. 4-5. There is a normative age at which the pattern of alternating feet should be achieved. The analysis of the task indicates that the efficient utilization of the balancing mechanism is prerequisite to this ability. Therefore the development of balance is prompted in this behavior.

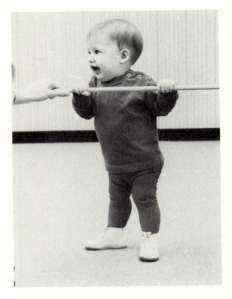

Fig. 4-6. Aiding a child who cannot stand erect.

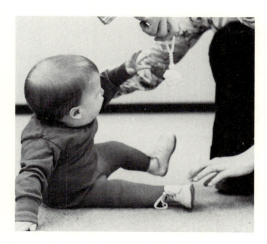

Fig. 4-7. This child needs greater balance to maintain a sitting position. Through task analysis of sitting, it can be seen that the placement of the hand indicates balance is a prerequisite to the sitting behavior. Task analysis can start with any skill at any level of development.

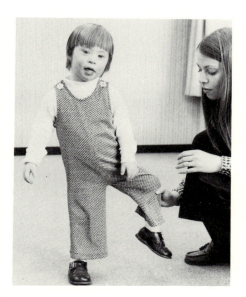

Fig. 4-8. Development of the balance mechanism should start early. A handicapped child 33 months of age begins a balance program.

ing letters or symbols such as "b" and "d" by activating the lateral balancing mechanisms. This will establish internal lateral perception, which is expressed externally with the child's vision.

A. *Task analysis*
1. Relate problem to development of laterality (internal awareness of right and left).[4]
2. Place in a lateral balance program (operational description of laterality).[4]
3. Diagnose current level of the learner's ability to balance (Figs. 4-7 and 4-8).

B. *The task*
Balance in a heel-to-toe position on a 1-inch stick for 5 seconds with eyes closed and hands on hips. (This is assuming that the child has not mastered this task.) This behavioral objective would be derived through assessment of current educational performance with subsequent determination of appropriate activity.

EXAMPLE B
I. Demonstrate the ability to stand in an upright position.

A. *Task analysis*
List all behaviors prerequisite to standing:
1. Control of the thoracic extensors of the spine
2. Control of the lumbar extensors of the spine
3. Muscular strength in the hips and knees
4. Counterbalance of gravitational forces to maintain balance

B. *The task*
After assessment for a hypothetical learner, a subtask might be to sit erect with legs extended and hands on the floor beside the hips for 10 seconds. (Many programs need to be constructed to achieve this terminal objective.)

Selection of appropriate curricular tasks

A systems curriculum must be capable of measuring the learning of each student along a developmental continuum (or of measuring the acquisition of skills not yet mastered in a behavioral inventory). The development of curricula is based on building blocks that consist of short-term instructional objectives that are discrete and unambiguous. The developmental instructional approach cannot be studied separately from the total curriculum. The application of such curricula through systems procedures can yield accountable learning results (data) for each learner, whether handicapped or not. This can be accomplished through behavioral inventories or through comparison of abilities along a developmental continuum. The selection and implementation of such a curriculum through a systems procedure has distinct advantages. These include the following:

1. The type of curriculum facilitates communication among professional and consumer advocates as to specifically what the child has learned and will learn.
2. The curriculum facilitates cooperative efforts among professional personnel through delineation of who is accountable for which of the behaviors needed to reach predetermined goals.
3. The curriculum provides for appropriate allocation of responsibility, time, facilities, and other resources among personnel.
4. The curriculum allows for the concept of mainstreaming through the process of individualization of instruction because each learner works on and moves through the curricula that he needs.

Incorporation of learning principles in the curriculum

Once target behaviors have been identified, it is possible to apply known learning principles to enable the learner to acquire new emerging behaviors. However, without programmed curricula to which assessment can be linked, there is little opportunity for the application of learning principles.

Sequential hierarchical curricula, mastered and unmastered,[1] tend to keep instructors informed as to which behaviors lie outside the current reservoir of each child's knowledge. Behavioral inventories are more difficult to interpret in the management of pupil information because one behavior may not be prerequisite to the acquisition of another. The charting of progression becomes much more difficult as the complexity of behavioral acquisition increases. The specification of what is to be learned in a systems curriculum provides immediate feedback to the learner as to whether or not he has mastered the task, enables self-reinforcement through known acquisition of task mastery, makes possible the analysis of task difficulty so behavior shaping procedures may be applied to the learner, and allows instruction to be directed toward the positive aspects of task mastery.

The intent of curricula designed for the developmental systems model is to allow reproducibility of the results achieved by the learner. The specification of such a curriculum as well as implementation procedures that allow for instructional reproducibility have several positive features, namely:

1. External evaluators can provide information on the procedures employed by the teacher and the results achieved by learners.
2. Evaluation of the procedures may be formulated.
3. Evaluation, followed by revisions of techniques in the training of teachers to implement the program, may be tested empirically.
4. Incorporation of suggestions from other teachers using the same or a similar system may be employed to improve instructional efficiency.

Placement profile

The placement profile sheet describes the strengths and weaknesses of each student in all units for which placement tests have been administered. It is an important means

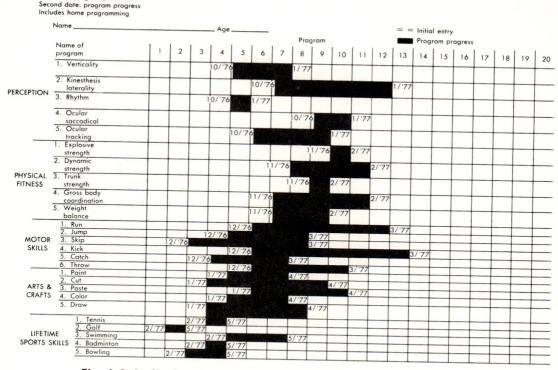

Fig. 4-9. Profile sheet for shifting criterion and shifting condition programs.

of determining which specific learning unit, element, or component has the highest priority for a specific learner. Utilizing the information received on each child, the teacher then selects those programs or units that are of highest priority to a particular child. The placement profile may also indicate the amount of time or the emphasis to be placed on a specific unit of work as compared to another (Fig. 4-9).

The placement profile sheet should contain the following information:

1. A vertical listing of the programs
2. The numbers of the activities in the programs indicated horizontally at the top of the page
3. The pupil's name
4. The student's birth date (to make comparison with normative data)
5. A graph of the entry level on each element of the program

6. The date on which each child entered

TYPES OF PROGRAMS USING THE DEVELOPMENTAL PROCESS

A program is built around a conceptual model of a skill that is analyzed into its component parts. Four types of programs can be used with this in mind. The *criterion shifting program* utilizes sequential behavioral objectives in which the standards of performance are continually raised. The *condition shifting program* allows sequential behaviors to emerge through shifting the conditions of the behavioral objective from a lesser to a greater difficulty. The *task analysis program* uses analysis of subtasks of a behavior in which there is a relationship of one part to another. The *pattern analysis program* uses analysis of movement behavior that is dependent on temporal-spatial relationships of elements of movement to form a pattern.

Program domain: Perceptual-motor

Justification of program: Two balls of different resiliency are dropped simultaneously (a 1-inch hard rubber ball with great resiliency and a 2-inch sponge rubber ball with less resiliency). This imparts variance in the height of the rebound and develops identification of different rates of speed of moving objects. The increment of distance between the balls that are dropped increases the span of perception that is important in sport, academic, and vocational skills.

Components developed by the program: Span of perception, hand-eye coordination

Type of program: Shifting criterion

Materials needed: Yardstick, 1-inch Superball, 2-inch sponge rubber ball

Communication code: Pictorial symbols:

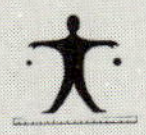

Equipment layout: Sufficient space to perform the task

Description of task: Place a yardstick on the floor in front of the body and drop the two balls on the floor so that the distance between the landing points of the balls can be measured. Arms start in front of shoulders and gradually increase in width during the ball drop.

Measurement system: Distance between the dropped balls

Task specifications:
1. The balls must be dropped from shoulder height.
2. The balls must be caught in the hands.

Fig. 4-10. Ball drop test, an example of a shifting criterion program.

Criterion shifting program

Fig. 4-10 illustrates an example of the criterion shifting program. In the ball drop, the wider the distance between the two dropped balls (which must be caught simultaneously on the rebound), the greater is the degree of difficulty. It can be stated that the smaller the area of focus, the more attention can be paid a specific aspect of a given environment.

Criterion shifting programs need to specify the task to be performed. These task specifications are taught and remain constant for the subsequent execution of tasks that follow; however, the criterion is shifted to make the standard of performance more or less difficult. It is likely, however, that children in such programs will practice the skill and record the best performance. If such a procedure is employed, learning principles are violated and

the end result is inefficient learning of the task at higher levels of performance (Fig. 4-11).

It is important in the implementation of programs of this type that the principles of programmed instruction be applied.

The following is a sample of the elements of a criterion shifting program. These aspects are contained in this type of program:
Name of program: Communicates the behavioral description of performance
Program domain: Classifies the program by major goals of instruction
Components developed: Specifies the worth of the program in achieving major goals
Type of program: Specifies the program as (1) shifting condition, (2) shifting criterion, (3) task analysis of a skill, (4) pattern analysis, or (5) developmental scale programming

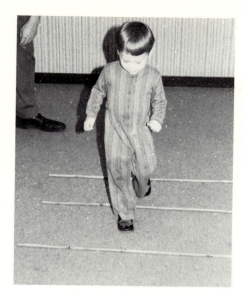

Fig. 4-11. In this shifting criterion program, the task, requiring that sequentially longer steps be taken, lengthens the stride and requires more efficient utilization of the balancing mechanism. The program is designed so that sequentially the sticks are moved a greater distance apart until the desired alteration in gait occurs.

Name of program: Broad jump

Program domain: Physical and motor

Justification of program: The broad jump is a significant program because it is (1) a normative measure for the construct of explosive strength and (2) a skill at the preschool levels that has the capability of measuring the phylogenetic development of the child. Therefore it is an important development task at most levels of development. Furthermore, it is a basic task that may be generalized into many aspects of sport skill performance. At the preschool levels of development, it involves (1) bilateral development, which later has implications for binocular fusion in the development of vision, and (2) elaboration of the posturing mechanism through its projection in front of the base.

Components developed by the program: Explosive strength
Type of program: Shifting criterion
Materials needed: Yardstick
Communication code: Pictorial symbols:

Equipment layout: There is a restraining line behind which the jump must be executed. Markers may be placed on the floor by the performer to indicate target distances that are to be attempted, commensurate with ability.

Criterion measure: Acquire a performance baseline on the jump and then require the pupil to jump 1 inch farther. The base level of performance should be determined for each child. The criterion measure for any jump for a specific child would be a specified distance indicated by the instructor above the base level, yet within the child's range of success in the near future.

Task specifications:
1. Place feet behind starting line.
2. Measure from the tip of the toe of the foot closest to the starting line.
3. Land on two feet.
4. Feet cannot move after they land.

Fig. 4-12. Broad jump test, an example of a shifting criterion program.

Table 4-3. Suggested measures for specific ability traits

Ability trait	Criterion
Strength	Increasing number of repetitions under standard conditions
Speed	Decreasing time it takes to run specified distance
Endurance	Increasing number of push-ups over specified time
Balance	Increasing length of time one can balance
Flexibility	Increasing range of motion of specific joint
Power or explosive strength	Increasing distance one can jump
Vision	Increasing span of vision on specific task

Materials: Materials needed to conduct the program

Communication code: Symbols that enable persons who are nonreaders to participate in the program

Equipment layout: Suggestions for management of the instructional area

Measurement: Way in which the activity is measured

Task specifications: Specification of the conditions (Fig. 4-12)

Criterion shifting programming provides the strongest type of measurement and thus unequivocably accountable data on the progress of children. However, its application to various types of tasks is limited. It is applicable to conversion of deficient ability prerequisites, as is suggested in Table 4-3.

Tasks that are most amenable to criterion shifting programs are those that relate to ability structures. More complex skills, which do not require high level of performance and are not specific tasks as ends in themselves, often need different types of programming.

Condition shifting program

Condition shifting programs have utility when teaching skills. The conditions of a model behavior are stated. From this model, task hierarchies are constructed and programs are formulated. Using bowling as an example, such conditions as the performer's distance from the pins, the distance apart that the pins are set, and the size of the ball can be changed to structure the task to fit the child's level of ability (Fig. 4-13).

The strength of condition shifting programming lies in the following:
1. There is variation in activity that tends to hold pupil interest.
2. There are subsequent activities with respect to difficulty that, if constructed appropriately, include something for most learners.
3. There is accommodation for children who function at low levels of development.
4. This form of curriculum facilitates the introduction of desired elements representing ability traits to be integrated into the activity of the program. More than one specific trait can be developed in a single activity.
5. The profiling procedure is not difficult.
6. Stick figures that represent the enactment of behavioral objectives of the program enable nonreaders to engage in self-instructional activity.
7. The units of gain can be computed in the program to indicate educational progress.
8. Pupils are aware of the progress that they are making in the program.

Task analysis program

Many physical education activities require a chain of tasks, all of which must be mastered to perform a routine. This type of curricular activity is best instructed through task analysis. Specific behaviors that are different from other behaviors in a routine are isolated for analysis. An assessment is then made to determine which behaviors in a routine have been developed to the point where successful participation by the handicapped child may be achieved. Those behaviors that are deficient receive further programming until all the behaviors in the routine are mastered.

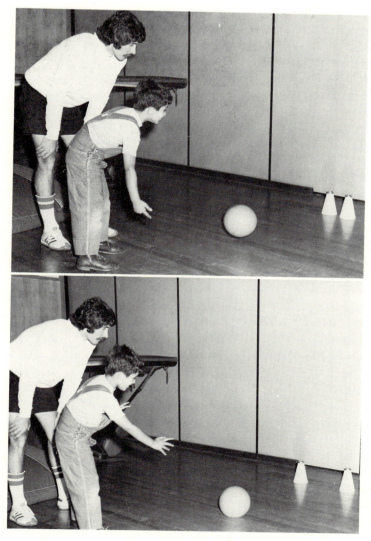

Fig. 4-13. A condition shifting program. In this bowling program, the hierarchies are (1) the bowler's distance from the pins, (2) the distance apart that the pins are set, (3) the number of pins that are knocked down, and (4) the number of pins that are set up and that are required to be knocked down. These variables can be manipulated. (Courtesy California State University, Audio Visual Center, Long Beach, Calif.)

TERMINAL OBJECTIVE: Demonstrate the ability to square dance to *Marching through Georgia* without error and subject to the criterion of mastery of all subtasks.

Square dance	Criterion for mastery
1. Locate your partner.	Find partner within 2 seconds after the call indicates to do so.
2. Place your hand on your partner's hip.	Extend arm, place hand on hip, and with other hand, grasp palm of partner's hand.
3. Place your inside foot next to your partner's.	Make sure the outer portion of your foot touches your partner's outer part.
4. Pivot on the inside foot and push off with the outside foot.	Make at least three pivots and no more than five pivots to one revolution.
5. Release your partner.	Take no longer than 2 seconds after the command.

EXAMPLE OF A BEHAVIORAL OBJECTIVE (from number 4 in the chart): Pivot on the inside foot and push off with the outside foot so there are at least three and no more than five pivots for each clockwise turn.

NOTE: This behavior could be broken down further as a physical or motor prerequisite that needed to be fulfilled before mastery of the task could be achieved. If the behavioral objective reaches the developmental level of the learner, all children (handicapped or not) can be included in the instructional process.

The boxed material above and on p. 85 are examples of a task analysis of a square dance routine and the standing broad jump.

Pattern analysis program

It is sometimes desirable to evaluate the qualitative aspects of performance. Therefore it may be desirable to derive a conceptual model of a pattern and then evaluate performance against that pattern. However, improvement in behavior toward the conceptual pattern does not necessarily mean that behavioral performance will result. The temporospatial relationships of the pattern may be as important as the pattern itself in acquiring behavioral results in a task.

Behavioral objectives may be generated through procedures employed with task analysis, pattern analysis, or programmed behavioral objectives in which either criterion or conditions for mastery have been shifted. Analysis of both curricular domain and learner ability within specified curricular areas is essential. Approaches that do not consider curricular content in relationship to learner assessment leave much to be desired with regard to meaningful decision making in the selection of experiences that will facilitate development of the handicapped in the instructional process.

NORMATIVE SCALES FOR DIAGNOSIS AND PROGRAMMING

Numerous researchers in growth and development have studied the chronological occurrence of motor behaviors on a normative continuum. These include Gesell (1954), Bayley (1951), Guttridge (1939), Wild (1938), and Wellman (1937). Most authorities classify behaviors according to the gross and fine motor domain. Gesell indicates that gross motor development proceeds in two directions: the cephalocaudal and proximodistal directions. Knowledge of the directions of development provides valuable information for developmental diagnosis of and subsequent programming for children who are in the early stages of development. Such information indicates which behaviors are part of the learner's

TERMINAL OBJECTIVE: Execute the basic skill of the standing broad jump appropriately as
defined by a conceptual model.

Broad jump	Criterion for mastery
Prepare for jump.	1. Retract arms at least parallel with torso at takeoff.
	2. Flex knees and hips between 45 and 90 degrees at takeoff and arms at 45-degree angle to jumping surface.
	3. Keep arms straight and in line with torso.
Take off.	4. Maintain knees extended to 180 degrees.
	5. Maintain hips extended to 180 degrees.
	6. Maintain ankles extended to 135 degrees.
	7. Hold body at 45-degree angle to floor.
Sustain flight.	8. Retract arms at least 45 degrees behind body before feet strike ground.
Make a landing.	9. Thrust arms forward so balance is maintained.
	10. Make legs reach forward and stay straight and maintain 45 degrees or less of flexion of trunk.
	11. Flex legs and hips to cushion landing.

EXAMPLE OF A BEHAVIORAL OBJECTIVE (from number 2 in the chart): Flex knees and hips
between 45 and 90 degrees at takeoff.

NOTE: This objective is stated in terms of an analyzed behavior that is part of the total
movement pattern, not in terms of the outcomes of behavioral performance, which involves
the total integration of the task.

repertoire and which have yet to be developed (Fig. 4-14). There may be some exceptions to the cephalocaudal and proximodistal principles, since there may be head-to-foot and shoulder-to-hand sweeps that are appropriate to advancing levels of maturity. These exceptions, however, do not impair the validity of the principle.

Motor development scales provide guidelines for curriculum construction and subsequent formulation of behavioral objectives. Developmental principles can be utilized in the formulation of curricula. One such principle is that children develop from the head to the foot (cephalocaudal). Rarick[8] indicates that there are definite cycles the child passes through in which he gains control over his axial skeleton in a cephalocaudal manner (Table 4-4).

Table 4-4. Cephalocaudal cycles of development*

Condition	Age (weeks)
Trunk in contact with supporting surfaces	0 to 29
Alternate flexion of legs	30 to 42
Movement to upright position in attempt to gain control over gravitational forces while standing	49 to 56
Full trunk extension and upright postural control, bilateral flexion and extension of legs	50 to 60

*From Rarick, G. L.: Motor development during infancy and childhood, Madison, Wis., 1954, University of Wisconsin. (Mimeographed.)

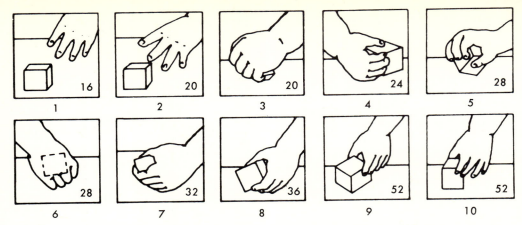

Fig. 4-14. Developmental progressions in grasping. (From Halverson, H. M.: Genet. Psychol. Monogr. **10**:107-286, 1931.)

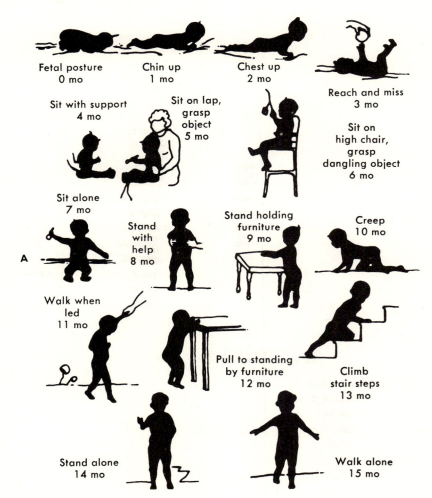

Fetal posture
0 mo

Chin up
1 mo

Chest up
2 mo

Reach and miss
3 mo

Sit with support
4 mo

Sit on lap, grasp object
5 mo

Sit on high chair, grasp dangling object
6 mo

Sit alone
7 mo

Stand with help
8 mo

Stand holding furniture
9 mo

Creep
10 mo

Walk when led
11 mo

Pull to standing by furniture
12 mo

Climb stair steps
13 mo

Stand alone
14 mo

Walk alone
15 mo

A

Fig. 4-15. A, Developmental sequence in bipedal locomotion. **B,** Comparison of data from Shirley and from *California infant growth study on median age of first passing of certain motor items.* (**A** from Shirley, M. M.: The first two years: a study of twenty-five babies, vol. II: intellectual development, Minneapolis, 1933, University of Minnesota Press; **B** from Bayley, N.: Monogr. Soc. Res. Child. Dev. **1**:1-26, 1935.)

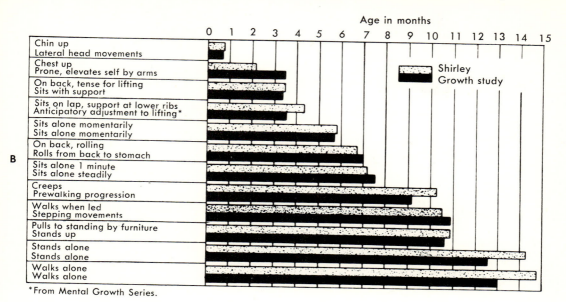

Fig. 4-15, cont'd. For legend see opposite page.

Shirley's[9] developmental scales indicate the sequence that leads to bipedal locomotion. Such information provides a guide to programming in order to assist cephalocaudal development. The chronological age norm associated with developmental progressions gives opportunities for the determination of acceleration rates as well as developmental lags of the children who have been assessed in these sequences (Fig. 4-15).

SERVING POPULATIONS VIA DEVELOPMENTAL PRINCIPLES

The direction of development (cephalocaudal and proximodistal) is most relevant to children at preschool ages and particularly to the motor development of children who are in the first year of life. Therefore persons who can benefit most from the application of these developmental principles are (1) normal children up to 1 year of age, (2) handicapped infants, and (3) profoundly mentally retarded children who have not developed beyond the first year of life according to chronological norms.

SUMMARY

The application of the developmental concept to the instructional processes of handicapped children now has a legal foundation. There are approved professional practices that require that the abilities and disabilities of the handicapped be assessed. These assessments are then paired with subsequent instruction that facilitates accountability of the educational progress of each child over a time frame. It is essential that replicative curricula and competent teachers be joined to deliver services that can be evaluated on the basis of their effectiveness. Specific types of curricula must be properly paired to the nature of the instructional tasks in order to achieve these goals.

REFERENCES

1. Auxter, D. M.: Perceptual-motor development programs for an individually prescribed instructional system, Slippery Rock, Pa., 1971, Slippery Rock State College.
2. Bayley, N. A.: The California Infant Scale of Motor Development, Berkeley, Calif., 1951, University of California Press.

3. Gagne, R. W.: Learning hierarchies, Educ. Psychol. 6:1-9, 1968.
4. Kephart, N. C.: The slow learner in the classroom, Columbus, Ohio, 1961, Charles E. Merrill Publishing Co.
5. Lindvall, C. M., and Bolvin, J. D.: Programmed instruction in the schools: an application of programming principles in individually prescribed instruction, sixty-sixth yearbook of the National Society of the Study of Education, Chicago, 1967, University of Chicago Press.
6. Miller, R. A.: Task description and analysis. In Gagne, R. M., editor: Psychological principles in system development, New York, 1962, Holt, Rinehart & Winston, Inc.
7. Miller, R. B.: Analysis and specification of behavior for training. In Glaser, R., editor: Training research and education, Pittsburgh, 1962, University of Pittsburgh Press.
8. Rarick, G. L.: Motor development during infancy and childhood, Madison, Wis., 1954, University of Wisconsin. (Mimeographed.)
9. Shirley, M. M.: The first two years: a study of twenty-five babies, vol. I: postural and locomotor development, Minneapolis, 1931, University of Minnesota Press.
10. Education of the handicapped act of 1975, P.L. 94-142, December 2, 1975, Washington, D.C., Weekly Compilation of Presidential Documents, vol. II, No. 49.
11. First consolidated concept paper under part B of the education of the handicapped act, P.L. 94-142, August 20, 1976, U.S. Office of Education, Bureau of Education for the Handicapped.

RECOMMENDED READINGS

Barsch, R. H.: Achieving perceptual-motor efficiency: an approach to learning, Seattle, 1967, Special Child Publications.
Broer, M. R.: Efficiency of human movement, Philadelphia, 1960, W. B. Saunders Co.
Bunn, J. W.: Scientific principles of coaching, Englewood Cliffs, N.J., 1955, Prentice-Hall, Inc.
Espenschade, A. S., and Eckert, H. M.: Motor development, Columbus, Ohio, 1967, Charles E. Merrill Publishing Co.
Gallahue, D. L., Werner, P. H., and Luedke, G. C.: A conceptual approach to moving and learning, New York, 1975, John Wiley & Sons, Inc.
Gesell, A.: The ontogenesis of infant behavior. In Carmichael, L., editor: Manual of child psychology, ed. 2, New York, 1954, John Wiley & Sons, Inc.
Getman, O. D.: The visuomotor complex in the acquisition of learning skills. In Hellmuth, J., editor: Learning disorders, vol. 1, Seattle, 1965, Special Child Publications.
Glaser, R., and Nitko, A. J.: Measurement in learning and instruction, working paper, Learning Research and Development Center, Pittsburgh, 1970, University of Pittsburgh Press.
Glassow, R. B., and Kruse, P.: Motor performance of girls age 6 to 11 years, Res. Q. 31:426-433, 1960.
Green, B. F.: A method of scalogram analysis using summary statistics, Psychometrics 21:79-88, 1956.
Guttman, L. A.: Basis for scaling quantitative data, Am. Sociol. Rev. 9:139-150, 1944.
Guttridge, M. V.: A study of motor achievements of young children, Arch. Psychol. 244:1-178, 1939.
Halverson, H. M.: An experimental study of prehension in infants by means of systematic cinema records, Genet. Psychol. Monogr. 10:107-286, 1931.
Halverson, H. M.: Studies of the grasping responses of early infancy, J. Genet. Psychol. 51:371-449, 1937.
Hay, J. G.: The biomechanics of sports techniques, Englewood Cliffs, N.J., 1973, Prentice-Hall, Inc.

Hendrickson, H.: The vision development process. In Wold, R. M., editor: Visual and perceptual aspects for the achieving and underachieving child, Seattle, 1969, Special Child Publications.

Hirst, C. F., and Michaelis, E.: Developmental activities for children in special education, Springfield, Ill., 1973, Charles C Thomas, Publisher.

Kibler, R. J., Barker, L. L., and Miles, D. T.: Behavioral objectives and instruction, Boston, 1970, Allyn & Bacon, Inc.

Lingoes, J. C.: Multiple scalogram analysis: a set theoretic model for analyzing dicotomous items, Educ. Psychol. Measurements 23:501-524, 1963.

McCaskill, C. L., and Wellman, B. L.: A study of common motor achievements at preschool ages, Child Dev. 9:141-150, 1938.

Miller, D. I., and Nelson, R. C.: Biomechanics of sports, Philadelphia, 1973, Lea & Febiger.

Nelson, R. C.: Biomechanics four, Baltimore, 1974, University Park Press.

Plagenhoef, S.: Patterns of human motion, Englewood Cliffs, N.J., 1971, Prentice-Hall, Inc.

Popham, W. J., editor: Instructional objectives, Skokie, Ill., 1969, Rand McNally & Co.

Resnick, L. G., and Wang, M. C.: Approaches to the validation of learning hierarchies, Paper presented at the eighteenth annual western regional conference on testing problems, San Francisco, May, 1969.

Stephens, B.: Training the developmentally young, New York, 1971, John Day Co., Inc.

Taber, J. I., Glaser, R., and Schaefer, H. H.: Learning and programmed instruction, Reading, Mass., 1965, Addison-Wesley Publishing Co., Inc.

Wellman, B. L.: Motor achievements of preschool children, Childhood Educ. 13:311-316, 1937.

Wild, M. R.: The behavior pattern of throwing and some observations concerning its course of development in children, Res. Q. 9:20-24, 1938.

PART TWO

KEY TEACHING AND THERAPY SKILLS

Part II of the text is designed to help the reader understand therapy skills that can be used with all types of inconvenienced persons of all age levels. Exercise, relaxation, fitness, nutritional status, and adapted sports and games are presented in this section.

5

EXERCISE THERAPY PROGRAMS
SELECTION ■ ASSIGNMENT ■ TEACHING

■ Remedial exercises play an important part in the adapted physical education program. In fact, carefully selected special exercises properly executed by students in *regular* physical education classes can do much to prevent bodily malalignment and to aid in the correction of deviations in posture, muscular imbalance, weak musculature, and poor general physical fitness. The values of performing regular exercises, when properly taught and assigned in the correct amount, are stated and substantiated in numerous texts on medicine, physiology of exercise, and physical education.

In general, exercise improves muscular strength and tone, can increase flexibility, produces increased efficiency in circulation and respiration, strengthens the heart muscle, and helps educate or reeducate the neuromuscular systems of the body so that we sit, stand, and move more effectively. Properly performed, exercises can aid in the correction of body deviations that are related to the neuromuscular joint systems and may aid in certain cardiorespiratory conditions.

THERAPEUTIC EXERCISE

The values of regular and therapeutic exercise have been established for many years. Since World War II, when such concepts as the need for early ambulation and preoperative and postoperative exercise

93

programs were reinforced, to the present time, during which great stress is being placed on cardiovascular fitness for both the normal and the subpar individual, there has been an increase in the acceptance of the value of exercise.

The following are selected factors that are important to therapeutic exercise:

1. Strength
   a. Muscle strength is increased with use and decreased with disuse.
   b. Muscle size increases (hypertrophy) with use and decreases (atrophy) with disuse.
   c. Heavy resistance increases muscle strength and size more rapidly than does light resistance.
   d. Isotonic exercises (involving muscular contraction and movement of a joint) increase strength, promote circulation and cardiovascular endurance, and maintain joint flexibility.
   e. Isometric exercises (involving muscular contraction, but no movement of the joint) increase strength and economize in the time spent in exercising, but contribute little to cardiovascular fitness and joint flexibility.
   f. DeLorme's Progressive Resistance Exercises (PRE) provide a system for exercising using the isotonic principle.[3, 4] This method employs the use of 10 repetition maximums (RM). The student selects a weight or any resistance that he can lift maximally 10 times in bouts or sets of three and he employs the following system: (1) first bout, 10 repetitions (reps) using one half the 10 RM load; (2) second bout, 10 reps using three fourths the 10 RM load; and, finally, (3) third bout, 10 reps using the full 10 RM load. There are many variations of the DeLorme method depending on the special requirements of the participant. If greater strength is needed, more resistance and less repetition should be used in each bout; conversely, if greater muscle endurance is needed, less resistance and a greater number of repetitions should be employed.
   g. The Hettinger-Müller research provides a system for exercises using the principle of isometric exercises.[6] Their work, although considered controversial by some researchers, has provided a rationale for using isometrics in the development of strength. They suggested that a single isometric contraction held for 6 seconds and executed once a week at three fourths the maximum effort will develop strength. This concept has direct implications for individuals who are recumbent and are not allowed isotonic movements, for the prevention of atrophy of a part, and for those individuals who may be subdeveloped and debilitated. Ordinarily, some modification of the procedure is employed when it is used in the adapted physical education class.
   h. Great strength is unnecessary in a muscle if proper balance is not maintained between antagonistic muscles.
   i. Strength is wasted if proper muscle, fascia, and joint flexibility is not maintained.

2. Flexibility
   a. Flexibility is maintained with normal use and is decreased with disuse.
   b. Body efficiency and grace are reduced as flexibility is decreased.
   c. Immobilized joints or restricted joint actions for long periods of time (consequences of casts, braces, or disuse) result in loss of flexibility.
   d. Stretching exercises are most effective when performed slowly and when aided by the pull of gravity.
   e. Sudden, rapid motions to induce stretch (bouncing or jerking against the muscles to be stretched) induce the "stretch reflex," which causes the affected muscle to tighten, and are thus less effective and may cause tearing.
   f. Actively contracting the muscle groups antagonistic to those that are being stretched aids flexibility through "reciprocal inhibition" (causes relaxation of the stretched muscle and is thus more effective for increasing flexibility).

3. Relaxation
   a. Relaxation principles and techniques are described in Chapter 6.

4. Endurance
   a. Endurance is increased when the rate of performance of an activity is increased.
   b. Endurance is developed by increasing the number of times an activity is performed.
   c. As endurance is increased, the rate and the repetitions must be increased to continue improvement.
   d. Endurance may be general (total cardiovascular system in the body).
   e. Specific (muscular) endurance is obtained through repetitious exercises for selected muscle groups.
   f. General (cardiovascular) endurance involving the total body is obtained by such activities as jogging,[1] walking, swimming, circuit training,[5] rope skipping, and bicycling.

To be effective for prevention or correction of body weakness or malalignment, exercises must be scientifically based, accurately taught, and properly learned. They must then be *practiced regularly*. Additional information on strength, endurance, and flexibility is found in Chapter 7.

Choice of exercises

The following points should be considered in the development or choice of an exercise:

1. What is the purpose of the exercise?
2. Does it accomplish that purpose?
3. Does it violate any principles of sound body mechanics?
4. What are the main joints involved?
5. What are the main muscle groups involved?
6. Is the exercise primarily for flexibility, strength, endurance, or coordination?
7. What is the intensity of the exercise: mild, moderate, or vigorous?
8. What elements of danger are involved? What cautions should be remembered in assignment and execution of the exercise?
9. Is the exercise good for more than one disability?
10. Can you measure student progress through this exercise?

Assignment of exercises to students

Since each individual has different needs and different problems, the student's exercise program will be most effective if it is designed specifically for him. Some important factors to consider in the selection of exercises for the student are the following:

1. What is the medical diagnosis and the recommendation of the physician?
2. What factors were discovered through physical education testing (posture and body mechanics examinations, fitness tests, neuromuscular tests, and perceptual-motor assessment)?
3. What are the interests of the student?

Selection of exercises for the individual should further consider the following points:

1. The type and extent of warm-up exercises needed should be considered; they should loosen, stretch, and warm up the parts to be concentrated on in the regular exercise workout.
2. All the areas to be exercised should be considered so that, when possible, exercises that aid two or more areas or conditions can be used and so that an exercise that may aid one condition, but may aggravate another, will not be used.
3. Exercises should be progressive, starting with stretching and loosening, then light active exercises, and, as the condition of the student permits, performance of active and resistive exercises.
4. The sequence of exercises should be from one body area to another. When all of the prescribed areas have been exercised once, they may be exercised a second and third time either by repeating the exercise program or by having more advanced exercises assigned by the instructor. Thus a student can work a part of the body vigorously, followed by a rest period for that body area while other body areas are exercised, returning to each body area with additional exercises later in the exercise period.
5. Relaxation may be an important part of the exercise program. If so, it should be scheduled as part of the workout. The student should be taught the techniques of progressive relaxation (Chapter 6).
6. The student should have a written exercise program showing progression, sequence, repetitions, resistance used, and, later, as the semester progresses, the goal toward which the student should work. A more detailed explanation of the use of an exercise card is presented later in this chapter.
7. Proper breathing during exercise is important. Holding the breath, especially during heavy lifting or vigorous exercises in which the handicapped person is straining to perform, should be done with an "open throat," accompanied by either inhalation or exhalation. This will prevent intra-abdominal strain that could

result in a hernia; helps to prevent the pooling of blood in the abdominal area when the breath is held during heavy lifting and strain activities; and prevents closing off the carotid artery, which may cause the Valsava effect. Regular breathing, like rhythmic isotonic exercise, promotes normal flow of the blood through the cardiovascular system.

Teaching of exercises

If an exercise is worth doing, it is worth doing well. Thus instruction must be clear and the student must be motivated to want to exercise and exercise correctly. Effective teaching of each exercise should help toward this end. Some points to be considered in teaching special exercises are the following:

1. An accurate demonstration and verbal description should be given by the teacher. Teach the "why" of the exercise as well as the "how" so that the student understands the reason for doing an exercise and doing it correctly.
2. The demonstration-explanation should take the student through each exercise step by step, that is, starting position, first move, second move, etc. The cadence or speed, the number of repetitions, the amount of resistance, and the precautions to observe in performing each particular exercise must be explained.
3. Important points about an exercise and the exercise program should be reviewed during the semester.
4. The instructor should observe the student's performance and make corrections frequently throughout the year.
5. The student should be given a reference for each exercise, that is, a written description and pictures or diagrams (Fig. 5-1). This will enable him to learn each exercise more accurately and to review his performance periodically throughout the school year.
6. The instructor should test the student and correct his exercise techniques by observation of his performance. Demon-

strations and written or verbal quizzes can be given to check the student on his knowledge of his exercises and exercise programs, reasons for assignment of particular exercises, and special values of each exercise.

7. It is desirable to limit the number of exercises taught at one time to three or four. More than this may serve to confuse the student.

Points to stress in doing a program of exercises include the following:

1. Do each exercise exactly right. The correct number of repetitions and the amount of resistance used are also important. The number of repetitions and/or the amount of resistance used should be steadily increased during the semester. Muscular endurance can be increased as the number of repetitions is increased. If strength and muscle size are the major objectives, repetitions may be reduced and the amount of resistance used steadily increased. The DeLorme system previously discussed is a plan that will promote both muscular strength and endurance and yet is a safe procedure to use in a rehabilitation setting.
2. Warm up and stretch first; then exercise and develop the desired parts.
3. In posture development programs, progress from recumbency exercises (to gain control of body segments with the aid of gravity) to sitting, then standing, and, finally, resistance exercises in which greater body control is necessary to perform the exercise properly.
4. Do exercises vigorously, hold correct positions momentarily, then relax and repeat. By using these techniques, both isotonic and isometric principles are used in the execution of an exercise.
5. Keep all body segments in good alignment throughout the exercise program, especially when resistive exercises are performed. This will help to reduce strain.
6. Complete the exercise program by "cooling down" by gradually reducing

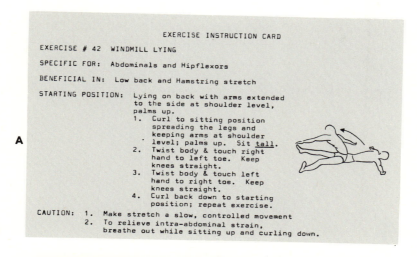

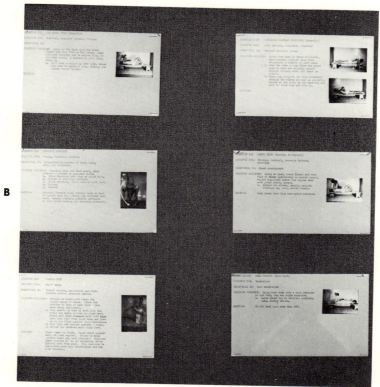

Fig. 5-1. Exercise instruction cards. **A,** Each card contains the name, number, description, and illustration of an exercise. **B,** Bulletin board displaying exercise cards for students to study and to check their performance.

		Weeks		Rec. Reps./Resist.	1	2	3	4	5	6	7	8	9	10	11	12	13	14	15

CALIFORNIA STATE UNIVERSITY, LONG BEACH
ADAPTED PHYSICAL EDUCATION EXERCISE CARD   Sect. No.   5
Name   Jill Jones   Date
Disabilities   Dysmenorrhea, Low physical fitness
Posture deviations   Kyphosis 2°, Pronated feet and ankles 3

Exercise objective	No.	Exercise name	Rec. Reps./Resist.	1	2	3	4	5	6	7	8	9	10	11	12	13	14	15
Warm up	2	Leg cross over																
	3	Windmill sitting	5 min.															
	10	Bicycles																
Dysm.	22	Cross-legged stretch	15 each side															
	23	Side stretch	5 each side															
	8	Mad cat	10															
Ky. 2°	4	Neck, back and shoulder flat	8															
	6	Neck flat at mirror	8															
	29	Chin lifts	12/15 lbs.															
Pron. 3°	12	Foot circling	10															
	15	Knee rotator	8															
	14	Foot curling	5 ea./1 lb.															
Low fit.	7	Abdominal curl	8															
	25	Four count wall wts.	12/3 wts.															
	28	Arm press	12/20 lbs.															
		Weekly grades																	

Fig. 5-2. Exercise assignment card.

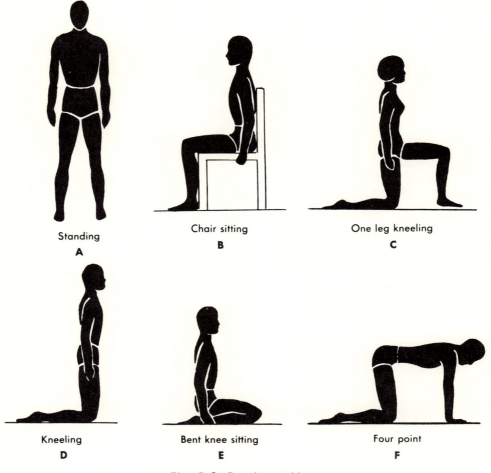

Standing
A

Chair sitting
B

One leg kneeling
C

Kneeling
D

Bent knee sitting
E

Four point
F

Fig. 5-3. Exercise positions.

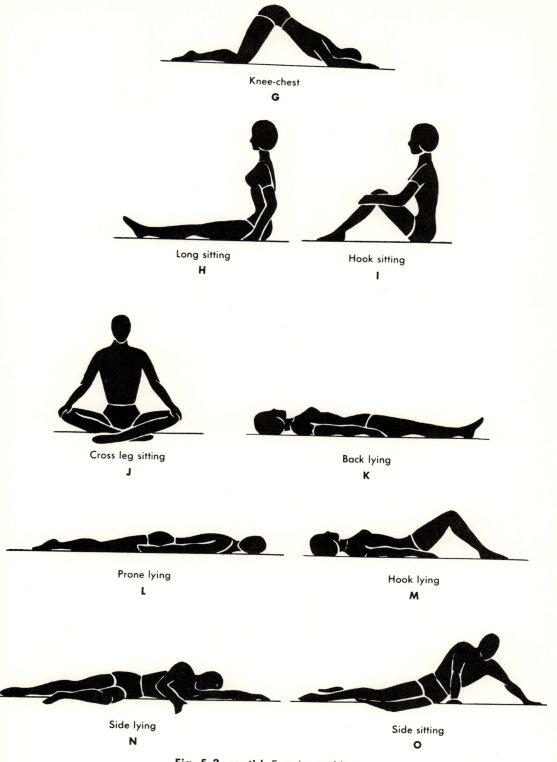

Fig. 5-3, cont'd. Exercise positions.

the intensity of the exercises to prevent blood engorgement in the muscles.

7. Keep an accurate record of performance (Fig. 5-2), including the sequence in which exercises are done, the number of repetitions, and the amount of resistance used. (This should be recorded by the student at least once each week and can be checked periodically by both the student and the teacher to note the progress being made.)

Correct positioning is essential for the proper execution of a particular exercise. Fig. 5-3 provides a key to standardizing therapeutic exercise starting positions.

Intensity of exercises

Exercises should be prescribed in terms of how vigorous they are. Two methods often used to consider and to describe the intensity of an exercise are discussed in the following paragraphs.

One classification of exercises, which grades them from easy to difficult, lists them as passive, assistive, active, and resistive. These terms are defined as follows:

1. A *passive exercise* is one in which the body part is put through the range of motion for the student. This enables him to maintain joint flexibility and produces some movement of the muscle mass. The student should be conscious of the attempted movement and should think about and try to execute the movement. The student may do passive exercises by moving the affected part with an unaffected part, a pulley arrangement, or other types of special exercise equipment. Passive exercises may also be performed for the student by the teacher, a therapist, or another student, using a "partner" system (Appendix I).

2. An *assistive exercise* is one in which the body part is moved for the student, but in which the student assists in the movement to the extent of his ability. Thus neuromuscular patterns are learned or relearned, muscle fibers are developed, and flexibility is retained or improved.

These exercises may be performed as described in paragraph 1.

3. An *active exercise* is one in which the student moves the body part himself and usually works against the counterforces of gravity. Many types of calisthenic exercises exemplify this type of action. Strength is developed, neuromuscular patterns are improved, and flexibilty is maintained. Retention or restoration of normal function is the desired result.

4. A *resistive exercise* is one in which the student exercises against some form of resistance. This may include the use of weights, springs, pulleys, dynamic tension, another person, water, or friction. The student strives to build greater strength in weak or subpar musculature than would normally be accomplished using active exercises. The student must be cautioned to increase resistance progressively, to exercise body parts through proper neuromuscular pathways, and to exercise through the full range of normal joint flexibility while engaged in resistive exercises.

Another similar plan for grading exercise in terms of difficulty is to consider the exercise in relation to gravity, that is, exercising with gravity as an aid, with gravity ruled out, against gravity, and with resistance greater than gravity.

Gravity as an aid in exercising

The easiest form of exercise is one in which gravity is used to assist the student in the movement of a body part. Examples of this type of exercise are those in which a body part is moved against the pull of gravity by good musculature, by a pulley, or by another person. The part is then helped in its return to the starting position by the weak musculature working with the assistance of the pull of gravity. Conscious effort must be made by the student to use the weak muscles or the exercise may become one of lengthening contraction of the already strong muscles and neglect of the muscles in need of mild exercise. More harm than good may then result.

Gravity ruled out

Ruling gravity out is usually accomplished by supporting the affected part so that it can be exercised without the interference of the pull of gravity. Supporting the part in a pool or ultilizing the support of a pulley or of another person allows the student to exercise the desired muscles with minimum interference from gravitational pull.

Against gravity

Antigravity exercises are more vigorous than the types previously described and involve the use of the affected parts against the pull of gravity. Standing erect involves the use of the extensor muscles of the body in opposition to the pull of gravity. Many of our traditional calisthenic exercises are of the antigravity type, either in their main movement or in the positions held by the other body segments to permit this main movement. Lifting the arms overhead while in the standing position or doing a sit-up or a leg-raise while recumbent exemplifies this type of exercise.

Resistance greater than gravity

Application of resistance greater than the pull of gravity involves the same principles described in the previous section of this chapter on resistive exercises.

The exercises to be assigned to students in an adaptive physical education class must be chosen with great care regarding the difficulty involved in their execution and the amount of work required. They must be graded carefully so that development occurs and improvement is made, but so that strain and injury are avoided. A safe number of repetitions for most exercises would be enough to involve a good workout for the affected muscles without undue fatigue or strain and without assuming an undesirable body position to accomplish the movement. *This is often the case when a student tries to do too many repetitions or use too much resistance.* Symptoms of overexercising, such as fatigue that lasts more than 5 hours, soreness the next day, or decreased range of motion the next day, may indicate a need for reexamination of the exercise program.

Students in an adapted physical education class who are assigned active or resistive exercises should be limited to 12 to 15 repetitions of the exercise (properly done) before progressing to a more difficult exercise or to the use of greater resistance. This minimizes the chance of strain or injury.

For the most part, it is wise to be conservative and careful in the assignment of the number of repetitions and the amount of resistance used by a student in his initial workout program. The teacher can easily increase the dosage as soon as the student's capacity for exercise has been determined.

EXERCISES FOR POSTURE CORRECTION

The assignment of exercises for the correction of body posture is largely a matter of selecting the proper exercises to develop certain of the antigravity muscles (see Fig. 9-34) and to enable the student to realign body parts through stretching and developing the proper antagonistic muscle groups. Proper neuromuscular patterns must be developed and the proprioceptive centers reeducated to enable the student to obtain the feeling of a well-balanced sitting, standing, and moving posture. Attention must be given both to the assignment and to the execution of exercises so that the body is not placed in positions of poor alignment and strain. Each exercise that is performed should contribute to the proper alignment of the body or one or more of its parts.

EXERCISES FOR REHABILITATION

The 40 key exercises described in the next section of this chapter can also be used as a nuclear set of exercises for rehabilitation of a variety of pre- or post-operative conditions or for therapeutic exercise programs to be assigned following illness, accident, or injury. (See subsequent discussion of exercise assignment information, p. 123.) To the exercises that are suggested for the rehabilitation of these special conditions, teachers or therapists can add others selected from other chapters of this text, from their own experience, or from standard texts covering these conditions. Exercise programs for special areas are discussed in other chapters, for example, the foot, ankle, and knee (Figs. 10-6 through 10-10), the hip and back (Figs. 10-15 through 10-18), and the shoulder (Figs. 10-20 through 10-23) are discussed in Chapter 10; exercises for tension reduction are given in Chapter 6; exercises for low vitality and fitness are contained in Chapter 7; exercises for chronic musculoskeletal disorders such as amputation, arthritis, hip afflictions, and spinal disabilities are discussed in Chapter 11; and exercise programs for cardiovascular problems are discussed in Chapter 12.

EXERCISE ASSIGNMENT SYSTEM

Since the problems and needs of students in an adapted physical education class are different, each student must have a program of exercise that is based on his needs and interests. Classes of adapted physical education often include 25 to 35 students, making individual assignment of and instruction in exercises a difficult problem. The following system of exercise assignment and technique of instruction is planned to facilitate assignment of individual exercise programs in sizable groups.[2]

These 40 exercises should form the nuclear group to be used for all types of cases found in an adapted physical education program, whether the student needs rehabilitation of body parts, improvement in physical fitness, attention to body mechanics, or an exercise program for some particular type of disability. Individual teachers or therapists will wish to add exercises to this series, strengthening areas

of special need in their program. These 40 exercises were selected from a set of 105 exercises that we have used extensively for the past 25 years.

The system consists of:

1. A list of exercises, each with a name and a number, arranged according to the type of exercise performed or the type of equipment used. (See section I, which follows immediately.)
2. An exercise assignment sheet that further categorizes the exercises into groups that can be assigned for some 50 special conditions, graded as to whether they are *specifically* for a condition or are of general value. They are further differentiated for use as a flexibility exercise or a developmental exercise. (See section II.)
3. Forty key exercises, described and illustrated. Since they have been chosen to include exercises for all parts of the body (both as stretches and as strengtheners), they can serve as the "backbone" of a set to be used by classes in adapted physical education. (See section III.)
4. Information on how to organize the class to allow for the selection of the proper exercises for each student, how to assign the exercises properly, how to work out proper progressions, and how to teach each student his individual exercise program using a small group method is presented in the section on selection of an exercise program for each student, which follows section III in the chapter.

Section I
Forty key exercises for adapted physical education

1. Supine stretch
2. Leg crossover
3. Windmill sitting
4. Neck, back, and shoulder flattener
5. Breaking chains
6. Neck flattener at mirror
7. Abdominal curl
8. Mad cat
9. Knee-chest curl

10. Bicycle
11. Heel cord stretch
12. Foot circling
13. Building mounds
14. Foot curling
15. Knee rotator
16. Quadriceps setting
17. Foot drag
18. Knee extension with boot
19. Tense and stretch
20. Elbow side falling
21. Horizontal ladder
22. Crosslegged stretch (modified from Billig)
23. Side stretch (Billig)
24. Head tilt (Billig)
25. Four-count wall weight
26. Shoulder rotator (wall weight)
27. Arm curl
28. Arm press
29. Chin lifts
30. Toe lifts
31. Arm crossovers
32. Shoulder shrugs
33. Towel wringing
34. Gripper
35. Wrist machines
36. Back stoop falling
37. Push-up
38. Chin-up or pull-up
39. Jumping jack with variations
40. Rope skipping

Section II
Exercise assignment information

Basic warm-up exercises

1. Supine stretch
2. Leg crossover
3. Windmill sitting
10. Bicycle
39. Jumping jack with variations
40. Rope skipping

Exercises for postural divergencies
Total body conditions

(S)* Sway Body sways, leans, and tilts are total
(L) Lean body conditions often resulting from
(T) Tilt some other deviation. The correction
of this deviation will often result in
the elimination of the sway, lean, or
tilt. Since the conditions may also be
caused by carelessness, habit, and
faulty body mechanics, the student
should be made conscious of correcting his total body malalignment as

*Letter abbreviations are for those conditions
shown in Fig. 5-46 on the posture examination
card and described in Chapter 9 and shown in
Figs. 9-34, B, and 9-35.

he corrects his special deviations
and improves his total body fitness.
Correcting total body alignment also
necessitates the reeducation of the
proprioceptive centers. Special symmetrical exercises that can be done
to improve body alignment and thus
correct a sway, lean, or tilt include
the following:
No. 1, supine stretch; No. 4, neck,
back, and shoulder flattener; No.
3, windmill sitting; No. 6, neck
flattener at mirror; No. 21, horizontal ladder; No. 25, four-count
wall weight; No. 39, jumping jack
with variations.
Exercises performed in front of a
mirror aid the student to see and
feel correct body alignment.

Head and neck conditions

(F) Forward head: No. 24, head tilt (stretch);
No. 4, neck, back, and shoulder flattener;
No. 5, breaking chains; No. 6, neck flattener at mirror; No. 29, chin lifts.
(T) Head tilt: No. 24, head tilt (stretch); No.
4, neck, back, and shoulder flattener; No.
5, breaking chains; No. 6, neck flattener
at mirror.

Chest conditions

(F) Flat chest: No. 4, neck, back, and shoulder flattener; No. 5, breaking chains; No.
6, neck flattener at mirror; No. 25, four-
count wall weight; No. 28, arm press;
No. 31, arm crossover; No. 29, chin lifts;
No. 21, horizontal ladder.
(H) Hollow chest: same as flat chest unless
especially prescribed by a physician.
(P) Pigeon breast: Prescription by physician.

Shoulder conditions

(F) Forward or round shoulders: No. 1, supine
stretch; No. 4, neck, back, and shoulder
flattener; No. 5, breaking chains; No. 6,
neck flattener at mirror; No. 29, chin lifts;
No. 25, four-count wall weight; No. 21,
horizontal ladder.
(L) Low shoulder: No. 1, supine stretch; No.
5, breaking chains; No. 6, neck flattener
at mirror; No. 21, horizontal ladder; No.
32, shoulder shrugs; No. 29, chin lifts.

Knee conditions

(K) Knock-knee: No. 10, bicycle; No. 15, knee
rotator; No. 14, foot curling; No. 17, foot
drag.
(B) Back knee: Develop hamstring muscles;
work on leg alignment at mirror to develop a balance of pull between quadri-

ceps and hamstring muscle groups; No. 10, bicycle; No. 17, foot drag.

Pelvic deviations

(L) Lateral tilt: Prescription by physician.

(R) Rotated pelvis: Prescription by physician.

(T) Anteroposterior pelvic tilts: Forward and backward.

(F) Forward pelvic tilt: No. 3, windmill sitting; No. 2, leg crossover; No. 4, neck, back, and shoulder flattener; No. 8, mad cat; No. 7, abdominal curl; No. 9, knee-chest curl; No. 5, breaking chains; No. 6, neck flattener at mirror.

(B) Backward pelvic tilt: Supine—double leg lift; prone—back arching; prone—double leg lifts; No. 36, back stoop falling; No. 25, four-count wall weight (with low back hyperextended).

Spinal deviations

(Ky) Kyphosis: No. 1, supine stretch; No. 4, neck, back, and shoulder flattener; No. 5, breaking chains; No. 6, neck flattener at mirror; No. 25, four-count wall weight; No. 29, chin lifts.

(Lo) Lordosis: No. 3, windmill sitting; No. 2, leg crossover; No. 22, crosslegged stretch; No. 4, neck, back, and shoulder flattener; No. 8, mad cat; No. 7, abdominal curl; No. 9, knee-chest curl; No. 5, breaking chains; No. 6, neck flattener at mirror.

(F) Flat: See exercises under backward pelvic tilt.

(Sc) Scoliosis°: Symmetrical exercises: No. 1, supine stretch; No. 4, neck, back, and shoulder flattener; No. 3, windmill sitting; No. 6, neck flattener at mirror; No. 25, four-count wall weight; No. 29, chin lifts; No. 38, chin-up or pull-up. Asymmetrical exercises: No. 1, supine stretch; No. 21, horizontal ladder; No. 20, elbow side falling; No. 19, tense and stretch.

Abdominal conditions

(Pt) Ptosis: No. 3, windmill sitting; No. 2, leg crossover; No. 6, neck flattener at mirror; No. 8, mad cat; No. 7, abdominal curl; No. 9, knee-chest curl.

Foot conditions

(L) Longitudinal arch: No. 10, bicycle; No. 11, heel cord stretch; No. 12, foot circling; No. 15, knee rotator; No. 14, foot curling; supination board or balance beam.

(M) Metatarsal arch: No. 10, bicycle; No. 11, heel cord stretch; No. 12, foot circling; No. 13, building mounds.

_____
°With approval of physician.

(P) Pronated ankles: No. 10, bicycle; No. 12, foot circling; No. 15, knee rotator; No. 14, foot curling; supination board or balance beam.

(TT) Tibial torsion (prescription of physician): No. 10, bicycle; No. 12, foot circling; No. 15, knee rotator; No. 14, foot curling.

Exercises for specific body areas and conditions

Foot and ankle

No. 10, bicycle; No. 11, heel cord stretch; No. 12, foot circling; No. 13, building mounds; No. 30, toe lifts; No. 39, jumping jack with variations; No. 40, rope skipping (Chapter 10).

Knee

No. 10, bicycle; No. 16, quadriceps setting; No. 18, knee extension with boot; No. 39, jumping jack with variations; No. 40, rope skipping (Chapter 10).

Shoulder

For general conditions: No. 5, breaking chains; No. 6, neck flattener at mirror; No. 26, shoulder rotator (wall weight); No. 25, four-count wall weight; No. 32, shoulder shrugs; No. 28, arm press; No. 31, arm crossovers; No. 29, chin lifts; No. 33, towel wringing; No. 37, push-up; No. 38, chin-up or pull-up; No. 21, horizontal ladder.

For postdislocation: No. 26, shoulder rotator (wall weight) (Chapter 10).

Hand, wrist, and elbow

No. 33, towel wringing; No. 35, wrist machines; No. 40, rope skipping; No. 29, chin lifts; No. 27, arm curl; No. 37, push-up; No. 38, chin-up or pull-up; No. 28, arm press; No. 31, arm crossover; No. 21, horizontal ladder (Chapter 10).

Low back and sacroiliac

For low back stretch and development of abdominal group; No. 4, neck, back, and shoulder flattener; No. 3, windmill sitting; No. 2, leg crossover; No. 22, crosslegged stretch; No. 7, abdominal curl; No. 9, knee-chest curl (Chapter 10).

Weak back

For low back and hip extensor development: No. 1, supine stretch; No. 4, neck, back, and shoulder flattener; No. 5, breaking chains; No. 6, neck flattener at mirror; No. 25, four-count wall weight; No. 32, shoulder shrugs; No. 29, chin lifts; prone back arches (Chapter 10).

Balance and coordination

No. 6, neck flattener at mirror; No. 25, four-count wall weight; No. 39, jumping jack with variations; No. 40, rope skipping; supination board or balance beam.

General muscle tone

No. 3, windmill sitting; No. 2, leg crossover; No. 7, abdominal curl; No. 10, bicycle; No. 25, four-count wall weight; No. 27, arm curl; No. 28, arm press; No. 31, arm crossover; No. 30, toe lifts; No. 40, rope skipping.

Dysmenorrhea

No. 1, supine stretch; No. 22, crosslegged stretch; No. 23, side stretch; No. 8, mad cat; No. 7, abdominal curl; No. 9, knee-chest curl; No. 6, neck flattener at mirror. (See Chapter 17 for complete discussion and for additional exercises.)

Exercises for special muscle groups

Erector spinae

No. 1, supine stretch; No. 4, neck, back, and shoulder flattener; No. 3, windmill sitting; No. 25, four-count wall weight; No. 29, chin lifts; No. 20, elbow side falling; No. 19, tense and stretch; prone back arches; No. 36, back stoop falling.

Abdominals

No. 4, neck, back, and shoulder flattener; No. 3, windmill sitting; No. 2, leg crossover; No. 8, mad cat; No. 7, abdominal curl; No. 9, knee-chest curl; No. 5, breaking chains; No. 6, neck flattener at mirror; No. 20, elbow side falling.

Rhomboid and trapezius

No. 4, neck, back, and shoulder flattener; No. 5, breaking chains; No. 6, neck flattener at mirror; No. 21, horizontal ladder; No. 25, four-count; wall weights; No. 32, shoulder shrugs; No. 29, chin lifts; prone back arches with hands in small of back.

Pectoral

No. 3, windmill sitting; No. 26, shoulder rotator (wall weight); No. 28, arm press; No. 31, arm crossovers; No. 33, towel wringing; No. 37, push-up; No. 40, rope skipping; No. 21, horizontal ladder.

Latissimus

No. 21, horizontal ladder; No. 25, four-count wall weight; No. 33, towel wringing; No. 38, chin-up or pull-up; No. 40, rope skipping; No. 5, breaking chains; No. 6, neck flattener at mirror.

Deltoid

No. 4, neck, back, and shoulder flattener; No. 5, breaking chains; No. 6, neck flattener at mirror; No. 25, four-count wall weight; No. 28, arm press; No. 31, arm crossover; No. 29, chin lifts; No. 37, push-up.

Biceps brachii

No. 40, rope skipping; No. 27, arm curl; No. 29, chin lifts; No. 33, towel wringing; No. 38, chin-up or pull-up; No. 35, wrist machines.

Triceps

No. 28, arm press; No. 31, arm crossovers; No. 37, push-up; No. 33, towel wringing; No. 25, four-count wall weight.

Forearm muscles

No. 27, arm curl; No. 33, towel wringing; No. 40, rope skipping; No. 35, wrist machines; No. 38, chin-up or pull-up; No. 28, arm press; No. 31, arm crossovers; No. 29, chin lifts; No. 21, horizontal ladder; No. 37, push-up.

Hip extensors

No. 10, bicycle; prone single and double leg lifts; No. 25, four-count wall weight; No. 40, rope skipping.

Hip flexors

No. 3, windmill sitting; No. 2, leg crossover; No. 9, knee-chest curl; No. 18, knee extension with boot.

Knee extensors

No. 10, bicycle; No. 16, quadriceps setting; No. 18, knee extension with boot; No. 39, jumping jack with variations; No. 40, rope skipping.

Knee flexors

No. 7, foot drag; No. 9, knee-chest curl; No. 10, bicycle.

Gastrocnemius and soleus

No. 12, foot circling; No. 11, head cord stretch; No. 22, crosslegged stretch; No. 30, toe lifts; No. 39, jumping jack with variations; No. 40, rope skipping.

Section III
Descriptions of forty key exercises for adapted physical education

1. Supine stretch (Fig. 5-4)

Specific for: General loosening and stretching of body

Beneficial in: Lateral curvatures of spine, kyphosis, forward shoulders, and low shoulder

Starting position: Lying on back on mat with legs extended:

1. Extend arms overhead and reach as far as possible; stretch so that heels reach down the mat as far from hands as possible. Do not arch the back.
2. Relax right leg and left arm and stretch crossways so that left heel and right hand are maximum distance apart. Repeat with opposite arm and leg.

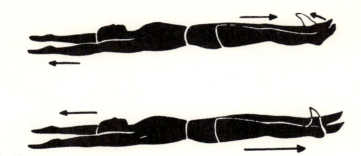

Fig. 5-4. No. 1, Supine stretch.

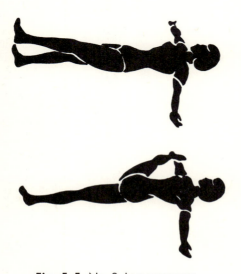

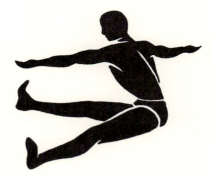

Fig. 5-6. No. 3, Windmill sitting.

Fig. 5-5. No. 2, Leg crossover.

3. Relax completely after each stretch and repeat as many times as required.

2. Leg crossover (Fig. 5-5)

Specific for: Low back and hip extensor stretch, warm-up and development of hip flexors, and abdominals

Starting position: Lying on back, arms extended at shoulder level, palms facing upward, heels pointed:

1. Flex left leg at hip to lift heel to rest on toes of right foot.
2. Twist body to right, bringing left foot across to floor, pause and stretch; then, keeping knee straight, slide foot toward right hand, stretch and return. (Keep heel pointed and legs straight.)
3. Do the same for right leg.

3. Windmill sitting (Fig. 5-6)

Specific for: Back stretch, hamstring stretch, and warm-up

Beneficial in: Abdominals and shoulder girdle

Starting position: Sitting on mat with arms extended sideward at shoulder level, palms up, legs spread wide apart, ankles plantar flexed:

1. Twist to right and bend forward with trunk so that fingers of left hand touch toes of right foot; stretch and hold. (Do a slow, controlled stretch.) Keep both legs straight.
2. Return to starting position and sit tall; then swing to left and repeat the exercise.
3. To increase the stretch of the back of the leg, dorsiflex the ankle.

4. Neck, back, and shoulder flattener (Fig. 5-7)

Specific for: Forward head, cervical lordosis, kyphosis, forward shoulders, and lordosis

Beneficial in: Abdominal strength and pelvic tilt

Starting position: Lying on back, knees drawn up, arms at side with palms down:

1. Inhale and expand chest as nape of neck is forced to mat by stretching tall and pulling chin in toward chest.
2. At the same time, flatten small of back to mat by tightening abdominal and buttocks muscles.

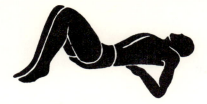

Fig. 5-7. No. 4, Neck and back flattener.

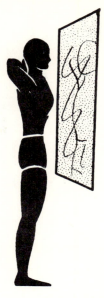

Fig. 5-9. No. 6, Neck flattener at mirror.

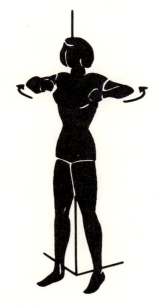

Fig. 5-8. No. 5, Breaking chains.

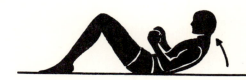

Fig. 5-10. No. 7, Abdominal curl.

3. Check with fingers to see if neck and back are flat on mat. Exhale.
4. As it becomes easier to flatten back, the exercise may be made more difficult and more beneficial by gradually extending legs until the low back cannot be maintained in a flattened position.

5. Breaking chains (Fig. 5-8)
Specific for: Forward shoulders
Beneficial in: Kyphosis, flat chest, forward head, lordosis, and shoulder development
Starting position: Standing, with back against corner of post or sharp edge of corner of a room, feet 6 inches apart; place fists together in front of chest with elbows at shoulder level:
1. Imagine you are breaking a chain by strenuously pulling fists apart, keeping elbows at shoulder level, pinching shoulder blades together. Inhale.
2. Tuck pelvis and press low back as close to wall as possible.

3. Hold position 10 seconds.
4. Relax and exhale.
Caution: Keep abdomen and buttocks tight and maintain body in starting plane during the exercise; when lordosis is present, the exercise may be done in sitting position with legs crossed in the tailor's position.

6. Neck flattener at mirror (Fig. 5-9)
Specific for: Forward head, kyphosis, forward shoulders, lordosis, and shoulder development
Beneficial in: Total anteroposterior postural deviations
Starting position: Standing tall in front of mirror, head up, chin in, elbows extended sideward at shoulder level, fingertips behind base of head:
1. Draw head and neck backward vigorously as fingers are pressed forward for resistance and elbows are forced backward (flattening upper back). Inhale.
2. Flatten low back by tucking the pelvis by

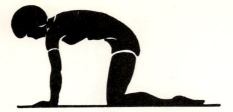

Fig. 5-11. No. 8, Mad cat.

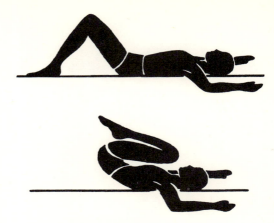

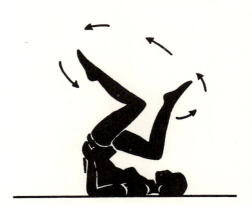

Fig. 5-12. No. 9, Knee-chest curl.

tightening the abdominals and hip extensors.
3. Hold; exhale; return to starting position. (Student can stand facing the mirror or with side of body toward mirror to check body position and to correct either antero-posterior or lateral posture deviations.)

7. Abdominal curl (Fig. 5-10)
Specific for: Ptosis (protruding abdomen), lordosis, and developing and shortening abdominals
Beneficial in: Forward pelvic tilt
Starting position: Lying on back, elbows at side of body and bent at 90 degrees, knees flexed, feet flat on floor:
1. Keep lower back flat on mat and, starting with head, curl body slowly forward and up to a 45-degree angle, lifting vertebra by vertebra off mat.
2. Uncurl slowly and with control.
Note: In all leg raising or trunk raising from the backward lying position, the student should exhale or count aloud as legs or trunk are raised to relieve intraabdominal pressure and strain.

8. Mad cat (Fig. 5-11)
Specific for: Lordosis and abdominal muscles
Beneficial in: Dysmenorrhea, arms, shoulders, shoulder girdle, and low back stretch
Starting position: Kneeling on all fours:
1. Hump lower back by tightening abdominal and buttocks muscles and drop head down while inhaling.
2. Lean forward by bending arms until forehead touches floor; keeping back humped, exhale and return to starting position.

9. Knee-chest curl (Fig. 5-12)
Specific for: Abdominal strength, ptosis, and lordosis
Beneficial in: Development of hip flexors and stretch of spinal extensors
Starting position: Lying on back with knees bent at right angles, feet flat on floor, arms straight out from shoulders, elbows bent 90 degrees, palms up:

Fig. 5-13. No. 10, Bicycle.

1. Bring knees toward chest while pulling with abdominal muscles and curl spine segment by segment off floor or mat; try to touch knees to chest or shoulders; hold, then uncurl to starting position.
Caution: See note on proper breathing for this exercise under description of exercise No. 7.

10. Bicycle (Fig. 5-13)
Specific for: General warm-up of foot and leg (for development and stretch)
Starting position: Lying on back, elbows at side of body, flexed at 90 degrees:
1. Bring knees to chest and roll up so that weight of body rests on shoulders and neck; place hands under hips for support and peddle on an imaginary bicycle with a large peddle sprocket.
2. Stress full motion in hip, knee, and ankle; alternately point toe and then heel to in-

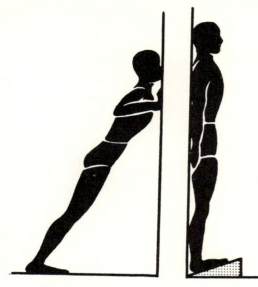

Fig. 5-14. No. 11, Heel cord stretch.

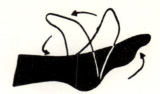

Fig. 5-15. No. 12, Foot circling.

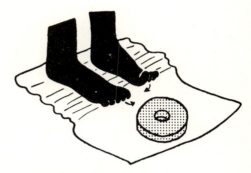

Fig. 5-16. No. 13, Building mounds.

crease flexibility of foot and ankle. Do slowly for increased flexibility, then rapidly for warm-up.

Caution: Those with arthritis of spine and cardiac problems should not roll up into inverted position on back of neck.

11. Heel cord stretch (Fig. 5-14)

Specific for: Stretch heel cord and back of leg
Beneficial in: Arms, shoulders, and shoulder girdle
Starting position: Standing at arm's length from wall, body inclined slightly forward, back flat, feet toed in slightly with hands on the wall, shoulder high and shoulder width apart, elbows slightly bent:
1. Bend arms until chest nearly touches wall. (Keep body in straight line; keep heels on floor to obtain heel cord stretch.)
2. Progressions: position self as before. Move feet back an inch or so, keeping heels on floor, and repeat exercise.
Note: Heel cord stretch board with back flattened against wall may be used as an advanced exercise.

12. Foot circling (Fig. 5-15)

Specific for: Metatarsal arch and toe flexors
Beneficial in: Flexibility and strength of foot and ankle and longitudinal arch
Starting position: Having removed shoes and socks, sitting on bench and fully extending knees, with toes pointed and heels resting on a towel on floor or mat:
1. With toes flexed, circle foot-in.

2. Circle foot-up, extend toes.
3. Circle foot-out, extend toes.
4. Circle foot-down while flexing toes, making full circle with foot and ankle; then repeat movements several times; rest. Value lies in obtaining full motion in each direction.
Caution: This exercise is contraindicated (never used) in hammer toes.

13. Building mounds (Fig. 5-16)

Specific for: Metatarsal arch and toe flexors
Beneficial in: Flexibility and strength of intrinsic muscles of feet and Morton's toe
Starting position: Sitting on bench, feet directly under knees, toes placed on end of towel:
1. Grip towel with toes and pull toward body, building a mound; pull with toes of both feet working together or pull alternately; heels must remain firmly on floor during exercise and pull on towel should be made to maximum toe flexion.
2. Repeat movements until end of towel or weight is reached.
3. When towel is to be flattened, shove its end back to former position with foot.
4. A weight may be placed on end away from body to increase resistance; when five repetitions can be done correctly, add more weight.

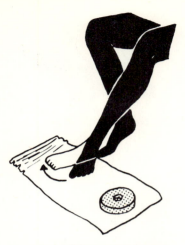

Fig. 5-17. No. 14, Foot curling.

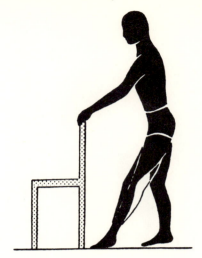

Fig. 5-19. No. 16, Quadriceps setting.

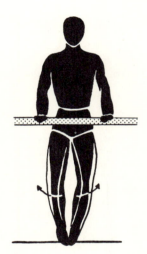

Fig. 5-18. No. 15, Knee rotator.

14. Foot curling (Fig. 5-17)

Specific for: Longitudinal arch, tibialis posterior muscle, and pronated ankle
Beneficial in: Tibial torsion
Starting position: Sitting tall on bench with thigh horizontal to floor, place left heel forward of knee about 6 inches, bring toes of right foot to rear and outside of left heel to serve as a brace; fold a towel lengthwise in thirds and place one end next to outside of left foot, extended to left:

1. Lift and turn foot to left, then press ball of foot forcibly on towel and rotate lower leg and foot to the right, pulling towel inward.

2. Repeat until towel is completely pulled across.
3. When exercise can be repeated five times, add a weight to far end of towel to add resistance.
Note: Do not substitute thigh adductors or rotators to pull towel across. Keep ball of foot and toes firmly on towel while pulling towel medially.

15. Knee rotator (Fig. 5-18)

Specific for: Knock-knees and tibial torsion
Beneficial in: Pronated ankle and longitudinal arch realignment
Starting position: Standing, holding onto stall bars, back of chair, etc., heels 3 inches apart, big toes together, with weight toward outside of feet:

1. Flex knees slightly and rotate knees outward vigorously as if to bring heels together against friction of the floor (but do not let them move); keep whole forepart of foot on floor so that a high, long arch is formed and kneecaps face outward.
2. Hold this position for 10 seconds.
3. Relax the foot and leg muscles by walking in place.
4. Repeat the exercise.

16. Quadriceps setting (Fig. 5-19)

Specific for: Stabilizing the knee anteriorly
Beneficial in: Stabilization of knee joint and improvement of muscle tone of the quadriceps muscle group (pre- and postoperatively)
Starting position: Standing with feet pointed straight ahead, one leg slightly in front of the

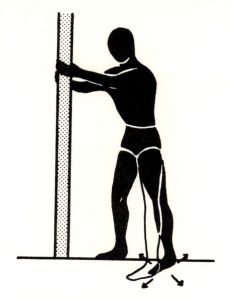

Fig. 5-20. No. 17, Foot drag.

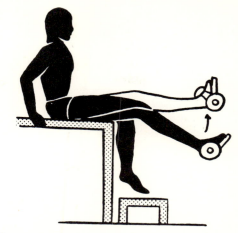

Fig. 5-21. No. 18, Knee extensor (with boot). A leg press machine or quadriceps machine can also be used for this exercise.

other with the knee straight, but not locked (may be done in sitting position if necessary):
1. Extend knee of front leg well backward.
2. Tense kneecap and raise it. Hold.
3. Relax muscles, allowing kneecap to drop to regular position.
4. Gradually increase amount of weight on foot.
Caution: When leg is tensed, hold contraction for a few moments and then relax muscles; more advanced exercises may include stair and hill climbing, running on smooth surfaces, and rope skipping.

17. Foot drag (Fig. 5-20)
Specific for: Reeducation of muscle groups, stabilizing knee and ankle joints, and improvement of muscle tone of whole leg and thigh
Starting position: Standing erect, feet pointed straight forward, knees slightly flexed, weight mostly on right foot:
1. Apply mild pressure to floor with bottom of left foot; then push it forward and backward, left and right and diagonally to form an "X", to greatest range of movement; cease movement at point of pain.
2. Circle foot clockwise and counterclockwise.
3. As condition improves, increase resistance by placing more weight on dragged foot.
Caution: Keep knees slightly bent and toes straight forward at all times, thus lessening strain on knee joint. Wear rubber-soled shoe to increase friction.

18. Knee extensor (with boot) (Fig. 5-21)
Specific for: Strengthening quadriceps muscle group
Beneficial in: Improvement of muscle tone of anterior thigh and hip flexors (if step 3 is added)
Starting position: Sitting on plinth or high bench with knee flexed and a weight on foot (boot or sandbag, *foot supported*):
1. Extend knee to straighten leg.
2. Hold, then lower slowly to supported position.
3. To increase strength of hip flexors, add the following movement: raise entire leg above horizontal, tensing leg muscle, sitting tall; lower slowly.
Caution: Be sure that exercise is done very slowly to ensure maximum development of whole front of thigh; climb stairs on every occasion, walk uphill, do road work on smooth surface. Exercises on a Universal Gym or with special isotonic exercise machines can be substituted.

19. Tense and stretch (Fig. 5-22)
Specific for: Scoliosis
Beneficial in: Torsion of trunk and low shoulder
Starting position: Standing tall (facing a mirror if possible):
1. Raise arm vertically over head, opposite from the way in which the spine curves (right arm for a left "C" scoliosis); rotate other hand and arm outward and vigorously press it into side of body (left arm for a left "C" scoliosis).

2. Hold position for 10 seconds. Lower arms to side and assume normal position.
3. Repeat exercise required number of times.

Caution: Be certain that back is maintained in straight position without twisting trunk; stand tall; do not let shoulders sag.

Note: Give only on prescription of physician unless exercise is done symmetrically, that is, to both sides.

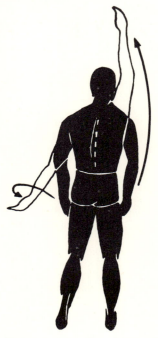

Fig. 5-22. No. 19, Tense and stretch. Dotted line indicates improved alignment resulting from exercise done in "keynote" position illustrated.

20. Elbow side falling (Fig. 5-23)

Specific for: Scoliosis and development of lateral flexors of trunk

Starting position: Resting on side toward convex side of spinal curve:

1. Rest on elbow toward curve; extend opposite arm, shoulder height, to side and lift hip completely off floor; hold with body supported on forearm and side of foot.
2. Lower hip to floor and rest.
3. Repeat.

Caution: Back must be in horizontal plane with neck, head, and back straight; upper leg may be placed in front of supporting leg for better balance.

Note: Give only on prescription of physician unless exercise is done symmetrically by doing the same exercise while resting on the opposite side of the body.

21. Horizontal ladder (Fig. 5-24)

Beneficial in: Total body stretch, scoliosis curves in spine, kyphosis and forward shoulders, low shoulder, and development of shoulder girdle muscles

Note: This exercise should be specified for each individual by the instructor; it may include climbing, hanging, stretching, swinging, etc. If horizontal ladder is mounted with one end higher than the other, asymmetrical exercises can be given for low shoulders, scoliosis, etc.

22. Crosslegged stretch (modified from Billig) (Fig. 5-25)

Specific for: Stretch of lower back, back of leg, and heel cord

Beneficial in: Lordosis and bent knees

Starting position: Standing on affected leg with knee fully extended, about 20 inches from and

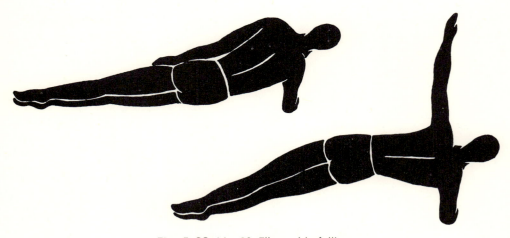

Fig. 5-23. No. 20, Elbow side falling.

with back to stall bars, chair, or bench, reach back and rest hand of affected side on stall bars for balance:

1. Then, with knee flexed, twine opposite leg tightly around front of affected leg; foot is placed in tiptoe position on floor, back and and to the outside of heel of affected leg.
2. Free hand is placed on opposite shoulder and, from this position, student bows forward at hips, reaching for heel of crossed-over

foot with elbow, at the same time dropping entire heel from tiptoe position to floor.

3. Execute five controlled stretches. Hold each stretch for 10 seconds; relax and repeat on opposite side.

23. Side stretch (Billig) (Fig. 5-26)

Specific for: Mobilization of hip and pelvis
Beneficial in: Dysmenorrhea (Chapter 17)
Starting position: Heels and toes together approximately upper-arm's distance from and with side to wall:

1. Place elbow against wall at shoulder level, elbow slightly ahead of line of shoulders, with forearm and hand resting on wall; heel of opposite hand is placed in back of hip joint (behind greater trochanter).
2. Keep shoulders in line with the elbow perpendicular to wall; do not allow them to shift forward. Keep knees completely extended and locked; strongly contract abdominal and gluteal muscles while shifting hips slightly forward and in toward wall, aiding this by pressure of the outside hand; push inside hip toward a point directly below hand that rests on wall.
3. Force the sideward and forward shift of hips toward wall far enough to produce a stretch on muscles and ligaments. Hold stretch position for 10 seconds. Repeat on opposite side.

24. Head tilt (Billig) (Fig. 5-27)

Specific for: Neck muscle stretching
Beneficial in: Muscle relaxation, remediation of neck strain, and muscle tension

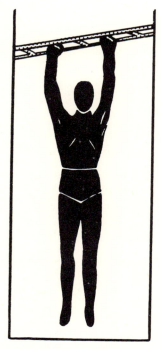

Fig. 5-24. No. 21, Horizontal ladder.

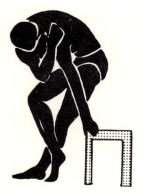

Fig. 5-25. No. 22, Crosslegged stretch (modified from Billig).

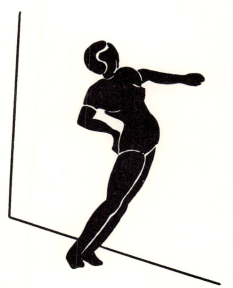

Fig. 5-26. No. 23, Side stretch (Billig).

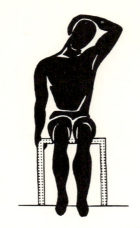

Fig. 5-27. No. 24, Head tilt (Billig).

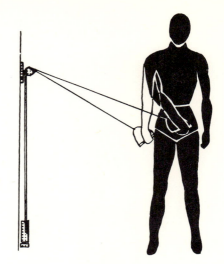

Fig. 5-29. No. 26, Shoulder rotator (wall weights).

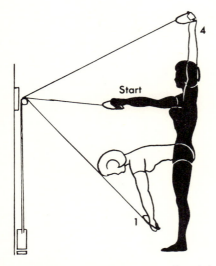

Fig. 5-28. No. 25, Four-count wall weight.

Starting position: Seated in a chair with hand on one side firmly grasping back leg of chair; head and neck are tilted laterally 45 degrees in the opposite direction:
1. Retract chin maximum distance possible and hold retracted (pulled in) throughout stretch.
2. Place free hand over head, covering ear, to forcibly continue tilt.
3. Pull to stretch, hold 10 seconds.
4. Repeat this stretching three times on each side three periods daily.

25. Four-count wall weight (Fig. 5-28)
Specific for: General conditioning of shoulders and upper back, kyphosis, and forward shoulders

Beneficial in: General fitness, back and hamstring flexibility, and abdominal strength
Starting position: Standing facing wall weights, holding handles straight forward at shoulder level:
1. Pull handles to toes, keeping legs and arms straight.
2. Return to standing position and pull handles back beyond sides of hips.
3. Return and pull handles out to side at shoulder level.
4. Return and pull handles straight overhead.
5. Return and repeat.
Caution: Keep body straight and tall throughout exercise; *do not* use more weight than can be handled while body is maintained in a good anteroposterior alignment; breathe freely.

26. Shoulder rotator (wall weights) (Fig. 5-29)
Specific for: Shoulder dislocation, pectoral muscles, and subscapularis
Beneficial in: General shoulder strength
Starting position: Standing with side toward wall weights, back straight and feet shoulder distance apart; grasp one or both handles with hand that is nearest weights:
1. Pull handle across in front of body with hand at hip level, elbow fully extended, body stationary.
2. Rotate arm inward (medial rotation) as far as possible as it is brought across body; hold; return.

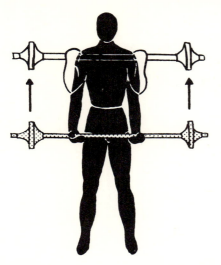

Fig. 5-30. No. 27, Arm curl (barbell or dumb-bell).

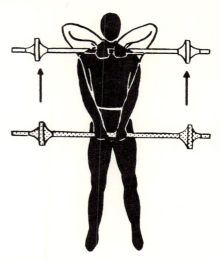

Fig. 5-32. No. 29, Chin lifts (barbell or dumb-bell).

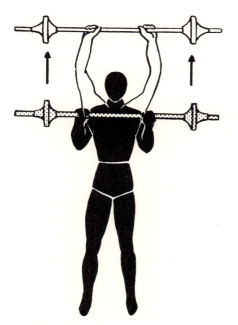

Fig. 5-31. No. 28, Arm press (barbell or dumb-bell).

27. Arm curl (barbell or dumbbell) (Fig. 5-30)
Specific for: Biceps, brachialis, and brachio-radialis
Beneficial in: Forearm and shoulder muscles
Starting position: Standing or sitting, weights held in front of body at thigh level, palms turned away from body:

1. Flex arms, keeping elbows close to, but not against sides, bringing weights to chest; hold and return slowly; reverse curl; repeat as described, except palms turned toward body in starting position.
2. Breathe freely.

28. Arm press (barbell or dumbbell) (Fig. 5-31)
Specific for: Triceps and deltoid
Beneficial in: General shoulder girdle and fore-arms
Starting position: Standing or sitting, palms facing away from body, weights at chest level:
1. Extend arms overhead; hold; lower slowly to back of neck. Extend arms; hold; return to starting position.
2. Stand tall with head up and chin in; do not arch low back excessively or strain to press too heavy a weight.
3. Breathe freely.

29. Chin lifts (barbell or dumbbell) (Fig. 5-32)
Specific for: Deltoid, biceps, trapezius, and levator
Beneficial in: Erector spinae and forearm mus-cles
Starting position: Standing or sitting, hands held close together, weights at thigh level, palms facing body, arms fully extended:
1. Inhale as you raise elbows upward and backward until weights touch chin; hold; exhale as weights are returned slowly to starting position.
2. Stand tall; raise elbows as high as possible; keep low back and abdomen flat.

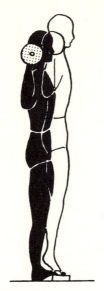

Fig. 5-33. No. 30, Toe lifts.

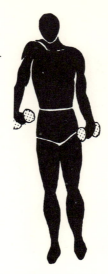

Fig. 5-35. No. 32, Shoulder shrugs (barbells or dumbbells).

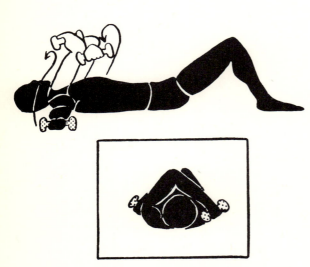

Fig. 5-34. No. 31, Arm crossover (dumbbells).

30. Toe lifts (Fig. 5-33)
Specific for: Ankle extensors (gastrocnemius, soleus)
Beneficial in: Heel cord stretch
Starting position: Standing, with weights supported by hands and held at back of neck, place toes and balls of feet on block of wood, mat, or other material raised 1½ to 2 inches higher than heels:
1. Stretch lower leg muscles and heel cord.
2. Raise up on forefoot until heels are higher than support and ankles are completely plantar flexed.
3. Hold; lower and repeat.
4. Keep body straight and stand tall throughout exercise.
Note: Leg press bar may be substituted.

31. Arm crossover (dumbbells) (Fig. 5-34)
Specific for: Pectoral, anterior deltoid, and triceps muscles
Beneficial in: Muscles of arm and shoulder girdle and stretch of anterior shoulder muscles
Starting position: Lying on back with knees flexed and feet flat on bench or plinth, arms extended directly out to either side at shoulder level, a dumbbell in each hand, palms up; let gravity stretch the anterior shoulder muscles:
1. Lift arms straight up (forward) over body, cross and bring them down to opposite side, bending elbow; return slowly, straightening elbow and then returning to starting position.
2. Exhale as arms cross; inhale as arms are stretched down and back.

32. Shoulder shrugs (barbell or dumbbell) (Fig. 5-35)
Specific for: Low shoulder, forward shoulders, trapezius, rhomboids, and levator
Starting position: Standing or sitting with arms down by either side, palms facing body, weight held at thigh level, arms fully extended:
1. Roll shoulders forward, upward, backward as you inhale; hold. Exhale while returning to starting position.
Caution: Keep head up, chin in, and back

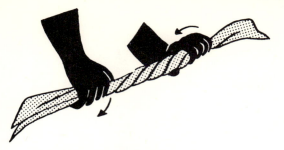

Fig. 5-36. No. 33, Towel wringing.

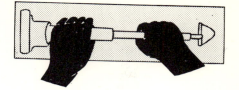

Fig. 5-38. No. 35, Wrist machines.

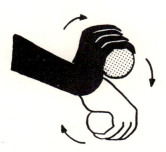

Fig. 5-37. No. 34, Gripper.

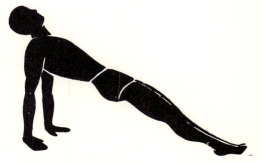

Fig. 5-39. No. 36, Back stoop falling.

straight; watch body alignment and shoulder position in mirror to check on body alignment.

33. Towel wringing (Fig. 5-36)

Specific for: Entire arm and shoulder strength
Beneficial in: Development of rotation of forearm and strengthening of entire arm, shoulder girdle, and grip strength
Starting position: Standing or sitting; fold towel lengthwise in four layers to avoid tearing:
1. Hold elbows close to sides and grasp near center of towel with both hands.
2. Twist towel as if wringing water from it, first in one direction and then in the other.
3. Repeat five times.
Caution: Keep arms at side, wring towel vigorously, and squeeze hard as if wet to obtain proper wrist action; keep shoulders back; sit or stand tall.

34. Gripper (Fig. 5-37)

Specific for: Strengthening hand and forearm
Beneficial in: Especially useful for improving muscle tone of all flexor muscle groups and decreasing joint limitations
Starting position: Either sitting or standing while grasping rubber doughnut or tennis or sponge ball:
1. Squeeze doughnut or ball hard while tensing

upper arm; while gripping, rotate wrist one direction and then the other; relax, repeat.
2. A handball may be substituted for the doughnut.
3. Advanced exercise: Use spring hand gripper.

35. Wrist machines (Fig. 5-38)

Specific for: Flexion, extension, abduction, adduction, rotation, and combinations of these wrist movements
Beneficial in: Hand and shoulder conditions
Note: Various types of wrist machines are available from commercial manufacturers, which enable the student to exercise with progressively greater amounts of resistance (Fig. 20-14); special exercise equipment can also be improvised by the instructor.

36. Back stoop falling (Fig. 5-39)

Specific for: Development of spinal and hip joint extensors, shoulder girdle, and arm strengthening
Starting position: Sitting on mat with legs extended and hands (palms down, fingers pointing toward feet) on mat just behind buttocks:
1. Extend arms and shoulders and straighten body, keeping head back, chin in, and back flat so that weight is supported on heels and hands.
2. Hold; return to starting position.

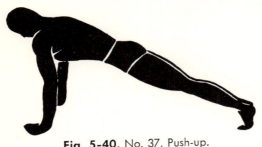

Fig. 5-40. No. 37, Push-up.

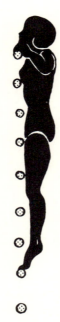

Fig. 5-41. No. 38, Chin-ups or pull-ups (stall bar or horizontal bar). Figure shows modified chin with toes on lower stall bar to help lift body.

3. Add alternate leg raises to increase difficulty of this exercise and involve hip flexors.

37. Push-up (Fig. 5-40)
Specific for: Shoulder girdle, anterior deltoid, triceps, and pectoral strength
Beneficial in: General conditioning and abdominals
Starting position: Lying face down with hands palms down on the mat directly beneath shoulders:
1. Push up by extending arms with body straight so that weight is supported on hands and toes.

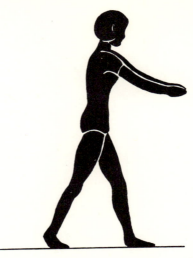

Fig. 5-42. No. 39, Jumping jack with variations.

2. Return only far enough to touch chest to mat and then push up again.
3. Keep head back, but chin in.
4. Modified push-up for girls is recommended as a lead-up skill (use knees, not toes for lower body support).

38. Chin-ups or pull-ups (stall bar or horizontal bar) (Fig. 5-41)
Specific for: Biceps, brachialis, and latissimus
Beneficial in: Shoulder girdle and pectoral, hand, wrist, and forearms
Starting position: Hanging on top rung facing stall bars, palms toward wall:
1. Keep body straight and relaxed while flexing arms to raise chin to top bar. (Horizontal bar may be used.)
2. Modified pull-up on stall bars: Ease weight on arms by climbing bars with toes; then slowly lower body under control.
Note: Do not swing or kick to aid in pull.

39. Jumping jack with variations (Fig. 5-42)
Specific for: General body warm-ups
Beneficial in: Improvement of coordination, rhythm, and timing
Starting position: Standing tall, arms down at sides:
1. Jump, spreading feet apart sideways while arms are swung sideward and hands brought together overhead (arms remain straight throughout).
2. Return to starting position. Variations:
   a. Spread feet forward and back instead of sideways.
   b. Spread feet forward and back, alternating left foot forward, then right foot forward.

c. Alternate spreading feet sideward, then forward and back, etc.

d. Bring hands together in front of body at shoulder level, arms straight (in coordination with various foot movements).

e. Bring hands together behind buttocks (in coordination with various foot movements).

f. Employ various combinations and patterns of these foot and hand movements.

g. Employ various rhythms: slow, medium,

fast, etc.; teacher leads first, then allows student to experiment with new patterns and rhythms. All of these variations can be done to music.

40. Rope skipping (Fig. 5-43)

Specific for: General body warm-up and improvement of endurance and strength

Beneficial in: Improvement of balance, coordination, and rhythm

Starting position: Standing, one end of jumping rope held in each hand, with rope adjusted so that it is slightly longer than necessary to enable student to jump through it and have it clear his head at the top of its swing. Variations:

1. Vary foot patterns to go with each swing of the rope: jump on both feet, jump on one foot only, jump on alternate feet (like running in place with one foot ahead of the other, stepping through each swing of the rope so that both feet are used during each turn).

2. Jump the same as in step 1, but perform two foot movements to each turn of the rope, then three movements, etc.

3. Employ hand and arm variation: turning rope once to each foot pattern, progressing to three or four turns for the advanced student; turning rope backwards and performing various foot patterns. (See Chapter 8 for added material on rope skipping.)

SELECTION OF INDIVIDUAL EXERCISE PROGRAM

The selection of the proper exercises for students in the class must be based on

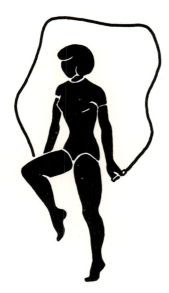

Fig. 5-43. No. 40, Rope skipping.

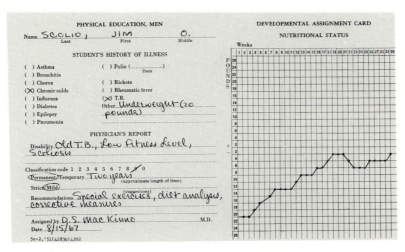

Fig. 5-44. Permanent record card including student's history of illness, physician's report, and body weight graph.

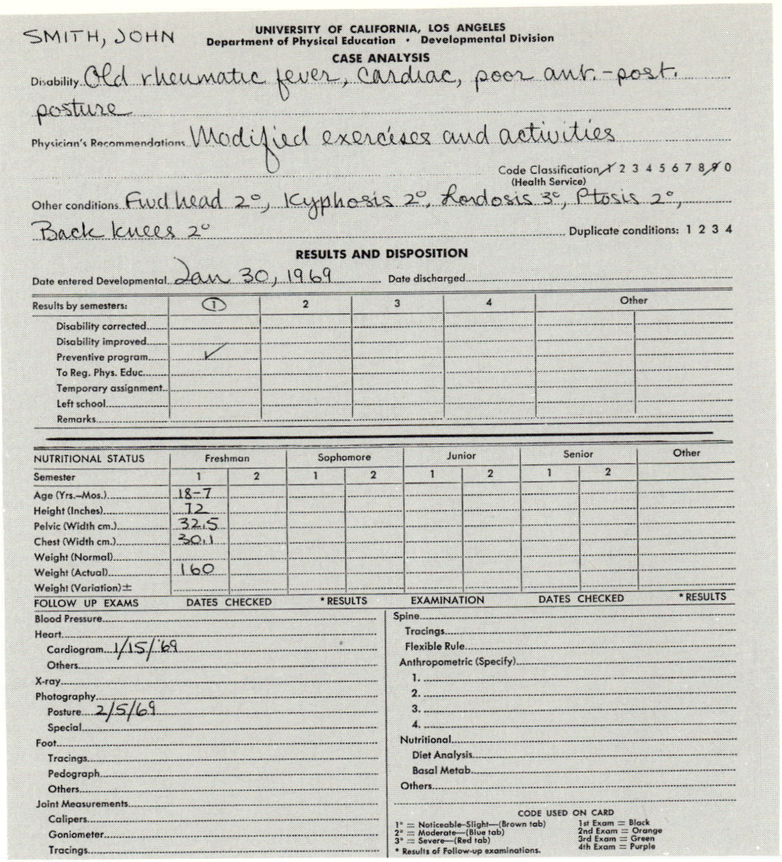

SMITH, JOHN

UNIVERSITY OF CALIFORNIA, LOS ANGELES
Department of Physical Education • Developmental Division
CASE ANALYSIS

Disability Old rheumatic fever, cardiac, poor ant.-post. posture

Physician's Recommendations Modified exercises and activities

Code Classification 1 2 3 4 5 6 7 8 9 0 (Health Service)

Other conditions Fwd head 2°, Kyphosis 2°, Lordosis 3°, Ptosis 2°, Back knees 2°

Duplicate conditions: 1 2 3 4

RESULTS AND DISPOSITION

Date entered Developmental Jan 30, 1969 Date discharged

Results by semesters:	1	2	3	4	Other	
Disability corrected						
Disability improved						
Preventive program	✓					
To Reg. Phys. Educ.						
Temporary assignment						
Left school						
Remarks						

NUTRITIONAL STATUS	Freshman		Sophomore		Junior		Senior		Other
Semester	1	2	1	2	1	2	1	2	
Age (Yrs.–Mos.)	18-7								
Height (Inches)	72								
Pelvic (Width cm.)	32.5								
Chest (Width cm.)	30.1								
Weight (Normal)									
Weight (Actual)	160								
Weight (Variation) ±									

FOLLOW UP EXAMS — DATES CHECKED — *RESULTS

Blood Pressure
Heart
Cardiogram 1/15/69
Others
X-ray
Photography
Posture 2/5/69
Special
Foot
Tracings
Pedograph
Others
Joint Measurements
Calipers
Goniometer
Tracings

EXAMINATION — DATES CHECKED — *RESULTS

Spine
Tracings
Flexible Rule
Anthropometric (Specify)
1.
2.
3.
4.
Nutritional
Diet Analysis
Basal Metab.
Others

CODE USED ON CARD
1° = Noticeable–Slight—(Brown tab)
2° = Moderate—(Blue tab)
3° = Severe—(Red tab)
* Results of Follow-up examinations.
1st Exam = Black
2nd Exam = Orange
3rd Exam = Green
4th Exam = Purple

Fig. 5-45. Adapted physical education case analysis (front side).

needs and interests. The needs are determined as a result of the physician's examination and recommendations (Figs. 5-44 and 18-2), the posture and body mechanics screening examination (Figs. 5-45 and 5-46), and any other assessment data available (physical fitness tests, tests previously performed on the student, etc.). The interest of the student can be ascertained from a written questionnaire (Fig. 5-47), oral consultation, or by having him indicate this information in writing. Considerable responsibility can be placed on students in secondary school and college in this respect. All these data are recorded on the adapted physical education appraisal form. One method that has been used successfully with classes in adapted physical education is described in detail in the following paragraphs.

Orientation procedures

After the completion of the physical examination, posture screening, fitness, perceptual-motor, and other types of diagnostic assessments, an orientation session is conducted for the students in the adapted physical education class. Departmental and class rules and regulations, general findings relative to the physical examination and other examinations (and what they mean to the student), and the types of activity programs available to the student should be explained. The adapted physical education appraisal form, containing general information about the

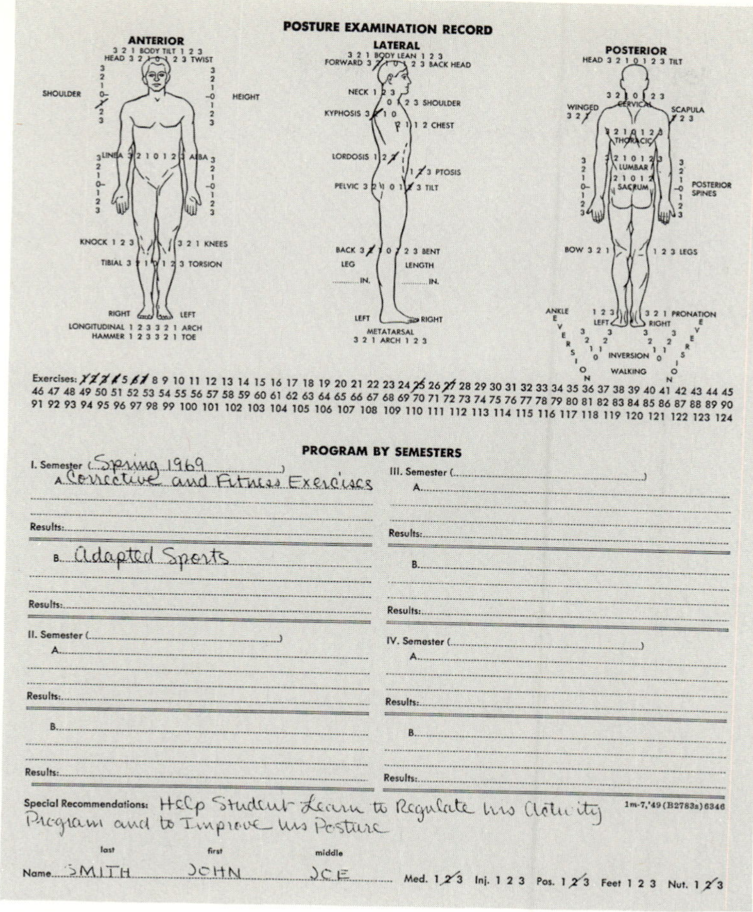

POSTURE EXAMINATION RECORD

ANTERIOR
3 2 1 BODY TILT 1 2 3
HEAD 3 2 1 0 1 2 3 TWIST
SHOULDER 3 2 1 0 1 2 3
HEIGHT 3 2 1 0 1 2 3
LINEA 3 2 1 0 1 2 3 ALBA
KNOCK 1 2 3 3 2 1 KNEES
TIBIAL 3 2 1 0 1 2 3 TORSION
RIGHT LEFT
LONGITUDINAL 1 2 3 3 2 1 ARCH
HAMMER 1 2 3 3 2 1 TOE

LATERAL
3 2 1 BODY LEAN 1 2 3
FORWARD 3 2 1 0 1 2 3 BACK HEAD
NECK 1 2 3
0 1 2 3 SHOULDER
KYPHOSIS 3 2 1 0
0 1 1 2 CHEST
LORDOSIS 1 2 3
1 2 3 PTOSIS
PELVIC 3 2 1 0 1 2 3 TILT
BACK 3 2 1 0 1 2 3 BENT
LEG ....IN. LENGTH ....IN.
LEFT RIGHT
METATARSAL
3 2 1 ARCH 1 2 3

POSTERIOR
HEAD 3 2 1 0 1 2 3 TILT
3 2 1 0 1 2 3 CERVICAL
WINGED 3 2 1 SCAPULA 1 2 3
3 2 1 0 1 2 3 THORACIC
3 2 1 0 1 2 3 LUMBAR
3 2 1 0 1 2 3 SACRUM
POSTERIOR SPINES 3 2 1 0 1 2 3
BOW 3 2 1 1 2 3 LEGS
ANKLE 1 2 3 3 2 1 PRONATION
LEFT RIGHT
EVERSION 3 2 1 0 INVERSION 0 1 2 3 EVERSION
WALKING

Exercises: 1 2 3 4 5 6 7 8 9 10 11 12 13 14 15 16 17 18 19 20 21 22 23 24 25 26 27 28 29 30 31 32 33 34 35 36 37 38 39 40 41 42 43 44 45
46 47 48 49 50 51 52 53 54 55 56 57 58 59 60 61 62 63 64 65 66 67 68 69 70 71 72 73 74 75 76 77 78 79 80 81 82 83 84 85 86 87 88 89 90
91 92 93 94 95 96 97 98 99 100 101 102 103 104 105 106 107 108 109 110 111 112 113 114 115 116 117 118 119 120 121 122 123 124

PROGRAM BY SEMESTERS

I. Semester (Spring 1969)
A. Corrective and Fitness Exercises
Results:
B. Adapted Sports
Results:

II. Semester (..........)
A.
Results:
B.
Results:

III. Semester (..........)
A.
Results:
B.
Results:

IV. Semester (..........)
A.
Results:
B.
Results:

Special Recommendations: Help Student Learn to Regulate his Activity Program and to Improve his Posture

1m-7,'49 (B2783s) 6346

Name: last SMITH first JOHN middle JOE   Med. 1 2 3 Inj. 1 2 3 Pos. 1 2 3 Feet 1 2 3 Nut. 1 2 3

Fig. 5-46. Adapted physical education case analysis (back side).

student's medical, postural, and fitness conditions, should be in the hands of the students during this orientation period so that they can relate the orientation information to their own needs for the special exercise and activity programs offered in the adapted class (Figs. 5-45 and 5-46).

After this general orientation session, the students should make a list, in order of importance, of those things that *they* want to concentrate on during the coming semester (individual objectives). These are reviewed with the student by the instructor so that important items are not missed and so that the conditions selected by the student are given the proper priority. (Programs for young children and severely handicapped persons are planned for them by the instructor or therapist.) Some adjustments and changes may need to be made at this time. The final choices, listed in the order of their importance, constitute the objectives of a particular student for the coming semester in his adapted physical education class (Fig. 5-2). A current trend is to state the objectives in behavioral or performance terms so that the student and instructor know exactly what the student must do to successfully accomplish his objectives. This should help in making student, instructor, and program evaluations and in arriving at a mark or

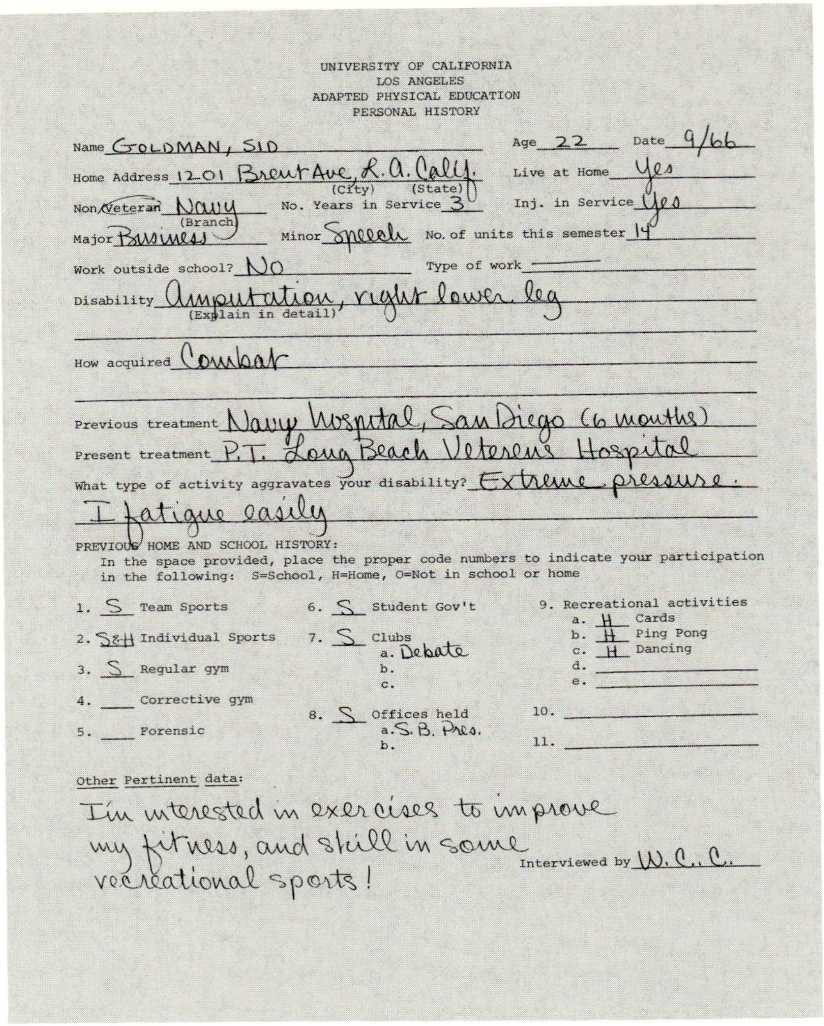

UNIVERSITY OF CALIFORNIA
LOS ANGELES
ADAPTED PHYSICAL EDUCATION
PERSONAL HISTORY

Name GOLDMAN, SID   Age 22   Date 9/66
Home Address 1201 Brent Ave, L.A. Calif.   Live at Home Yes
                (City)   (State)
Non/Veteran Navy   No. Years in Service 3   Inj. in Service Yes
        (Branch)
Major Business   Minor Speech   No. of units this semester 14
Work outside school? No   Type of work _____
Disability Amputation, right lower leg
        (Explain in detail)

How acquired Combat

Previous treatment Navy Hospital, San Diego (6 months)
Present treatment P.T. Long Beach Veterens Hospital
What type of activity aggravates your disability? Extreme pressure.
I fatigue easily

PREVIOUS HOME AND SCHOOL HISTORY:
   In the space provided, place the proper code numbers to indicate your participation
   in the following: S=School, H=Home, O=Not in school or home

1. S Team Sports   6. S Student Gov't   9. Recreational activities
                                                        a. H Cards
2. S&H Individual Sports 7. S Clubs   b. H Ping Pong
                              a. Debate   c. H Dancing
3. S Regular gym   b.   d. _____
                             c.   e. _____
4. ___ Corrective gym
                           8. S Offices held   10. _____
5. ___ Forensic   a. S.B. Pres.
                             b.   11. _____

Other Pertinent data:

I'm interested in exercises to improve
my fitness, and skill in some
recreational sports!   Interviewed by W.C.C.

Fig. 5-47. Adapted physical education personal history questionnaire.

grade for each person in a school situation, for example, the instructor and student might agree on objectives to be accomplished by the student by the end of the semester.

For example, a student (a 16-year-old boy) assigned to an adapted physical education class (or to a therapist) for a special program for asthma, for kypholordosis, and for rehabilitation of a postoperative knee condition might have the following performance objectives:

For asthma

1. Demonstrate that he can walk/run 1 mile in 6 minutes by the end of the semester.

2. Show his ability to exhale vigorously using three different techniques to encourage forced exhalation while blowing a Ping Pong ball 5 feet across the top of a table.

For kypholordosis

1. Show a decrease of at least ¼ inch in each of his two curves as measured on the conformator.

2. Write one paragraph each on the correction of kyphosis and lordosis, including information on gravitational

pull, flexibility, and muscle development necessary to effect a correction of each condition. This assignment is to be judged and evaluated by the instructor as to accuracy and completeness as compared to information given in a specified standard text.

For postoperative knee condition
1. Demonstrate the ability to perform the knee extensor exercise (No. 18) correctly, making 15 repetitions with 15 pounds of resistance by the end of the eighth week of the semester.
2. Increase the girth of the affected thigh to at least that of the unaffected one by the end of the semester.

ASSIGNMENT OF INDIVIDUAL EXERCISE PROGRAMS

The priority list of needs and interests (objectives) worked out by the student and the teacher, together with the results of all the examinations and recommendations of the physician, enables the teacher to plan an individual activity program. Since the teacher has available all the necessary information, this can be done in his office or home prior to the next meeting of the class. This enables the student to start on his individual exercise or activity program at the earliest possible time.

The mechanics of this operation can be simplified for the teacher by having the student do some of the basic clerical work. As soon as the student and teacher have agreed on the student's objectives, the student can write them in the proper place on his exercise or activity card (Fig. 5-2). The rest of the information needed on the card can also be filled out (name, disability, etc.) by the student so that it is ready for the teacher to write in the assigned exercises.

Using the exercise assignment information (section II, p. 103), the teacher then selects the exercises that will best meet the needs and interest of each student. He lists these in proper order on the exercise card. A suggested starting dosage (repetitions, resistance, time, etc.) should also be re-corded in the first column of the card by the instructor. An exercise program, which would require approximately 30 minutes, should include from 10 to 12 exercises. Since persons teaching adapted physical education full time may have as many as five classes of 25 students each, they may find it necessary during their first session of exercise program planning to limit the number of exercises for each student to one or two key exercises for each of the conditions listed. Other exercises can then be added to the program when the teacher has more time after the first class meeting. This basic exercise program can be modified and the number of repetitions and the amount of resistance adjusted by the instructor as the exercises are being taught and, again throughout the year, as the student finds that his suggested program is too easy or too difficult.

TEACHING OF EXERCISE PROGRAMS

Students should report to class dressed for activity on the class period after the orientation and planning period previously discussed. Each student should be given his exercise card, which lists his individual exercise program and suggests a starting number of repetitions for each of them. To enable all the students to learn these exercises quickly and to facilitate teaching a variety of individual exercises to a group of 25 students, the following system of organization for the class has proved successful:
1. The instructor first teaches the four or five exercises that have been most frequently assigned as warm-up exercises. Each student does only those assigned to him on his card. He either sits and observes or practices an exercise he has already learned while exercises are being taught that are not on his program.
2. By a quick show of hands (or by compiling the information while assigning the exercises), the teacher can determine how many students have each of the 40 key exercises on their exercise card. Usually 10 or 12 of the key exer-

cises will appear on a majority of the students' exercise cards. These exercises are taught in the order of frequency of assignment as soon as the warm-ups have been learned. Other exercises are similarly taught until the instructor comes to the special exercises assigned to only one or two students. By then, most of the class will have learned the majority of their exercises and thus can be busily engaged in their workout while the instructor teaches the exercises that are assigned less frequently.

3. When all the students have learned their complete programs, attention should be given to doing the exercise routine in the proper sequence. The usual order is as follows: (1) warm-up exercises; (2) the first exercise assigned under the first condition (objective), which is usually either the least difficult one or a stretch exercise; (3) the first exercise assigned under the second condition, and so on, until the first exercise for each of the areas has been completed; (4) the student then proceeds to the second exercise in each area (a more difficult exercise), until all exercises are completed, thus allowing for concentration on one body area at a time, followed by a rest period for each body area while another is being exercised; (5) if additional time exists after completing an exercise program, the student can go back and review certain key exercises that are of special *value* or can repeat exercises that are of special *interest* to him. No exercise should be attempted by the student unless it is included on his exercise card.

4. Students can also check the written descriptions and study the diagrams of the exercises, which should be posted on the bulletin board or made available to the students for study. This will enable them to do the exercises correctly and to better understand what each exercise is designed to do (Fig. 5-1).

5. After all the exercises have been taught, the teacher should circulate from student to student to check on correct performance of exercises, to further explain how and why the exercise is done, to add to or change exercise programs when necessary, and to evaluate and grade the students on their performance.

The combination of this individual method of exercise assignment and instruction with other more formal methods of class or group assignment and instruction is discussed in Chapter 19. Explanations of other special exercises and systems of organizing exercise programs for selected disabilities are found in the chapters in which particular disabilities are discussed. The reader should consult the index for exercise and activity programs for specific conditions. Chapters 4, 6, 7, 9, 10, 11, 12, and 13 and the appendix include such materials.

EXERCISES IN WATER

There are many advantages to including aquatic exercises and activities in an adapted physical education program. Aquatic exercises are discussed in this section whereas aquatic activities, games, and sports are covered in Chapter 8. Some of the special values of offering a unit in swimming and water therapy include the following:

1. Often exercises that cannot be done elsewhere can be performed in the water, since it is quite easy to rule out the effect of gravity and therefore exercises can be more accurately graded according to their severity.

2. Students who have the support of the water or who use floating devices while walking or swimming in water have the amount of pressure on joints reduced and are able to walk and perform activities in the water before they could be attempted against the pull of gravity in the exercise room.

3. Swimming provides good all-around exercise for musculature.

4. Swimming provides a release of tension and may even promote relaxation if the

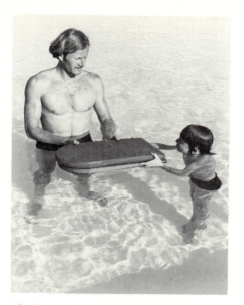

Fig. 5-48. Walking with aid of buoyancy, kickboards, and instructor. (Courtesy California State University, Audio Visual Center, Long Beach, Calif.)

water is sufficiently warm (82° to 86° F in a regular pool and 90° to 100° F in a therapeutic pool).

5. Swimming activities are generally fun for all students, but they are especially desirable for students in the adapted physical education program, since they can be adapted for almost any disability, thus providing physical and skill development not possible in many other types of physical activities.

The buoyancy of the body and its parts in water makes many types of movements and activities much easier in water than under the direct influence of gravitational pull. A person standing in water up to his chin has minimal weight to bear and can stand and walk much earlier in the rehabilitation period than he would be able to out of the water. Walking in progressively shallower water, using support as needed, is an excellent activity to lead up to locomotion activities in the ward, the clinic, and the

gymnasium. Walking forward, backward, and sideward using different patterns of movement will help build muscle strength, body balance, and coordination necessary for locomotion.*

The therapist or teacher should carefully consider the changes that must be made in assigning therapeutic exercises in water as contrasted with exercises for similar body parts used in the ward or gymnasium. Each person and each of his limbs must be considered individually for they will have different degrees of buoyancy. The body as a whole may float, but the legs and arms *individually* may be less buoyant and will sink unless supported.

If a progressive resistance exercise (PRE) system is to be effected in water, factors such as buoyancy and water resistance must be carefully considered, for example, if a passive exercise is desired for the hip flexors and the patient's legs are nonbuoyant, he should be placed near the surface of the pool in the prone position so that the weight of the leg will pull it down into the flexed position. If the legs are buoyant, however, the patient should assume a half-sitting supine position to allow buoyancy to lift the leg to the surface and cause the hip joint to flex.

If a mildly active exercise is desired, the student should be placed on his side with his leg supported by the clinician, a tube, or a buoy. The leg can then be slowly flexed and extended from the hip by the student without the influence of either buoyancy or gravity. The same movement can become a more active exercise by increasing its speed. A resistance exercise will result if the tube or buoy on the ankle is retained, the student is turned face down (prone), and hip flexion is performed against the resistance of the flotation device. Resistance can be made greater by increasing the amount of buoyant material used at the

---

*For suggested activities and exercises, see Assignment 12 in Crowe, W. C., Arnheim, D. D., and Auxter, D.: Laboratory manual in adapted physical education and recreation, St. Louis, 1977, The C. V. Mosby Co.

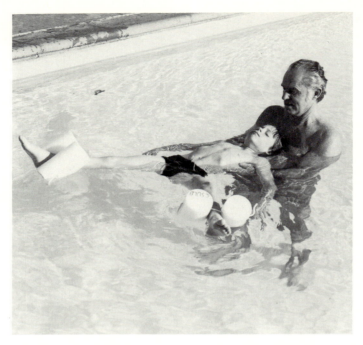

Fig. 5-49. Hip abduction and adduction with instructor and flotation support. (Courtesy California State University, Audio Visual Center, Long Beach, Calif.)

ankle or by increasing the speed of movement of the leg.

There are ways to increase or decrease resistance in water. Resistance is reduced if a part is moved slowly through the water and if it is as streamlined as possible (presents its narrowest side). Resistance is increased by presenting broad surfaces of the body to the water, by wearing rough, absorbant materials on a part (a sweat suit), and by increasing the speed of the movement (the resistance increases according to the square of the speed; a movement that is twice as fast creates a resistance four times as great).

Adjustments similar to those described earlier can be made to enable a person to exercise all body segments using progressive resistance exercise techniques. A series of exercises that can be modified by using these techniques is presented in the *Laboratory Manual in Adapted Physical Education and Recreation,* as previously mentioned.

Types of support for aquatic exercises

Many types of support can be given to maintain the patient or student in a given position while he performs his exercise program. Some of these include a water plinth; a support table, the parallel walking bars (in a therapeutic pool); the steps; the ladder; the gutter; a large kickboard; a water mat; and the therapist, the teacher, the aide, or another student in a regular pool. Most areas of the body can also be exercised quite specifically by the more advanced swimmer while he is floating or maintaining either a vertical or a horizontal position in the pool with minimal finning or sculling motions.

Materials that can be used as flotation devices for the limbs include life jackets; inner tubes (from trucks, cars, bicycles, or wheel toys); styrofoam rings, tubes, and squares with ropes or straps for attachment; water mats; and kickboards of various types and sizes.

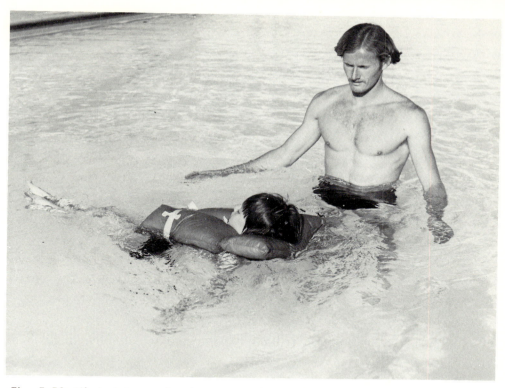

Fig. 5-50. Life jacket as a flotation support. (Courtesy California State University, Audio Visual Center, Long Beach, Calif.)

Persons representing many different types of disabilities will benefit from a well-planned aquatic exercise program. For many it is important to have water as warm as 90° to 95° F, if this is possible, and to have protection from the cold when entering and leaving the pool. Outside temperature should be 5° warmer for the aged, for persons with arthritis, for those with spinal cord injuries or cerebral palsy, and for persons in relaxation programs. With other types of disabilities and for younger and more active persons, temperature is not as critical, but in most cases, the disabled individual will be more comfortable and relaxed and the attention span will be longer if the individual does not become chilled.

Swimming as a general therapeutic activity

Swimming generally accepted strokes such as the crawl, elementary backstroke, breast-stroke, and sidestroke is an excellent way to promote general cardiovascular fitness and to develop the general musculature of the body. Whether this is good for persons with various types of disabilities should be carefully weighed by the physician, the therapist, and the physical education teacher. To have persons with already weak musculature swim the regular strokes commonly taught in our school and recreation programs may develop already strong musculature to the detriment of those muscles that most need to be developed. Students should be carefully studied to see if special therapeutic exercises are needed or if they should be taught to swim one or more of the traditional swimming strokes, possibly with some modification of the standard technique, so that swimming as an activity will not negate the advantages of the rehabilitation program.

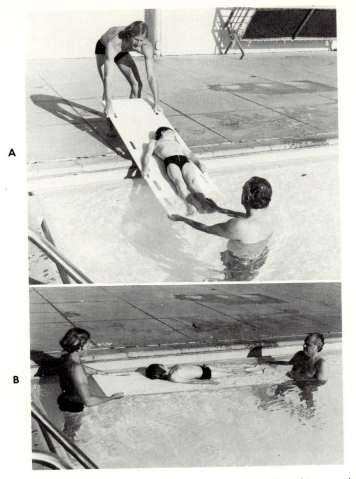

Fig. 5-51. Assisting with pool entry. **A,** Sliding method. **B,** Lifting method. (Courtesy California State University, Audio Visual Center, Long Beach, Calif.)

Severely handicapped persons may have to be lifted into and out of the pool. Hospitals often have electric lifts. In school and recreational pools, teachers, clinicians, and recreation leaders may have to improvise their own procedures. Safety and patient comfort must be considered (Fig. 5-51).

REFERENCES

1. Bowerman, W. J., and Harris, W. E.: Jogging, New York, 1967, Grosset & Dunlap, Inc.
2. Crowe, W. C., et al.: Developmental syllabus. Unpublished, University of California at Los Angeles, 1950.
3. DeLorme, T. L.: Restoration of muscle power by heavy resistance exercises, J. Bone Joint Surg. **27:**645-667, 1945.
4. DeLorme, T. L., and Watkins, A. C.: Progressive resistance exercises, New York, 1951, Appleton-Century-Crofts.
5. Morgan, R. E., and Adamson, G. T.: Circuit training, New York, 1958, Sportshelf and Soccer Associates.
6. Müller, E. A.: The regulation of muscular strength, J. Assoc. Phys. Ment. Rehabil. **11:** 41-47, 1957.

RECOMMENDED READINGS

Adams, W. C., and McCristal, K. J.: Foundations of physical activity, Champaign, Ill., 1968, Stipes Publishing Co.

The Alliance: Physical activity programs and practices for the exceptional individual, third national conference, Long Beach, Calif., 1974, The Office of the Los Angeles County Superintendent of Schools, Division of Special Education.

The Alliance: Physical activity programs and practices for the exceptional individual, fourth national conference, Los Angeles, Calif., 1975, The Office of the Los Angeles County Superintendent of Schools, Division of Special Education.

Arnheim, D. D.: Area I physical activity: general stretching. In Larson, L. A., editor: Encyclopedia of sport sciences and medicine, New York, 1971, Macmillan Publishing Co., Inc.

Barney, S., Hirst, C., and Jensen, R.: Conditioning exercises: exercises to improve body form and function, St. Louis, 1972, The C. V. Mosby Co.

Barrett, M., et al.: Foundations for movement, Dubuque, Iowa, 1968, William C. Brown Co., Publishers.

Berger, R. A.: Optimum repetitions for the development of strength, Res. Q., 33:334, 1962.

Billig, H. E., Jr., and Lowendahl, E.: Mobilization of the human body, Stanford, Calif., 1949, Stanford University Press.

Carr, D. B., et al.: Sequenced instructional programs in physical education for the handicapped, Los Angeles City Schools Special Education Branch, Physical Education Project, P.L. 88-164, Title III, December 1970.

Christina, R.: The relationship of kinesthesis to physical education, Phys. Educ., 24:167-168, 1967.

Cooper, K. H.: Aerobics, New York, 1972, Bantam Books, Inc.

Cooper, K. H., and Cooper, M.: Aerobics for women, New York, 1973, Bantam Books, Inc.

Corrective physical education, Los Angeles, 1958, Los Angeles City Schools.

Cratty, B. J.: Movement behavior and motor learning, ed. 3, Philadelphia, 1973, Lea & Febiger.

Davis, E. C., Logan, G., and McKinney, W.: Biophysical values of muscular activity, Dubuque, Iowa, 1965, William C. Brown Co., Publishers.

Digennaro, J.: Individualized exercise and optimal physical fitness, Philadelphia, 1974, Lea & Febiger.

Doolittle, L., and Paschal, J.: The effect of rope jumping program upon cardiovascular efficiency, Calif. Assoc. Health Phys. Educ. Rec. J. 30:11, 1968.

Drury, B. J.: Posture and figure control through physical education, Palo Alto, Calif., 1966, National Press Books.

Exercise and fitness, Washington, D.C., 1964, American Association for Health, Physical Education, and Recreation.

Fait, H. F.: Special physical education, Philadelphia, 1972, W. B. Saunders Co.

Falls, H. B., Wallis, E. L., and Logan, G. A.: Foundations of conditioning, New York, 1970, Academic Press, Inc.

Glass, J.: Exploring movement, Freeport, New York, 1966, Educational Activities, Inc.

Guide for programs in physical education and recreation for the mentally retarded, Washington, D.C., 1968, American Association for Health, Physical Education, and Recreation.

Guidelines for adapted physical education, Harrisburg, Pa., 1966, Department of Public Instruction, Commonwealth of Pennsylvania.

Hackett, L. C., and Jenson, R. G.: A guide to movement explorations, Palo Alto, Calif., 1967, Peek Publications.

Hayden, F. J.: Physical fitness for the retarded, Toronto, 1964, Metropolitan Toronto Association for Retarded Children.

Huber, J. H., and Vercollone, J.: Using aquatic mats with exceptional children, J. Phys. Educ. Recr. 47:44, 1976.

Jokl, E.: Nutrition, exercise, and body composition, Springfield, Ill., 1964, Charles C Thomas, Publisher.

Kendall, F. P.: A criticism of current tests and exercises for physical fitness, Phys. Ther. 45: 187-197, 1965.

Keogh, J.: Motor performance of elementary school children, Los Angeles, 1965, Department of Physical Education, University of California.

Kraus, H.: Therapeutic exercise, Springfield, Ill., 1963, Charles C Thomas, Publisher.

Kraus, H., and Raaf, W.: Hypokinetic disease, Springfield, Ill., 1961, Charles C Thomas, Publisher.

Krusen, F. H., editor: Handbook of physical medicine and rehabilitation, Philadelphia, 1971, W. B. Saunders Co.

Larson, L. A.: Fitness, health, and work capacity, New York, 1974, Macmillan Publishing Co., Inc.

Licht, S.: An exploration and analytical survey of therapeutic exercise, Am. J. Phys. Med. 46:1, 1967.

Licht, S., and Johnson, E. W.: Therapeutic exercise, Baltimore, 1965, Waverly Press, Inc.

Lilly, L. J.: An overview of body mechanics, Palo Alto, Calif., 1967, Peek Publications.

Logan, G., and Dunkelberg, J.: Adaptations of muscular activity, Belmont, Calif., 1964, Wadsworth Publishing Co., Inc.

Lowman, C. L.: Analysis of exercises commonly misused, Phys. Educ. 24:115-116, 1967.

Lowman, C. L.: Technique of underwater gymnastics, Los Angeles, 1937, American Publications, Inc.

Massey, B. H., et al.: The kinesiology of weight lifting, Dubuque, Iowa, 1959, William C. Brown Co., Publishers.

Mathews, D. K., Kruse, R., and Shaw, V.: The science of physical education for handicapped children, New York, 1962, Harper & Row, Publishers.

Metheny, E.: Body dynamics, New York, 1952, McGraw-Hill Book Co.

Moffroid, M. T., and Whipple, R. H.: Specificity of speed of exercise, Phys. Ther. **50**:1692-1699, 1970.

Mott, J. A.: Conditioning and basic movement concepts, Dubuque, Iowa, 1968, William C. Brown Co., Publishers.

Mueller, G. W., and Christaldi, J.: A practical program of remedial physical education, Philadelphia, 1966, Lea & Febiger.

Myers, C. R., Golding, L. A., and Sinning, W. E.: The Y's way to physical fitness, Emmaus, Pa., 1973, Rodale Press.

Oermann, K. C., Young, C. H., and Mitchell, J. G.: Conditioning exercises, games, tests, Annapolis, Md., 1960, U.S. Naval Institute.

Olson, E. C.: Conditioning, Columbus, Ohio, 1968, Charles E. Merrill Publishing Co.

O'Shea, J. P.: Scientific principles and methods of strength fitness, Reading, Mass., 1969, Addison-Wesley Publishing Co., Inc.

Perceptual-motor foundations: a multidisciplinary concern, proceedings of the perceptual-motor symposium sponsored by the Physical Education Division, American Association for Health, Physical Education, and Recreation, Washington, D.C., 1969, American Association for Health, Physical Education, and Recreation.

Physical education for high school students, ed. 4, Washington, D.C., 1970, American Association for Health, Physical Education, and Recreation.

Physical fitness in business and industry, Washington, D.C., 1972, President's Council on Physical Fitness and Sports.

Planned motor activities for special groups, Los Angeles, No date, Los Angeles County Department of Parks and Recreation.

Practical guide for teaching the mentally retarded to swim, Washington, D.C., 1969, American Association for Health, Physical Education, and Recreation.

Rathbone, J., and Hunt, V.: Corrective physical education, Philadelphia, 1965, W. B. Saunders Co.

Royal Canadian Air Force: Royal Canadian Air Force exercise plans for physical fitness, New York, No date, Essandess Special Editions.

Ruff, W. R.: Physical conditioning through weight training, Palo Alto, Calif., 1966, National Press Books.

Rusk, H. A.: Rehabilitation medicine, ed. 3, St. Louis, 1971, The C. V. Mosby Co.

Seligman, T., Randel, H. O., and Stevens, J. J.: Conditioning program for children with asthma, Phys. Ther. **50**:641-648, 1970.

Shepard, R. J.: Endurance fitness, Toronto, 1969, University of Toronto Press.

Sigerseth, P. O.: Physical activity: general flexibility. In Larson, L. A., editor: Encyclopedia of sport sciences and medicine, New York, 1971, Macmillan Publishing Co., Inc.

Swimming for the handicapped, instructor's manual, Washington, D.C., 1960, American National Red Cross.

Techniques and methods for handicapped youth, first national conference, Los Angeles, Calif., 1973, The Office of the Los Angeles County Superintendent of Schools, Division of Special Education.

Vitale, F.: Individual fitness programs, Englewood Cliffs, N.J., 1973, Prentice-Hall, Inc.

Williams, M., and Worthington, C.: Therapeutic exercise, Philadelphia, 1957, W. B. Saunders Co.

6

TENSION CONTROL

■ Tension is described by Cratty[5] as being the overt muscular contraction caused by an emotional state or increased muscular effort. Nervous tension is a product of our hectic times and often stems from anxiety. The anxious person is one who tends to worry and has an abnormal amount of undefined fear. The anxiety state may be manifested in pathological systemic conditions. With continued anxiety and emotional stress, there may arise psychosomatic disorders.

Selye[17] suggested the existence of a general adaptation syndrome (GAS) that occurs in animals and humans when they are subjected to continual emotional stress. The GAS is composed of three consecutive stages: the *alarm reaction*, which represents normal bodily changes caused by emotion; the *resistance to stress*, or one's adjustment to the alarm reaction, which requires considerable energy resources; and the *exhaustion stage*, in which the energy storehouse is used up. The exhaustion stage may lead to the death of single cells, organs, organ systems, or the entire organism. The pathological conditions of hypertension, rheumatism, arthritis, ulcers, allergies, and other conditions have been described by some authorities as possibly caused by stress. The overanxious individual has a high level of cerebral and emotional activity, coupled with nervous muscular tension that may eventually lead the individual to the exhaustion stage and perhaps to psychosomatic disorders. It is commonly accepted in medicine that chronic stress may lead to one or more disease states.[17]

It is desirable for all individuals to be able to consciously control their tension levels. It is particularly important for persons having high degrees of tension attributable to some emotional or physical problem to be able to attain a relaxed state at will. Pain and nervous distress are accentuated and compounded by disorders of the mind and body. Characteristically, individuals with cardiovascular, respiratory, or rheumatic—as well as other—conditions need to develop the ability to reduce their tension levels.

Of extreme importance to all physical educators is the ability to instruct their students in the skill of recognizing abnormal tensions and reducing them. It is even more important for adapted physical educators, who deal directly with individuals with special problems, to have as part of their credentials the ability to recognize overt signs of abnormal muscular tension levels and to teach ways of overcoming them.

RELAXANTS

Relaxation is an elusive and much sought state that most individuals in all cultures generally or on given occasions desire to experience. There are many current practices in the United States designed to achieve the relaxed state. Many may be considered healthful, whereas other modes may be deleterious to the mind and body.

Pills, powders, and drinks

The American public annually pays millions of dollars, both legally and illegally, for the purchase of medicinal agents and alcoholic beverages consumed with the express purpose of reducing an uncomfortable sense of tension and attaining a state of euphoria or peace of mind. Drug abuse is an ever pressing problem in the world today.[8] Individuals seeking relief from painful anxieties and feelings of inadequacy attempt escape through drugs that alter neural activity. Common categories of those agents used for relaxation and alteration of the personality are psychotomimetic drugs, narcotics, analgesics, sedatives, ataractics or tranquilizers, and depressives.

Psychotomimetic drugs. Psychotomimetic or hallucinogenic agents such as LSD (lysergic acid diethylamide) and mescaline are often used by individuals who are dissatisfied with their present life and are seeking the peace of mind and understanding that comes with an expanded consciousness. The psychotomimetic used in very small doses produces a toxic psychosis that may cause perceptual distortions of any one or all of the senses. Users of such hallucinogens may end up with a "bad trip" resulting in altered behavior, which is manifested in irrationality and uncommon fears.

Narcotics. Derivatives of opium, especially morphine, are used medically for their sedative and analgesic actions. Unfortunately they are also sought for their euphorigenic properties, particularly found in heroin. Addicts of opiates and opiate-like narcotics are attempting to relieve emotional pain that is found in daily anxieties and hostilities that are difficult to cope with.[8]

Marijuana, unlike the opiates, is not considered physiologically addicting. Its sole source is the plant *Cannabis sativa*. When smoked, the marijuana leaf may produce euphoria, sedation, and hallucinations in the user. The user may display an altered consciousness, expressing feelings of lightness, gaiety, and detachment from reality.

Analgesics. Salicylates are used in a number of compounds that may be applied to the body externally or internally. Acetylsalicylic acid (aspirin) represents the most common compound. The salicylate has the ability to reduce inflammation and pain. As a pain reliever, it has a definite effect on the musculoskeletal system. Although it does not produce sedation or euphoria, as do the opiates, there is recent indication that aspirin has some tranquilizing qualities. It might be speculated that aspirin's great use as a tension reducer is attributable not to its tranquilizing effects, but mainly to its ability to relieve muscular discomfort that is below the pain threshold level.[4]

Sedatives. Barbiturates are considered hypnotic and sedative drugs and are widely used by individuals for sleep or (in smaller dosages) for calming effects. The physiological effects of the barbiturate are not well understood; however, there are some indications that a general depression of the central nervous system takes place. Barbiturates are highly habit-forming and are addicting to the user. The chronic user of barbiturates is in a constant state of severe depression, which manifests itself in numerous personality changes.

Tranquilizers. Tranquilizers, or ataractics, have become increasingly prominent in medicine and in the patent drug industry. Used for tension and anxiety, tranquilizers affect the sympathetic nervous system by suppressing synaptic stimuli. The main use of ataractics in medicine has been in the areas of behavioral disorders and mental disease. The hyperirritable patient who becomes tranquilized is more amenable to psychotherapy. For much of the general public, tranquilizers have increasingly become a crutch for coping with daily stress.

Depressives. Ethyl alcohol has been used systemically for centuries as a generalized depressant and has hypnotic qualities. It is believed to block the synaptic connections of nerve impulses in the central nervous system, producing varying degrees of depression. Alcohol is an anesthetic to man's higher faculties and thus brings about a state of temporary relaxation. Depression of the higher brain centers results in diminished control of emotional behavior and decreased movement control.

Rituals, systems, and methods

The majority of persons in the world practices various methods of achieving relaxation in daily life. Some methods may be very beneficial to health, whereas others, as mentioned before, may be deleterious to health. Some methods may be momentary, whereas others are more lasting and involve an established routine or ritual. Western civilization utilizes many such techniques, for example, imagery, physical therapy, psychology and religion, and exercise.

Imagery. Imagery involves word symbolization or auditory stimulation to evoke mental pictures that are both pleasing and relaxing, for example, while in a comfort-able position, a person can imagine himself either floating on a cloud or becoming increasingly heavy as he gradually sinks deeper and deeper. Listening to soothing music of a slow tempo may result in a state of calm or viewing a beautiful landscape painting may conjure the feeling of quiet and peace.

Physical therapy. To achieve a relaxed state, Americans utilize many methods that come under the classification of physical therapy. Some common methods are the use of the sauna or steam bath, hydromassage, hot water soaks, and massage.[18] For example, the Finnish sauna bath has been used for centuries as a means to decongest engorged muscles after exercise and to increase relaxation in tense musculature. The European practice of repeatedly heating the body to temperatures of 185° F for 15 minutes and following this with a cool shower is fast becoming a popular technique in America. It invokes a euphoric feeling of physical well-being and relaxation. Many resort hotels and spas are now offering sauna baths and hydromassage in small warm-water pools, followed by an envigorating dip in a large cool swimming pool. Hydromassage is a popular form of relaxing the body. The water is agitated around the body by means of a machine that forces jets of water from various openings in the pool. The pressures applied to the body by the water soothe nerve endings, providing the recipient with a sense of reduced muscular tension.

Since recorded history, some form of manual massage has been used as a means of bringing about a physiological response. Defined as the systematic manipulation of the soft tissues of the body, massage may be applied in numerous ways: mechanical vibrators, rollers, agitated water, or, most commonly, the laying on of hands. Many experts indicate that hands, when controlled by a knowledgeable operator, offer the most efficient way to apply massage. Through physiological, mechanical, and psychological effects, massage can produce relaxation. The most frequently used technique is effleurage, which allows the hands to glide lightly over the body in a slow rhythmical pattern, passively reducing muscular tension.

Psychology and religion. The tenets of psychology and religion often try to aid individuals who are disturbed in seeking peace within themselves. Millions of books are sold with such themes as achieving self-renewal, overcoming personal conflicts, or attaining peace in a tension-filled world.

Recently, individual Americans have become interested in following some of the Eastern religions and philosophies whose foundations are set in inner contemplation and meditation. There are various forms of meditation, most of which begin by having the subject assume a comfortable posture and then focus on some external or internal object. Transcendental meditation employs a mantra, a specific single sound or short phrase that is repeated over and over. Focusing on an object or making a continuous sound helps the meditator avoid distracting thoughts that creep into his consciousness. Scientific research has determined that meditation can significantly reduce mental anxiety and muscular tension.[13] A recent meditation approach that blends both Eastern and Western concepts is titled "the relaxation response."[3] This method uses the three basic elements found in most meditation and conscious relaxation techniques: (1) proper posture, (2) dwelling on an object or sound, and (3) the assumption of a passive attitude. In the relaxation response, the participant sits quietly in a comfortable chair with his eyes closed; progressively relaxes his muscles, starting with the feet and moving up the body; and then breathes through his nose, saying "one" to himself on each inhalation and expiration for 10 to 20 minutes.

One of the most significant biomedical advances in recent times has been the development of biofeedback methods. Through training, individuals can increase their alpha brain waves, which predominate in the mentally relaxed state.[12] Using machines that monitor the brain waves and are designed to make a sound when alpha waves are present, the subject learns to control anxiety and bring about mental and physical relaxation at will.[12]

For many individuals, hypnosis is a means of reducing anxieties and muscular tension psychotherapeutically. Hypnosis has been defined as "an artificially induced passive state in which there is increased amenability and responsiveness to suggestions and commands, provided that these do not conflict seriously with the subject's own conscious or unconscious wishes." Under hypnosis, various suggestions about relaxation can be made to the subject, dealing with such things as reducing worry, anxiety, or fear; decreasing pain; and relaxing muscles.[14, 15]

Exercise. Most persons would agree that the body senses a reduction in tension after any physically fatiguing activity.[11] Electromyographic studies show that neuromuscular tension levels decrease significantly with vigorous exercise, particularly in individuals having high tension levels; however, effects are usually transitory.[6]

Other forms of exercise that result in a relaxed state are specifically rhythmical motion, muscle stretching, and the physical exercise system of hatha-yoga, known as āsana. Music and rhythm are used extensively for the purpose of initiating coordinated movement and relaxation. Synchronization of specific movement patterns, as expressed through kinesthesia, is the basis for skilled activity. Rathbone[16] indicates that rhythmical exercise relieves the feeling of fatigue and residual tension. Activities that have as their basis a continuous or even sequence of movement, such as walking, dancing, swimming, or bicycle riding, result in reduced tension. Muscle stretching, which is designed to increase joint flexibility, also tends to reduce tension within the musculotendinous unit. It is logical therefore to presume that an articulation that is unencumbered by tight restricting tissue will also be one that is capable of relaxation. Stretching the body helps overcome the discomfort of stiffness and allows the various body segments to relax. Research indicates that a steady progressive stretch tends to decrease the myostatic reflex and reduce muscle tension, whereas the ballistic or jerky stretch increases the tension state. Many of the āsanas of hatha-yoga tend to improve joint range of motion. Each yoga posture is executed slowly and deliberately. It is considered by devotees that relaxation occurs as the mind and body become harmonious.

CONSCIOUS CONTROL OF MUSCULAR TENSION

By far the most useful and beneficial means of reducing muscle tension is through conscious control.[7] Abnormal hypertonicity can be decreased by willed inhibition of neural pathways. By relaxing the neuromusculotendinous unit, a person can also diminish excitement of other nervous areas such as in the higher and lower brain centers.

The technique of tension recognition requires the development of a keen kinesthetic perception of hypertonicity, as has been proposed by Jacobson.[9, 10] This method includes the achievement of awareness of residual tension by progressively engaging in muscular contraction of decreasing intensity until an acute sensitivity is developed. Jacobson's system starts with muscles of the left upper extremity and moves to the right upper extremity, followed by the left lower extremity, right lower extremity, abdominal muscles, respiratory muscles, back, pectoral region, shoulder muscles, and facial muscles. An example of Jacobson's technique[10] is as follows: (1) the subject relaxes a body part for about 5 minutes; (2) the subject keeps eyes closed; (3) the subject stiffens the body part slowly and smoothly; (4) when tension is perceived in the active muscle group, the subject gradually lets the tension go out of the part slowly and smoothly; and (5) during the early stages of learning progressive relaxation, the act of muscle tensing requires several minutes, whereas the releasing of tension takes upward of 10 to 15 minutes as the subject consciously seeks less and less tonicity.

MUSCLE TENSION REDUCTION

To the physiologist, relaxation indicates a complete absence of neuromuscular activity (zero).[9] The relaxed body part does not resist stretch, but reflects the lengthened state of muscle fibers. An overt sign of relaxation is a limp and completely motionless body part. Through relaxation of overly tense muscles, a number of positive effects can occur. Some of these effects may be seen in respiration, circulation, and neuromuscular coordination.

Respiration. The reduction of tension in the thorax and muscles of respiration allows for a greater capacity of inspiration and expiration. With this increased capacity, there is a more efficient exchange of oxygen and carbon dioxide within the body. For individuals with breathing disorders, relaxation of the thoracic mechanism allows for a greater respiratory potential.

Circulation. Relaxation of tense skeletal muscles allows the blood to circulate unimpeded by constricted blood vessels to all the bodily tissues. A person with cardiovascular disease is greatly aided when he can reduce his own muscular tension level at will. Blood pressure may be reduced by diminishing outside resistance, which subsequently decreases the strain on heart and blood vessels.

Neuromuscular coordination. In order for the body to move uninhibited, there must be a smooth synchronization of muscles. Differential relaxation or controlled tension attributable to the reciprocal action of agonist and antagonist muscles provides for coordinated movement without undue fatigue. Individuals who, as a result of neuromuscular or cerebral problems, express poor coordination must learn to relax tense muscles differentially in order for their purposeful movement to be smooth, accurate, and enduring.

IMPLICATIONS FOR PHYSICAL EDUCATION

Learning to relax is a motor skill and must be considered an important part of the total program of physical education. As a skill, relaxation must be taught and practiced for competency. Too often, teachers of physical education are concerned with gross movement activities alone. To lie down when tired or to practice relaxation when tense or overanxious is considered unmanly or a waste of time by many male teachers. This narrow point of view eliminates consideration of a very important aspect of the field of physical education. Relaxation is of special importance to many atypical as well as typical students.

A number of positive benefits can be accrued by the disabled child who has conscious control of his tension level. He can expect to conserve needed energies and obtain better control of his emotions (fears and anxieties become less intense). Sleep comes easier, the acquisition and conduction of motor skills are enhanced, pain and physical discomfort become less intense, and the ability to learn may be improved. Relaxation therefore becomes a vital tool in the total machinery of the educational process.

Teaching a system of relaxation

The adapted physical education instructor can teach a variety of relaxation techniques depending on time and available conditions. As has been described earlier in this discussion, imagery and tension recognition provide a convenient means of learning to relax. Both may be combined and used with success in the typical 30-minute physical education period.

Identifying abnormal tension areas in the body requires the performance of a series of muscle contractions and relaxations. In this modified system of progressive relaxation, muscle contractions should be performed gradually and slowly for 30 seconds and then a "letting go" of the tension should be made for 30 seconds in an attempt to obtain a "negative" state. The

pupils are continually reminded to tense only those muscles the instructor indicates. An attempt is made by the pupil to keep all other body areas relaxed while contracting a single part. Special consideration is given to those areas of the body of which it is difficult to "let go," for example, the low back, the abdominal, the shoulder, the neck, and the eye regions. After the guided session, the student makes a record of those areas that he found difficult to relax. Eventually, with diligent practice, the student will have to tense and relax only those areas he finds difficult to relax. In doing so, he can achieve at will a general decrease of muscular tonus throughout the entire body.

Preliminary requirements

In order for the student to develop a keen perception of tension and learn to relax, the instructor should make provisions for a number of environmental and learning factors that may strongly affect the ability to reduce body tension.

Room. The room in which relaxation exercises are conducted should have a comfortable temperature (between 72° and 76° F); it should be well ventilated with no chilling drafts. The light may be dimmed or turned off and signs may be posted outside to prevent interruption of the relaxation lesson.

Dress. The student should wear comfortable, warm, loose-fitting apparel and no shoes.

Equipment. In actuality, very little equipment is needed to teach relaxation. Ideally, five small pillows or rolled up towels and a firm mat are all that is required. A pencil and paper should be available and in close proximity to each student in order to record personal reactions following the session.

Positioning. Although a person can learn to relax standing or sitting, the ideal position for tension recognition is lying supine on a firm mat with each body curve comfortably supported by a pillow or towel (Fig. 6-1). Contour support is afforded the curves of the cervical and lumbar verte-

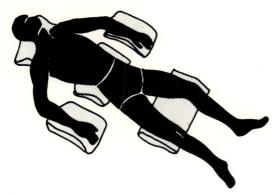

Fig. 6-1. Basic position for tension reduction exercises.

brae; each forearm is supported, resulting in a slight bend to each elbow; and the knees, like the elbows, are maintained in a slightly flexed position with thighs externally rotated. By affording minimal support to the body curves and limbs, free muscle contraction can take place while the individual is in a comfortable, relaxed position. If, however, equipment is not available for joint support, a flat mat surface will suffice.

Sound. A number of techniques utilizing sound may be used by the teacher to aid the student in acquiring the right frame of mind for relaxing. Soft music playing in the background may be beneficial. If music is not available, the monotone pattern of a metronome clicking at 48 or fewer beats/minute may be helpful. Most important, however, whether there is sound equipment or not, is the voice of the instructor, which should be quiet, slow, rhythmical, and distinct.

Breathing. During the relaxation session, the student is instructed to take slow, deep inhalations and make long, slow exhalations. Gradually, through breath control, the student consciously tries to let go of his total bodily tensions. As relaxation occurs, breathing becomes increasingly slow and shallow.

Using imagery. The tension recognition technique involves two distinct phases: a *contraction phase*, whereby the subject contracts a particular muscle or group of mus-

cles to sense tension and a *letting go phase*, whereby the subject seeks a complete lack of tension or negativeness. To aid the pupil in the second phase, the teacher encourages the use of imagery. The student is told to imagine the things that are most relaxing to him. Imagining that he is in a warm bath, that he is floating on a cloud, or that his body is very heavy may help a student to relax. Children at the elementary school level have keen imaginations and respond readily to such suggestions as that they imagine their bodies as snowmen on a hot day or butter in a hot pan.

Sleep. The pupil should be instructed that developing awareness of tense body areas and the ability to relax consciously without falling asleep is the main purpose of the exercise session. However, if sleep does occur during the session, it should be considered a positive reaction.

Procedure

There are a number of ways the instructor can proceed. The teacher can instruct the pupils by having them start with contracting their facial muscles and then moving downward to finish in the lower limbs or, conversely, by having them move from foot to head. If less time is available, using large muscle groups and progressing to the smaller muscles of the body is another alternative. Whatever the technique used, the goals are the same and the teacher will soon develop a style that seems to work best.

Because of the limited amount of time available in the physical education period, many sessions may be required before adequate desired results are reached. A home program should be encouraged for those persons who find it difficult to let go of tension.

Directions to the student

For expediency in the physical education setting, each muscular contraction and each relaxation phase is conducted for approximately 30 seconds, providing a total of 1 minute for each step. During the intro-

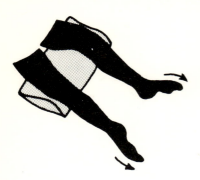

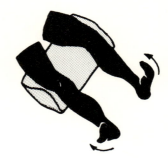

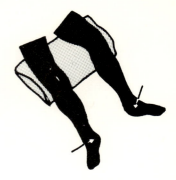

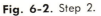

Fig. 6-2. Step 2.   **Fig. 6-3.** Step 3.   **Fig. 6-4.** Step 4.

ductory session, the muscle contraction should be intense enough to cause a degree of fatigue. For each subsequent session, the tension becomes less and less, requiring a greater perceptual sensitivity. *The following is a sample of a relaxation session given to a group of students in a typical school setting.*

Step 1. Lie still for a minute and stare at an object on the ceiling. Do the eyes feel as though they are getting heavy? As this occurs, gradually let them close. Take five deep breaths, inhaling and exhaling slowly. Think of all the joints of the body as being very relaxed.

Step 2. Curl the toes down and point both feet downward toward the end of the mat (Fig. 6-2). Feel the tension in the bottoms of the feet and behind the legs. Do not reinforce the contraction by biting down hard with the teeth or holding the breath. Remember, while tensing one area of the body, all other parts should be relaxed. Now, release the muscle contractions slowly, trying to let go to a complete relaxed state. Feel the body getting extremely heavy and sinking into the mat.

Step 3. Curl the toes and both feet back toward the head (Fig. 6-3). Sense the tenseness on the tops of the feet and legs. Remember not to reinforce the movement by tensing other parts of the body. Breathe easily and relax. Let go of the muscle contraction, allowing the feet and ankles to go limp slowly.

Step 4. Leaving the legs in their original position, with the knees slightly bent, press down against the mat with the heels, attempting to curl the legs backward (Fig. 6-4). Feel the tension in the back of the thighs and buttocks. Remember, while holding this contraction, all other parts of the body (ankles, legs, chest, back, arms, and face) should be at ease. Relax, slowly feeling the discomfort of tension completely leave the body.

Step 5. Remain in the same position as in step 4 and straighten the legs to full extension (Fig. 6-5). Feel the tightness in the tops of the thighs. Do not reinforce this tightness. Now, let go. Breathing should come easily and in a relaxed manner and a profound sense of heaviness should be present throughout the body.

Step 6. With the legs and thighs in their original resting position, draw the thighs up to a bent (flexed) position, with the heels raised off the mat about 3 inches (Fig. 6-6). The tension felt should be primarily in the bend of the hip. Try not to reinforce this with other muscle groups. Return slowly to the starting position and then let go to negative again.

Step 7. Forcibly rotate the thighs outward (Fig. 6-7). Feel the muscle tension in the outer hip region. Remember, be conscious of any other tension creeping into various parts of the body. Now, slowly relax the hip rotators. Go limp.

Step 8. Rotate the thighs inward (Fig. 6-

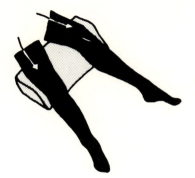

Fig. 6-5. Step 5.

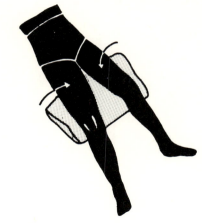

Fig. 6-8. Step 8.

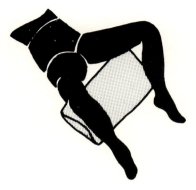

Fig. 6-6. Step 6.

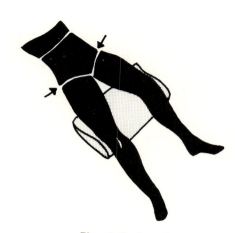

Fig. 6-9. Step 9.

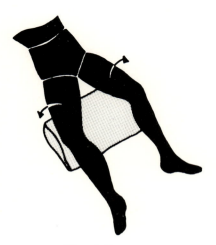

Fig. 6-7. Step 7.

8). Feel the muscle tension deep in the inner thighs. Relax slowly, let go of all tension, and let the thighs again rotate outward. Sense the body sinking deeper into the mat.

Step 9. Squeeze the buttocks (gluteal muscles) together tightly and tilt the hips backward (Fig. 6-9). The only muscular tension that should be felt is in the buttocks and low back region. Again, be acutely aware of other tensions that may be occurring in the body: the feet, legs, thighs, low back, abdominal muscles, chest, neck, upper back, arms, and face. Now, let go of the contraction and try to sense the joints becoming extremely loose.

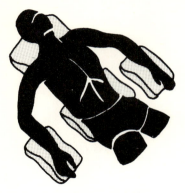

Fig. 6-10. Step 10.

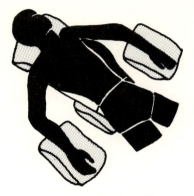

Fig. 6-11. Step 11.

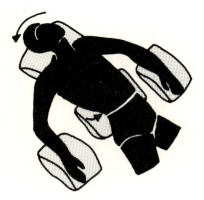

Fig. 6-12. Step 12.

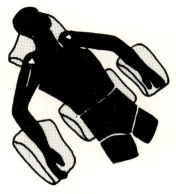

Fig. 6-13. Step 14.

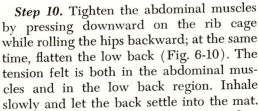

Step 10. Tighten the abdominal muscles by pressing downward on the rib cage while rolling the hips backward; at the same time, flatten the low back (Fig. 6-10). The tension felt is both in the abdominal muscles and in the low back region. Inhale slowly and let the back settle into the mat.

Step 11. Inhale and exhale slowly and as deeply as possible three times (Fig. 6-11). A general tension should be felt throughout the rib cage. After the last forced inspiration and expiration, return to normal quiet breathing and sense the difference in tension levels.

Step 12. Accentuating the curve of the neck (cervical spine), press the head back and lift the upper back off the mat (Fig. 6-12). The tension felt should be in the back of the neck and upper back. Settle slowly back to the mat.

Step 13. Next, pinch the shoulders back, squeezing the two shoulder blades (scapula bones) together. Tension is felt in the back of the shoulders. Release the contraction slowly and fall easily back to the mat. Be aware of any residual tension that might remain after returning to the mat.

Step 14. Leaving the arms in their resting position, lift and roll shoulders inward so that tension is felt in the front of the chest (Fig. 6-13). Do not reinforce this by contracting other muscles. Now, allow the shoulders to drop back to the mat in a resting position. Feel the tension leave the chest.

Step 15. Spread and grip the fingers of both hands. Do this three times (Fig. 6-14). The tension felt is in the hands and forearms. As the fingers are gripped and spread, be sure not to lift the elbows off the mat.

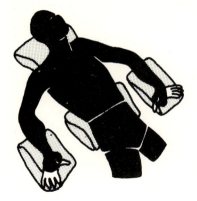

Fig. 6-14. Step 15.

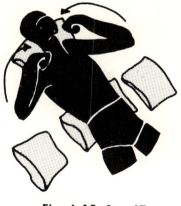

Fig. 6-15. Step 17.

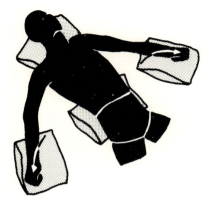

Fig. 6-16. Step 18.

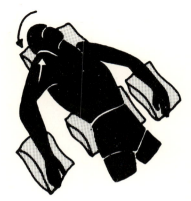

Fig. 6-17. Step 19.

After the third series, let hands and forearms fall limply back to their support.

Step 16. Make a tight fist with both hands and slowly curl the wrists back, forward, and to both sides. Tension should primarily be felt at the fist, wrist, and forearm. After these movements, allow fingers and thumbs to open gradually and go to zero.

Step 17. Make a tight fist with both hands and slowly bend (flex) the forearms at the elbows against the upper arms, at the same time lifting the arms at the shoulders (Fig. 6-15). Tension is felt in the front part of the forearms, in the biceps regions, and in the front part of the shoulders. After the flexion of the shoulders, the arms should be slowly uncurled and returned to their original resting position; relax each segment separately until the arms become limp, motionless, and negative.

Step 18. Make a tight fist with both hands, stiffen the arms, and press hard against the mat (Fig. 6-16). Tension should be felt in the forearms and the back of the upper arms and shoulders. Hold the pressure against the mat for 30 seconds and then release slowly.

Step 19. Shrug the right shoulder; then bend the head sideward (laterally flex neck), touching the ear to the elevated shoulder (Fig. 6-17). The only tension that should be felt is in the upper right shoulder and the right side of the neck. Release the contraction, slowly returning the neck and shoulder to their resting positions.

Step 20. As in step 19, shrug the left

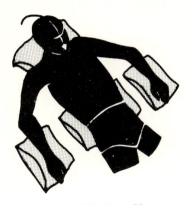

Fig. 6-18. Step 21.

shoulder; then laterally flex the neck, touching the ear to the elevated shoulder. The only tension that should be felt is in the upper left shoulder and the lateral muscles of the neck. Release the contraction, slowly returning the neck and shoulder to their resting position.

Step 21. Bend the head forward, touching the chin to the chest (Fig. 6-18). Tension is felt in the front of the neck. Relax and slowly return the head to a resting position. Continue to concentrate on the body as being extremely heavy and at a zero state.

Step 22. Lift eyebrows upward; wrinkle the forehead. Feel the tension in the forehead region. Let the face go blank.

Step 23. Close the eyelids tightly and wrinkle the nose. Tension is felt in the nose and eyes. Let the face relax slowly. Concentrate on the tension leaving the face.

Step 24. Open the mouth widely as if to yawn. Feel the tension in the jaw. Now, let the mouth close slowly and lightly.

Step 25. Bite down hard and then show the teeth in a forced smile. Tension should be felt in the jaw and lips. Slowly allow the face to return to a blank expression. Be sure not to tense other parts of the body when contracting the facial muscles.

Step 26. Pucker the lips hard as if to whistle. Sense tension at the edge of the mouth. Let the tension melt away.

Step 27. Push the tongue hard against the roof of the mouth. Let go. Push the tongue against the roof of the mouth again as hard as possible. Relax. Push the tongue against the upper teeth. Relax. Sense the contraction of the tongue muscles. As you do this exercise, try not to use any other body parts. Relax.

Step 28. Lie very still for a short while and try to be conscious of those body areas that were difficult to relax. Move slowly and take any position desired. Relax and rest.

Teacher evaluation

Although the most accurate indication of abnormal tension is by electromyographic tests, subjective evaluation still has its place for the physical education instructor. Tension is easily observable through mannerisms such as extraneous movements or muscle twitches (eye twitches, fingers movements, stiffness, changes of body position, or playing with hands and vocal sounds of all kinds). The instructor should test muscle resistance by lifting the students' arms or legs after the relaxation session. Limbs that have a residual tension do not feel limp or lifeless; they tend to feel stiff and unyielding. The instructor tells the students that they will be tested for relaxation at the end of the session. The following four factors may be made apparent by the tests: (1) whether the student assists the movement, (2) whether the student resists the movement, (3) whether the student engages in positioning body parts, or (4) whether the student ideally displays a complete lack of tension.*

Student evaluation

After the exercise session, the students are asked to answer questions about their personal reactions, writing their answers on a sheet of paper by their side. Some suggested questions could be the following:

1. What was your general reaction to the

---

*See also Crowe, W. C., Arnheim, D. D., and Auxter, D.: Laboratory manual in adapted physical education and recreation, St. Louis, 1977, The C. V. Mosby Co.

session? Was it good, bad, or indifferent?

2. Were you comfortable for the whole 28 minutes? If not, what disturbed you?
3. Did you sense the tensions and relaxations at all times? If not, why not?
4. Were there areas of the body that you just could not continually relax? What were they?

Questions such as these help the student identify his reactions to the relaxation period. It may require a number of sessions for the student to identify tense regions of his body accurately. As he learns to relax individual parts, the student will gradually be able to relax larger and larger segments until he will eventually be able to relax the whole body at will.

RELAXING THE PHYSICALLY IMMATURE

Conscious control of muscular tension for the physically immature individual is usually very difficult. A program of relaxation training must be commensurate with the subject's developmental and maturational level. Before a training program can be effectively instituted, the subject must understand what tension and relaxation are and how they are contrasted. The concept of relaxation can be taught by having the individual pretend his arms are like rubber bands, that he is melting like a very hot snowman, or that he is a rag doll that cannot stand up. Another good technique to develop the concept of tightness and looseness is to have the participant stiffen his whole body for about 30 seconds and then gradually let go of the tension by pretending to be a pat of butter melting in a very hot pan (Fig. 6-19). Following this activity, the instructor can introduce to the individual questions such as "How does it feel to be relaxed?" or "Doesn't it feel better to be relaxed than stiff and tense?" Once the subject perceives the difference between tensing and releasing tension, the instructor can begin to develop a skill program that gradually takes the student from a total body to a segmental relaxation program.[1]

DIFFERENTIAL RELAXATION

Decreasing and increasing muscular tension levels at will requires varying degrees of coordination (Fig. 6-20). All skilled movement requires differential relaxation. A technique that has been found beneficial in training individuals to selectively control specific muscles is known as the "muscle tension recognition and release method."[1,2] This technique starts with the subject tensing and letting go of the entire body and proceeds to "bilateral body control" in which the subject learns control of

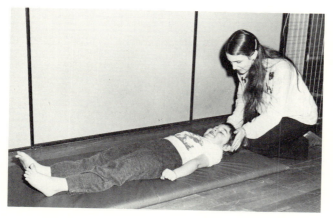

Fig. 6-19. Stiffening the entire body to learn the difference between muscle tension and relaxation. (Courtesy California State University, Audio Visual Center, Long Beach, Calif.)

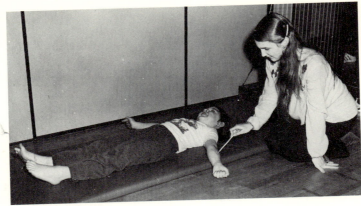

Fig. 6-20. Learning to differentiate specific body areas by tensing and relaxing on command. (Courtesy California State University, Audio Visual Center, Long Beach, Calif.)

both upper limbs and then of both lower limbs. Following successful demonstration of bilateral limb control, the subject advances to "unilateral body control," whereby muscular tension is increased on one side of the body and completely released on the other, for example, tensing the right arm and leg and relaxing the left arm and leg. From unilateral control, the subject progresses to "cross lateral body control," which involves tensing the opposite arm and leg. The last stage of differential relaxation training is the isolation and relaxation of specific body parts at will. In general, differential relaxation training is a useful tool for developing total body control, increasing body awareness, and reducing anxiety. However, this technique cannot force maturation and should be limited to the particular developmental level of the individual.

REFERENCES

1. Arnheim, D. D., and Pestolesi, R. A.: Developing motor behavior in children: a balanced approach to elementary physical education, St. Louis, 1973, The C. V. Mosby Co.
2. Arnheim, D. D., and Sinclair, W. A.: The clumsy child: a program of motor therapy, St. Louis, 1975, The C. V. Mosby Co.
3. Bension, H.: The relaxation response, New York, 1975, William Morrow & Co., Inc.
4. Collier, H. O. J.: Aspirin, Sci. Am. **209**:96-108, 1963.
5. Cratty, B. J.: Movement behavior and motor learning, Philadelphia, 1973, Lea & Febiger.
6. deVries, H. A.: Physiology of exercise, ed. 2, Dubuque, Iowa, 1974, William C. Brown Co., Publishers.
7. Frederick, A. B.: Tension control, J. Health Phys. Ed. Rec. **38**:42-44, 78-80, 1967.
8. Goth, A.: Medical pharmacology: principles and concepts, St. Louis, 1974, The C. V. Mosby Co.
9. Jacobson, E.: Progressive relaxation, Chicago, 1938, The University of Chicago Press.
10. Jacobson, E.: Self-operation control, Philadelphia, 1964, J. B. Lippincott Co.
11. Larson, D., editor: Encyclopedia of sports science and medicine, New York, 1971, Macmillan Publishing Co., Inc.
12. Melzack, R.: The promise of biofeedback: don't hold the party yet, Psychol. Today **9**:18-22, 80-81, 1975.
13. Naranjo, C., and Ornstein, R. E.: On the psychology of meditation, New York, 1971, The Viking Press, Inc.
14. Powers, M.: Advanced techniques of hypnosis, ed. 4, Hollywood, Calif., 1956, Wilshire Book Co.
15. Powers, M.: A practical guide to self-hypnosis, Hollywood, Calif., 1963, Wilshire Book Co.
16. Rathbone, J. L.: Relaxation, Philadelphia, 1969, Lea & Febiger.
17. Selye, H.: The stress of life, New York, 1956, McGraw-Hill Book Co.
18. Tappan, F. M.: Massage techniques, New York, 1961, Macmillan Publishing Co., Inc.

7

UNDERDEVELOPMENT AND LOW PHYSICAL VITALITY

■ One of the primary objectives of physical educators is to develop in their students the physical characteristics necessary to perform the activities of daily living without undue fatigue and to function with optimal competency in the performance of motor skills.

The problem of physical underdevelopment and low vitality is a major concern of physical education, involving a great number of persons having physical and mental as well as emotional problems. Chronically ill persons with debilitating conditions are par-

ticularly prone to low physical vitality and development. Individuals with cardiorespiratory conditions such as chronic bronchitis and various heart defects (Chapter 12) are particularly prone to poor physical fitness and are a special challenge to the instructor in adapted physical education. The mentally limited as well as many normal individuals are often lacking in the important factors of fitness necessary for success at play and in many common activities of daily living (Chapter 15).

MOVEMENT EFFICIENCY

Of utmost importance to the student in an adapted physical education class is the ability to move as efficiently as possible. Inherent in movement efficiency is *motor fitness*, which can be defined as the ability to effectively perform movement activities that require strength, flexibility, and endurance. All human movement requires relative levels of muscular strength, joint flexibility, and stamina as well as the ability to use these motor components in activities requiring balance and coordination.[2, 24] *Motor fitness* refers to tasks that require neuromuscular coordination for task performance and involve temporospatial coor-

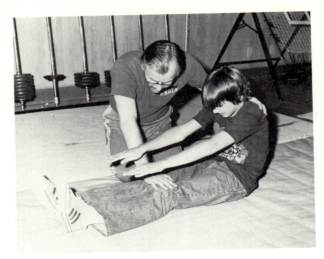

Fig. 7-1. Testing extent flexibility. (Courtesy California State University, Audio Visual Center, Long Beach, Calif.)

dination of many large muscles. Generic skill (running, jumping, and throwing) is included in this group. *Physical fitness*, on the other hand, includes components that are less complex with regard to skilled performance than is motor fitness in that, by and large, refined neuromotor integration is not required to successfully perform tasks. Such components are generally described as strength, flexibility, and endurance.

Operational definitions of the physical components, adapted from Fleishman,[18] are as follows:

1. *Extent flexibility:* Ability to stretch muscles as far as possible (Fig. 7-1)
   EXAMPLE: Toe touch activities
2. *Static strength:* Maximum force that a subject can exert for a brief period, where the force is exerted continuously to this maximum (Fig. 7-2)
   EXAMPLE: Pulling against dynamometers

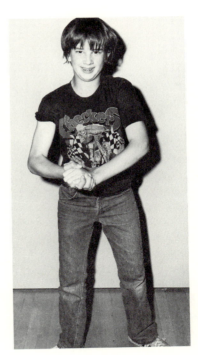

Fig. 7-2. A display of static muscle exertion. (Courtesy California State University, Audio Visual Center, Long Beach, Calif.)

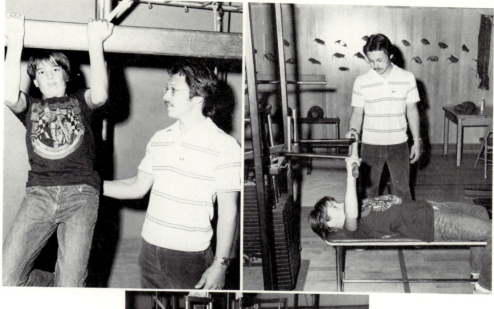

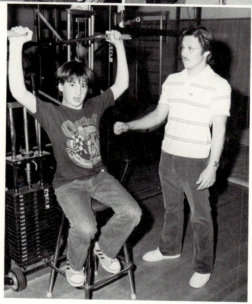

Fig. 7-3. Activities requiring dynamic strength. (Courtesy California State University, Audio Visual Center, Long Beach, Calif.)

3. *Dynamic strength:* Ability to exert muscular force repeatedly and move one's own approximate body weight (Fig. 7-3)

EXAMPLES: Chinning, dips on parallel bars, push-up activities (activities 18, 25, 26 to 32, and 35 to 38 in Chapter 5)

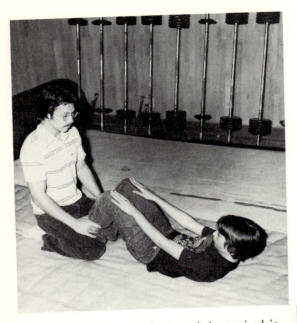

Fig. 7-4. Dynamic trunk strength is required in sit-ups. (Courtesy California State University, Audio Visual Center, Long Beach, Calif.)

4. *Trunk strength:* Dynamic strength specific to the trunk muscles, particularly the abdominals (Fig. 7-4)
   EXAMPLES: Sit-ups, knee-chest curls
5. *Stamina:* Capacity to continue maximum effort requiring prolonged muscular exertion over time
   EXAMPLES: Distance running, rope jumping, bench stepping, bicycling (Fig. 7-5)

The following are descriptions of components that are included in the motor fitness areas:

1. *Dynamic flexibility:* Ability to make rapid flexing or extension movements in which the resiliency of the muscles in recovery from distortion is critical
   EXAMPLES: Activities 10, 39, and 40 in Chapter 5

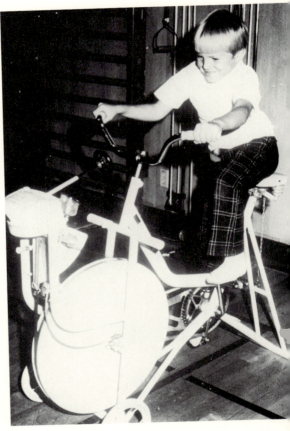

Fig. 7-5. Stamina building through bicycling. (Courtesy California State University, Audio Visual Center, Long Beach, Calif.)

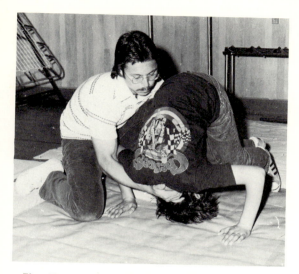

Fig. 7-6. A forward roll requires dynamic flexibility. (Courtesy California State University, Audio Visual Center, Long Beach, Calif.)

2. *Explosive strength:* Ability to expend a maximum of energy in one or a series of explosive acts (Fig. 7-6)
   EXAMPLES: Broad jump, high jump, shot put, 50-yard dash, and shuttle run (American Alliance for Health, Physical Education, and Recreation test) (Fig. 7-7)
3. *Gross body coordination:* Ability to coordinate the simultaneous actions of different parts of the body while making gross body movements
   EXAMPLE: Rope jumping

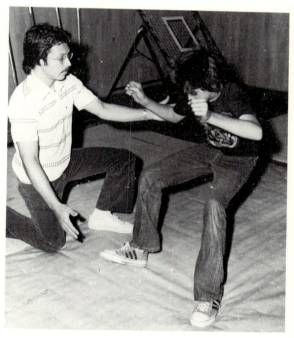

Fig. 7-7. Completing a standing broad jump, which illustrates the use of explosive strength. (Courtesy California State University, Audio Visual Center, Long Beach, Calif.)

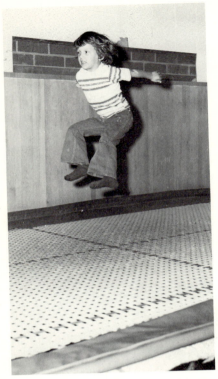

Fig. 7-8. Developing gross body equilibrium through trampoline jumping. (Courtesy California State University, Audio Visual Center, Long Beach, Calif.)

4. *Gross body equilibrium:* Ability of the individual to maintain his equilibrium despite forces pulling him off balance when he must depend on vestibular and kinesthetic cues (Fig. 7-8)

EXAMPLES: Walking a balance beam or jumping on a trampoline

When programs for the physically subfit are implemented, it is desirable to be more comprehensive with regard to programming for general physical and motor fitness components. Therefore programs for the subfit should be comprehensive so that the results of the program can be generalized to many physical and motor aspects of life.

There are many physical and motor fitness test batteries in the physical education literature. The Fleishman test battery is one that pairs tasks with tests of a specific component. Thus it is a comprehensive test battery because the factor analysis from which the tests come is comprehensive. This is not the case with other test batteries such as the PFI Oregon short form, the Kraus-Weber test, and the American Alliance for Health, Physical Education, and Recreation test.[11]

SYSTEMS APPROACH

A systems approach starts by asking the question, "What are the objectives that need to be achieved by the students?" In this approach, the question to be answered is, "What are the components of physical and motor fitness that can be developed in an individual?" Once this question is answered, a concrete plan for interrelating program objectives, diagnosis, and remediation can be made.

The systems approach is concerned with isolating different components of physical and motor development, measuring current levels of functioning of these components in an individual, and then pairing them with specific activities directly related to assessment of physical and motor components. This systematic approach usually generates a profile of abilities for each child, showing differing needs and abilities. Thus it provides information that aids the instructor in making decisions in the selection of appropriate activities according to a specific pupil's need.

If a systems approach is to be employed in developing physical and motor fitness, it is necessary to know what physical and motor components can be developed in an individual. The establishment of a taxonomy is the first step in developing such a systematic approach. A taxonomy, in this case, is a means of categorizing diverse physical actions in such a way that useful relationships among activities are established. It simplifies and identifies the way in which individuals possess traits in common and yet differ in characteristics and it is extremely useful in describing performance on a wide variety of tasks.

The development of a taxonomy makes it possible to formulate goals, select tests relevant to those goals, and then more precisely specify activity objectives for individuals according to target deficiencies. Thus if the instructor makes use of taxonomy, through the systems approach he may do the following: (1) generate a profile of abilities in components of the taxonomy and (2) select appropriate activities according to each child's need. Thus each child, regardless of his developmental status and disability, works toward the acquisition of skills commensurate with his abilities.

Before a taxonomy can be justified, there must be evidence that supports discrete identifiable physical and motor properties existing within each component. Factor analysis studies tend to describe the ways in which individuals may be different. This statistical technique assists in the classification of motor tasks into components and thus enables the construction of a taxonomy. Such components are discussed in the following pages.

Strength

Strength is that factor of motor fitness that allows a person to overcome a resistance through muscular exertion. There are three discrete components of strength: (1) explosive strength, (2) static strength, and (3) dynamic strength. Explosive strength is apparent in those activities requiring movement, speed, and sudden changes in direction, for example, in running through an obstacle course or in throwing an object for distance. Static or isometric strength requires little muscle shortening and is necessary in overcoming a heavy resistance. Dynamic strength, on the other hand, is the component found in repeated muscle contractions.

Normal muscle capacity is maintained at a level that is in keeping with our daily activities. Consequently, children who are in the habit of minimal physical activity may develop subaverage strength or continue in a condition of low vitality. However, through proper training, the general strength of the body may be increased. This is usually done by providing a training stimulus greater than the normal daily stress requirement of a particular muscle or group of muscles. The traditional method of strength training is through the application of the overload principle, in which the training stimulus exceeds the demands of daily activity. For best results, training should be pushed to the point of fatigue. This enhances the total effect of training more effectively than if training is interrupted prior to the fatigue point.[22] A general axiom in strength training that generally yields good results for increasing muscular strength would be: "Greater work effort rather than long duration of effort." To make optimal gains in strength training, it has been recommended that the training stimulus be increased at least every 14 days, for the overload effect is not as great unless resistance is increased periodically. In the case of weaker children, the training effects will be great at first; however, with the acquisition of greater strength, slower progress will be made.[22]

Some muscle groups are more susceptible to strength training than are others. Muscle groups that are used most strenuously in day-to-day activity are those that respond less readily to strength training. Among them are the muscles of the forearm and the arm, whereas the gastrocnemius, gluteal, and hip extensor muscles respond more favorably to stimulus training.[22] In accord with this concept is the fact that atrophied muscles respond five or six times more favorably to strength training than well-trained groups of muscles. Stated in another way, the trainability of muscle groups shows a direct relationship to their use in the activities of daily living (Chapter 5).[22]

Flexibility

Flexibility is the range and degree of motion through which one extremity can move in relation to another. It is generally agreed that varying degrees of flexibility are required for efficiency of joint movement and motor performance. Although the optimal amount of flexibility for successful performance is not clearly understood, there seems to be a consensus that each activity has it own desirable amount of flexibility.[14] When considering just how much flexibility is needed by the individual, all eventualities should be taken into consideration. A highly elastic and mobile body should allow for sudden uncommon or unexpected movements.

There is no single factor that determines the differences in the flexibility of one individual as compared to another. Variance in flexibility can be attributable to heredity, a difference in joint structure, the extent of elasticity in connective tissue that is found throughout the body, the extent of reciprocal coordination and muscular tension, and muscle viscosity. Thus there is no single factor that accounts for the ability of a joint to move through a given range.

Although it is generally thought that its elasticity changes as the body grows older, studies indicate that flexibility varies more with individual movement habits and growth patterns than with age.[3] It can be concluded therefore that in order to maintain or increase body mobility and joint range of movement, an individual must engage in a great variety of gross and fine motor activities that involve a full range of movement of the joints employed.

Two common types of exercise for increasing flexibility are the ballistic and static, or gradual, stretching techniques. In the ballistic technique, a rebounding movement is initiated that is controlled and slowly employs the principle of reciprocal muscle action. Consequently, moving muscles pull the body part into a stretch position while the opposing set of muscles relaxes. To avoid the possibility of injury to the musculotendinous unit, stretching by the ballistic method is not carried to the point of discomfort. The student is cautioned against engaging in lunging and uncontrolled movements. Static, or gradual, stretching, on the other hand, discourages the bobbing action of the ballistic technique by maintaining the stretch position

for a period of 30 seconds or longer. The participant is instructed to stretch a little beyond the point of discomfort. Logan and Egstrom[26] studied the effects of static and ballistic stretch on the sacrofemoral angle and concluded that both types of exercise were equally effective. However, in a comparison of ballistic and static stretching, deVries[16] indicates that static stretching tends to decrease the chances of muscle strains in preactivity warm-up (Chapter 5).

Physical stamina

Physical stamina refers to a person's ability to engage in continuous activity. Two primary components stand out as being necessary for "staying power" in any physical endeavor, namely, dynamic strength and cardiorespiratory endurance. Both components are closely interrelated. Muscle strength and endurance must be considered as being on a continuum, ranging from one muscle contraction to repeated muscle contractions and sustained type of activities. Efficiency of the cardiorespiratory system, on the other hand, is an individual's capacity to use oxygen during physical activity.[7, 8]

Well-constructed programs of physical activity can be of significant value to children who are lacking in cardiovascular fitness. There is evidence that systematic muscular exercise leads to an increase in height and weight as well as to an increase in the function of the vital organs of children. Another value of physical exercise programs in assisting children who are physically unfit is in the area of producing organic changes in the lungs and circulatory system, improving their function in normal living.

It is the hope of the physical educator that favorable attitudes toward physical exercise can be instilled in all students. It is commonly held that exercise is one of the factors deterring the onset of hypokinetic disease, primarily of the cardiovascular system. Exercise reduces hypertension, which is often caused by anxiety and emotional stress; serves as an outlet for nervous tension; and helps maintain the elasticity of the blood vessels. However, it is necessary to realize that there is no royal road to fitness, for it requires time and energy. In the development of cardiovascular fitness, each bout of exercise must be a little stronger than the previous one; in this way, each bout will lead to progressive efficiency of the cardiovascular system. (See discussion of cardiovascular fitness in Chapters 5 and 12.)

Postural fitness

As will be disussed in detail in Chapter 9, good body alignment is essential for efficient movement. Faulty posture and poor body mechanics produce an imbalance in muscle strength and extensibility that results in the expenditure of more energy than necessary in the performance of a motor activity. Moreover, faulty posture either causes or results from distortions in body awareness and inaccurate sense of body position.

Coordinated movement

Motor fitness is essential for coordinated movement to take place. In order for an individual to achieve success in a great variety of physical activities, there must be present an effective interweaving of all the various factors of motor fitness. Awkward movement behavior implies asynchronous and inefficient muscle action.[2]

APPRAISING MOTOR FITNESS

It is of the utmost importance that great care be taken in the selection of tests that evaluate the status of an individual student wth respect to subdevelopment in physical and motor areas. The purpose of a test may be classifying, grading, or diagnosing physical and motor deficiencies. In setting up a program of developmental activities or establishing adapted physical education programs, it is important to ensure that evaluative tests be of a diagnostic nature. A test enables the physical educator to assess current status, set up programs for the student on the basis of the diagnostic test,

measure current progress in the program, and, in many instances, provide motivation for continuing the activities of the program.[43]

Criteria for the selection of evaluation measures are as follows:

1. The test should relate to fundamental diagnosed factors that can be improved through the adapted physical education program.
2. The test must reflect a philosophy of the local adapted physical education program with respect to those dimensions of physical and motor development that are of value to those who implement and administer the program.
3. Tests in the battery should be carefully evaluated so that no two tests measure the same factor. The tests should cover as many different areas of motor and physical development as possible.
4. Those tests should be selected that have the best scientific foundation. Some of the information that should be known about the test includes its reliability, the consistency with which the same results are acquired, its validity (does the test measure what it claims to measure?), the norms that make it possible to compare the test results with a comparable random sampling of population, and the feasibility of its administration (the amount of time and equipment required and the degree of difficulty in administering the test).

Selected tests for classification, grading, and diagnosing physical and motor deficiencies are discussed specifically in Chapters 2, 5, 7, 9, 11, and 12.

PROGRAM FOR MOTOR FITNESS

Besides the developmental exercises found in Chapter 5, which are designed for specific body areas and conditions, the adaptive physical educator can employ the circuit training concept to increase a student's level of physical development and vitality.

It is well established that a progressive resistive exercise program is the best method for the development of muscular strength and that an interval training program of running, swimming, rope skipping, and bicycle riding is best for the development of circulorespiratory endurance. Therefore the conditioning system that best meets the needs of both strength and circulorespiratory endurance is the circuit training method.[8] Circuit training has the potential to fulfill specific diagnosed areas of deficiencies among students through the selection of carefully arranged exercises. Each numbered exercise in a circuit is called a station. Therefore there can be many stations throughout a particular gymnasium with persons of varying deficiencies routed to the stations that have exercises prescribed to meet each one's particular deficiency. The circuit training system is extremely adaptable to a great variety of situations and has the potential to meet individual differences that happen to be present within a particular class. The advantages of a circuit training system in developing *subaverage* physical and motor factors are the following: (1) it can cope with most diagnosed deficiencies, (2) it has the potential of applying the progressive overload principle, and (3) it enables a large number of performers to train at the same time and yet meets the individual needs of each performer.

Circuit training usually involves the introduction of a time element into training, which often forces the participant to perform at submaximal levels. However, this need not be entirely the case. Each performer can be assigned a specific circuit in which he performs a prescribed number of repetitions at each station. If one wishes to develop both cardiovascular and strength variables, the load may be of a submaximal nature so that the person may continuously engage in exercise as he moves from station to station. However, if the strength component is a more desirable outcome for some students, then fewer repetitions with a large dosage should be achieved before the person moves to the next station. After one circuit lap has been completed, it

is at the discretion of the instructor to move the student through a second or third lap, depending on the total dosage desired for a given student. The advantages of the circuit system are as follows:

1. It is adaptable to a number of varying situations.
2. It can be used by 1 or 100 persons and fits almost any time requirements.
3. Progression is assured.
4. A person always works at his present capacity and then progresses beyond that.
5. It provides a series of progressive goals, which is a powerful motivating force for a person to do better.
6. It may utilize variables such as load, repetition, and time and consequently it may develop motor and physical developmental characteristics that have been identified by diagnostic testing.
7. It has the possibility of providing a vigorous bout of exercise in a relatively short period of time.
8. Any number of stations can be constructed to meet any identifiable need.
9. The student knows what he is required to do because the construction of an individualized program.

Regardless of the system of training used in the developmental program, it should always be kept in mind that the primary goal of the system is to meet the individually diagnosed needs of each child in the program through planned progressive exercise. If this principle is applied, chances are that the program will be beneficial to the physical and motor development of the child.

Fig. 7-9 shows the implementation of a circuit program. This circuit program consists of 10 different exercises at separate stations, each performed according to a prescribed number of repetitions and load. It must be remembered that there are as many stations possible as there are exercises or areas of subdevelopment. The illustration shows five different levels at each station, permitting four steps of progression. Individuals subjectively select a

Name of exercise	Developmental levels*				
	I	II	III	IV	V
	Wt.	Wt.	Wt.	Wt.	Wt.
Two arm curl	40	50	55	60	65
Military press	50	60	65	70	75
Deep knee bends	70	80	85	90	95
Dead lift (straight leg)	70	80	85	90	95
French curl (or dip) with dumbbell	10	15	20	25	30
Situps (time)	--	--	--	--	--
Bench step-ups (time)	--	--	--	--	--
Bench press	55	60	65	75	85
Lateral raises (dumbbell)	5	10	15	20	25
Pushups (time)	--	--	--	--	--

*When 10 repetitions are reached, advance to the next developmental level.

Fig. 7-9. A suggested circuit training program.

starting level and then gravitate to the level that will optimally challenge their ability. Whenever the individual is able to meet the prescribed number of repetitions (10 in this case), he moves on to the next level. Progression depends on the individual's ability to meet the set number of repetitions, which will enable him to move on to the next progressive level. At each station, it is desirable to place on the wall a card naming the item and showing the five levels of performance. The load and number of repetitions initially should be selected to meet the capabilities of the average student in the class; however, the circuit can be adapted to suit individuals who find loads either too heavy or too light. Also, it must be remembered that it is not necessary for each student to participate at each of these 10 stations. It may be administratively unfeasible to have each child participate in a 10-station circuit. Therefore each student may be routed to four, five, or six stations (whatever the case may be) according to his need. Any station may be devised that meets a physical or motor need of children and a progressive program may be established.

SELECTED FITNESS PROBLEMS

As mentioned earlier in this chapter, the problem of underdevelopment and low physical vitality is closely associated with a great number of organic, mental, and emotional problems discussed throughout this book. However, three major problem areas transcend most, namely, malnutrition, anemia, and aging.

Malnutrition

The term "malnutrition" means poor nutrition, whether there is an excess or a lack of nutrients to the body. In either instance, the individual who is malnourished is one who has relatively low physical vitality and may be underdeveloped, along with having other serious disadvantages.[5]

Underweight

It is important that the cause of physical underdevelopment be identified. One of the causes for physical underdevelopment may be a lack of physical activity, which, consequently, does not provide opportunity for the body to develop to its physical potential. However, there are some children who are physically underdeveloped partially because of undernutrition. When a person's body weight is more than 10% below the ideal weight indicated by standard age and weight tables, this may indicate that undernutrition is a cause. Tension, anxiety, depressions, and other emotional factors may restrict a person's appetite, causing insufficient caloric intake and weight loss. Impairment to development of the body may also ensue. In culturally deprived areas, diets in some instances may be deficient in proper nutrition, either as a result of insufficient food, idiosyncrasy, and lack of appetite because of some organic problem. It is necessary to remember that proper nutrition and exercise go hand in hand in growing children and that one without the other may cause lack of optimal physical development. The role of the physical educator in dealing with the underweight person is to help establish sound living habits with particular emphasis paid to proper diet, rest, and relaxation. The student should be encouraged to keep a 5-day food intake diary, after which, with the help of the teacher, a daily average of calories consumed is computed. After determining the average number of calories taken in, the student is encouraged to increase his daily intake by eating extra meals that are both nutritious and high in calories.*

Overweight

Many persons in the United States are overweight. Obesity, particularly in adults, is considered one of the great current medical problems because of its relation to cardiovascular and other diseases. The frequency of overweight among male pa-

tients, as reported by Master, Jaffe, and Chesky,[29] was nearly 40% in patients with angina pectoris, coronary insufficiency, and hypertension and nearly 50% in those with coronary occlusions as compared with approximately 20% in the populations used as controls.

Overweight may be defined as any excess of 10% or more above the ideal weight for a person and obesity is any excess of 20% or more above the ideal weight.[28] Obesity constitutes pathological overweight that requires some means of correction. There are several factors that must be considered in determining whether a person is overweight. Among these are sex, weight, height, age, general body build, bone size, muscular development, and accumulations of subcutaneous fat.

In the past, there has not been sufficient attention given to the diagnosis of the large number of overweight children in our modern society. Research on the incidence of overweight children in our schools has indicated estimates of 10% or more.[31] The incidence therefore is of such significance that attention to prevention and remediation should be provided by public school doctors, nurses, and health and physical educators in our schools.

Overweight persons have a greater tendency than normal or underweight individuals to contract diseases of the heart, circulatory system, kidneys, and pancreas. They also have a predisposition to be afflicted with structural foot conditions and joint pathology because of their increased weight and a lack of motor skill to accommodate the excess weight.

The basic reason for overweight is that the body's food and caloric consumption is more than the physical activity or energy expended to utilize them. Consequently, the excess energy food is stored in the body as fat, leading to overweight. In many instances, overeating is a matter of habit. Thus the body is continually in the process of acquiring more calories than needed to maintain a normal body weight.

Overweight and obesity have many

---

*See also Crowe, W. C., Arnheim, D. D., and Auxter, D.: Laboratory manual in adapted physical education and recreation, St. Louis, 1977, The C. V. Mosby Co.

causes. Among them are (1) caloric imbalance from eating incorrectly in relationship to energy expended in the form of activity; (2) dysfunction of the endocrine glands, particularly the pituitary and the thyroid, which regulate fat distribution in the body; and (3) emotional disturbance.

There is impressive evidence that obesity in adults has its origin in the individual's early childhood obesity. There seems to be a substantial number of overweight adults whose difficulty in controlling their appetite stems from childhood.[41] Obesity has been considered by some to be related to various crises of childhood. Some of these crises have been identified at the 3-year-old level, at which time a child reaches out for family satisfaction; at the 6-year-old level, at which time the child begins school; between the ages of 8 and 14 years when prepuberty and adolescence start; and again between the ages of 15 and 17 years when the drive for social adjustment and acceptance begins.[28] There is also evidence that the social environment in which a child is reared may have some bearing on obesity. Gurney[20] found that 73% of the children he investigated were obese when both parents were overweight, 41% when only one parent was obese, and 10% when both parents were of average weight. In the preschool years, thinness rather than obesity is the general developmental characteristic of a child. However, during the early school years and up to early adolescence, children seem susceptible to excess fat deposition.

A prevalent belief among some authorities is that a great portion of obesity is caused by emotions. They theorize that children at the age of 7 years are particularly susceptible to obesity from overeating in order to compensate for being unhappy and lonely. Evidently, eating may give comfort to the child. This particular period is significant because it is the period in life when the child is transferring close emotional ties from the family to peer relationships. In the event that children do not successfully establish close friendships with other children, they feel alone. Therefore a compensatory mechanism of adjustment is eating, which gives comfort. Eating may also be used as a comfort when the child has trouble at home or at school.

Personality characteristics of the obese. In many instances, obesity reflects other personality traits. The obese child often gives the appearance of being advanced physically because of increased body size and physical maturation. In addition, although commonly having intelligence comparable with that of his peers, the obese child, in many instances, exhibits characteristic that are of an immature nature socially and emotionally. It is not uncommon for the obese child to dislike the games played by his peers, for his obesity handicaps him in being adept at the games in which his peers are adequate. This child is often clumsy and slow, the object of many stereotyped jokes, and incapable of holding a secure social position among other children. Consequently, he becomes oversensitive and unable to defend himself and thus may withdraw from healthy play and exercise. This withdrawal from activity decreases the energy expenditure needed to maintain the balance that combats the obesity. Therefore in many instances, obesity leads to sedentary habits. It is often difficult to encourage these children to participate in forms of exercise that permit great expenditure of energy.

Obesity may be an important factor as a child forms ideas about himself as a person and about how he thinks he appears to others. The ideas that he has about himself will be influenced by his own discoveries, by what others say about him, and by the attitudes they show toward him. If the child finds that his appearance elicits hostility, disrespect, or negative attention from parents and peers, these feelings may affect his self-concept. Traits described by his parents and peers may affect his inner feelings and may be manifested in his behavior, for children often assess their worth in terms of their relationships with peers, parents, and other authority figures. The evaluation of these persons is instrumental in the formulation of the child's concept of worth.

When the child passes from the child-centered atmosphere of the home into the competitive activities of the early school years, social stresses are placed on him. He must demonstrate physical abilities, courage, manipulative skill, and social adeptness in direct comparison with other children of his age. The penalties for failure are humiliation, ridicule, and rejection from the group. Obesity places a tremendous social and emotional handicap on a child. Therefore it is of utmost importance that educators be concerned with his particular condition and give these children all possible assistance and guidance in alleviating obesity or adjusting to it.

Evaluating obesity. There are many ways that overweight or obesity can be determined; some of these are highly technical methods requiring sophisticated equipment, whereas others are relatively simple, but less valid. Some of the least recommended means of measuring fatness are the normative age, sex, and height/weight tables. These tables do not normally allow for the person who may have a preponderance of muscle tissue in place of fat or for those with wide frames and/or heavy skeletal structures. The most accurate method of determining fatness, which can easily be used by the adaptive physical educator, is the direct application of anthropometric measurement such as the Pryor width-weight technique and the skin fold measurement approach.[35]

The Pryor method predicts body weight based on an individual's skeletal structure. By ascertaining the lateral diameter of the chest at the nipple line and the width of the pelvis at the iliac crest (Fig. 7-10) and then comparing these measurements to the height and age of the individual, a predicted weight is determined.[35] Fig. 7-11 shows the Pryor method in predicting weight for boys 2 to 6 years of age.

Skin fold measurement provides both a simple and accurate method of assessing quantitatively the fat content of the human body.[39] It is applied to locations on the

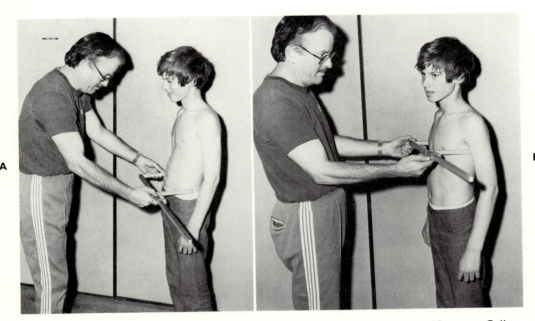

Fig. 7-10. Determining lateral diameter of the pelvis, **A,** and chest, **B.** (Courtesy California State University, Audio Visual Center, Long Beach, Calif.)

body where a fold of skin and subcutaneous fat can be lifted between the thumb and the forefinger so that it is held free of the muscular and bony structure. The skin fold caliper has become an evaluation tool for universal comparability of fat fold measurements. The accepted national recommendation is to have a caliper designed so as to exert a pressure of 10 gm/mm² on the caliper face. The contact surface area to be measured should be in the neighborhood of 20 to 40 mm². The skin fold measurement to be obtained should be picked up in standard fashion. The recommended method is to pinch a full fold of skin and subcutaneous tissue between the thumb and forefinger, at a distance of about 1 cm from the site on which the caliper is to be

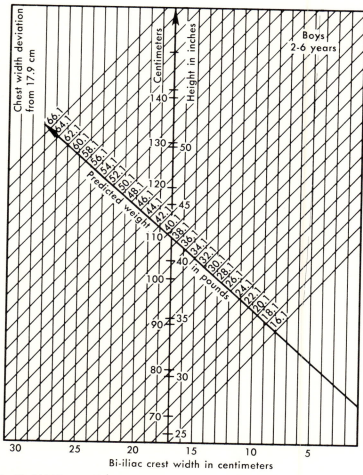

1. Find bi-iliac width at bottom of graph.
2. Follow the vertical channel indicated, up to standing height.
3. Take nearest slant axis to predicted weight.
4. Correct for chest width if necessary. (Go up 1 unit or down 1 unit for each centimeter that the chest measurement exceeds or falls short of the mean at the top of the graph.)

Fig. 7-11. Predicting weight for boys 2 to 6 years of age through the use of the Pryor method.

placed, and then to pull the fold away from the underlying muscle.[39]

The calipers are then applied to the fold about 1 cm below the fingers so that the pressure on the fold at the point measured is exerted by the faces of the calipers and not by the fingers. The handle of the caliper is then released and a recording is made to the nearest 0.5 mm. When skin folds are thick, the recording should be made 2 or 3 seconds after the caliper pressure is applied.

Although the skin fold at the triceps site has been thought by many to adequately represent total body fat, it is advisable, for the greatest accuracy, to take measurements at several additional body sites (Table 7-1).

Table 7-1. Obesity standards for white Americans*†

| Age (years) | Skin fold measurements (mm) | |
	Men	Women
5	12	14
6	12	15
7	13	16
8	14	17
9	15	18
10	16	20
11	17	21
12	18	22
13	18	23
14	17	23
15	16	24
16	15	25
17	14	26
18	15	27
19	15	27
20	16	28
21	17	28
22	18	28
23	18	28
24	19	28
25	20	29
26	20	29
27	21	29
28	22	29
29	23	29
30-50	23	30

*Minimum triceps skin fold thickness in millimeters indicating obesity. Figures represent the logarithmic means of the frequency distributions plus one standard deviation.
†Adapted from Seltzer, C. C., and Mayer, J.: Postgrad. Med. **38**:101-107, 1965.

Durnin and Rahaman,[17] for example, used four sites for their study of body fat content of 13- to 34-year-old persons: (1) the biceps, (2) the triceps, (3) the subscapular, and (4) the suprailiac areas (Table 7-2). Their method of taking skin fold measurements was as follows:

1. All subjects were seated.
2. Only measurements of the right side were taken.
3. The *biceps* were measured over the midpoint of the muscle (Fig. 7-12) while the forearm was resting supinated on the subject's thigh.
4. The *triceps* were measured at a point half the distance between the olecranon and acromion process while the arm was hanging vertically (Fig. 2-5, A).
5. The *subscapular* region was measured just below the tip and to the lateral side of the inferior angle of the scapula (Fig. 2-5, B).
6. The *suprailiac* region was measured just above the iliac crest at the midaxillary line (Fig. 2-5, C).

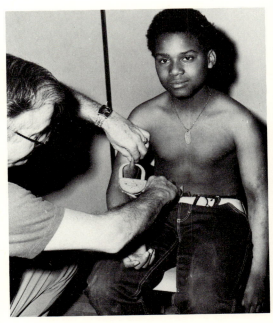

Fig. 7-12. Biceps skin fold measurement.

Table 7-2. Measurements required to determine total skin fold thickness at four skin fold sites (biceps, triceps, subscapular, and suprailiac)*

Body build	Skin fold measurement (mm)			
	Men	Women	Boys	Girls
Thin				
Mean	24.0	31.2	22.4	33.3
Standard deviation	7.1	6.3	5.3	9.5
Intermediate				
Mean	34.7	39.9	29.7	36.2
Standard deviation	15.7	10.0	7.6	8.8
Plump and obese				
Mean	57.2	66.0	43.2	49.0
Standard deviation	21.4	22.7	13.2	13.6

*Adapted from Durnin, J. V. G. A., and Rahaman, M. M.: Br. J. Nutr. **21**:681-689, 1967.

Table 7-3. Percentages of fat corresponding to the total of skin fold measurements at four sites (biceps, triceps, subscapular, and suprailiac)*

Total skin fold measurement (mm)	Body fat (%)			
	Men	Women	Boys	Girls
15	5.5	—	9.0	12.5
20	9.0	15.5	12.5	16.0
25	11.5	18.5	15.5	19.0
30	13.5	21.0	17.5	21.5
35	15.5	23.0	19.5	23.5
40	17.0	24.5	21.5	25.0
45	18.5	26.0	23.0	27.0
50	20.0	27.5	24.0	28.5
55	21.0	29.0	25.5	29.5
60	22.0	30.0	26.5	30.5
65	23.0	31.0	27.5	32.0
70	24.0	32.5	28.5	33.0
75	25.0	33.5	—	—
80	26.0	34.0	—	—
85	26.5	35.0	—	—
90	27.5	36.0	—	—
95	28.0	36.5	—	—

*From Durnin, J. V. G. A., and Rahaman, M. M.: Br. J. Nutr. **21**:681-689, 1967.

Durnin and Rahaman studied thin, intermediate, and obese adolescent boys and girls from the ages of 13 to 16 years and young adult men and women from the ages of 21 to 34 years. They also approximated the percentages of the subjects' body fat based on the four skin fold sites (Table 7-3).

Implications for physical education. Since overweight children are often handicapped in performing the activities of the physical education program efficiently, it is not uncommon for them to dislike many of these activities. Often, as a result of their lack of ability to participate in the program, they are the objects of practical jokes and disparaging remarks made by other children. Exposed to such an environment, the obese and overweight boys and girls become unhappy and ashamed and often withdraw from the activity to circumvent emotional involvement with the group.[27] It is of the utmost importance for the physical educator to attempt to create an environment that will enable the obese child to have successful experiences in the class, thus minimizing situations that could degrade the child's position as a person of positive worth. His assignment therefore might be either in an adapted class or in a regular class, depending on which would meet his needs more adequately. The physical educator is also challenged with regard to developing attitudes on the part of the nonhandicapped majority. Consequently, proposing the acceptance of children with differences to the normal group is an important and worthwhile goal of the physical educator.

There can be no one program for the remediation of children who are overweight. It is necessary that the true cause of the problem be found. When the cause of overweight or obesity is known, there are available several avenues of treatment; they are as follows:

1. Control of the diet by reduction of caloric intake
2. Medical treatment in the case of a glandular dysfunction
3. Counseling when emotional causes are at the root of the problem
4. Counseling on the consequences of obesity to the total personality
5. A program of exercise within the capacity of the child to increase energy expenditure in order to balance the caloric intake
6. Disruption of sedentary ways of living

It is sound reasoning in combating obesity and overweight to attempt to change living patterns in terms of physical activity and diet rather than to go into crash programs for fast reduction of weight. The habits of everyday living are of longer range than the crash programs and more value will be accrued by this type of living in the long run.

Obese and overweight students should be guided into activities that can be safely performed and successfully achieved. This will tend to encourage them to participate in more vigorous activities.[9, 31] Some of the activities that can be used to combat obesity are general conditioning exercises, dancing, rhythms, and sports and games based on ability and a chance for success. Much can be done for these children with personal guidance, encouragement, and selection of the proper developmental experience for the individual child.

A program for obese students is currently underway at Slippery Rock State College in Pennsylvania. The student is given therapeutic support in sustaining an individual exercise program and a low-calorie diet. One of the innovations that has assisted the program is a weekly weigh-in in which a projected number of pounds is scheduled to be reduced in a given week. The value of this weigh-in is that it projects a precise goal for the student to achieve each week. It is hoped that sustained reduction over a 15-week semester may afford opportunities for establishing eating and exercising patterns that will carry on beyond the semester. To date, the program has produced weight reduction of up to 25 pounds in an individual case. The general approach to the exercise program in which the student engages is one of progression. Exercises based on calculated energy expenditures are initiated with slight progression ensured in the program with each successive day of attendance. Activities that constitute the program are walking, jogging, bicycle riding, rope jumping, swimming, stair and hill climbing, and stepping up on and down from a bench. The main purpose of these exercise programs is to sustain moderate activity over a period of time in order to expend calories. If the student can be induced to engage in more than one exercise bout a day, this is of greater value.

Anemia

Anemia is a condition of the blood in which there is a deficiency of hemoglobin, which delivers oxygen to body tissues. This deficiency of hemoglobin may be a result of the quantity contained in the red corpuscles of the blood or a reduction in the number of red corpuscles themselves.

The physical education teacher should be aware of the characteristics that anemic persons display. In many instances, the anemic person appears to be pale because his blood is not as red as it is in typical persons. The person with anemia tires easily because of impaired oxidation in the muscles, and he also may become short of breath. Consequently, in many instances, the rate of breathing is increased. As a rule, children with anemia fatigue more easily than do typical children, are often unable to make gains in physical strength, and are impaired in learning motor skills.

Some of the symptoms that may give rise to suspecting anemia are an increased rate of breathing, a bluish tinge of the lips and nails (because the blood's color is not as red), headache, nausea, faintness, weakness, an inability to withstand the onset of fatigue, and a lack of strength.

Causes

There are many diverse reasons for the occurrence of anemia. The following are some of the main ones: (1) great loss of blood; (2) decreased blood production within the system; (3) diseases such as malaria, septic infections, and cirrhosis of the liver; (4) poisons such as lead, insecticides, and arsenobenzene; and (5) chronic dysentery, intestinal parasites, and diseases associated with endocrine deficiency and vitamin deficiencies. Anemia is symptomatic of a disturbance that in many cases can be remedied. Inasmuch as there are several varieties of anemia, the method of treatment is dependent on the type of anemia present.

Types

There are several forms of anemia. *Chlorosis* is a form of anemia that is characterized by a reduced amount of hemoglobin in the corpuscles and usually occurs in young women at about the time of puberty. Anemia can be caused by excessive hemorrhage, in which case the specific gravity of the blood is reduced because there is a

greater proportion of fluid in comparison with corpuscles in the blood. Occurring less often than chlorosis, *pernicious anemia* is characterized by a decrease in the number of red corpuscles. It can cause changes in the nervous system, along with loss of sensation in the hands and feet. In *aplastic anemia,* the red bone marrow that forms blood cells is replaced by fatty marrow. This form of anemia can be caused by radiation, radioactive isotopes, and atomic fallout. Certain antibiotics may also be a causative factor. *Iron deficiency anemia* is a form of anemia that afflicts millions of American women. It is caused by insufficient iron to replace that which is lost during each menstrual period. One prevalent type of anemia among blacks is *sickle cell anemia*. This type afflicts 8% of all blacks in the United States. Jones, Shainberg, and Byer[23] indicate that 50% of the blacks afflicted with this disease die before they reach the age of 20 years.

Treatment

The various forms of anemia require different treatments. Chlorosis may be remedied or cured by increasing the amount of iron-bearing foods in the diet. However, pernicious anemia requires the intramuscular injection of liver extracts. Aplastic anemia may be corrected by transplanting bone marrow from healthy subjects and by utilizing the male hormone testosterone, which is known to stimulate the production of cells by the bone marrow if enough red marrow is present for the hormone to act on. In the case of iron deficiency anemia, treatment consists of improving the iron content of the diet or taking diet supplements that contain iron. Vitamin B_{12}, which is important for bone marrow activity, is also an important ingredient in treating pernicious anemia. This is true because the gastric juice appears to be missing the substance, produced in the lining of the stomach, that promotes the absorption in the intestine of vitamin B_{12}, which is stored in the liver and released as required for the formation of red blood cells in the bone marrow.[37]

Implications for physical education

The final decision regarding the nature of physical education activities for a child with anemia should be made by medical personnel. A well-conceived and supervised physical education program can be of great value to the child who has anemia. Exercise stimulates the production of red blood cells through the increased demand for oxygen. However, to be beneficial, an activity must be planned qualitatively with regard to the specific anemic condition. It is worthwhile to note that it is not uncommon for children who have anemia to be retarded in the development of physical strength and endurance. Identification of the anemic condition and its cure often may result in significant gains in physical fitness and muscular endurance. The alert physical educator conceivably will be able to assist in the identification of anemia and thus to refer the student to medical authorities who may, in turn, alleviate the condition. Anemia that is undiagnosed may have social implications because of the possibility of curtailment in motor skill and physical development and may set the child apart from his peers in social experiences.

Aging

The science that studies aging man is called *gerontology*, whereas the field of *geriatrics* is concerned more specifically with diseases and management of old age.[1]

Aging in man is relative. Chronological age, the age in years, is a poor indicator of the stage of man's total development. Aging per se does not progress or decline at an even rate. There is great variability in anatomical, physiological, and psychological aging. Consequently, a man may have a chronological age of 50 years, the heart and arteries of a man age 30 years, and a mental vitality of age 25 years.

Therefore aging must be considered a dynamic biological process of growth and development and not merely degeneration

or organic regression.[15] Physiological aging, in general, produces a loss of the essential functioning substances of organs and the gradual degeneration of the organ systems to the less specialized fibrous connective and fatty tissues. The collagenous substances within the connective tissues of the body, such as those found in tendons and ligaments, become hardened and inelastic. Organs that undergo aging lose their ability for normal nutrient and metabolic transfer between the cellular structures and blood. Microscopic degeneration resulting in cellular death spreads and progresses to organs and subsequently to an entire organ system. Senescence occurs when the death rate of cells is greater than the rate of their respective reproduction.

Problems in aging

The cardiovascular system (CVS) is vital to the normal functioning of the entire body. Aging affects the CVS efficiency and subsequently results in alterations in the rate and efficiency of oxygen nutrient utilization. With age, connective tissue and fat content increases within inner surface membranes and cavities of the heart. The senile heart moves from an oblique to a more upright position. Valves become inelastic, resulting in a tendency toward dilation and muscular incompetency in the heart, with subsequent arrhythmia. Coronary arteries supplying the heart become thickened at their innermost lining (intima). Blood vessels, particularly arteries, display age by their inelasticity and thinning muscular walls. Stretched arteries become more twisted in their course. Degeneration and the collection of fat deposits further weaken artery walls. After structural arterial change comes a functional rise in systolic blood pressure and a lowering of diastolic pressure. The aging person's lungs gradually become inelastic, smaller, and, in general, less viable. Chest excursion may be hampered by the rigidity of the thorax as a result of the calcification of cartilaginous tissue. An inability to inhale or expand the chest fully produces lowered vital capacity and a decreased breathing capacity.

With senescence comes a number of musculoskeletal changes, primarily degeneration and atrophy of muscle fibers and resultant strength loss, cartilage calcification, and softening of bony structures through absorption of mineral matter *(osteoporosis)*. Joint changes also occur, resulting in articular degeneration and eventually arthritis. Disuse is the reason given for accentuated osteoporosis and muscular atrophy. Evidence indicates that strength diminishes very slowly during the mature adult period and increases its rate of decline after the fifth decade.

Gross brain size diminishes with age; microscopic studies show degeneration of the nerve ganglion cells as well as the highly specialized supporting elements of the nervous system. Anderson and Langton[1] indicate that with brain atrophy and cellular degeneration there occurs increased cerebrospinal fluid, thickened dura mater, and a decrease of general blood circulation with a resultant decrease in metabolism. Such alterations are manifested in slower learning and motor response, inability to visually accommodate near points (presbyopia), and a decrease in auditory acuity.

Organs of internal secretion, such as thyroid, pituitary, and adrenal glands, start a definite regression as aging progresses. Bodily functions controlled by the endocrine glands, such as basal metabolism rate (BMR) and resistance to infection, decline with age. Also the reproductive organs decline rapidly and cease to function at about 50 years of age for the female and 65 years of age for the male. Increasing age brings with it a decrease in androgenic hormones and increases in the speed of atrophy of muscular tissue and internal organs.

Wolff[42] summarized the basic findings of scientific investigation on the changes produced in aging as the following:

1. An increase in connective tissues
2. A gradual loss of connective tissue elasticity
3. A disappearance of nervous system cells
4. A reduction of normal cells
5. An increase in the amount of fat
6. A decrease in the ability to use oxygen
7. A decrease in blood volume while resting
8. A decrease in vital lung capacity
9. A decrease in muscle strength
10. A decrease in the amount of hormones and endocrine excretion

All adults are affected to some degree by pathological aging. A number of factors cause an individual's aging process to be either atypically slow or prematurely fast, namely, heredity, general adaptation to stress, and particular style of living. An individual's constitutional inheritance affects the aging process because it passes on deficiencies or the predisposition for certain diseases. Heredity also helps determine one's ability to adapt to life's stresses. Selye's[36] "general adaptation syndrome" (GAS) indicates that each individual is born with a given store of genetic energy that must be considered in the process of adaptation. Worry, fatigue, and constant muscular tension, together with improper physical activity, may constitute a life-style that would tend to exhaust genetic energies and result in premature aging.

As a person grows older, there is increased susceptibility to the condition of tissue deterioration. In general, the most common degenerative diseases are considered to be those of the heart, arteries, and kidneys. Anderson and Langton[1] described arteriosclerosis, hypertension, nephritis, and heart disease as a degenerative quartet. Arteriosclerosis, cancer, arthritis, rheumatic disorders, nervous diseases, and mental breakdowns are considered the most prevalent aging disorders.

Many authorities have attributed premature aging and degenerative diseases, primarily in the area of the cardiovascular system,[9, 19] to American living practices. A cause has not been singled out, but rather there appears to be a multitude of causes. The main ones might be listed as hypoactivity, overweight, excessive cigarette smoking, and worry.[29]

Over 100,000 Americans die each year from some major disease of the heart and/or blood vessels, not to mention those who are permanently disabled by such disease. This number accounts for about one half of the deaths that occur annually in the United States. Besides cardiovascular disease, the adult population suffers from untold orthopedic, emotional, and metabolic disorders that may be attributed directly or indirectly to contemporary life-styles.

Exercise and aging

To prevent involution, atrophy, and ultimate cellular and organ deaths, tissue stimulation must occur. Mateeff[30] states that "exercise is that vital factor that alone is capable not only of stopping the processes of involution and atrophy but also of reversing them, which promotes and brings into play the processes of self-repair and self-renovation at the molecular level in organisms of the aging." Exercise engaged in in a planned and progressive manner can produce such positive gains as increased strength and skeletal muscle hypertrophy, hypertrophy of the heart with the resultant training effect of decreased heart rate, increased ability to expend energy, more efficient use of oxygen, a greater vital capacity, and improved body suppleness from increased joint mobility.[32] Bortz[6] indicated that physical activity helps delay the diminution of sex hormone excretion

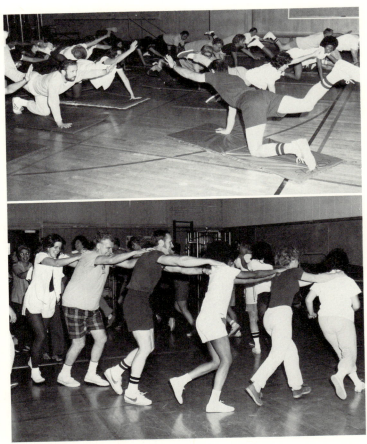

Fig. 7-13. An adult exercise program. (Courtesy Faculty Fitness Club, California State University, Long Beach, Calif.)

(Fig. 7-13). Activity therefore can maintain the anabolic protein-building qualities of the sex glands and concomitant muscle strength. Many physically active older persons express a higher level of vitality, ability to sleep, mental capacity, and desire for socialization than their sedentary counterparts.

To offset many of the problems of premature aging, preventive conditioning adapted physical education programs have been emerging in the United States, primarily in YMCA's, colleges, universities, municipal recreation departments, and private organizations. However, the government, insurance companies, and industries have been slow to respond to this need because of a lack of concrete evidence that preventive measures can be applied to the subfit adult. In these medically supervised programs, adults can remedy or offset the debilitating influences of inactivity.

As discussed previously, aging progresses at varying speeds in different persons and in different organs within the same person. However, the organ system that should be of the greatest concern to the average American today is the cardiovascular system. The reason for this concern is the degeneration that occurs in this system after 20 years of age. The total peripheral vascular resistance increases 1.7%/year, heart work output decreases 0.6%/year, and resting cardiac output and maximum work rate decrease about 1%/year.[38]

It has been pointed out that the fit, as compared to the unfit, individual has the ability to deliver oxygen to his body as it is required. On the other hand, an unfit person experiences a greater energy demand than physical capacity to deliver it.

Recent research studies and clinical observations point to the fact that regular physical activities may contribute to fitness by preventing obesity and by decreasing the possibility of premature coronary heart disease. Exercise for the mature adult increases the individual's potential for withstanding the stresses of life.[24, 29] Most authorities agree that the cardiovascular bene-

fits from exercise are as follows:

1. Improved oxygen economy of the heart
2. More effective parasympathetic and sympathoinhibitory counterbalances
3. Slower heart rate at rest and less acceleration during effort
4. Faster heart deceleration after exercise
5. Reduction of peripheral blood vessel resistance
6. Increased residual blood volume of the heart
7. Improved coronary blood flow as a result of increased collateral capillarization of heart muscle
8. Prolongation of coagulation time and a lowering of the serum cholesterol level

Although there are positive signs that exercise may be beneficial to the cardiovascular system, proof must come through further research. Studies have attempted to obtain definitive information from programs designed to *intervene actively* in living patterns of subjects who are either postcoronary patients or who are considered high-risk subjects, as determined by an electrocardiograph stress test. Such tests are administered by a cardiologist who determines whether there are ischemic heart changes after exercise. Test results serve as a useful index for the amount of exercise in which an individual can safely engage.[3, 21]

Implications for physical education

With the increased awareness of the deleterious effect of inactivity on the sedentary adult population, physical education has emerged with new importance. Through the efforts of many disciplines, the public is beginning to realize that proper exercise can be a deterrent to many characteristics of premature physiological aging as well as to their concomitant diseases.

Recent research and studies have resulted in new concepts about the type of physical fitness activities best suited for adults. Rhythmical, continuous, and sustained activities can serve as preventive conditioners. Activities that are explosive in nature tend to place an abnormal demand on the heart and vascular system and should be avoided until the individual reaches an appropriate fitness level. Isotonic exercise is preferable to isometric exercise, particularly in cases of cardiovascular disease history. Isometric exercise may result in irregular heartbeats, premature ventricular contractions, and abnormally fast heartbeats in heart disease patients.

A multidisciplinary approach has resulted from medicine's concern for premature cardiovascular disease and the positive effects of proper exercise. The physician, physical educator, applied physiologist, and many other professional persons are lending their particular skill to help solve the problem of adult physical fitness. With the implementation of many medically oriented adult physical education programs, there is an increased need for trained adapted physical education teachers who understand the problems and needs of the adult population. Establishing individualized physical education programs for adults is one of the greatest challenges of our times.

REFERENCES

1. Anderson, C. L.: Health principles and practice, ed. 6, St. Louis, 1970, The C. V. Mosby Co.
2. Arnheim, D. D., and Pestolesi, R. A.: Developing motor behavior in children: a balanced approach to elementary physical education, St. Louis, 1973, The C. V. Mosby Co.
3. Astrand, I.: Clinical and physiological studies of manual workers 50-64 years old at rest and during work, Acta Med. Scand. **162:** 155, 1958.
4. Billing, H. E., and Lowendahl, E.: Mobilization of the human body, Stanford, Calif., 1949, Stanford University Press.
5. Bogert, L. J., et al.: Nutrition and physical fitness, ed. 9, Philadelphia, 1973, W. B. Saunders Co.
6. Bortz, E. L.: Creative aging, New York, 1963, Macmillan Publishing Co., Inc.
7. Clarke, H. H.: Circulatory-respiratory endurance improvement, Phys. Fitness Res. Digest Ser. 4, No. 3, Washington, D.C., President's Council on Physical Fitness and Sports.
8. Clarke, H. H., editor: Development of muscular strength and endurance, Phys. Fitness Res. Digest Ser. 4, No. 1, Washington, D.C., 1973, President's Council of Physical Fitness and Sports.
9. Clarke, H. H.: Exercise and fat reduction, Phys. Fitness Res. Digest Ser. 5, No. 2, Washington, D.C., 1975, President's Council on Physical Fitness and Sports.
10. Clarke, H. H.: Joint and body range of movement, Phys. Fitness Res. Digest Ser. 5, No. 4, Washington, D.C., 1975, President's Council on Physical Fitness and Sports.
11. Clarke, H. H.: Physical fitness testing in schools, Phys. Fitness Res. Digest. Ser. 5, No. 1, Washington, D.C., 1975, President's Council on Physical Fitness and Sports.
12. Clarke, H. H.: Strength development and motor-sports improvement, Phys. Fitness Res. Digest Ser. 4, No. 4, Washington, D.C., 1974, President's Council on Physical Fitness and Sports.
13. Clarke, H. H., editor: Towards a better understanding of muscular strength, Phys. Fitness Res. Digest Ser. 4, No. 1, Washington, D.C., 1973, President's Council on Physical Fitness and Sports.
14. Clarke, H. H., and Carter, G. H.: Oregon simplification of the strength and physical fitness indices, Res. Q. **30:**3-10, 1959.
15. Course syllabus: principles and practice of geriatric rehabilitation, New York, 1960, New York College, Metropolitan Medical Center, Physical Medicine and Rehabilitation Department.
16. deVries, H. A.: Warm-up effects of relaxation and stretching techniques upon gross motor performance. Unpublished doctoral dissertation, University of Southern California, 1961.
17. Durnin, J. V. G. A., and Rahaman, M. M.: The assessment of the amount of fat in the human body from measurements of skin fold thickness, Br. J. Nutr. **21:**681-689, 1967.
18. Fleishmann, E. A.: The structure and measurement of physical fitness, Englewood Cliffs, N.J., 1963, Prentice-Hall, Inc.
19. Guild, W. R.: How to keep fit and enjoy it, New York, 1967, Cornerstone Library, Inc.
20. Gurney, R.: Hereditary factors in obesity, Arch. Intern. Med. **57:**557-561, 1956.
21. Haskell, W. L., and Fox, S. M.: The possible place of stress testing to discover and physical activity to prevent, coronary heart disease, South. Med. J. Assoc. **59:**642-647, 1966.
22. Hettinger, T.: Physiology of strength, Springfield, Ill., 1961, Charles C Thomas, Publisher.
23. Jones, K., Shainberg, L., and Byer, C.: Principles of health science, New York, 1975, Harper & Row, Publishers.
24. Kraus, H., and Hirschland, R. P.: Minimum muscular fitness in school children, Res. Q. **25:**178-188, 1954.

25. Kraus, H., and Raab, W.: Hypokinetic disease, Springfield, Ill., 1961, Charles C Thomas, Publisher.
26. Logan, G. A., and Egstrom, G.: Effects of slow and fast stretch on the sacrofemoral angle, Paper presented to AAHPER Southern District Convention, April, 1955, Albequerque, N.M.
27. Lourie, R. S.: A pediatric-psychiatric viewpoint on obesity, Pediatrics **20:**552-556, 1957.
28. Marks, H. H.: Influence of obesity on morbidity and mortality, Bull. N.Y. Acad. Med. **36:**196-313, 1960.
29. Master, A. M., Jaffe, H. L., and Chesky, K.: Relationship of obesity to coronary disease and hypertension, J.A.M.A. **153:**1449-1501, 1953.
30. Mateeff, D.: Problems of the fight for longevity, Quest, 1964.
31. Mayer, G.: Obesity in school children, Nutr. Rev. **15:**233, 1957.
32. Mayer, J.: Middle-aged man must exercise, Postgrad. Med. J. **40:**127-132, 1966.
33. Morgan, R. E., and Adamson, G. T.: Circuit training, London, 1961, G. Bell & Sons, Ltd.
34. Pryor, H. B.: Charts of normal body measurements and revised width-weight tables in graphic form, J. Pediatr. **68:**615-631, 1966.
35. Pryor, H. B.: Width-weight tables, ed. 2, Stanford, Calif., 1936, Stanford University Press.
36. Selye, H.: The stress of life, New York, 1956, McGraw-Hill Book Co.
37. Stecher, P. G., et al.: The Merck index, ed. 8, Rahway, N.J., 1968, Merck & Co., Inc.
38. Stein, J.: Adaptation of the internal system to general exercises and calisthenics, Phys. Educ. **17:**1-6, 1960.
39. U.S. Public Health Service: Obesity and health, Washington, D.C., 1966, U.S. Government Printing Office.
40. Vodala, T. M.: Individualized physical education program for the handicapped child, Englewood Cliffs, N.J., 1973, Prentice-Hall, Inc.
41. Wilkes, E. T.: A survey of three hundred obese girls, Arch. Pediatr. **77:**441-452, 1960.
42. Wolff, K.: The biological, sociological, and psychological aspects of aging, Springfield, Ill., 1959, Charles C Thomas, Publisher.
43. Youth fitness test manual, Washington, D.C., 1965, American Association for Health, Physical Education, and Recreation.

RECOMMENDED READINGS

Behnke, A. R., and Wimore, J. H.: Evaluations and regulations of body build and composition, Englewood Cliffs, N.J., 1974, Prentice-Hall, Inc.

Bowerman, W. J., and Harris, W. E.: Jogging: a physical fitness program for all ages, New York, 1967, Grosset & Dunlap, Inc.

Clarke, H. H.: Muscular strength and endurance in man, Englewood Cliffs, N.J., 1966, Prentice-Hall, Inc.

Cooper, K. H.: Aerobics, New York, 1970, Bantam Books, Inc.

Guthrie, H. A.: Introductory nutrition, ed. 3, St. Louis, 1975, The C. V. Mosby Co.

The healthy life: special report, New York, 1966, Time-Life Books.

Williams, S. R.: Nutrition and diet therapy, ed. 2, St. Louis, 1973, The C. V. Mosby Co.

8

MODIFYING SPORTS AND GAMES

■ No program of adapted physical education should be considered complete unless it includes provision for modifying sports and games. Many persons have traditionally thought of the adapted physical education program as consisting of only special exercises done daily by the students enrolled in a special class. Although the special exercise program is highly desirable and is needed by many of the students in an adapted program, there are many reasons that it is desirable to include a program of modified sports and games for these students. Some of the reasons for including adapted sports activities in the program are the following:

1. There are many students assigned to an adapted physical education class who are unable to correct an existing condition, but who also are unable to participate in regular physical education. A program of adapted sports would be ideal for such students.

2. Students in the adapted physical education program need activities that have carry-over value. They may continue exercise programs in the future, but they also need training in carry-over types of sports and games that will be useful to them in later life.

3. Adapted sports activities may have a therapeutic value if they are carefully structured for the student.

4. Adapted sports and games should help the handicapped individual learn to handle his body under a variety of circumstances.

5. There are recreational values in games and sports activities for the student who is facing the dual problem of getting a good education and overcoming some

type of handicap; some of his special needs can best be met through recreational kinds of activities.

6. A certain amount of emotional release takes place in play activities and this is important to the student with a disability.

7. The adapted sports program, whether it is given every other day or several weeks out of the semester, tends to relieve the boredom of a straight exercise program. No matter how carefully a special exercise program is planned and organized, it is difficult to maintain a high level of interest if the students participate in this kind of activity on a daily basis for one or more semesters.

Not all students in the adapted physical education program need to have special games and sports activities conducted as a part of this program. Some students will be able, for part of their time in school, to attend regular classes in physical education because these classes meet the special needs and interests of these students. This practice should be encouraged in the school so that there is a free exchange of students between the so-called regular physical education classes and the special classes in adapted physical education. Sometimes students in regular physical education classes who sustain an injury or come back from an illness need to have a special exercise or a special activity program. When cooperation exists between the medical service and the teachers of the adapted and the regular physical education classes, these students are assigned to the adapted class for their physical education so that they can profit from the special attention received there.

When one hears the title "adapted games and sports," two kinds of activities might very well come to mind: (1) there are certain kinds of physical education activities that lend themselves especially well to activity programs for students who have some kind of a physical handicap and (2) almost any activity that can be engaged in by a student in a regular physical education class in public or private schools can be modified to the special needs of students. Actually, in its broadest sense, the adapted sports and games program should include both these categories. Each of them is discussed in some detail in the following sections of this chapter.

MODIFICATION OF GAMES AND SPORTS FOR ADAPTED PHYSICAL EDUCATION CLASSES

Practically all games and sports in which students regularly participate in physical education classes in our schools can, with minor modifications, be made safe and interesting for students in the adapted class. A general rule to consider might be that the rules, techniques, and equipment of a game or activity should be changed as little as possible when modified for the adapted physical education students who are participating in it. It should, however, retain as many of the elements of the regular game or activity as possible. Some of the ways that regular physical education and sports activities can be modified are the following:

1. The size of the playing area can be made smaller, reducing the amount of activity proportionately.

2. Often, larger balls or larger pieces of equipment can be introduced so that the game is easier or so that the tempo of the game is slowed down.

3. For other types of games and sports, a smaller, lighter ball or striking implement may be necessary (plastic or styrofoam balls and plastic bats) or an object that is easier to handle (a bean bag or Nerf ball) can be substituted.

4. More players can be added to a team, reducing the amount of activity and the responsibility of individuals in a game.

5. Minor rule changes can be made while as many of the basic rules of the contest or game as possible are retained.

6. The amount of time allowed for play can be reduced by providing shorter quarters or the total time for a game or contest can be reduced.

7. An attempt can be made to avoid "head-lining" by any one player. In games such as softball, soccer, and football, players can be required to rotate positions frequently so that all the participants will have an opportunity to perform various kinds of activities and play various positions (as long as a particular position or activity would not be contraindicated for any one of the participants).

8. The number of points required to win a contest can be reduced.

9. Free substitutions can be made, allowing the students alternately to participate and then have a rest period while the contest continues.

Any or all of these modifications can be made in a game or contest in order to modify it for selected students in the adapted physical education program (Fig. 8-1).

In addition to these modifications of games and sports, it is also possible to provide activities similar to those being engaged in by the regular physical education classes by using many of the sports fundamentals that are involved and by practicing them in drill types of activities. Examples would be playing such games as "twenty-one," "two on two," "around the world," or taking free throws as lead-up activities to basketball. Working on punting, passing, running pass patterns, and place kicking may be done in preparation for participation in football. Pitching, batting, throwing, catching, fielding, and games such as "over the line" can be played as lead-up activities for softball. Serving, stroking, volleying, and the like can be practiced as lead-up activities for tennis. In all cases, these activities serve as modifications of a sport or game, provide interesting activities for the student, and ensure similar kinds of drills to those being engaged in by the regular physical education student. They also help the adapted physical education students become more skillful in various activities, so that when they return to a regular class or are able to participate in the whole game or sport, they are able to do so with a reasonable degree of success.

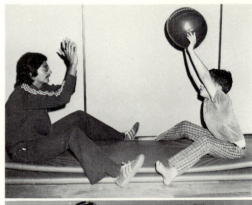

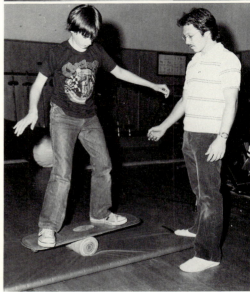

Fig. 8-1. Modifying activities for indoor classes. **A,** Medicine ball. **B,** Balance board. **C,** Combatives. **D** and **E,** Rebound activities. (Courtesy California State University, Audio Visual Center, Long Beach, Calif.)

SAFETY ASPECTS OF THE PROGRAM

Adapted physical education instructors must constantly be aware of any situation in the adapted activity program that would be hazardous to students in their classes. They must also be alert to any situation that would tend to aggravate the condition of any of the students. For these reasons, each activity must be assigned to a student on an individual basis, predicated when-

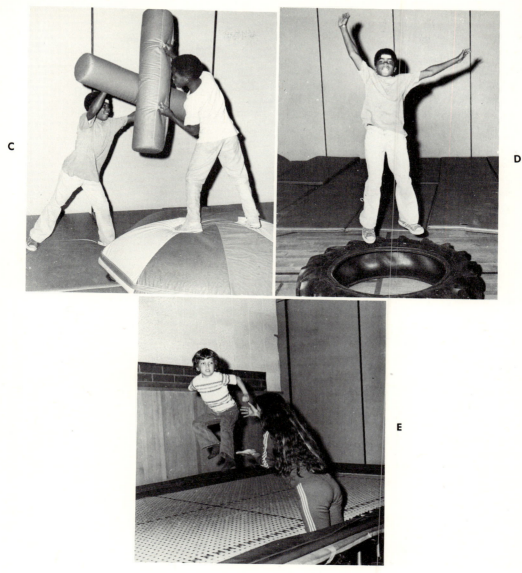

C

D

E

Fig. 8-1, cont'd. For legend see opposite page.

ever possible on the student's interest, but, more important, based on the good judgment of the physical education teacher and on the recommendations of the physician. All students in the program must be cautioned to watch for certain signs indicating that they or their classmates are involved in the wrong activity or that they are overdoing in any of their activity programs. Students should be instructed to stop an activity and report to the instructor if any of the following conditions are noted: (1) pain in any part of the body, (2) dyspnea (shortness of breath), (3) abnormal amount of flushing about the face, (4) feeling of general systemic fatigue, or (5) cyanosis (blueness of the lips).

If students are observed to have these conditions or if they report them to the instructor, their activity program must imme-

Table 8-1. Suggested activities, games, and sports for adapted physical education classes

	Hindman[9]		Chapman[3]
	Book I	Book II	
Indoor games			
QUIET GAMES			
Card games			212-213
Concentration (2 players)	140		
Authors (4-8 players)	141		
Go fish (3-6 players)	142		
Wild eights (crazy eights) (2-4 players)	143		
Card cutting			221
Paper and pencil games			
Ticktacktoe (2 players)	147		
Battleship (2 players)	149		206-208
Table games			
Pyramid (2 players)	151		
Checkers (2 players)			
Dominoes (2 players)	92, 212		
Chess (2 players)			
Crokinole (carom) (2-4 players)	195		
Box hockey (2 players)			
Shuffleboard (table or floor) (2-4 players)	210-212		
Croquet (2-4 players)			
ACTIVE GAMES			
Races and relays			
Head-balance race (or relay)	165		
Ping-Pong race (or relay)	166		
Paper clip relay (5-8 players on team)	174		
Arch pass relay (4-8 players on team)	178		
Car (pencil) relay (4-8 players on team)	180		
Hand clasp relay (4-8 players on team)	181		
Folding chair relay (4-8 players on team)	183		
Through-the-hoop relay (4-8 players on team)	184		
Sitting through-the-hoop relay (4-8 players on team)	184		
Rubber band relay (4-8 players on team)	185		
Over-and-under relay (8-20 players)			248-249
Throwing objects			
Balloon throw (shot put) (any number)	186		
Balloon hammer throw (any number)	186		
Playing card throw (any number)	186		220
Soda straw throw (javelin) (any number)	187		
Ball blow (asthma) (any number)	188		
Indoor lawn bowling (2-6 players)	193		
Indoor quoits (2-4 players)	194		
Bean bag board (2-4 players)	200		219, 238
Magic-square toss (2-4 players)	202		
Ball-board (2 players)	204		
Ring toss (2-4 players)			250

Eisenberg[6]	Pomeroy[13]	Fait[7]	Arnheim and Pestolesi[2]	Van Hagen, Dexter, Williams[16]	Anderson, Elliot, LaBerge[1]	Ercapep[5]
363						
443						
432-434				465		
439-440				908-909 583-585		
		235-241	229-241	427-432		GR 1-23
				491-492		
379			239			
				593	183	GR 26
421-422		235-241				GTC 1-24
387-388						
387-388						
387-388						
387-388						
423	316					
426-429	309			536-538		
426-427		237		536-538		
				536-538		
422-423	316					GTC 5

Continued.

Table 8-1. Suggested activities, games, and sports for adapted physical education classes—cont'd

	Hindman[9]		Chapman[3]
	Book I	Book II	
Indoor games—cont'd			
GAMES FOR ADAPTED ROOM			
Elementary school			
Tag with variations (5-20 players)		10-27	
Posture tag (5-20 players)		24	
Pom-pom pullaway with variations (10-20 players)		39-44	
Snatch-the-handkerchief with variations (10-20 players)		56-58	245
Hop scotch and variations (5-20 players)			
Swat tag with variations (15-30 players)		65, 81	239
Circle rush (10-25 players)		89	
Circle squat with variations (10-25 players)		175	
Simon says with variations (10-25 players)		177	251-252
Follow the leader (2-25 players)			246
Statues (10-20 players)			
Secondary school and college			
Rec-room shuffleboard (2 players)	210-212		
Table shuffleboard (2 players)	212		
Tenpins (bowling) with variations (2 players)		184	
Medicine ball (2-20 players)			262
Stall bar activities			265-266
Steal the bacon (15-30 players)			252-253
Swat tag with variations (15-30 players)		65, 81	239
Follow the leader with variations (2-20 players)			246
Wastebasket basketball (4-20 players)			
Outdoor games and sports			
Games of low organization			
Dodge ball with variations (15-30 players)		112-119	244-245
Around the world (2-8 players)		224	
Twenty-one with variations (2-8 players)		224-229	268-269
Punt drive (association football) (4-20 players)		246-247	
Tetherball (2 players)		268-270	253-254
Parachute play			
Games and sports			
Field hockey with variations (12-22 players)		403-408	
Football variations		367-368, 397-400	275
Basketball variations (2-10 players)		362-365	257-258, 291-2
Table tennis with variations (2-4 players)		280-282	267-268
Bowling			272
Shuffleboard with variations (2-4 players)		216-220	262-263
Golf with variations			259-260
Archery (archery golf)		202	
Goal hi			258-259
Volleyball and Newcomb with variations (4-20 players)		250, 254-260	269-270
Softball with variations (4-20 players)		311-329	273-274

Eisenberg[6]	Pomeroy[13]	Fait[7]	Arnheim and Pestolesi[2]	Van Hagen, Dexter, Williams[16]	Anderson, Elliot, LaBerge[1]	Ercapep[5]
463-469		229-241	224-227 227-239	410	238	GFC 1-15 GFC 14
475						
466		239				GL 11
467						GPG 3, 4 GCF 40
336		238	239 226	486-487	153	
341				411		
	308	239	233	421		
439-440				908-909		
439				908		
449		242	234	641		GCF 42
467						
373						
480		234 243-244	231-243 244 255 255 257	409, 683-684 799-800 671-672	189 283 283 256	GTC 17-21 GB 7 GB 9
444	320	244-246	245 200-201	588, 917	197	GPG 12
		298-301	257-260	752-774 659-661, 745-751, 756-761, 792- 799	243-265	GT 1-6
		290-293	247-256	661-668, 678-679 720-749	274-300	GB 1-13 GR 29-31
343	321	281-286		789-791	208-211	
311		265-266		634, 889		
439	317	286-288		892-894		
	313	268-276				
	310	262-265				
				649-652		
	323	301-303	248, 254-255	801-811	311-332	GV 1-9
	321	294-298	248-249, 260-263	566-581	353, 369, 190	GBA 1-21

Continued.

Table 8-1. Suggested activities, games, and sports for adapted physical education classes—cont'd

	Hindman[9]		Chapman[3]
	Book I	**Book II**	
Outdoor games and sports—cont'd			
Games and sports—cont'd			
Paddle tennis		278-280	
Tennis with variations (2-4 players)		261-262, 270-278	275
Croquet (roquet) (2-6 players)		199-201	240-242
Horseshoe pitching (2-4 players)		203	261-262
Quoits (2-4 players)		206	
Lawn bowling with variations (2-4 persons)		207-213	256
Handball with variations (2-4 players)		283-288, 295	
Deck tennis (quoitennis) (2-8 players)		252-253	256-257
Badminton (2-4 players)		262-266	254-255
Aerial darts (2-4 players)		266-268	
Soccer with variations (2-24 players)			273
Kickball with variations (2-24 players)			247-248
Pateca (2-4 players)			
Track and field			
AQUATIC GAMES AND ACTIVITIES			
Water games			
Swimming			274
Baseball type (4-20 players)		322-323	
Basketball type (4-20 players)		370	270
Water polo (4-20 players)			275-276
OUTDOOR EDUCATION			
Boating and canoeing			
Fishing			
Camping, hiking, and nature study			
Rhythm and dance			88-116
Square dance			106-116
Social dance			98-102
Folk dance			104-106
Fundamental rhythms			
Creative rhythms			
Running and jogging			

diately be reevaluated and reassignment or modification of their activity programs may be necessary.

SELECTED ADAPTED GAMES

A large selection of interesting games geared to the interest and ability levels of various age and disability groups can be found in a number of standard sources in the library. These will often be listed under the categories of games or recreational activities recommended for the elementary, the junior and senior high school, or the college age level; according to the type of activity involved, for example, *quiet games, low organization games,* and *active games;*

Eisenberg[6]	Pomeroy[13]	Fait[7]	Arnheim and Pestolesi[2]	Van Hagen, Dexter, Williams[16]	Anderson, Elliot, LaBerge[1]	Ercapep[5]
	312 316	275-278		669-670 411, 653, 853-854 764-768	200	GPG 8, 11
485		257		549-552, 561 868-870 561, 855-860	208-211 198-199 321, 332	
	310	278-281				
	323	241	250, 255	773-788	222-250	GS 1-7, GR 32
486-487			249		212-218	
		270-272	257	484-485	339-347	GTF 1-10
489-493 84, 490	317-320			152-153		
	310 312	329-337		875-876		
236 494-540		257-259 259 256-257 254-256	218-223 208-218 205-206 206-208	191-197 204 211, 214 207-210, 931	440-446 412-438 377-384 385-398	RF 1-18 RSD 1-24 RFD 1-44 RF 19-25
			257	172-175		PFA 10, 11 PFC 3-5

or according to the type of activity area needed, for example, table games, indoor games, and outdoor games. Some authors have even organized their adapted sports and games according to disabilities so the teacher can find recommended activities under such headings as cardiac conditions, asthma, or cerebral palsy. Many of these games can be used as described, but others will have to be modified for use in the adapted program. Careful study of these references and a little ingenuity on the part of teachers will enable them to select a number of these games for inclusion in the program (Table 8-1).

Adapted games and sports are generally

offered in one of several activity areas in the physical education plant: the adapted physical education room, the gymnasium, the blacktop area, the fields, the pool, or the dance studio.

Indoor games
Games in the adapted room

A program of games in the adapted room can be used to motivate students before or after their regular exercise program. Often, contests and relays can be organized to include some of the actual exercises and activities that the students participate in during their regular exercise program. A typical lesson in the adapted physical education room might consist of the following activities: a short formal warm-up for all students led by the instructor, followed by 15 minutes of special and group exercises done by individuals and small groups of students in the class, and then a 10-minute game and activity period under the general direction of the teacher.

A few examples of the kinds of activities that might be given in this type of a situation follow. A posture relay might be conducted with squads chosen by the instructor according to their special abilities or limitations. The students would run a traditional type of relay, but would be walking with headboards or books balanced on their heads, thus working for good balance and good body mechanics as they participate in the relay. A game of swat tag with students deployed in a circular formation could be used in a similar way. This is a very popular kind of activity for a boys' class in adapted physical education. A pigeon-toe walk relay might be given that involved short distances, but required that the student throw the foot into an over-corrected position while involved in this lap of the relay. There might be relays for students to pick up marbles with the toes and drop them into a box, using an activity similar to an exercise that they might have in the exercise program for their feet. Over-the-head and under-the-leg passing relays are popular as is passing a volleyball, basketball, or medicine ball back over and through a squad line. Another activity that has proved to be quite successful is to have an interesting obstacle course set up in the adapted physical education room. Students then move through each obstacle, performing an exercise or stunt or demonstrating a skill as required (Fig. 8-2). Many games that can be played in a small space and indoors can be selected from one of the standard game books. Such selections should be appropriate for the age level, the interest level, and the capacities of the students in the adapted class. Lists of such games and activities are included in Table 8-1.

Games in other areas

Other games that require more space or more height than would be found in the adapted room may be offered in the gym, in the apparatus room, in the multipurpose room, on a blacktop area, in the pool, in the dance studio, or on the athletic fields. Whenever possible, it is desirable to have the students in the adapted class participate in a variety of activities outdoors (Fig. 8-3). Games of low organization lend themselves to this kind of activity and prove to be very popular with the students in the adapted class. Many of these games require no special type of floor or deck space and involve the use of equipment that is readily available from the regular physical education program. Lead-up activities for football, basketball, speedball, volleyball, soccer, softball, hockey, and the like can also be offered.

Special area for adapted sports

It is also possible for a special adapted sports area to be constructed to provide the kinds of activities that would lend themselves particularly well to students in a program of this nature. Special areas for adapted sports are described in Chapter 20. These special areas allow for participation in a variety of activities all concentrated in one area so that they can be supervised by one adapted physical educa-

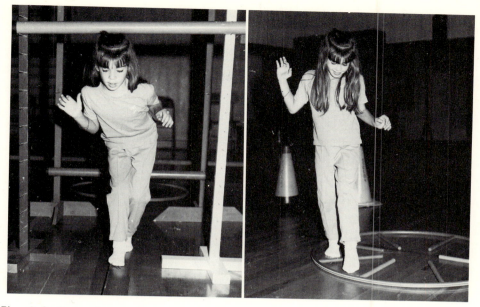

Fig. 8-2. Parts of a perceptual-motor obstacle course. (Courtesy California State University, Audio Visual Center, Long Beach, Calif.)

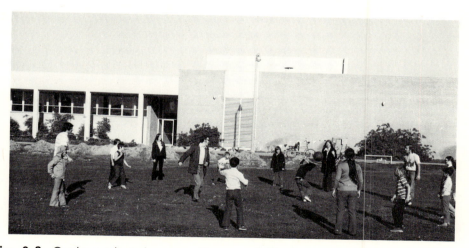

Fig. 8-3. Outdoor adapted games. (Courtesy California State University, Audio Visual Center, Long Beach, Calif.)

tion instructor. Paddle tennis, modified volleyball, croquet, shuffleboard, horseshoes, deck tennis, and table tennis provide interest and activity for the adapted physical education students. These activities usually do not have to be modified for students in the program and they are less frequently offered in the regular physical education program.

MODIFYING GAMES AND SPORTS FOR SELECTED DISABILITIES

Since most physical, mental, and emotional handicaps are quite individual in

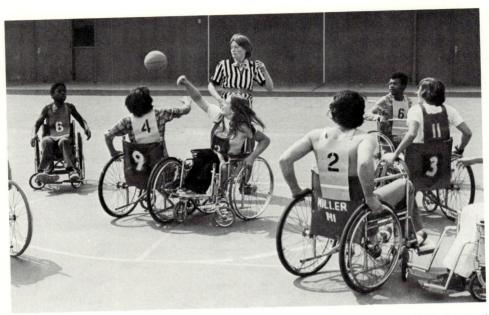

Fig. 8-4. Wheelchair basketball. (Courtesy Lyonel Avance, Los Angeles City Unified School District, Special Education Division, Los Angeles, Calif.)

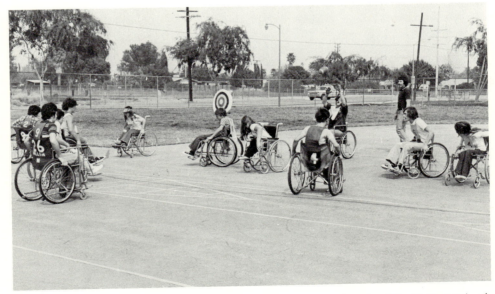

Fig. 8-5. Wheelchair football. (Courtesy Lyonel Avance, Los Angeles City Unified School District, Special Education Division, Los Angeles, Calif.)

terms of what the person can and cannot do, only selected examples of how a variety of activities can be modified will be offered in this chapter. Complete texts have been written on this subject and these and other references are recommended for further study in Table 8-1 (Figs. 8-4 and 8-5).

Aquatics

1. Provide a device (metronome, music, etc.) that emits a sound or signal so that the blind or visually handicapped person retains his orientation while in the pool.
2. Teach the person with one arm to swim the side stroke with his remaining arm on the lower side of the body to allow him to retain his balance and breathe without difficulty.
3. Teach those with partial loss of locomotion to move in the swimming pool, where body weight is minimal and muscle reeducation and body locomotion can take place during a carefully graded exercise and/or activity program.

Team sports

1. *Volleyball.* A volleyball game is modified for a senior high school adapted class by changing it as follows: Nine players are permitted on each team, a serve can be helped over the net by a teammate for selected players, and two players are permitted to catch and then throw the ball in place of a proper pass. All other rules and techniques are the same as for a regular game.
2. *Softball.* A junior high school class of girls are playing "over the line," an adaptation of softball. The rules are modified as follows: A runner is provided for one of the girls, the line over which the ball must be hit is moved closer to the batter for three of the girls, and seven players are permitted on each team.

Dual sports

1. *Badminton.* Four students in wheelchairs and four students with mild cardiac disorders in a college adapted class are scheduled for a game of badminton with four players on each side. Those in wheelchairs play up front; each is backed up by his cardiac teammate. Players do not rotate and each side is permitted two side outs before relinquishing the serve. The serve is alternated between the short man and the deep man. Only the serving team scores.
2. *Table tennis.* A game of table tennis is modified so a boy on crutches can compete with a boy with one arm. The only changes necessary are that the crutch walker plays only one side of his half of the table. The amputee serves by balancing the ball on his paddle, throwing it up in the air and striking it for the serve. If the ability level is still different, a handicap can be applied to the score until competition is equalized.

Individual sports

1. *Archery.* Archery can be modified in many ways to meet the special needs of boys and girls in adapted physical education classes. Blind students need a raised pointer along the ground or floor to direct them toward the target. They also need a rack to guide them in the placement of their front and back hands (to aid in giving direction and also to show how far to pull). Students with loss of strength in one hand may need to have the bow strapped to that hand. The arrow can then be properly drawn and released with the other hand. Students with leg involvement can have other students retrieve their arrows and they can shoot from crutches or a wheelchair.
2. *Bowling.* Most children and adults can be taught to bowl, regardless of their physical handicap. Bowling can be set up in the gymnasium, on the green, or at regulation bowling alleys. Adaptations for a wheelchair bowler might consist of utilizing a smaller or lighter ball or, in cases of bilateral hand and arm weakness, holding a special chute in the patient's lap, from which the ball is

rolled to hit the pins. Wheelchair bowlers and those with problems of ambulation can use a preliminary arm swing rather than the traditional walking approach to increase the momentum and accuracy of their delivery.

Dancing and rhythms

Participation in rhythmic activities provides an important recreational outlet for many disabled persons and often provides therapeutic values as well. Many students with neuromuscular problems, including some types of cerebral palsy, can benefit from rhythmic exercises and may also profit from various types of dancing. Increased relaxation, coordination, and timing are often experienced during rhythmic activities performed to the tempo of a metronome, record, or tape or to sound patterns provided by other students using drums, tambourines, and rhythm sticks (see Fig. 20-17). Some adaptations may be necessary to protect the individual as he participates in various types of rhythmic activities. These include the following:

1. Many activities are extremely vigorous and stimulating and should be contraindicated for the severely handicapped. Time limits and scheduled rest periods should be provided for others.
2. Certain groups, such as the mentally retarded, may need a considerable amount of individual attention during rhythmic activities and progress may be very slow until fundamentals are learned.
3. Placement of the student should be carefully considered in relation to his ability to hear the music, see the demonstration, and imitate a skill or move about easily in a dance pattern (either square or modern).
4. Psychological and emotional needs of the student may be better satisfied in rhythmic types of activities than in many other adapted activities. The proper type and amount of activity must be carefully selected by a competent and understanding teacher.

SELECTED ADAPTED SPORTS

Many students in the adapted physical education program can participate in selected sports offered in the regular physical education program and, if schedules permit, may be allowed to participate in these activities in one of the regular physical education classes (mainstreaming). However, since this often is not possible, it is necessary for adapted physical education teachers to organize their own programs of sports activities, which are similar to those being engaged in by the regular physical education classes, so that their students will have the opportunity to engage in as many of the regular activities as possible. These sports activities should be offered in the appropriate activity area, using equipment as similar as possible to that being used by the regular classes and with only minor adaptations in the rules of the contest when necessary. Since a class in adapted physical education is usually small, an excellent opportunity exists for individual instruction. These students will thus be able to bring their skills to a relatively high performance level. Compared to opportunities for specialized instruction in the larger regular physical education classes, those in adapted physical education have a decided advantage.

Swimming activities and therapeutic exercises in the pool

Students in an adapted physical education program often can profit from either a swimming improvement or a therapeutic exercise program specifically designed to meet their needs in the swimming pool. Although swimming facilities are usually heavily scheduled, it is often possible for the teacher of adapted physical education to offer a unit on swimming either between regular classes or by using the shallow end of the pool or a smaller teaching pool if one is available. It is important to remember that each student in an adapted class must be considered individually in relation to a program of swimming activities. Teaching some of the students regular swimming strokes and aquatic games and activities might very well aggravate conditions that already exist. Thus already strong muscles would be overstrengthened at the expense of weak ones. It is therefore necessary that some students either be taught adaptations of the regular swimming strokes or activities or be provided with a therapeutic exercise program that is designed to help them strengthen their weak areas.[11]

Adapting sports and games for use in the pool

Adapting therapeutic exercises for use in a pool is covered in Chapter 5. Adapting sports and games and choosing perceptual-motor activities for use in an aquatics program are presented in the following sections of this chapter.

Shallow-water activities

Water volleyball. Water volleyball is an excellent activity for its recreational, fitness, and teamwork values. Modification of rules and techniques should be based on the abilities of the players involved and might include any of the following:
1. Allow for an assist on the serve (or a substitute server).
2. Reduce the size of the playing area and increase the number of players (since it is very difficult to move from place to place and cover more than a minimal area).
3. Allow more flexibility in passing techniques (four or more passes allowed on a side and standard bump pass not required).
4. For the severely handicapped, use a lighter ball.
5. Allow players to use flotation devices, if necessary. (If inner tubes are used, the valve stems should be removed or taped down to prevent injury to players.)

Water polo. Water polo allows walking, running, swimming, and passing to advance the ball toward the opponents' goal. The ball is not out of bounds until it actually passes across the edge of the pool, that is, the ball can strike the pool edge and rebound into the pool and it is still in play. Other modifications of rules and techniques may include any of the following:
1. Use a larger, lighter ball.
2. Allow those who need them to use flotation devices; the ball may then be carried in the tube for a maximum of five arm strokes.
3. Allow no player contact.
4. Allow no more than five walking or running steps to be taken before the ball is passed or shot.
5. Increase the number of players and reduce the size of the playing area.
6. On the pool deck, use regular playground benches turned on their sides, with the legs turned toward the pool, as goals.

Water basketball. Water basketball allows for walking, running, swimming, and passing to advance the ball toward the opponents' basket. The ball is not out of bounds until it passes completely across the pool edge. Other modifications of rules and techniques may include any of the following:
1. Use a smaller, lighter ball.
2. Allow those who need them to use flotations devices; the ball may then be carried in the tube for a maximum of five arm strokes.
3. Allow no player contact.
4. Allow no more than five walking or running steps to be taken before the ball is passed or shot.
5. Increase the number of players and reduce the size of the playing area, if necessary.
6. Offensive players cannot shoot from closer than 8 feet from the basket.
7. Mount regular basketball backboards and baskets on frames that sit on the pool deck at either end of the playing area. The baskets should be placed so that they are 12 to 18 inches above the water's surface. Another adaptation is to place tires on the side of the pool or inner tubes in the pool to serve as baskets.

Deep-water activities

All the games described in the previous section can be played in deep water, but some further modifications may be necessary.

Water volleyball. A possible modification of rules for deep-water volleyball may be as follows:

1. Serves may be made from a sitting position on the side or an overhand pass type serve, which may be assisted over the net, may be allowed.
2. A small court size or a large number of players is necessary, since each player can only cover an area a little less than his reach in each direction.
3. All types of passes are permitted and the number of passes and repeat hits should be increased (this improves the game and allows for rallies to take place).
4. All or a portion of the players may use flotation devices, life jackets, inner tubes, etc.
5. A lighter ball may be used.
6. The net should be suspended with its top about 3 feet above the water surface; a paddle tennis or badminton net may be used in place of the regulation volleyball net.

Water polo. A possible modification of rules for water polo in deep water may be as follows:

1. All or part of the players may use flotation devices.
2. Players using a tube for a flotation device may carry the ball in their tube for not over five arm strokes before they must pass the ball or shoot.
3. Players with life jackets and those swimming freely may not use more than five arm strokes before they must pass the ball or shoot.
4. No player contact should be allowed, that is, the ball only should be played.
5. The size of the playing area may need to be reduced or the number of players increased according to the abilities of the contestants.

Water basketball. Suggested modifications for deep-water basketball will be the same as those for water polo in deep water.

Perceptual-motor activities in the pool

A variety of perceptual-motor activities can be included in aquatic programs. Activities can be planned so that the participants will be able to keep their heads above the water at all times; underwater activities can be planned in which participants look at or retrieve objects that are either at the bottom of or are suspended in the water. In addition to the motor activity involved, considerable learning can take place if the objects in the pool are of different shapes and colors, if they have numbers or letters printed on them, and if the clinician or teacher includes conceptual development as a part of each appropriate activity. Some of the different types of equipment that can be used in the aquatic program are described in the following sections.

1. Balls of different sizes and weights can be thrown, pushed, sunk, or, in some cases, used to support the student. They can be employed in a variety of games and activities (Fig. 8-6).
2. Hoops, like hula hoops (of various colors and sizes), normally float on the surface and can be used as targets in throwing activities; the student can be positioned inside or outside of them. They can be weighted on one side so as to float vertically, thereby serving as a tunnel through which to dive and swim or they can be weighted so as to sink to the bottom to be stood in, to be walked around, to serve as a target, or to be dived for and brought to the surface.
3. Floating plaques of various sizes, shapes, and colors can be used with the previously described equipment either as targets or to be thrown into a target. Students can be asked to identify plaques of different sizes, shapes, or colors or with given numbers or letters on them; to arrange several of them in various patterns; or to pass them to

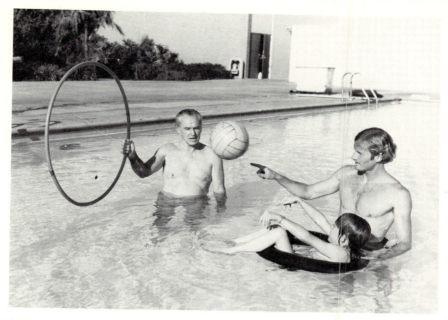

Fig. 8-6. College instructor and teacher-in-training provide aquatic skills instruction. (Courtesy California State University, Audio Visual Center, Long Beach, Calif.)

another person in a specified order. Plaques can also be weighted so as to float suspended in the water or so as to sink to the bottom of the pool.

4. Face masks, snorkels, fins, and swim gloves may also be used where appropriate to assist vision in the water, to aid persons with breathing problems, or to facilitate movement through the water.

5. Flotation devices such as life jackets, inner tubes (automobile, motorcycle, bicycle, etc.), styrofoam blocks, kickboards, and the like can also be used either to support an individual or one of his limbs or for many of the activities previously described. A flotation device may provide for many new and different types of experiences for persons with a variety of disabling conditions and often will serve as a vehicle to help these persons overcome fears and apprehensions associated with learning to swim. Such items as life jackets and inner tubes may facilitate participation in a variety of aquatic activities and sports.

Excellent materials and activities involving therapeutic exercises, water games, and activities in the pool are offered by Lowman,[11] Daniels,[4] Fait,[7] Mathews, Kruse and Shaw[12] and in a manual by the American National Red Cross.[15]

Rope skipping

Rope skipping is an excellent activity to include in the adapted physical education program. It involves exercise for a large number of the muscles of the body; it is helpful in the development of balance and coordination; and it is an excellent activity for the development of muscular endurance and cardiovascular efficiency. Since many students in the adapted program spend much of their time performing special exercises, endurance type activities such as rope skipping, jogging, and swimming should be a part of their total physical education experience whenever they can be tolerated.

Manufactured ropes with handles, some with special swivel action that facilitates

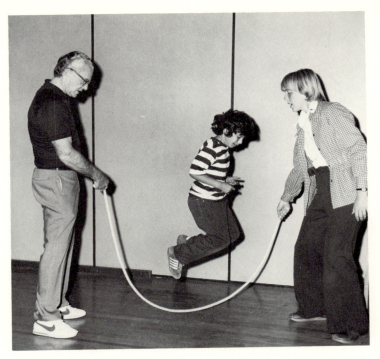

Fig. 8-7. Rope skipping. (Courtesy California State University, Audio Visual Center, Long Beach, Calif.)

turning the rope rapidly, can be purchased or ropes can be cut from lengths of ¼- or ⅜-inch diameter clothesline or nylon rope. The latter ropes are quite satisfactory and several different lengths can be cut to accommodate the various lengths needed by the students in the class. Longer lengths of rope can be used in cases in which two persons turn one or two ropes for another person to jump (Fig. 8-7). The more advanced jumper can even jump a single short rope while jumping the long rope turned by others.

Students of all ages may have some trouble in learning to skip rope. It requires patience and practice to become proficient. It is such an interesting, challenging activity that time limitations may have to be placed on certain students so that they do not overdo. Students who are under par or who experience cardiovascular insufficiency may need to have a modified program of rope skipping set up especially to meet their needs and limitations. Using heavier, slower turning ropes, with definite allotted time periods (interspersed with required rest periods), these students may be allowed to participate in rope skipping without overexertion on the approval of their physicians.

A student can learn the basic footwork involved in skipping rope simply by jumping in place on both feet at the same time; on one foot at a time, using the same foot; and on one foot at a time, alternating the feet. The hand, wrist, and arm motion can be practiced by taking both handles of the rope in one hand. Rotating the hand and wrist with the hand held down by the side of the hip, the center of the rope can be swung in a large arc in a plane parallel to the direction the student is facing. This should be practiced with each hand separately if the student is having trouble with the hand and wrist motion.

The student is then ready to put these

two drills together and learn various patterns of jumping with a rope. Probably the easiest pattern to learn is to execute one single jump with each turn of the rope so that as the rope nears the feet, the student jumps just enough to clear it and to allow it to continue its swing over his head. The rope can either be turned to the front or to the rear and both types of rope skipping should be learned. The following are other types of rope jumping:

1. Jumping two times to each turn of the rope (This can be done on one or both feet.)
2. Alternating feet with each turn of the rope as in running in place
3. Jumping with one foot in front of the other so that the student "rocks" over the rope first with one foot and then with the other (either foot can be put forward in this drill)
4. Spinning the rope twice for each jump
5. Crossing the hands in front of the body as the rope swings over the head so that the jump is made with each hand placed by the opposite hip and then uncrossing the hands prior to the next jump

6. Jumping on both feet with one ankle crossed over the other
7. Jumping forward and back or side to side over a line drawn on the floor

All these styles of jumping can be executed while the rope is swung either forward or backward and all should be practiced both ways until perfected.

After these patterns have been learned, they can be worked into numerous combinations to challenge those of all ability levels in the program.[2, 5, 8]

SUGGESTED ACTIVITIES, GAMES, AND SPORTS FOR ADAPTED PHYSICAL EDUCATION CLASSES

The activities, games, and sports listed and classified in Table 8-1 are described in detail either in standard texts on recreation, games, and stunts; in specific texts for some of the better-known sports and games; or in special sources on recreation for the handicapped. Two or three references are given for each activity presented in the chart in order to facilitate finding descriptions of the activities. Additional information about sports and games can

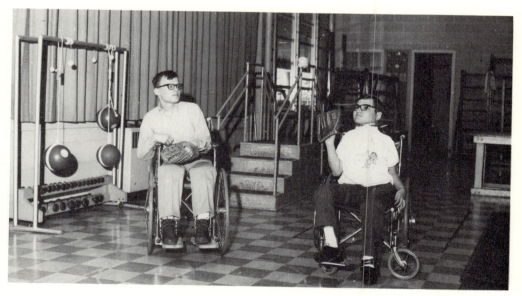

Fig. 8-8. Sports activities for children in wheelchairs. (Courtesy Dr. Julian Stein, Washington, D.C.)

be found in Stafford,[14] Hunt,[10] Pomeroy,[13] and Fait.[7]

Many of the games and sports listed can be used in an adapted class without any modification. In many cases, modified forms of the activity are suggested in the text. Any game can be modified as much as desired by applying the techniques suggested earlier in this chapter (Fig. 8-8).

The full reference for each book cited in Table 8-1 appears in the reference list at the end of the chapter. Additional information on adapting activities is given in Chapters 12, 14, and 16.

REFERENCES

1. Anderson, M. H., Elliot, M. E., and LaBerge, J.: Play with a purpose, New York, 1966, Harper & Row, Publishers.
2. Arnheim, D. D., and Pestolesi, R. A.: Developing motor behavior in children: a balanced approach to elementary physical education, St. Louis, 1973, The C. V. Mosby Co.
3. Chapman, F. M.: Recreation activities for the handicapped, New York, 1960, The Ronald Press Co.
4. Daniels, A. S., and Davies, E. A.: Adapted physical education, ed. 3, New York, 1975, Harper & Row, Publishers.
5. Educational Research Council of America: Physical education program guide, Columbus, Ohio, 1969, Charles E. Merrill Publishing Co.
6. Eisenberg, H., and Eisenberg, L.: Omnibus of fun, New York, 1956, Association Press.
7. Fait, H. F.: Special physical education, Philadelphia, 1972, W. B. Saunders Co.
8. Fitness for children through hopscotch, rope skipping, peg board, Sacramento, Calif., 1957, California State Department of Education.
9. Hindman, D. A.: Complete book of games and stunts, Englewood Cliffs, N.J., 1959, Prentice-Hall, Inc.
10. Hunt, V. V.: Recreation for the handicapped, Englewood Cliffs, N.J., 1955, Prentice-Hall, Inc.
11. Lowman, C. L.: Technique of underwater gymnastics, Los Angeles, 1937, American Publications, Inc.
12. Mathews, D. K., Kruse, R., and Shaw, V.: The science of physical education for handicapped children, New York, 1962, Harper & Row, Publishers.
13. Pomeroy, J.: Recreation for the physically handicapped, New York, 1964, Macmillan Publishing Co., Inc.
14. Stafford, G. T.: Sports for the handicapped, Englewood Cliffs, N.J., 1950, Prentice-Hall, Inc.
15. Swimming for the handicapped: instructor's manual, Washington, D.C., 1960, American National Red Cross.
16. Van Hagen, W., Dexter, G., and Williams, J. F.: Physical education in the elementary school, Sacramento, Calif., 1941, California State Department of Education.

RECOMMENDED READINGS

Abernathy, K., et al.: Jumping up and down, San Rafael, Calif., 1970, Academic Therapy Publications.

Adams, W. C., Daniel, A., and Rullman, L.: Games, sports, and exercises for the physically handicapped, Philadelphia, 1972, Lea & Febiger.

Boehm, D. A.: The family game book, New York, 1967, Doubleday and Co., Inc.

Bond, G.: An adapted surfing device. Unpublished master's thesis, California State University, Long Beach, 1974.

Borst, E., and Mitchell, E.: Social games for recreation, New York, 1959, The Ronald Press Co.

Bowerman, W. J., and Harris, W. E.: Jogging, New York, 1967, Grosset & Dunlap, Inc.

Brownell, C. L., and Moore, R. B.: Recreational sports, Mankato, Minn., 1969, Creative Educational Society, Inc.

Carr, D. B., et al.: Sequenced instructional programs in physical education for the handicapped, P.L. 88-164, Title III, Dec., 1970, Los Angeles, 1970, Los Angeles City Schools Special Education Branch, Physical Education Project.

Chaney, C., and Kephart, N. C.: Motoric aids to perceptual training, Columbus, Ohio, 1968, Charles E. Merrill Publishing Co.

Clark, D. E.: Physical education: a program of activities, St. Louis, 1969, The C. V. Mosby Co.

Counselman, J. E.: The science of swimming, Englewood Cliffs, N.J., 1969, Prentice-Hall, Inc.

Cowart, J., and Dressel, M.: Sport adaptions for a student without fingers, J. Phys. Educ. Rec. 47:46, 1976.

Cratty, B. J.: Development games for physically handicapped children, Palo Alto, Calif., 1969, Peek Publications.

Cratty, B. J.: Movement behavior and motor learning, ed. 3, Philadelphia, 1973, Lea & Febiger.

Cratty, B. J., and Breen, J. E.: Educational games for physically handicapped children, Denver, 1972, Love Publishing Co.

Crowe, W. C., Arnheim, D. D., and Auxter, D.: Laboratory manual in adapted physical education and recreation, St. Louis, 1977, The C. V. Mosby Co.

Dauer, V. P.: Dynamic physical education for

elementary school children, Minneapolis, 1972, Burgess Publishing Co.

Designs for dance, Washington, D.C., 1968, American Association for Health, Physical Education, and Recreation.

Donnelly, R., et al.: Active games and contests, New York, 1958, The Ronald Press Co.

Drowatzky, J. N.: Physical education for the mentally retarded, Philadelphia, 1971, Lea & Febiger.

Fredrick, A. B.: 212 ideas for making low-cost physical education equipment, Englewood Cliffs, N.J., 1963, Prentice-Hall, Inc.

Graham, D., and Ingersol, J. B.: Helping adolescents get moving: the reality therapy approach, J. Phys. Educ. Rec. 46:32-33, 1975.

Guide for programs in physical education and recreation for the mentally retarded, Washington, D.C., 1968, American Association for Health, Physical Education, and Recreation.

Hackett, L. C.: Movement exploration and games for the mentally retarded, Palo Alto, Calif., 1970, Peek Publications.

Harris, J. A.: Fun O' File, Minneapolis, 1970, Burgess Publishing Co.

Hayes, S.: The use of rhythmical activities in adapted physical education. Unpublished master's thesis, University of California at Los Angeles, Los Angeles, 1957.

How we do it book, ed. 3, Washington, D.C., 1964, American Association for Health, Physical Education, and Recreation.

Huber, J. H., and Vercollone, J.: Using aquatic mats with exceptional children, J. Phys. Educ. Rec. 47:44, 1976.

Klafs, C.: Rhythmic activities for handicapped children. Unpublished doctoral dissertation, University of Southern California, Los Angeles, 1957.

Kratz, L. E.: Movement without sight, Palo Alto, Calif., 1973, Peek Publications.

Kraus, R.: Recreation leader's handbook, New York, 1955, McGraw-Hill Book Co.

Latchaw, M.: A pocket guide for games and rhythms for the elementary school, Englewood Cliffs, N.J., 1958, Prentice-Hall, Inc.

Lawrence, C. C., and Hackett, L. C.: Water learning, Palo Alto, Calif., 1975, Peek Publications.

Merrill, T.: Activities for the aged and infirm: a handbook for the untrained worker, Springfield, Ill., 1967, Charles C Thomas, Publisher.

Moran, J. M., and Kalakian, L. H.: Movement experiences for the mentally retarded or emotionally disturbed child, Minneapolis, 1974, Burgess Publishing Co.

Mulac, M. E.: Games and stunts for school, camp, and playground, New York, 1969, Harper & Row, Publishers.

Physical activities for the mentally retarded (ideas for instruction), Washington, D.C., 1968, American Association for Health, Physical Education, and Recreation.

Physical activity programs and practices for the exceptional individual, third national conference, Long Beach, Calif., 1974, The Alliance for Health, Physical Education, and Recreation.

Physical activity programs and practices for the exceptional individual, fourth national conference, Los Angeles, 1975, The Alliance for Health, Physical Education, and Recreation.

Pomeroy, J.: "Recreation unlimited": an approach to community recreation for the handicapped, J. Phys. Educ. Rec. 46:301, 1975.

Practical guide for teaching the mentally retarded to swim, Washington, D.C., 1969, American Association for Health, Physical Education, and Recreation.

Schmais, C.: What is dance therapy? J. Phys. Educ. Rec. 47:36, 1976.

Shivers, J. S., and Fait, H. F.: Therapeutic and adapted recreational services, Philadelphia, 1975, Lea & Febiger.

Smith, H.: Water games, New York, 1967, The Ronald Press Co.

Stein, J. U.: Special olympics instructional manual, Washington, D.C., 1972, American Assocation for Health, Physical Education, and Recreation and the Joseph P. Kennedy, Jr. Foundation.

Stoner, W. T.: Trampoline lesson plans for teaching trampoline, Whittier, Calif., 1973, Remedial Physical Education, Lowell Joint School Districts.

Williams, A. M.: Recreation in senior years, New York, 1962, Associated Press.

Witengier, M.: An adaptive playground for physically handicapped children, Phys. Ther. **50:** 821-826, 1970.

PART THREE

PROGRAMMING FOR SPECIFIC PROBLEMS

An understanding of specific types of disabilities found in adapted physical education classes at the elementary, secondary, and college levels of instruction should prepare the teacher of persons with these disabilities to be better able to apply assessment procedures, to set reasonable performance objectives, and to plan appropriate exercise and activity programs for these students.

9

POSTURE AND BODY MECHANICS

■ An individual's posture, in a large measure, determines the impression that he makes on other persons. Good posture gives the impression of enthusiasm, initiative, and self-confidence, whereas poor posture often gives the impression of dejection, lack of confidence, and fatigue. We know that faulty posture does not necessarily indicate illness; however, we also know that good posture and body mechanics help the internal organs assume a position in the body that is favorable to their proper function and that allows the body to function most efficiently mechanically. Good posture should not be confused with the ability to assume static positions in which the body is held straight and stiff and during which good alignment is achieved at the sacrifice of the ability to move and to function properly. Possibly, "good body mechanics" would be a better term to use in describing the proper alignment and use of the body during both static and active postures.

The term "body mechanics" is sometimes defined as the static and the functional relationships between the parts that make up the body and the body as a whole. Regardless of what we call it, there is general agreement that the human body operates best when its parts are in good alignment and are maintained so while sitting, standing, walking, or participating in a variety of occupational and recreational types of activities. It is important to remember that there is no such thing as a normal posture for an individual. Certain anatomical, ethnological, and mechanical principles have been developed over the years that aid physicians, therapists, and physical educators in the identification of faulty body mechanics both in static and in moving postures. Proper body mechanics and posture help individuals keep their bodies in proper balance with as small an expenditure of energy as possible and with the minimum amount of strain.[5, 9, 10]

The center of gravity of the human body is located at a point where the pull of gravity on one side is equal to the pull of gravity on the other side. This center of gravity (higher in men than in women) falls in front of the sacrum at a point ranging from approximately 54% to 56% of the individual's height when standing. The center of gravity is changed any time the body or its segments change position.

In the upright standing position, the human body is relatively unstable. Its base of support, the feet, is small; its center of gravity is high; and it consists of a number of bony segments superimposed on one another, bound together by muscles and ligaments at a large number of movable joints. Any time the body assumes a static or dynamic posture, these muscles and ligaments must act on the bony levers of the body to offset the continuous downward pull of gravity.

Whenever the center of gravity of the body falls within its base of support, a state of balance exists. The closer the center of gravity is to the center of the base of support, the better will be the balance or equilibrium. This has important implications for the individual both in terms of good posture and as it relates to good balance for all types of body movement. The body is kept well balanced for activities in which stability is important, whereas it may be purposely thrown out of equilibrium when movement is desired, speed is to be increased, or force is to be exerted on another object.[1, 12]

As the human being matures, balance for both static and dynamic positions becomes more automatic. An individual develops a feel for a correct position in space so that little or no conscious effort is needed to

regulate it and attention can be devoted to other factors involved in movement patterns. This feeling for basic postural positions as well as for dynamic movement is controlled by certain sensory organs located throughout the body. The eyes furnish visual cues relative to body position. The semicircular canals of the inner ear furnish information on body equilibrium. Receptors in the tendons, joints, and muscles also contribute to the individual's ability to feel the body's position in space. The loss or malfunction of any of these sense organs requires that major adjustments be made by the individual to compensate for its loss. Such adjustments are part of the functions performed by the physician–physical educator–therapist team.[1, 4]

It therefore is important for physicians, teachers, and parents to include, as part of the training of children and youth, the proper use of the body and, whenever necessary, programs for the correction of defects in posture and body mechanics. There are many causes of poor posture and poor body mechanics. Included among these are such factors as environmental influences, psychological conditions, pathological conditions, growth handicaps, congenital defects, and nutritional problems. Any one of these may have an adverse effect on the posture of the growing child, the adolescent, or the adult.

Environmental factors that may cause poor posture include such things as improper shoes, narrow or short socks, clothing that does not fit the growing youngster properly, and overfatigue and overwork, especially with the growing child and adolescent. Also of concern are improper seating, including chairs, tables, and desks and other insufficient objects of furniture, including short or sagging beds and poor mattresses. Some types of toys that cause asymmetrical development may have an adverse effect on the posture of the child. Examples are scooters, skateboards, skating on one skate—in fact, the unilateral use of any type of toy. Psychological problems that may lead to postural deviations include such things as egotism, shyness, modesty, hypersensitiveness, and depression. Pathological conditions, too, often lead to both functional and structural postural deviations. Some of these are faulty vision and hearing; various cardiovascular conditions; tuberculosis; arthritis; and neuromuscular conditions resulting in atrophy, dystrophy, and spasticity. Growth handicaps include some of the following types of conditions: weaknesses in the skeletal structure and in the muscular system, growth divergencies of various sorts, fatigue, and glandular malfunctions. Congenital defects include such things as amputations, joint and bone deformities, spina bifida, clubfoot, and the like (Chapters 10 and 11). Nutritional problems include underweight, overweight, and poor nourishment.

GOOD POSTURE AND BODY MECHANICS

Before we identify some of the deviations in posture and the methods used to determine the presence and severity of these conditions, it might be beneficial to look rather carefully into the matter of what constitutes good posture and good body mechanics in various body positions.

Good posture might be defined as a position, or positions, that enables the body to function to the best advantage with regard to work done, health, and appearance.[11]

Standing posture

In the standing position, the body should be held erect and well balanced, but not in a stiff or posed manner. The feet should be approximately parallel and a comfortable distance apart. The weight of the body should be equally distributed over the feet and borne on the heel, along the lateral side of the bottom of the foot, and across the total ball of the foot with the assistance of the five toes. The legs should be straight, but not stiff. The pelvis should be balanced over the top of the legs with the lower abdomen kept flat and with a normal amount of anteroposterior curvature in the lower back. The upper back

should also have a normal amount of anteroposterior curvature; the shoulders should be held level and comfortably balanced with the head high, chin in, and the lobe of the ear directly over the center of the tip of the shoulder. The chest should be held high, but not stiff. The shoulder blades should be flat against the back of the rib cage; the arms should hang comfortably at the sides. Looking at the individual from the front or rear view, the pelvis should be level, the shoulders level, the spine straight, and the head erect above the shoulders.

A side view of the person would show the following segments balanced and superimposed directly above one another: a point 1½ inches anterior to the external malleolus, a point just posterior to the patella, the center of the hip, the center of the shoulder, and the lobe of the ear (Fig. 9-1). This test for body alignment, called the plumb line or gravity line test for standing posture, is described in a later section of this chapter.

Sitting posture

The position of the body while sitting is similar to the position of the body while standing, that is, the head is held erect, the chin is kept in, normal anteroposterior curves are maintained in the upper and lower back, and the abdomen is flat. The hips should be pushed firmly against the back of the chair. The thighs should rest on the chair and help support and balance the body. The feet should be flat on the floor or the legs comfortably crossed at the ankles. The shoulders should be relaxed and level with the chest kept comfortably high (Fig. 9-2).

Correct posture in walking

The basic position of the body in walking is similar to that of the standing posture, but all parts of the body are also involved in moving through space. The toes face straight ahead or toe out very slightly as the leg swings straight forward; the heel strikes the ground first, with the weight

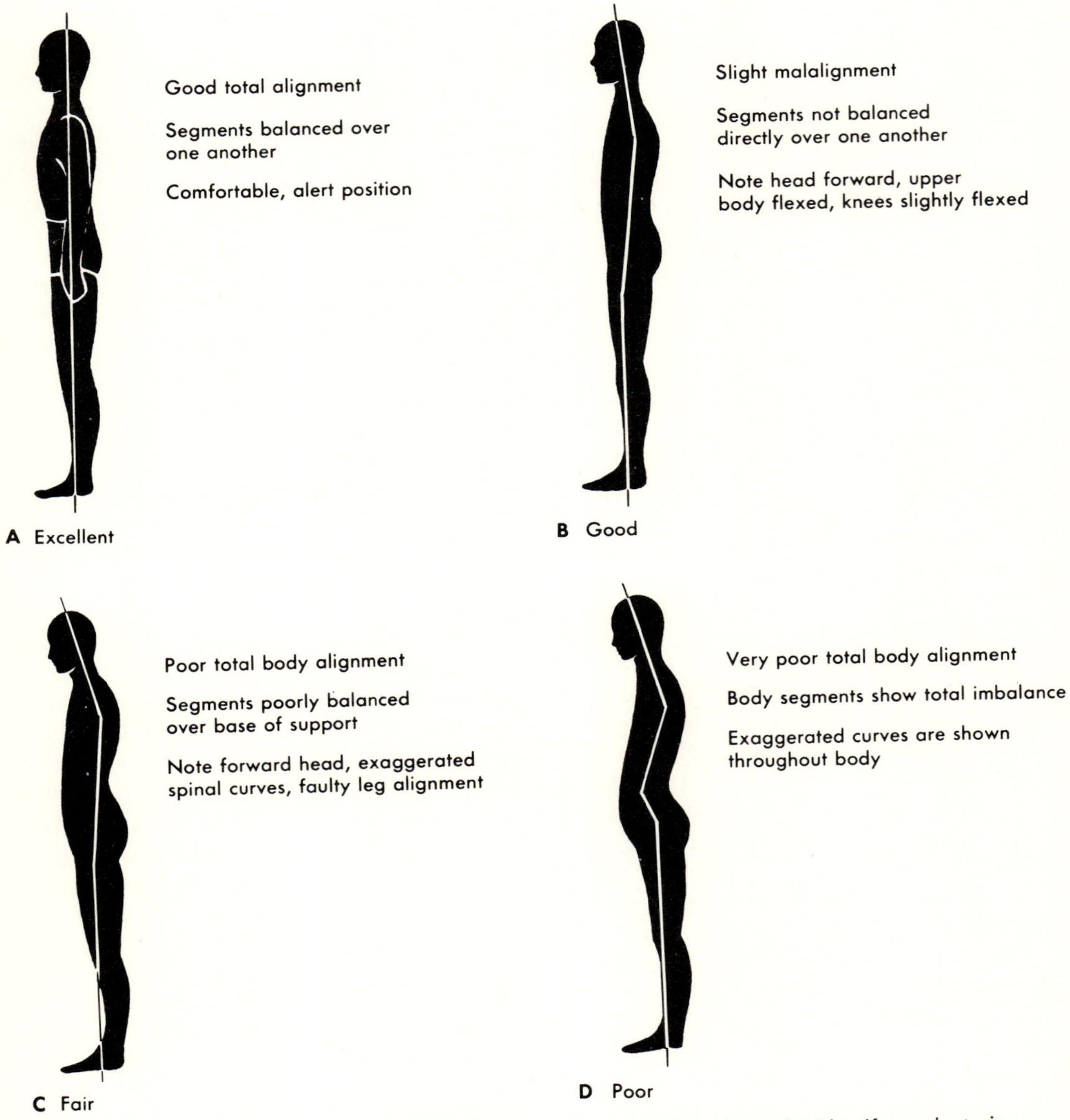

Good total alignment

Segments balanced over
one another

Comfortable, alert position

A Excellent

Slight malalignment

Segments not balanced
directly over one another

Note head forward, upper
body flexed, knees slightly flexed

B Good

Poor total body alignment

Segments poorly balanced
over base of support

Note forward head, exaggerated
spinal curves, faulty leg alignment

C Fair

Very poor total body alignment

Body segments show total imbalance

Exaggerated curves are shown
throughout body

D Poor

Fig. 9-1. Four-figure system for rough assessment of posture (used to identify students in need of a more discriminating type of posture examination).

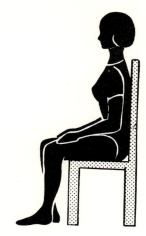

Fig. 9-2. Good sitting posture.

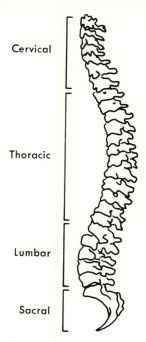

Fig. 9-4. Normal spine.

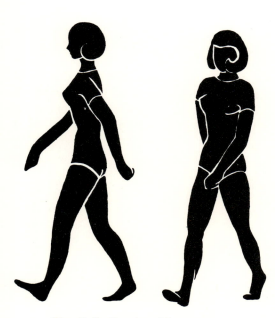

Fig. 9-3. Good walking posture.

the legs. The head is held erect with the chin tucked in a comfortable position. The chest is held high, the shoulder blades are flat against the rib cage, and the shoulders are held even in height (Fig. 9-3).

The spinal column

Viewed from the front or rear, the spinal column should be straight. However, when the spine is viewed from the side, or lateral view, curves normally exist in various vertebral segments. The cervical spine is slightly hyperextended, stretching from the base of the skull to about the top of the thoracic vertebrae. The dorsal or thoracic spine is flexed throughout the length of the thoracic vertebrae. The lumbar curve is hyperextended throughout the length of the lumbar vertebrae and the sacral curve is flexed and extends throughout the sacral and coccygeal vertebrae. These curves are present in the spinal column to help the individual maintain balance and to absorb shock and they should be considered normal unless they are exaggerated (Fig. 9-4).

being transferred along the lateral side of the bottom of the foot. The weight is then shifted to the forward part of the foot and balanced across the entire ball of the foot. The step is completed with a strong push from all the toes. The upper body should be held erect with the arms swinging comfortably in opposition to the movement of

POOR POSTURE ALIGNMENT PATTERNS

Postural deviations are ordinarily noted during examination of the individual from the lateral, anterior, and posterior views. In conducting a posture examination, it is considered best to perform the examination from the base of support upward. Thus if deviations are noted at one level, they can be checked to see if compensatory deviations have occurred in areas above that particular level.

Postural deviations
Foot and ankle

Postural deviations of the foot and ankle can be observed while the student is standing in the upright position or participating in activities that involve walking or running. The evaluation of the foot should be made by observing it from the anterior, lateral, and posterior views and should involve both a walking and a static examination of the feet. The number of individuals with deviations of the foot is large at all age levels and the number of persons who suffer with painful feet increases with increasing age. Muscles and joints of the foot and ankle become weakened from age and misuse. Pain associated with faulty mechanics in the use of the feet also begins to show up with increased age. The good mechanical use of the feet throughout life plus other factors such as good basic health, the maintenance of a satisfactory level of physical fitness, proper choice of shoes and socks, and proper attention to any injury or accident to the foot should serve as preventive measures to the onset of weak ankles and feet in later life.

The foot consists of seven irregularly shaped tarsal bones bound together by strong ligaments to make up the posterior half of the foot. These bones articulate anteriorly with five metatarsal bones, long and narrow in shape, which, in turn, are joined distally with the 14 phalanges that make up the toes (Fig. 9-5). The tarsal bones articulate with the distal end of the tibia through the talus bone to form the ankle joint. When the individual is standing in the upright position, the body weight is transferred from the tibia, through the talus, into the calcaneus and the navicular bones. The body weight is

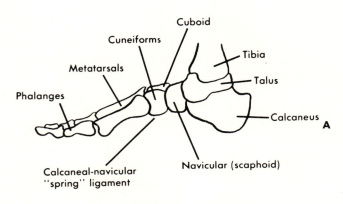

Medial aspect

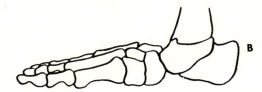

Fig. 9-5. Bones of the foot. **A,** Normal foot. **B,** Flatfoot.

transferred anteriorly in the foot through the three cuneiform bones and the cuboid bone, located just anterior and lateral to the navicular (scaphoid), then, through these bones to the metatarsals, and, finally, to the phalanges. The total body weight is borne on the heel and the forepart of the foot with the weight fairly well distributed across the heads of the five metatarsal bones. The first metatarsal bone and the two sesamoid bones located just under its distal head assume a slightly greater portion of the total weight on the anterior part of the foot. The bottom surfaces of the toes should also rest on the floor and should be active in helping support the foot both in the standing position and while walking.

The foot consists of a longitudinal arch that extends from the anterior portion of the calcaneus bone to the heads of the five metatarsal bones. The medial side of the longitudinal arch is usually considerably higher than the lateral side, which, as a general rule, makes contact throughout its length with the surface on which it is resting (Fig. 9-6, A to C). This is particularly true when the body weight is being supported on the foot. The longitudinal arch is sometimes described as two arches, a medial and a lateral arch, extending from the anterior aspects of the heel to the heads of the metatarsal bones. However, it is currently most frequently described as one long arch that is dome shaped and higher on the medial than on the lateral side. On the forepart of the foot, in the region of the metatarsal bones, a second arch can be distinguished that runs across the forepart or ball of the foot. This arch, called the transverse or metatarsal arch, is slightly dome shaped, being higher at the proximal ends of the metatarsal bones than at the distal ends. It often is considered a continuation of the dome-shaped long arch described previously and thus we have just one dome-shaped arch of the foot (Fig. 9-6, D and E).

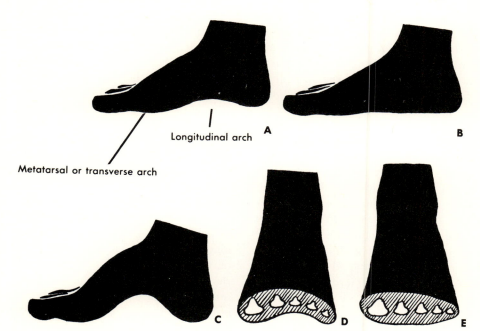

Fig. 9-6. Arches of the foot. **A,** Normal foot. **B,** Pes planus. **C,** Pes cavus. **D** and **E** are cross-sections of the arch. **D,** Normal metatarsal arch. **E,** Flat metatarsal arch.

Although these arches are described and named differently in the literature and there appears to be a difference of opinion in relation to the importance of their height, there is substantial agreement about the need for correct structure and placement of the bones, the importance of the strong ligamentous bands that help hold the bones in place to form the arches of the foot, and the need for good muscular balance between antagonistic muscles that support the foot. All these factors have an important effect on the position of the foot under both weight-bearing and non–weight-bearing conditions. A foot is considered strong and functional when the following conditions are present:

1. The foot is pain free.
2. The bones are properly placed and bound together by strong ligamentous bands (especially the calcaneonavicular ligament and the long plantar ligament).
3. The feet have adequate muscle strength (especially the posterior tibial muscle and the long flexor muscles of the toes) to support the longitudinal arch of the foot.
4. The bones have strong ligamentous and fascial bindings and well-developed small intrinsic muscles of the foot are present to maintain proper strength of the arch in the metatarsal region (Chapters 5 and 10).

In addition to considering the structure of the foot and ankle, it is also necessary to consider such other factors as the range of movement in the foot and ankle; the support of the body by the foot and ankle; and the effect that various positions of the foot, ankle, knee, and hip have on the mechanics of the foot itself. A consideration of the various movements possible in the foot and ankle, together with a description of the terminology used to describe these movements, should help clarify the discussion of those deviations of the foot and ankle that are presented in more detail in later portions of this chapter. The ankle joint is a hinge joint and therefore only dorsiflexion and plantar flexion are possible. The numerous articulations between the individual tarsal bones and between the tarsal and metatarsal bones allow for inversion and eversion of the foot and for abduction and adduction of the foot.

Movements of the foot are as follows:

Dorsiflexion: Movement of the top of the foot in the direction of the knee

Plantar flexion: Movement of the foot in the opposite direction, in the direction of the sole of the foot

Inversion: Tipping the medial edge of the foot upward or *varus* (walking on the outer border of the foot)

Eversion: Tipping the lateral edge of the foot upward or *valgus* (walking on the inner border of the foot)

Adduction: Turning the whole forepart of the foot in a medial direction

Abduction: Turning the forepart of the foot in a lateral direction

Pronation: Combination of tipping the outer border of the foot up and toeing out (eversion with abduction)

Supination: Combination of tipping the inner edge of the foot upward while toeing in (inversion with adduction)

It should also be remembered that it is possible to turn the foot into a toed-in and toed-out position by rotating the lower leg when the knee is bent and by rotating the whole leg at the hip when the knee is straight. Thus when an individual toes in or toes out while walking or standing, the examiner must determine whether this is the result of a foot deviation or a rotation of the leg (Fig. 9-7). Many foot and ankle deviations are closely linked to alignment problems occurring in the leg above the region of the ankle.

Pes planus. Pes planus, or flatfoot, refers to a lowering of the medial border of the longitudinal arch of the foot. The height of this side of the longitudinal arch may range anywhere from the extremely high arch known as *pes cavus*, to the so-called normal arch, and down to a position in which the medial border lies flat against the surface on which the individual is standing. When this side of the foot is

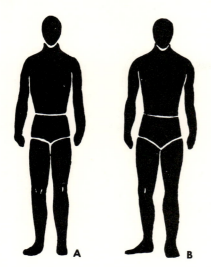

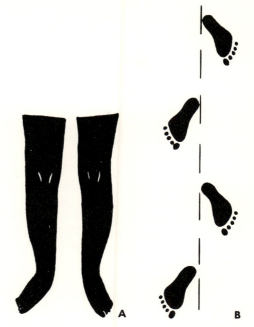

Fig. 9-7. Abduction of the foot and leg. **A,** Abduction of the foot. **B,** Toeing out of the foot resulting from outward rotation of the hip joint. Note difference in position of patella.

Fig. 9-8. Improper walking. **A,** Toeing out and walking across medial border of the foot. **B,** Footprints show outward rotation or splay-foot position while walking.

completely flat, the medial border of the foot may even assume a rather convex appearance to the observer (Fig. 9-6, *A* to *C*). Pes planus may be the result of faulty bony framework, faulty ligamentous pull across the articulations of the foot, an imbalance in the pull of the muscles responsible for helping to hold the longitudinal arch in its proper position, or racial differences. The specific cause may often be linked to improper alignment of the foot and leg and to faulty mechanics in the use of the foot and ankle. When the foot is held in a toed-out or abducted position while standing and walking, there is a tendency to throw a disproportionate amount of body weight onto the medial side of the foot, thus causing stress on the medial side of this arch.

Over a period of time, this stress may cause both a gradual stretching of the muscles, tendons, and ligaments on the medial aspect of the foot and a tightening of like structures on the lateral side. When the individual walks with the foot in the abducted or toed-out position, these same factors are again accentuated and, in addi-

tion, there is a tendency for the individual to rotate the leg medially in order to have it swing in alignment with the forward direction of the step. When the leg is swung straight in line with the direction being traveled and with the foot toed out, the individual will walk across the medial side of the foot with each step (Fig. 9-8). This not only weakens the foot, but also predisposes the individual to a condition called tibial torsion. Since the individual is walking with the leg in basically correct alignment, but with the foot abducted and/or toed out, malalignment results. Thus when the foot and leg alignment are examined, it will be found that when the legs and kneecaps face straight forward, the feet are in the abducted position; when the feet are aligned in a position parallel to one another, the kneecaps are facing in a slightly medial direction (tibial torsion). This may produce strain and possibly cause a lowering of the medial side of the longitudinal arch.

Correction of pes planus must involve a reversal of the factors and conditions just described. The total leg from the hip through the foot must be properly re-aligned so that the weight is balanced over the hip, the knee, the ankle, and the foot itself. The antagonistic muscles involved must be reoriented so that those that have become stretched (tibial muscles) are developed and tightened and those that have become short and tight (peroneal muscles) are stretched; thus the foot is allowed to assume its proper position. The muscles on the lateral side of the foot must be stretched (peroneal group). The gastroc-nemius and soleus muscles, which some-times become shortened in the case of flatfoot, exert an upward pull on the back of the calcaneus bone, thus adding to the flattening of the arch. These muscles must also be stretched whenever tightness is indicated. The major muscle group that must be shortened and strengthened is the posterior tibial muscles, which are extreme-ly important in terms of supporting the longitudinal arch, along with help from the long and short flexor muscles of the toes. The individual must also be given foot and leg alignment exercise in front of a mirror in order to observe the cor-rect mechanical position of the foot while exercising, standing, walking, and actively using the feet. (See Chapter 5 for special exercises.)

Such activities as walking in soft dirt, on grass, or in sand with the foot held in the proper position can do much to help strengthen the foot and realign it with the ankle and hip. Emphasis here should be on walking straight over the length of the foot, placing the heel down first, with the weight being transferred along the outer border of the foot and with an even and equal push-off from the forepart of the foot and the five toes. In actual practice, the great toe should be the last toe to leave the surface on the push-off.

Pes cavus. Pes cavus is a condition of the foot in which the longitudinal arch is abnormally high. This condition is not found as frequently in the general popu-lation as is pes planus. If the condition is extreme, the student is usually under the special care of an orthopedic physician. Special exercises are not usually given for the high arch unless the person has con-siderable associated pain, requiring special corrective procedures recommended by the physician (Fig. 9-6, *C*).

Pronation of the foot. Since the ankle joint is a hinge joint allowing only plantar flexion and dorsiflexion, pronation of the ankle—as it is sometimes called—is ac-tually a condition of pronation of the foot. As described previously, this is a combina-tion of abduction of the foot itself and eversion. Since pronation involves ever-sion, the medial border of the foot is lowered as it is in the flat longitudinal arch. When this condition occurs, the for-ward part of the foot is also abducted, a condition caused by a shifting of the cal-caneus bone downward and inward. This also changes the relationship of the talus to the other tarsal bones so that the tarsal metatarsal and the metatarsal phalangeal articulations must adapt, thus causing the abduction of the forepart of the foot[8] (Fig. 9-9). The reverse of this condition, one that involves inversion and adduction of the forepart of the foot, is called supina-tion of the foot.

Viewed from the front of the individual being examined, the pronated foot is char-acterized by the turning of the forepart of the foot outward, by the lowering of the

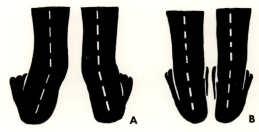

Fig. 9-9. Faulty foot and ankle positions. **A,** Foot and ankle pronation. **B,** Supinated foot.

medial side of the longitudinal arch, by the prominence of the scaphoid or navicular bone, and by the prominence of the internal malleolus of the ankle. From the posterior view, the same conditions of the forepart of the foot are present, the internal malleolus will be prominent, and the Achilles tendon bows inward or medially (Helbing's sign). Correction of pronation of the foot is similar to that described for pes planus or flatfoot. Special exercises are described in Chapter 5.

Proper foot and leg alignment. Proper foot and leg alignment has been mentioned previously in rather general terms. More specifically, when properly aligned, the leg should be straight and the foot should be facing straight forward or in a slightly toed-out position. A plumb line held so that it hangs in line with the anterior inferior spine of the ilium passes through the center of the patella, the center of the ankle, and the second toe of the foot. When viewed from the rear, the gravity line should pass through the center of the knee, the leg, and the calcaneus bone. The Achilles tendon must appear straight with no curvature.

Metatarsalgia. Two types of metatarsalgia may be recognized in a thorough foot examination. The first is a general condition, involving the transverse (metatarsal) arch, in which considerable pain is caused by the pressure of the heads of the metatarsal bones on the plantar nerves. The second type, Morton's toe, is more specific and is discussed in a later portion of this chapter.

Metatarsalgia in general may be caused by undue pressure being exerted on the plantar surface of the foot by the heads of the metatarsal bones. This pressure ultimately causes inflammation and therefore results in pain and discomfort. Its causes relate to such factors as wearing shoes or socks that are too short or too tight, wearing high-heeled shoes for long periods of time, and participating in various types of occupational or athletic endeavors that place great stress on the ball of the foot.

The mechanism of injury may result in a stretching of the ligaments that bind the metatarsophalangeal joints together and therefore pressure is exerted on the nerves in this area. Correction involves the removal of the cause, if this is possible, and the assignment of special exercises to increase flexibility of the forepart of the foot. Exercises are then assigned to strengthen and shorten the muscles on the plantar surface, which may aid in maintaining a normal position in the metatarsal region. The physician may prescribe special shoes or suggest that an arch support or metatarsal bar be worn to support the metatarsal region of the foot to help reduce pain (Fig. 9-6, *D* and *E*).

Morton's toe. Morton's toe, often called "true metatarsalgia," is more specific than the general breakdown of the metatarsal arch described previously. The onset of true metatarsalgia is often abrupt and the pain associated with it may be more intense than that found in general metatarsal weakness. In true metatarsalgia, the fourth metatarsal head is severely depressed, sometimes resulting in a partial dislocation of the fourth metatarsophalangeal joint. The abnormal pressure on the plantar nerve often produces a neuritis in the area, which, in turn, causes intense pain and disability. Treatment consists first of the removal of the cause of the condition. The orthopedic physician will advise which procedure will follow this. A second type of Morton's toe is characterized by the presence of a second metatarsal bone that is longer than the first metatarsal bone.

Hammer toe. In hammer toe, the proximal phalanx of the toe is hyperextended, the second is flexed, and the distal phalanx is either flexed or extended. This condition will often result from having worn socks or shoes that are too short or too tight over a prolonged period of time or congenital causes. (Fig. 9-10). Tests must be made to see whether the condition has become structural. If the condition is functional in nature and the affected joints can be

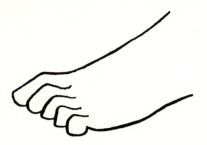

Fig. 9-10. Hammer toes.

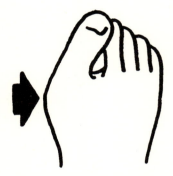

Fig. 9-11. Hallux valgus.

stretched and loosened, corrective measures may be taken to reorient the antagonistic muscle pull involved in this deviation. The first step, however, must be the removal of the cause and, in severe cases, an orthopedic physician should be consulted relative to special bracing, splinting, or surgery for correction of this condition.

Hallux valgus. Shoes or socks that are too short, too narrow, or too pointed or a faulty metatarsal bone can cause a deviation of the toe known as hallux valgus. In this condition, the great toe is deflected toward the other four toes at the metatarsophalangeal joint (Fig. 9-11). The exposed medial side of the metatarsophalangeal joint is thus subject to undue pressure and irritation from the shoes and the result is often a bunion in this region of the foot. As irritation continues, the body's natural defense is to deposit calcium over the metatarsophalangeal joint and under the bunion. This increases the size of the joint and also the amount of

pressure that occurs in this area of the foot. Correction of this condition must first involve consultation with a physician and usually requires the removal of the calcium deposit and the bunion. Further corrective measures would be to prescribe proper socks and shoes to allow sufficient room for the great toe to be held in the normal straight position. As an added precaution, both the standing and walking positions of the foot should be analyzed to determine whether the foot is being used in proper alignment. If the foot is not properly aligned and is toeing out excessively, remedial measures should be taken to correct this alignment in order to prevent a further aggravation of hallux valgus.

Lateral posture examination

Deviations in the foot and ankle were discussed in detail in an earlier section of this chapter.

The knee. The instructor's eyes, in examining the student from the side, move upward from the foot and ankle through the knee. Common deviations that may be noted in the position of the knee consist of either a hyperextended knee *(genu recurvatum)* or a hyperflexed knee. The normal position of the knee should be straight, but not stiff. It is possible to correct both forward and backward knee by realigning the pull of the muscles that control its flexion and extension and by reorienting the student to the proper position of the leg. Bent and "back" knee, respectively, often will be associated with flat lower back and lordosis of the lumbar spine (Fig. 9-12).

The pelvis. The normal pelvis is inclined forward and downward at approximately a 60-degree angle when a line is drawn from the lumbosacral junction to the symphysis pubis. Any variation in this angle, with the pelvis tipping (tilt) downward and forward, would usually result in a greater curve of the lumbar spine; by the same token, a variation in the angle, with the pelvis tipping upward and backward, would tend to produce a flatness in the lumbar area. Since the sacroiliac joint is

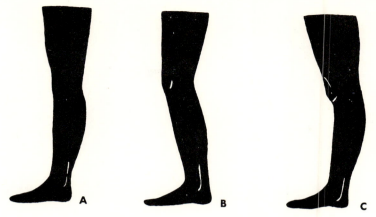

Fig. 9-12. The knee. **A,** Normal. **B,** Bent (flexed). **C,** Hyperextended.

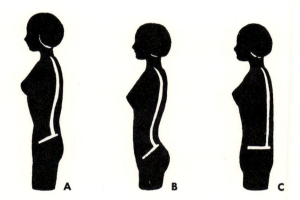

Fig. 9-13. Pelvic positions. **A,** Normal. **B,** Forward (downward) pelvic tilt. **C,** Backward (upward) pelvic tilt. Note position of spine as pelvic position changes.

basically an immovable joint and only a minimum amount of motion takes place at the lumbosacral joint, pelvic inclination and lumbar spinal curves are closely linked (Fig. 9-13). Since exaggerated spinal curves may limit normal motion in the low back, both lordosis and flat low back require special attention.

Lordosis. Lordosis is an exaggeration of the normal hyperextension in the lumbar spine. It is usually associated with tight musculature in the lower erector spinae or sacrospinalis muscle group, tightness in the iliopsoas and rectus femoris muscle groups, and either weak or stretched abdominal muscles. Correction of this condition would therefore necessitate stretching and loosening the lower erector spinae, the iliopsoas, and the rectus femoris muscles, together with assigning exercises designed to shorten and tighten the abdominal muscle group. It may also be important to develop muscular control of the gluteal and hamstring groups, which can exert a downward pull on the back of the pelvis. It is necessary to remember, however, that the development of the gluteal and hamstring groups can help the individual assume a correct position while stretching, while exercising, and even while in the static standing position, but that these muscles must be relaxed when the individual wishes to walk, move, or run. It is then necessary for the abdominal mus-

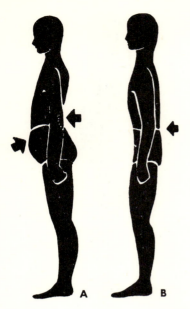

Fig. 9-14. A, Ptosis and lordosis. **B,** Flat back.

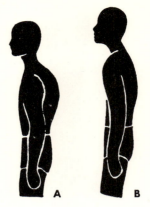

Fig. 9-15. A, Kyphosis. **B,** Forward or round shoulders.

cles to hold the front of the pelvis up and to maintain the desired curvature in the lower back. A condition called *ptosis* (visceroptosis) is often associated with a forward pelvic tilt and lordosis. This condition is characterized by a sagging of the lower abdominal muscles and a protrusion of the lower abdominal area. It can also be corrected by shortening, tightening, and strengthening the abdominal muscle groups (Figs. 9-13, *B*, and 9-14, *A*).

Flat lower back. A flat lower back condition can develop when the pelvic girdle is inclined upward at the front, thereby decreasing the normal curvature of the lumbar spine. Often associated with this condition are tight hamstring and gluteus maximus muscles with weakened and stretched iliopsoas and rectus femoris muscles, coupled with weakness in the lumbar section of the erector spinae muscle group. A flat back can be corrected by stretching and increasing the flexibility of the hamstring and gluteal muscles and by developing, shortening, and tightening the iliopsoas, the rectus femoris, and the erector spinae groups (Fig. 9-14).

In the correction of both lordosis and flat low back, the individual student must learn to reorient his standing position by learning to feel what it is like to stand with the body in the correctly aligned position. It is helpful for the student to practice this corrected position while standing with his side to a regular or three-way mirror in which he can observe his body in the correct mechanical position. A gravity line painted on the mirror or a plumb line hung down the length of the mirror will assist the student in realigning his body (Figs. 9-13, *C*, and 9-14, *B*).

Kyphosis. Kyphosis is an abnormal amount of flexion in the dorsal or thoracic spine. An extreme amount of kyphosis is called *humpback.* This condition ordinarily involves a weakening and stretching of the erector spinae and other extensor muscle groups in the dorsal or thoracic regions, along with a shortening and tightening of the antagonist (pectoral) muscles on the anterior side of the chest and shoulder girdle (Fig. 9-15, *A*). Its correction is effected largely by stretching the anterior muscles of the chest and shoulders (Fig. 20-8) so that the spinal extensor and shoulder girdle adductor muscle groups can be developed, strengthened, and shortened in order to pull the spine back into a more desired position. Often associated with kyphosis, but not necessarily found with it,

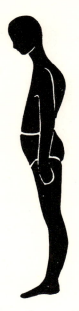

Fig. 9-16. Fatigue slump with kypholordosis.

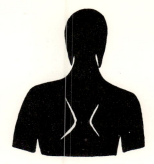

Fig. 9-17. Winged scapula.

are forward or round shoulders, flat chest, and winged scapula.

Forward or round shoulders. Forward or round shoulders is a condition involving an abnormal position of the shoulder girdle. This condition usually exists when the anterior muscles of the shoulder girdle (pectoral muscles) become shortened and tightened and the retractors or adductors of the shoulder girdle (rhomboids and trapezius muscles) become loose, weak, and stretched. It is often associated with a flat chest and kyphosis. The basic correction of this condition is to stretch and loosen the anterior muscles of the chest and shoulder girdle and to develop, strengthen, and shorten the adductor muscles of the shoulder girdle (Fig. 9-15, *B*).

Students with either kyphosis or forward shoulders should also practice standing and sitting in good alignment in front of a mirror to get the feeling of what it is like to hold the body comfortably in proper balance. When the correct position becomes easy and natural, the student will no longer have to rely on the mirror and the visual cues associated with its use.

Kypholordosis. Kypholordosis is a com-

bination of the two deviations described previously: that of kyphosis in the upper back and lordosis in the lower portion of the spine (Fig. 9-16). Often, one of these deviations is a compensation for the other and involves the body's attempt to keep itself in balance. Correction of kypholordosis consists of the same basic principles that are involved in correcting the individual conditions described previously; however, time can often be saved in the exercise program by assigning certain exercises that would be beneficial for the correction of both conditions. The exercise assignment sheet in Chapter 5 lists exercises that can be assigned to aid in the correction of all these conditions.

Flat upper back. A flat upper back would be the opposite of a kyphotic spine and would involve a decrease or absence of the normal anteroposterior spinal curve in the dorsal or thoracic region. Exercises and activities that would be beneficial for this condition include stretching the posterior muscles of the upper back to allow their antagonists on the anterior side of the body to be developed and shortened (Chapter 5).

Winged scapula. Winged scapula is a condition that involves the abduction or protraction of the shoulder blades (the medial border of the affected scapula being a greater distance from the spinal column than normal). A projection of the medial border of the scapula posteriorly and a protrusion of the inferior angle are other concomitants of this condition (Figs.

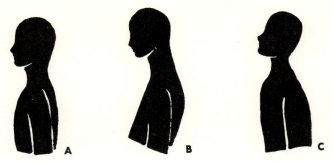

Fig. 9-18. Forward head and cervical lordosis. **A,** Normal head position. **B,** Forward head. **C,** Cervical lordosis.

9-17 and 20-24). It is a very common condition among young children, who exhibit it especially when their arms are raised forward to the shoulder level. This results from lack of shoulder girdle strength; ordinarily, the condition will be outgrown as the child begins to participate in hanging and climbing activities for the development of the muscles of the shoulder girdle. In the adolescent and the young adult, the condition is one that involves unequal pull of the antagonist muscles of the shoulder girdle; corrective measures may be necessary to correct it. In general, the procedure to follow would be to stretch and loosen the anterior muscles of the shoulder girdle and to develop the retractors or adductors of the scapula, involving both the trapezius and the rhomboid muscles. Developmental exercises for the serratus anterior muscle also are necessary, since it has a major responsibility for keeping the scapula in the correct position flat against the rib cage.

Forward head. Forward head is one of the most common postural deviations. It often accompanies kyphosis, forward shoulders, and lordosis. Two factors are involved in analyzing the causes of and in correcting forward head. The extensors of the head and neck are often stretched and weakened because of the habitual malposition of the head in the forward position. Correcting this condition involves bringing the head into proper alignment, with the chin "tucked" so that the lower jaw is basically in line with the ground and so that the chin is not tipped up when the head is drawn back. This involves reorientation of the head and neck so that the individual knows what it feels like to hold the head in the correct position. The antagonist muscles involved must be reeducated to hold the head in a position so that the lobe of the ear approximates a position in line with the center of the shoulder (Fig. 9-18, *A* and *B*).

Cervical lordosis. Cervical lordosis may result from an attempt to compensate for other spinal curves occurring at a lower level in the spinal column or from incorrect procedures in attempting to correct a forward head. The spinal extensors are often tight and contracted so that the head is tilted well back and the chin is tipped upward (Fig. 9-18, *C*). As in the case of forward head, a reeducation of the antagonistic muscles and the proprioceptive centers involved is necessary so that the lower jaw is held in line with the ground. In the correction of cervical lordosis and forward head, the student must learn to assume the proper position and must exercise in front of a mirror in order to assist himself in recognizing the correct position (Fig. 9-18, *A*). Special exercises for the correction of cervical lordosis and forward head are found in Chapter 5.

Posterior overhang (round swayback or "debutante slouch"). In posterior over-

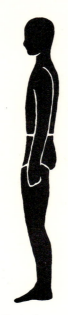

Fig. 9-19. Posterior overhang.

Fatigue slump. Fatigue slump is a term used to describe a rather complete breakdown in the alignment of the total body. Students, from the upper elementary school grades through the first year or two of high school, are especially susceptible to this condition (both physically and emotionally). These early adolescent years are times of physical, emotional, and mental stress that may often result in a general "sagging" of the whole body. The student will often have all of the following postural deviations: back knees, forward pelvic tilt, lordosis, kyphosis, forward shoulders, and forward head. The student may also have some lateral deviations such as a low shoulder and a head tilt.

Since part of the cause of fatigue slump may be linked to a period of rapid growth of bone, joint, and muscle, symmetrical development may not occur. Corrective measures for fatigue slump must include a consideration of both physical and emotional factors. Students must be motivated to want to work toward the correction of their posture. Motivation for boys should include such factors as strength and motor proficiency, whereas girls may be more interested in body poise and esthetics. This may be a very individual matter at this age level; motivation must be based on individual needs and interests. The actual physical correction of the fatigue slump is a twofold matter involving the realignment of antagonistic muscle groups throughout the body and the development of a feeling for sitting, standing, and moving with the body properly aligned. Realignment techniques previously described and exercises given in Chapter 5, especially those that develop the antigravity (extensor) muscles of the body and stretch their antagonists, should be assigned. The student should also work on body alignment (sitting, standing, and moving) in front of a mirror or with a competent person observing him so that he can develop a feeling for his newly acquired correct posture. Correction of total body malalignment is difficult and requires a vigorous exercise

hang, the upper body sways backward from the hips so that the center of the shoulder falls in back of the gravity line of the body. To compensate for this position, the hips and thighs may move forward of the gravity line, the head may tilt forward, and the chest may be flat. Correction of a posterior overhang involves a reorientation of the total body so that its several parts are returned to a position of alignment. The student is instructed to work in front of a mirror and align himself with a gravity marker on the mirror. Alternatively, he may have his posture checked and corrected by the instructor. His exercise program includes a reeducation of the antagonistic muscles so as to enable him to return the body to a position of balance. Those muscle groups needing special attention are the abdominal muscles, the antagonist muscle groups responsible for anteroposterior alignment of the tilt of the pelvis, the adductor muscles of the shoulder girdle, and the extensor muscles of the upper spine. The student must stand tall, with chin tucked and abdomen flat, to correct this condition (Fig. 9-19).

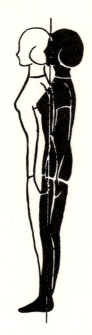

Fig. 9-20. Forward and backward leans.

regime, coupled with sufficient self-discipline to overcome whatever emotional and mental factors are contributing to the problem (Fig. 9-16).

Body leans. When viewed from the side, the total body may lean a considerable distance either forward or backward of the line of gravity. When the total body, from foot to head, is in good alignment, but leans forward or backward from the ankle so that the lobe of the ear is positioned either anterior or posterior to the gravity line, the condition is considered to be a total body lean (Fig. 9-20). If body leans are not corrected, as the individual attempts to compensate for the lean and bring the body back to a balanced standing position, they often will be transferred into one or more of the postural conditions discussed previously. Correction of the forward or backward lean of the total body is largely a matter of reorientation of the proprioceptive centers of the body to enable the individual to feel when he is standing with his body in correct alignment. Checking the body against a gravity line or a plumb line

hung vertically down the face of the three-way mirror is an excellent way for the student to see whether he has a forward or backward deviation and to recognize the feel of standing with the body in the correct position. Symmetrical exercises can then be assigned so that the student can develop the flexibility and strength necessary to hold the body in correct alignment.

Anterior and posterior posture examinations

Deviations of the foot and ankle that would be noted in examining a student from the anterior or posterior view were discussed in an earlier section of this chapter.

The knee. Three conditions involving the knee and the upper and lower leg may be noted when a student is examined from the anterior or posterior view. Bowlegs and knock-knees are recognized from either of these two views, whereas tibial torsion is more easily identified when the student is examined from the anterior view.

Bowlegs (genu varum). Bowlegs can be identified by examining a student with a plumb line, by comparing alignment of the leg with one of the vertical lines of the posture screen, or by having the student stand with the internal malleoli touching and the legs held comfortably straight. In the latter test, if a space exists between the knees when the malleoli are touching, the individual may be considered to have bowlegs. Unless this is either a functional condition in the young child (which may be outgrown) or a condition related to hyperextending the knees and rotating the thighs in order to separate the knees, corrective measures ordinarily must be prescribed by an orthopedic physician. Hyperextended and rotated knees causing a bowleg can be corrected by having the student assume the correct standing position and by developing proper balance in the pull of the antagonistic muscles of the hip and leg (Fig. 9-21, *C*).

Knock-knees (genu valgum). Knock-knees can be identified as described in the sec-

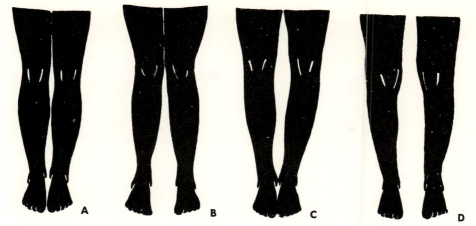

Fig. 9-21. Faulty leg alignment. **A,** Normal. **B,** Knock-knees. **C,** Bowleg. **D,** Tibial torsion.

tion on bowlegs; however, in this case, when the inner borders (medial femoral condyles) of the knees are brought together, a space exists between the internal malleoli. Knock-knees may be related to pronation of the ankle and weakness in the longitudinal arch. Correction involves realignment of the antagonist muscles of the leg and foot, which control proper alignment. This usually involves developing the outward rotators of the thigh and shortening and tightening the structures that traverse the medial side of the leg at the knee; those on the lateral side should be stretched. Correction of this condition will also involve realignment of the foot, the ankle, and the hip (Fig. 9-21, *B*). Knock-knees also may be related to tibial torsion.

Tibial torsion. Tibial torsion, or twisting of the tibia, is identified by examining the student from the anterior view. When his feet are pointed straight ahead, the individual with tibial torsion will have one or both of the kneecaps facing in a medial direction or when the kneecaps are facing straight forward, the feet are rotated in a toed-out position (Fig. 9-21, *D*). Correction of this condition involves realignment of the total leg, with emphasis being placed on the regions of the ankle, knee, and hip. The outward rotators of the hip and the thigh must be developed, whereas muscles

on the medial and lateral side of the foot and ankle must be properly stretched and strengthened to obtain proper alignment. Special exercises for these problems of leg alignment are described in Chapter 5.

Lateral pelvic tilt. A lateral pelvic tilt, in which one side of the pelvis is higher or lower than the other side, can be observed during both the anterior and the posterior posture examinations. These conditions can be evaluated by marking either the anterior superior iliac spines or the posterior superior iliac spines of the ilium and then observing their relative height through the grids of a posture screen. The height of the pelvis can also be evaluated by placing the fingers of the examiner on the uppermost portion of the crest of the ilium and observing the relative height of the two sides of the pelvis (Fig. 9-22). A lateral pelvic tilt may result from such things as unilateral ankle pronation, knock-knees, bowlegs, a shorter long bone in either the lower or upper portion of one leg, structural anomalies of the knee and hip joint and deviations in the pelvic girdle, or a scoliotic spine, all of which are discussed in Chapters 10 and 11. Before an exercise program for a lateral pelvic tilt is initiated, its cause must be determined by a physician, who may then suggest either symmetrical or asymmetrical exercises to realign the pelvic

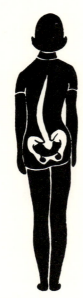

Fig. 9-22. Lateral pelvic tilt.

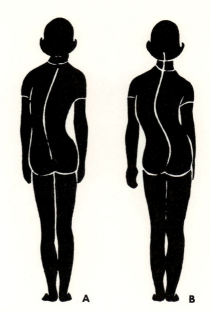

Fig. 9-23. Scoliosis. **A,** Total left C curve. **B,** Regular S curve.

level. The position of the pelvic girdle as viewed from the anterior or posterior view has very definite implications for the position of the spinal column as it extends upward from the sacrum. A lateral tilt of the pelvis will be reflected in the spinal column above it, since the sacroiliac and the lumbosacral joints are semi-immovable. The resulting lateral spinal curvatures are discussed in the next section of this chapter. Lateral tilt of the pelvis may also be related to a twisting of the pelvic girdle itself. This is a complicated orthopedic problem involving, in addition to the pelvis, resultant manifestations in both hip joints, the legs, and the vertebral column. Such cases should be referred to the orthopedic physician for treatment and for advice relative to a special exercise program.

Scoliosis. Scoliosis is a rotolateral curvature of the spine. When viewed from the front or from the rear, a scoliotic spine has a curvature to one side; in advanced stages, it may curve both to the left and to the right. Scoliosis curves are ordinarily described in relation to their position as the

individual is being viewed from the rear. A curvature is described as a simple C curve to the left or right. In a more advanced stage, compensation above or below the original curve may occur and the resulting curvature is described as a regular S curve or a reverse S curve. Examples of scoliotic curves are shown in Fig. 9-23.

Initially, a lateral deviation of the spine may involve only a simple C curve to the left or right in any segment of the spine, depending on the cause of the problem, the resulting change in soft tissues, and the pull of the antagonist muscles. These curves are often functional in nature and thus are correctable through properly assigned stretching and developmental exercises under the guidance of a physician. Untreated spines will often become progressively worse, involving permanent structural changes.

Scoliosis is often caused by asymmetry of the body. Lateral pelvic tilt, low shoulder, asymmetrical development of the rib cage, or lateral deviation of the linea alba may be involved in a "cause *or* effect" relationship with a rotolateral curve of the spine. Evidence of this would be found in one or more of the following bodily changes:

1. When the thoracic vertebral column is displaced laterally, the rotation of the vertebral bodies is in the direction of the convexity of the curve.
2. Lateral bending of the spine is accompanied by a depression and protrusion of the intervertebral discs on the concave side, with a greater separation between the sides of the vertebrae on the convex side of the lateral curve.
3. There is an imbalance in the stability and pull of the ligaments and muscles responsible for holding the vertebral column in its normal position. Muscles and ligaments on the concave side become tight and contracted, whereas those on the convex side become stretched and weakened. Muscle atrophy may occur.
4. Changes in the rib cage involve a flattening and depression of the posterior aspects of the ribs on the concave side, with a posterior bulging of the ribs on the side of the convex spinal curve. The opposite is true of the anterior aspect of the chest. There the ribs on the concave side are prominent, whereas, on the convex side, they are flattened or depressed.

The treatment of scoliosis is rather specific, depending on the cause of the condition and the resulting changes in the spinal column. Students with scoliosis must be referred to an orthopedist for examination and recommendations relative to stretching and developmental exercises. These may be either symmetrical or asymmetrical in nature. Some orthopedic physicians believe that the treatment of scoliosis should be very specific and will indicate the types of asymmetrical exercises that should be engaged in by the student. Others subscribe to the theory that the cause of scoliosis should be eliminated if possible, but that only symmetrical types of exercise should be assigned for this condition. Both types of exercise for scoliosis are presented in Chapter 5.

Since scoliosis of the spine is a very complicated and difficult type of condition to diagnose and treat, it is necessary for the adapted teacher or therapist to rely on the advice of the physician relative to the types of activities and exercises that should be prescribed for the student. Since lateral spinal curves are accompanied by a certain amount of rotation of the spine, a great deal of skill is required to diagnose and treat the condition correctly. Recommendations relative to types of games, sports, and activities should therefore be indicated by the examining physician. Although scoliosis is usually recognized when the student is examined from the posterior view, the student with scoliosis often will also exhibit certain characteristics of asymmetry when checked from the anterior view. These include asymmetry of the rib cage and a lateral deviation of the linea alba.

Scoliosis in young girls. During the last several years, the importance of identifying and treating scoliosis in young girls between the ages of 9 and 13 or 14 years has been stressed by orthopedic physicians. Early detection by physical education teachers, therapists, and nurses and immediate referral to a physician who *specializes* in scoliosis treatment may prevent permanent deformity in many of these young persons.

Treatment may consist of utilization of casts or braces (Fig. 9-24) combined with a special exercise program assigned by the physician. Exercise programs without the cast or brace are not usually recommended. Cases that are not discovered early may require surgery with spinal fusion or the insertion of rods along the vertebral column to straighten the severely curved spine (Fig. 9-25).

Physicians at the Los Angeles Orthopedic Hospital and the Orange County Orthopedic Hospital in California have successfully treated large numbers of young girls and have spearheaded campaigns to provide for early diagnosis of this serious problem.

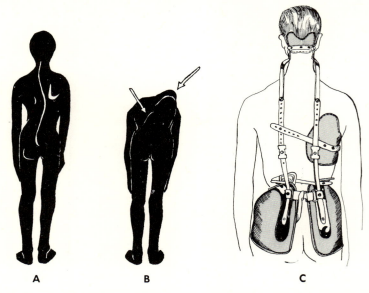

Fig. 9-24. Scoliosis. **A,** Rotolateral curve. **B,** Rotation viewed from Adams position. **C,** Milwaukee brace.

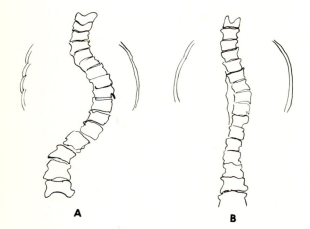

Fig. 9-25. Severe scoliosis. **A,** Before surgery. **B,** After surgery and corrective procedures.

Treatment of patients with severe scoliosis (Chapter 5 includes specific exercises for scoliosis) may include any or all of the following:

1. Removal of the cause, if possible.
2. Assignment of symmetrical exercises, especially for the abdomen, back, and hip regions.
3. Promoting mobilization of tightness in soft tissue in the trunk, shoulder girdle, and hip region.
4. Giving asymmetrical exercises to tighten muscles on the convex side of the curves on the recommendation of an orthopedic physician.
5. Recommendation of traction of the spine by the physician.
6. Assignment of exercises to increase the strength and the anteroposterior balance and alignment of the spine.
7. Specific prescription of any derotation exercises by the physician.

Physical educators who specialize in adapted physical education should inform those teaching regular physical education, the school nurse, and other health-related personnel of the importance of screening young persons for scoliosis and other body mechanics problems early enough to involve them in preventive programs under the guidance of a physician who specializes

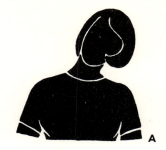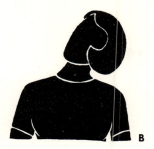

Fig. 9-26. Faulty head positions. **A,** Head tilt. **B,** Head twist.

in the diagnosis and care of scoliosis and other serious orthopedic problems.

Shoulder height. It is rather common for an individual to have one shoulder higher or lower than the other. This condition usually results from asymmetrical muscle or bony development of the shoulder girdle or lateral curvature in the spinal column. Correction of an abnormal curve in the spine may result in the shoulders returning to a level position, although corrective exercises may be required in the process. When the cause is muscular in origin, correction is a relatively simple matter of developing the strength of the weaker or lower side and stretching the contracted side. This also involves a reorientation of the student's feeling for the correct shoulder and body alignment. Exercise for a low or high shoulder should be done in front of a regular or three-way mirror to enable the student to learn to feel the position of the body when it is being held in proper alignment. (See Chapter 5 for special exercises.)

Head tilt or twist. When viewed from the anterior or posterior view, the head may be either tilted directly to the side or tilted to the side with a concomitant twisting of the head and neck (Fig. 9-26). In either case, it is necessary to reorient the student to the proper position of the head. Very often, deviations in the position of the head and neck are compensatory for other postural deviations located below this area. The correction of these conditions should accompany the reorientation and correction of the position of the head itself.

The correction of the head position will involve reeducating the antagonist muscles responsible for holding the head in a position of balance, plus reorienting the student in terms of holding the head in the correct position. This will involve the appropriate proprioceptive centers and balance organs. The exercise program for correction of the condition should be rather specific in terms of those muscle groups that are stretched and developed. Moreover, the exercise program should be practiced with the individual standing in front of a mirror so that he can not only visualize the correct position but also develop the feeling of holding the head in correct alignment. Selected exercises used in stretching and developing muscles that control the position of the head are presented in Chapter 5. A discussion of torticollis (wryneck) is included in Chapter 10.

Body tilt. Another deviation that may be noted in the anterior and posterior posture examination is a problem of body alignment in which the total body is tilted to the left or right of the gravity or plumb line (Fig. 9-27). Standing with the body tilted to the side causes increased strain on the bones, joints, and muscles and may result in compensation being made to bring the body back into a position of balance over its base of support. Often, this compensation results in the hips and shoulders being thrown out of alignment, leading to the development of a lateral curvature in the spine. Correction of this condition involves an analysis of the causative factors of the

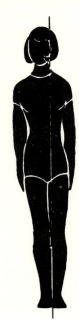

Fig. 9-27. Body tilt.

tilt, such as unilateral flatfoot, pronated ankle, knock-knee, or short leg. On the other hand, standing out of balanced alignment may be habitual with the student. Before correction of the lateral body tilt can be accomplished, unilateral deviations must be corrected. Specific suggestions for the correction of a weak foot, ankle, or knee are contained in another section of this chapter. Together with these specific corrective measures, exercises should be given to the student for body tilt. Exercises and activities that involve the symmetrical use of the total body and that will help the student learn to stand with the body in correct alignment and balance are needed. Exercising in front of the mirror will give the student a visual concept of the feeling of standing with the body in a balanced position, which should help him to effect a correction of a lateral tilt of the body. (Special exercises are described in Chapter 5.)

TESTS AND MEASUREMENTS FOR POSTURE AND BODY ALIGNMENT

Tests and measurements can be used in adapted physical education to evaluate student improvement, to aid in instruction, to determine whether body parts are properly aligned, and to motivate students to work toward correction of body malalignment. Some of the tests and measurements traditionally used in adapted physical education programs are not high in validity and reliability, but may still be of some use in identifying deviations, in helping the instructor explain malalignments to students, and in motivating students to work toward self-improvement. If any or all of these values are obtained from testing the students, it should be a worthwhile part of the total program.

Tests and measurements can be made more useful if instructors carefully observe the following matters in their testing procedures:

1. Obtain the best testing equipment possible.
2. Keep all equipment in correct working condition.
3. Use correct testing procedures.
4. Use the same piece of testing equipment on successive tests, if possible.
5. Have the same tester administer each successive test.
6. Test under similar conditions, for example, before a workout each time, at the same time each day, or at the same time in each period.
7. Record all information accurately and indicate the date that the test was given.
8. Determine accurately the location of landmarks used in measurement.
9. Attempt to standardize all procedures and provide a written description of these procedures so that they can be followed on each occasion by any teacher or tester who administers the test.

Tests for the foot
Podiascope

Description. The podiascope is a device used to observe the plantar surface of the foot under weight-bearing conditions. It consist of a wooden box (usually made of ¾-inch thick plywood) approximately 14 inches square with the top surface of ¾-inch thick plate glass. The front side is

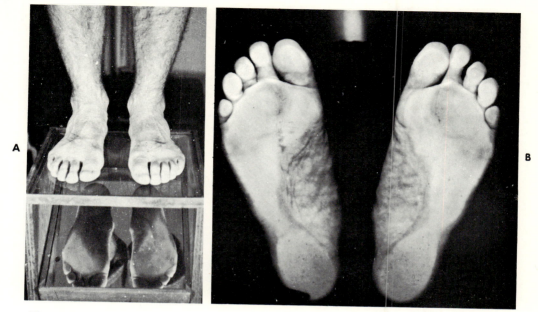

Fig. 9-28. The podiascope examination. **A,** Subject standing on podiascope. **B,** Photograph of feet through podiascope.

left open. Inside the box, under the glass and facing toward the open side, is an adjustable mirror slanting downward at approximately a 45-degree angle. The mirror is mounted on a piece of wood and made adjustable so that its back edge can be moved up and down to facilitate viewing the bottom of the foot from various angles in front of the podiascope or when it is placed in front of a wall mirror so that the student can view his own feet (Fig. 9-28).

Instructions for use. The podiascope is placed on a bench or table. The glass top is thoroughly cleaned and the student stands on the glass facing toward the open side. The instructor, seated so as to be able comfortably to look into the mirror, can then observe the reflection of the bottoms of the students' feet. After approximately 1 minute of standing on the glass, the weight-bearing surfaces of the feet begin to show up as pale white areas, whereas the nonweight-bearing areas are pink in color. The examiner will then be able to observe the following:

1. The shape of the longitudinal arch
2. The height of the longitudinal arch
3. The areas of stress on the bottom of the foot (indicated by darker colorations and calluses that occur from abnormal pressures during weight bearing)
4. Whether the toes are bearing their share of the weight, whether they are straight, and whether the second toe projects forward a greater distance than the great toe
5. Heavy callous formation along the medial side of the great toe and on the lateral side of the heel, indicating abnormal use of the foot
6. Callous formation in the metatarsal arch region

These calluses may reflect pressuse of one metatarsal bone or may be large, reflecting pressure across the total transverse arch. Pressure or stress may result from the poor mechanical use of the foot caused by functional or structural deviations or from activities that produce heavy friction to the foot, that is, dancing, cross-country running, and basketball.

Uses and limitations. The podiascope can

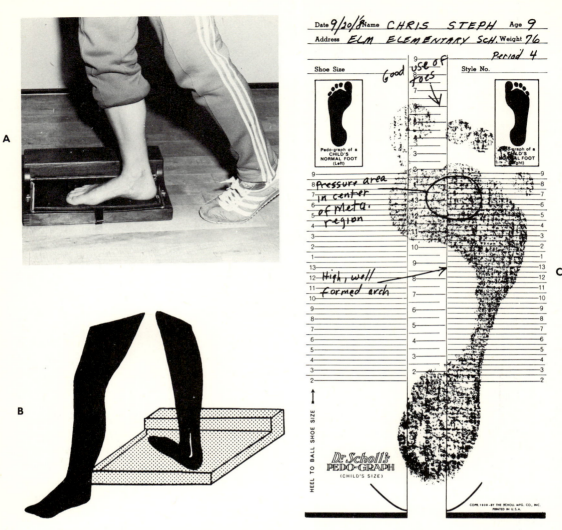

The following handwritten annotations appear on the pedograph chart (C):

Date 9/20/8 Name CHRIS STEPH Age 9

Address ELM ELEMENTARY SCH. Weight 76

Period 4

Shoe Size   Good use of toes   Style No.

Pressure area in center of Meta. region

High, well formed arch

Dr Scholl's PEDO-GRAPH (CHILD'S SIZE)

HEEL TO BALL SHOE SIZE

Fig. 9-29. Footprint examinations. **A,** Making a pedograph print. **B,** Student stepping on large-sized pedograph. Note badly abducted foot position. **C,** Pedograph print with markings used to show findings from the podiascope examination. (**A,** Courtesy California State University Audio Visual Center, Long Beach, Calif.)

be used to examine the longitudinal and transverse arches of the foot while weight bearing and to check for areas of stress and strain on the foot. By placing the podiascope in front of a regular or three-way mirror, the student can observe the foot problems that have been discovered and described to him by the instructor. A permanent record can be made of the podiascope findings by photographing the bot- tom of the foot through the glass. If photography is not used, a permanent record of the examination can be recorded on a pedograph print by the instructor (Fig. 9-29).

Pedograph

Description. A pedograph is an ink print that is made of the bottom of the foot under weight-bearing conditions. This print is made by placing either a special or a blank piece of paper directly beneath a rubber sheet whose underside has been inked. The student is then instructed either to step on the rubber sheet with his full weight or to take a walking step across the pedograph so that a permanent print of the foot under weight-bearing conditions is recorded. The William M. Scholl Company, Chicago, Ill., commercially produces a pedograph machine for use by the general public. A device of this type is satisfactory for school use; however, similar equipment can be constructed by the adapted physical education teacher or the maintenance or industrial arts department of the school (Fig. 2-29).

Instructions for use. The footprint machine is placed on the floor directly in front of the student, with the paper placed under the rubber sheet. The student is then in-

structed to step on the print with the full body weight being borne as in normal use. The print of the foot can be taken as the individual steps directly on and off the rubber sheet or it can be taken as the individual takes a normal walking step across it. The latter would indicate his pattern of weight bearing during normal walking; however, to permit the individual freedom in the placement of his foot, the pedograph must be larger than the Scholl pedograph. To accommodate the foot in whatever position is usual for the student, a 14- by 16-inch space is needed.

Uses and limitations. Although the pedograph does not indicate deviations as clearly as the podiascope, it will furnish a permanent print for study and for comparison during later examinations. If a pedograph print is made prior to the time the podiascope examination is performed, information that is obtained from the podiascope examination can be recorded by the instructor on the pedograph print. This can be done by writing explanatory notes on the pedograph or by circling areas of special significance on the print, for example, abnormal patterns of weight bearing, prominent calluses, and poor alignment of the toes and feet (Fig. 9-29, *C*).

The pedograph print can also be used to record the results of a foot tracing made to show the amount of medial displacement of and pronation in the foot and ankle. The procedure for making a foot tracing is described in detail in this chapter in the section discussing the ankle (Fig. 9-30).

Height of the longitudinal arch test

Description. The height of the longitudinal arch of the foot seems to be of interest to some doctors, therapists, and physical educators, especially if the measurement of its height is one that compares the arch under weight-bearing and nonweight-bearing conditions. The functional flatfoot may be a painful flatfoot and the height of the arch, in this case, will often show considerable difference when weight-bearing

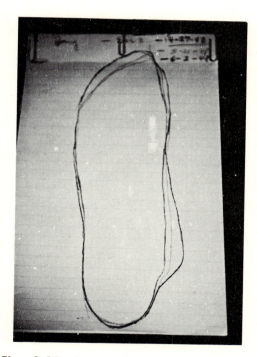

Fig. 9-30. Foot tracing. Note improvement shown in successive examinations (lines on medial side of foot move progressively toward the midline of the foot) as leg, foot, and ankle are realigned. (See Fig. 20-26.)

and nonweight-bearing measurements are compared.

Instructions for use. The test involves measurements made of the height of the scaphoid bone. The instructor first marks, with either a skin pencil or a ballpoint pen, the farthest medial projection of the scaphoid or navicular bone with a dot or a short line parallel to the floor. The student is then asked to place his foot on a flat surface without bearing weight on it and the instructor measures the distance from the supporting surface to the mark on the scaphoid bone. The student then places his weight on the foot and the height of the mark is again measured. The difference in the height of the mark is compared with the scale found in Fig. 9-37.

Uses and limitations. The height of the long arch test can be used with students who have functional flatfoot and for those with ankle pronation. It is a relatively easy test to administer; however, difficulty may be encountered in finding the medialmost projection of the bone on some subjects.

It should be remembered that there is no direct relationship between the height of the arch and the strength of the foot. Many persons with very low arches, or even with flatfeet, are free of pain and also highly successful in terms of athletics and other physical endeavors. However, measurement of the height of the arch and examination of the foot for proper mechanics can provide information that is useful to the instructor in the assignment of special exercises to strengthen the foot, for recommendations relative to good mechanics in the use of the foot, and for such other matters as recommending proper footwear and special care of the feet.

Tests for the ankle

The ankle joint is a hinge joint, capable of only two fundamental motions: dorsiflexion and plantar flexion. However, because of its close connection with the bones of the foot and because it is superimposed directly above the foot bones, certain foot deviations are also reflected in the position of the ankle. It is therefore necessary in doing a complete foot examination not only to examine the foot, but also to examine the structures located above it, including the ankle, the knee, and the hip.

Foot and ankle tracings

Description. Lowman, Colestock, and Cooper[9] described a technique of making a tracing around a person's foot with a pencil that is held perpendicular to the surface on which the person is standing. The pencil thus reflects indentations and prominences around the edge of the foot as the tracing is made. The tracing will also show other projections above the region of the sole of the foot such as the medial aspect of the scaphoid bone, the position of the medial malleolus, and the position of the lateral malleolus. Young[10] devised a small block arrangement with a pencil inserted so that the block slides in a position perpendicular to the sheet on which the tracing is made and the mark made by the pencil reflects more accurately the foot and ankle position described previously (Figs. 9-30 and 20-22).

Instructions for use. The student assumes his normal standing position, with his feet about 6 inches apart, either on pedograph prints previously made of his feet or, if preferred, on two blank pieces of paper. The instructor then traces an outline around the foot, making sure that the front edge of the tracer is kept in firm contact with the foot and that the pencil is recording properly on the paper. The lower surface of the tracer is kept flat on the paper as it slides around the edge of the foot. To standardize procedures, the same tracer, with a different colored pencil in the tracer, should be used each time an individual is retested. Thus the second tracing can be made on the same paper and directly compared with the first. When this is done, it is important to compare the complete tracing of the foot on each of the examinations so that if, during a second examination, the total foot is shifted to the medial or lateral side of the position taken during the first tracing, the individual reading the tracing will not suspect that improvement or change has taken place. When the foot is placed in the same position each time and the medial side of the tracing moves toward the center of the foot on successive tests, that is, less prominence of the scaphoid bone and internal malleolus, improvement in pronation and alignment is indicated (Fig. 9-30).

Uses and limitations. Foot tracings can be used to show the student deviations in the foot and ankle position that have been observed by the instructor during the posture and foot examination. Of particular importance are such factors as abduction of the forepart of the foot, medial protrusion of the scaphoid bone, and medial displacement of the internal malleolus, all of which will show up rather clearly in the tracing. Seeing this illustration of the deviation and then observing how changes can take place when the muscles are reeducated so that the inside of the foot and arch are realigned should serve as motivation for students to work toward improvement of pronation of the feet and ankles and abduction of the feet. Special exercises for realigning the foot and the ankle are presented in Chapter 5.

Achilles tendon test

Description. The Achilles tendon test is usually conducted as part of a total posture examination; however, it must also be a standard procedure for all foot examinations. This test is made from the rear of the student and involves viewing the alignment of the heel cord of the individual while he is standing in his normal position. It can be made by viewing the student while he stands behind the posture screen, by using a plumb line for comparison, or by simply viewing the heel cord and estimating the degree of straightness or the amount of inward curve that is present in the Achilles tendon.

Instructions for use. The individual to be tested stands with his back turned toward the instructor, who stands 5 to 10 feet be-

hind him. The instructor then uses the vertical lines of the posture screen, a plumb line, or his own judgment to determine whether the heel cord is straight. The Achilles tendon of a properly aligned foot and ankle will not curve inward or outward. However, an individual who has pronation of the ankles will often reflect a bowing inward of the heel cord (Helbing's sign); conversely, a person with supinated feet will display outward bowing. When ankle pronation is present, the inner malleolus will be more prominent and the scaphoid bone will protrude in a medial direction. The forepart of the foot may also be turned out and the medial side of the foot may be depressed (Fig. 9-9).

Tests for knock-knees and bowlegs

Description. Tests for knock-knees and bowlegs are used to determine whether the individual's legs are straight or whether either knock-kneed or bowlegged and the approximate extent of either of the latter conditions.

Instructions for use. The individual is asked to assume a normal standing position while his general leg alignment is observed from the front and rear. He then is requested to slide his legs together until either the inner sides of the condyles of the knee or the medial malleoli touch. If the inner sides of the knees come together first and the ankle bones are still separated, a knock-knee condition exists. The extent of this deviation can be determined by measuring the distance between the internal malleoli. If, on the other hand, the internal malleoli touch and the medial condyles of the knees are separated, a bowleg condition exists. This condition can be measured by determining the distance between the inner sides of the knees. Inside calipers can be used to measure the amount of deviation or, if this equipment is not available, the instructor can measure the approximate distance with a tape measure or with small pieces of wood that have been cut for this purpose in various predetermined widths ranging from ½ to 3 inches.

Uses and limitations. The amount of knock-knee or bowleg can also be estimated while the individual stands behind a posture screen by observing the leg alignment in relation to the vertical lines of the grid. If heavy fat pads exist on the medial side of the leg just above the knee, it may be difficult to obtain an accurate measurement with either of these two tests. Consequently, the individual is instructed to bring the inner sides of the condyles of the knees together firmly on the pronation test. When a measurement of the distance between the inner sides of the knees is made, it should be made with enough pressure to eliminate the effect of the musculature and the fatty pads that may be present in this region. Tests for alignment of the total leg are described in the following section.

Tests for leg alignment

Description. The alignment of the leg can be evaluated from the anterior, lateral, or posterior view. Each of these positions will give the examiner an opportunity to look for certain basic factors related to good segmental balance and alignment in the foot, ankle, knee, and hip.

Instructions for use. These examinations can be made with the individual standing behind a posture screen, using the vertical lines of the screen or a plumb line as a reference. When the examination is made from the anterior view, the student is instructed to stand in his normal posture facing the examiner. After they have been located for the student by the instructor, the anterosuperior spines of the ilium are marked with a skin pencil or the student is instructed to hold his index finger on these points. The instructor then moves to a position 5 to 10 feet away from the student and holds the gravity line out at full arm's length in order to sight through it, observing certain pertinent landmarks on the student. When the gravity line falls just medial to the anterosuperior spine of the ilium, it should pass down the leg through

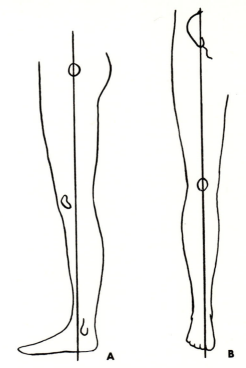

Fig. 9-31. Leg alignment tests. **A,** Lateral view examination. **B,** Anterior view examination.

the center of the knee, the center of the ankle joint, and then through a point between the first and second toes of the foot (Fig. 9-31, *B*). Any deviation from these positions could indicate a knock-knee or bowleg, respectively, depending on whether the plumb line fell lateral to or medial to the correct position at the center of the knee. A pronated or supinated ankle or an abducted or adducted foot would likewise be identified according to its relationship to the plumb line.

After the student has been examined and his normal standing position evaluated, the instructor can have him make whatever corrections are necessary to bring the foot, ankle, knee, and hip into proper alignment. The correctly aligned position is then practiced while standing, walking, and running.

When the gravity line examination is made to determine anteroposterior deviations in leg alignment, the student is viewed through the posture screen or evaluated with the plumb line from a position directly to his side. The student is asked to assume his normal standing position and certain landmarks are checked by the instructor against the gravity line. This runs through the center of the hip (approximately through the center of the greater trochanter of the femur bone), just posterior to the kneecap, and about 1 to 1½ inches anterior to the outer ankle bone (external malleolus) or approximately in line with the center of the scaphoid (navicular) bone (Fig. 9-31, A). Any deviation from this alignment indicates either that the individual has a forward or backward lean of the total body or a deviation in the region of the knee in which there is either abnormal hyperextension or hyperflexion. These conditions can be described to the student and efforts can be made to realign the body in order for him to assume correct balance. He should then exercise the appropriate muscles and practice this new position until it becomes natural to stand with the legs in proper alignment (Fig. 9-12).

Uses and limitations. These tests are usually given in connection with, or in addition to, the general posture examination. They should supplement the general examination and should call particular attention to problems that exist specifically in the leg and foot. Measurements on this test are not precise and will be dependent on the subjective judgment of the instructor. However, the plumb line or the posture screen serves as a good point of reference from which to make fairly accurate judgments. Exercise programs for the various conditions that might be discovered in these examinations are described in Chapter 5.

Tests of the pelvic girdle
Anteroposterior deviations

Description. Tests for an increased pelvic angle, sometimes called a forward (downward) pelvic tilt, and for an upward (backward) tilt of the pelvis are made

while the person is examined from the lateral view. Several tests are available for use by the instructor. The first test compares the position of the anterosuperior spine of the ilium with the symphysis pubis. In correct pelvic alignment, these two landmarks fall on the same vertical line. If the anterosuperior spine of the ilium falls in a plane anterior to the line of the symphysis pubis, the student has a condition described as a *forward* (anterior) or *downward* pelvic tilt, whereas the reverse would be described as a *backward* (posterior) or *upward* pelvic tilt.

A second test involves a comparison of the position of the anterosuperior spine of the ilium with the posterosuperior spine of the ilium. In this case, the two landmarks fall on the same horizontal line. If the anterosuperior spine of the ilium falls in a plane that is lower than the posterosuperior spine, the individual has an *increased forward* (anterior) or *downward* pelvic tilt. If the reverse is true, he has a *decreased backward* (posterior) or *upward* pelvic tilt.

The third test is called the pelvic angle test. This consists of locating the lumbosacral joint and the symphysis pubis and drawing an imaginary line connecting these two segments. The angle that results when this line joins a horizontal plane of the body can be compared by the instructor with the so-called normal angle of 50 to 60 degrees of pelvic inclination[12] (Fig. 9-32).

Uses and limitations. Any one of these tests can be used to help determine the amount of pelvic inclination that exists in the student being examined. A completely objective evaluation of pelvic inclination is difficult to make for several reasons. The individual may be very heavy, with large fat pads anteriorly and posteriorly that make it difficult to make any evaluation of either the pelvic position or the pelvic angle. The individual may be wearing bulky clothes that cover the region of the pelvis and low back and therefore make visual inspection difficult. The individual

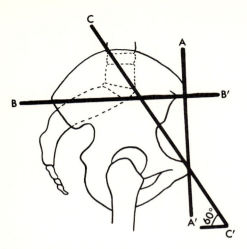

Fig. 9-32. Anteroposterior pelvic tilt examinations. *A-A'*, Anterosuperior spine and symphysis pubis in vertical alignment; *B-B'*, Anterosuperior spine and posterosuperior spine in horizontal alignment; *C-C'*, Line connecting lumbosacral joint with symphysis pubis forms a 50- to 60-degree angle with a horizontal line.

may also have a very large buttock region or a large anterior overhang of the lower abdominal region, which makes a subjective evaluation very difficult to make. Usually one set of the measurements described previously can be obtained while the individual is examined and they will allow the instructor to make a more accurate evaluation. The relationship between the tilt of the pelvis, the alignment of the upper leg and knee, and the lower portion of the spine has been discussed in an earlier portion of this chapter. It is important to check the amount of pelvic inclination of any student with bent or back knee or with lordosis or flat lower back. For a more objective evaluation of pelvic tilt, an x-ray examination is necessary.

Lateral deviations

Description. Lateral tilt of the pelvis can be evaluated from either the anterior or the posterior view. Usually the examination is made from both views in order to verify that a lateral tilt exists and to

look for torques in the pelvis. These tests are usually made by evaluating the individual with the horizontal lines of the posture screen.

Instructions for use. For the anterior examination, the anterosuperior spines of the ilium are either marked with a skin pencil or located by the instructor and the student is instructed to place one index finger on each spine. The student then stands behind the posture screen with his feet placed an equal distance to either side of the center (gravity) line of the screen. The instructor then steps back 10 to 12 feet from the screen, directly at its center, and sights through the screen to determine whether the anterosuperior spines fall on the same horizontal line. The posterior examination is conducted in the same manner, with the posterosuperior spines of the ilium being marked and the individual checked from the posterior view. The amount of deviation in the height of the spines can then be estimated and recorded on the student's posture examination form (Fig. 9-38, *C*).

If the instructor so desires, a measuring tape can be used to check the distance from the floor to the anterosuperior spine of the ilium on each side in order to determine whether the leg lengths are identical. Individual segments of the leg can also be measured in an attempt to determine where any deviation in length exists, for example, measuring the distance from the internal malleolus to the patella or to the anterosuperior spine on each side. Another technique that can be used to determine how much difference there is in the height of the sides of the pelvis involves the use of leg length blocks. These blocks are approximately 12 inches long and 3 inches wide and vary in thickness from 1/8 to 1 1/2 inches at 1/4-inch intervals. Any one or combination of these blocks can be placed underneath the foot of the leg on the low side of the pelvis until the pelvis is level, as viewed through the grids of the posture screen. If the student stands on this board with his back to the posture screen, any resulting improvement in the lateral alignment of the spine can be observed. If the student wears a lift in his shoe, but does not have one for his gym shoes, these same blocks can be placed under the foot while he is exercising in the adapted physical education room. Students with marked deviations in the height of the pelvis or with pain associated with pelvic tilt should be referred to an orthopedist for a more extensive examination, for recommendations relative to the need for a lift in the shoe, and for advice on special exercises and activities.

Other tests of the pelvic girdle

Jorris[6] devised an instrument, called the "tilt-o-meter," with which anteroposterior and lateral pelvic tilts can be measured. Where it is possible to locate the same landmarks as were described previously, it is possible to use the Jorris tilt-o-meter to obtain an evaluation of the amount of tilt of the pelvis.

Total body examinations
Plumb line tests

Description. A plumb line can be held by the instructor or can be hung so that it falls between the person being examined and the instructor. It is used as a vertical line or reference to check both the anteroposterior and the lateral body alignment of the student. Certain surface landmarks on the body that align with the gravity lines of the human body have been located by kinesiologists and engineers. These surface landmarks can be used as points of reference in conducting examinations designed to see how well the body is balanced and how well its segments are aligned in the upright position.

Lateral view. From the lateral view (anteroposterior deviations), starting at the base of support and working up the body, the gravity line should fall at a point about 1 to 1½ inches anterior to the external malleolus, just posterior to the patella, through the center of the hip at the ap-

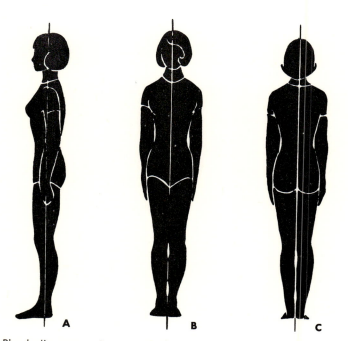

Fig. 9-33. Plumb line tests. **A,** Lateral examination. **B,** Anterior examination. **C,** Posterior examination.

proximate center of the greater trochanter of the femur, through the center of the shoulder (acromial process), and through the lobe of the ear.

Anterior view. From the anterior view (lateral deviations), the gravity line should fall an equal distance between the internal malleoli and between the knees; should pass through the center of the symphysis pubis, the center of the umbilicus, the center of the linea alba, the center of the chin, and the center of the nose; and should bisect the center of the upper portion of the head.

Posterior view. The landmarks to be checked in the posterior examination (lat-

eral deviations) would include the following: the same points in the region of the ankle and the knee, the cleft of the buttocks, the center of the spinous processes of the spinal column, and the center of the head. The plumb line does not provide as many points of reference as does the posture screen, since only one vertical line is available to be used as a reference for all anteroposterior and lateral postural deviations (Fig. 9-33). The posture grid provides both vertical and horizontal lines to be used as reference points for evaluating all segments of the body in relation to their contribution to a well-balanced, comfortable standing position, which is maintained by proper use of the antigravity muscle groups of the body (Fig. 9-34).

Posture screen

Description. A posture screen consists of a rectangular frame, mounted on legs so that it stands upright and laced with string so that a 2-inch-square grid pattern (4- and 6-inch squares are recommended by some) crosses the frame. The vertical lines are parallel to a center (gravity) line and the horizontal lines are exactly at right angles to the gravity line. The center line is usually of a color different from that of the other strings. This makes it easy to identify and to use in comparison with the landmarks described previously. It is possible to have a conformator built into the side of the posture screen, thus allowing the teacher with limited budget and space to have two pieces of apparatus in one. The conformator will be described later under the discussion of anteroposterior curvature of the spine (Figs. 9-40 and 20-24).

Instructions for use. The student should wear as little clothing as possible during the posture examination. Tight-fitting trunks for boys and girls, with a halter type of top for girls, are suggested. Neither shoes nor socks should be worn. It is almost impossible to administer an accurate examination if such landmarks as the ankle bones, kneecaps, spines of the pelvis, spi-

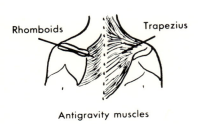

Antigravity muscles

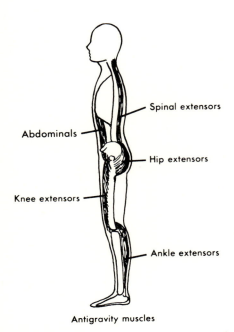

Antigravity muscles

Fig. 9-34. Antigravity muscles involved in maintaining erect posture.

nous processes of the vertebrae, medial borders of the scapula, and linea alba cannot be observed.

The posture screen should be checked for proper alignment with a plumb line to be sure that the gravity line is actually true and that the screen is also plumb when viewed from the side. It is then necessary to locate a point, about 18 inches from the posture screen, where the student will be centered properly behind the gravity line. This point is determined by having the instructor move to a position 10 to 15 feet away from the posture screen and standing in alignment with the center string while holding a plumb line out in front. Sighting through the plumb line and the center line of the screen, a point can be marked on the floor 18 inches behind the screen. This point will be in alignment with the instructor and the center line itself. Thus when the student stands behind the screen with the internal malleoli 1½ inches behind this point, it is possible to evaluate the posture from the anterior, posterior, and lateral views in relation to the center line of the screen (Fig. 9-35).

A posture screen may be used to give quick superficial screening examinations to identify students in need of special posture correction programs or it may be used to give a very thorough examination to those students who have been screened previously and identified as being in need of special programs for the correction of their posture and body alignment.

A posture examination is much more meaningful to the student and far more useful to the teacher if the findings are carefully recorded by the examiner (especially during review of the material obtained in the examination prior to setting up an exercise or activity program or when involved in doing a reevaluation of the pupil several months after the original examination). The examination record must provide space for the instructor to record the findings of the examination quickly and accurately. Provisions should be made for recording the severity of each of the conditions identified in the examination. The findings of successive examinations can also be recorded on the same form. An example showing a three-way figure with the proper labels and with numbers to indicate the severity of the conditions discovered is shown in Fig. 9-36, *B*. With this kind of prepared examination form, the instructor can very quickly identify deviations observed through the posture grid and can record them on the card by drawing a diagonal line through the number that indicates the severity of the condition: first degree, slight; second degree, moderate; and third degree, severe (Fig. 9-37). No other writing is necessary unless the instructor identifies something that does not appear on the chart or wishes to

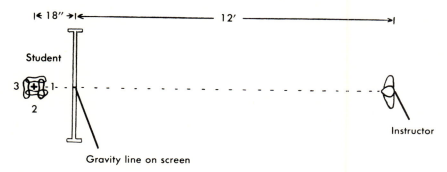

Fig. 9-35. Alignment of posture screen as viewed from above. *1,* Anterior, *2,* lateral, and *3,* posterior examinations.

California State University, Long Beach
MEN'S PHYSICAL EDUCATION DEPARTMENT

Adapted physical education appraisal

Name _____ Age _____ Date _____
          Last   First   Middle

Year in school _____

Physical disability (Be exact, give dates.) (This information is obtained from the student or parent.)
_____
_____
_____

Other disabilities and injuries discovered (Be exact, give dates.) _____
_____
_____

Results of physical examination (This information is obtained from the physician.)

Classification   A   B   C   1   2   3   4   5   6   7   8   9   0   _____
_____
_____

Recommendation of physician _____
_____

Assignment in adapted physical education class   Temporary   Permanent   Strict   Mild
_____

Nutritional status information _____

	Examination number	1	2	1	2

Pryor index _____   Behnke index _____
  Age (years, months) _____   Weight (normal) _____
  Height (inches) _____   Weight (actual) _____
  Pelvis width (cm) _____   Weight (variation) _____
  Chest width (cm) _____
  Weight (normal) _____   Other tests _____
  Weight (actual) _____   _____
  Weight (variation) _____

Skin fold measurements (mm) _____
  Triceps _____ = %   Biceps _____ = %
  Scapular _____ = %   Suprailiac _____ = %

Body type (Sheldon) _____

Endomorph	Mesomorph	Ectomorph
1 2 3 4 5 6 7	1 2 3 4 5 6 7	1 2 3 4 5 6 7

Follow-up examinations

Examination	Dates checked	Examination	Dates checked
Blood pressure _____		Anthropometric measurements (Specify.) _____	
Heart _____		1. Girth _____	
Cardiogram _____		2. _____	
Others _____		3. _____	
X-ray films _____		4. _____	
Photography _____		Nutrition _____	
Posture _____		Diet analysis _____	
Divergency _____		Basal metabolism _____	
Foot _____		Other tests _____	
Tracings _____		_____	
Pedograph _____			
Podiascope _____			

Joint measurements _____   **Code used on this appraisal sheet**
  Calipers _____

Severity of condition	Record of examinations
Goniometer _____ 1 degree = Noticeable to	First examination—Black pencil
Tracings _____ slight	Second examination—Blue pencil
Spine _____ 2 degree = Moderate	Third examination—Red pencil
Tracings _____ 3 degree = Severe	Fourth examination—Green pencil
Conformator _____	

A

Fig. 9-36. Adapted physical education appraisal. **A,** Front. **B,** Back. See text for explanation of appraisal of scoliosis conditions marked with an asterisk.

POSTURE EXAMINATION USING POSTURE SCREEN WITH 2-INCH GRIDS

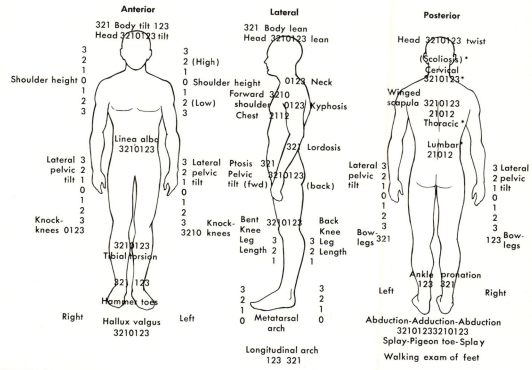

Anterior

321 Body tilt 123
Head 3210123 tilt

3
2
1
Shoulder height 0
1
2
3

Linea alba
3210123

Lateral 3
pelvic 2
tilt 1
0
1
2
3

Knock-
knees 0123

3210123
Tibial torsion

321 123
Hammer toes

Right   Hallux valgus
3210123

Lateral

321 Body lean
Head 3210123 lean

3
2 (High)
1
0 Shoulder height   0123 Neck
1
2 (Low)   Forward 3210
3   shoulder   0123 Kyphosis
                Chest 2112

                321 Lordosis

3 Lateral   Ptosis 321
2 pelvic   Pelvic
1 tilt   tilt (fwd) 3210123   (back)
0
1
2
3
Knock-   Bent 3210123   Back
3210 knees   Knee   Knee
                Leg   3   3 Leg
                Length 2   2 Length
                        1   1

3   3
2   2
1   1
0 Metatarsal   0
    arch

Left   Longitudinal arch
                123 321

Posterior

Head 3210123 twist

(Scoliosis) *
Cervical
3210123 *

Winged
scapula 3210123
                21012
Thoracic *

                Lumbar*
                21012

Lateral 3   3 Lateral
pelvic 2   2 pelvic
tilt 1   1 tilt
0   0
1   1
2   2
3   3
Bow-   Bowlegs 321   123 legs

                Ankle pronation
                123 321

Left   Right

Abduction-Adduction-Abduction
3210123 3210123
Splay-Pigeon toe-Splay

Walking exam of feet

B

SUMMARY OF FINDINGS
Medical 123 Injuries 123 Posture 123 Feet 123 Nutrition 123

REMARKS:
Recommendations:

A. Student's interest toward improvement:

B. Corrective exercises: (indicate nos. assigned)
1 2 3 4 5 6 7 8 9 10 11 12 13 14 15 16
17 18 19 20 21 22 23 24 25 26 27 28 29
30 31 32 33 34 35 36 37 38 39 40

C. Other exercises assigned:

D. Remarks and disposition of student:

Fig. 9-36, cont'd. For legend see opposite page.

DEGREE OF DEVIATION CHART
Individual posture examination using
a posture screen with 2-inch grids

Anterior view		Lateral view		Posterior view	
Condition	Degree of severity	Condition	Degree of severity	Condition	Degree of severity
Body tilt	1 inch = 1 degree	Body lean	1 inch = 1 degree	Head twist	Subjective evaluation
Head tilt	½ inch = 1 degree	Head lean	½ inch = 1 degree	Scoliosis (see cervical,	½ inch = 1 degree at each
Shoulder height	½ inch = 1 degree	Forward shoulders	Subjective evaluation	thoracic, lumbar)	spinal level
Linea alba	½ inch = 1 degree		(check tip of shoulder	Winged scapula	Subjective evaluation and mea-
Lateral pelvic tilt	½ inch = 1 degree		with gravity line)		sure distance between
(anterior, su-		Kyphosis	Subjective evaluation and		scapulae
perior spines			/or conformator	Lateral pelvic tilt (com-	¼ inch = 1 degree
of ilium)		Chest	Subjective evaluation	pare postero superior	
Knock-knees	½ inch = 1 degree	Lordosis	Subjective evaluation and	spines of ilium)	
(measure at			/or conformator	Bowlegs (measure at the	½ inch = 1 degree
the ankles)		Ptosis	Subjective evaluation	knees)	
Tibial torsion	Subjective evalua-	Pelvic tilt	Mark anterior and poste-	Ankle and foot pronation	Subjective evaluation, Helbing's
	tion		rior spines of ilium and		sign, and foot tracer
Hammer toes	Subjective evalua-		compare height	Abduction (splay foot) or	Subjective evaluation and foot
	tion	Bent and back knee	Subjective evaluation	adduction (pigeon toe)	tracer
Hallux valgus	Subjective evalua-		re: gravity line	Longitudinal arch	Height of scaphoid bone
	tion	Metatarsal arch	Subjective evaluation or		¼ inch = 1 degree
Leg length	Measure legs or use		pedograph print and		
	leg length boards		podiascope		
	and posture				
	screen				

Fig. 9-37. Individual posture examination degree of deviation chart. These figures were developed over a 10-year period for use with college men at the University of California at Los Angeles and California State University at Long Beach.

record special information to be used at a later time. Successive examinations can be made on the same posture form by using different colored pencils to indicate second, third, or fourth examinations. In this way, improvement can be shown through the use of the cumulative record. Other information that can be recorded on this card is discussed in detail in Chapter 18.

Anterior view. The student is instructed to stand directly behind the posture screen with the internal malleoli of the ankles placed 1½ inches posterior to and an *equal* distance from the + mark on the floor. (See Fig. 9-35.) This will place the student in the proper position so that the surface landmarks of the body will fall in correct alignment in relation to the center (gravity) line of the screen. The student is then instructed to stand as he would normally. The instructor should take a position about 10 to 15 feet back from the posture screen and in direct line with the center line. The posture examination record can be mounted on a clipboard held by the examiner or a lectern can be used to hold

the forms so as to facilitate recording the findings. Since the feet serve as the base of support, it is important to examine the student from the base of support upward in checking for proper body alignment. Specific examinations for the foot, ankle, knee, and leg have been covered in preceding sections of the chapter; they will be reviewed very briefly in this section, largely in terms of their influence on posture and the alignment of the rest of the body.

The feet should be checked to see if they are pointed straight forward or toeing in or out. The longitudinal arch should be higher on its medial than on its lateral side. The inner and outer malleoli should be about equal in prominence and the scaphoid bone should not project unduly medially. The ankles and knees should be straight, with the kneecaps facing directly forward when the feet are held in the straight forward position. The height of the kneecaps and the anterosuperior spines of the ilium should be even. The gravity line passes midway between the ankle

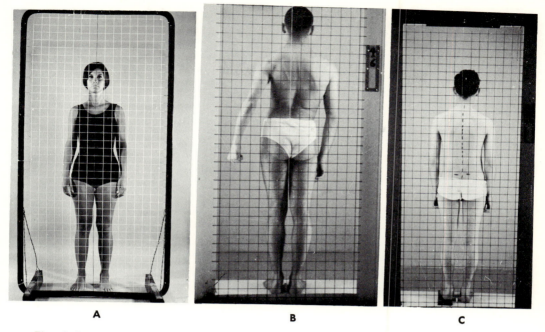

Fig. 9-38. Posture examinations with a posture screen. **A,** Anterior view examination. **B,** Structural scoliosis. **C,** Functional scoliosis. Note spinal alignment when a leg lift board is placed under the left foot.

bones, between the knees, and then falls directly through the umbilicus, the linea alba, the center of the chin, and the center of the nose. As the instructor's eyes move up the body from the region of the pelvis to the shoulders, the symmetry of the sides of the body must be checked. Any abnormal curvature or creasing on one side of the trunk (not found on the other side) should lead to a more careful examination to determine whether a lateral sway or tilt of the body or a lateral curvature of the spine exists. Lateral spine curvature must be checked if any deviations in the position of the umbilicus or of the linea alba exist or if there are any apparent differences in the depth of the sides of the chest.

In the boy's examination, the nipple level is compared and, with both boys and girls, the heights of the creases made where the arms join the body should be checked to be sure that the two creases on either side are symmetrical. It is also neces-

sary to check to see if one arm hangs closer to the trunk than the other (Fig. 9-38, *B*). The shoulder height must be checked to see if the shoulders are level. If the pelvis is found to have a lateral pelvic tilt or if a high or low shoulder is noted, the student is then checked for a lateral curvature of the spine. Although lateral curvatures will not occur with all the previously noted conditions, these types of conditions may serve as possible indicators of such a problem. The examiner next checks the head position to be sure that it is held in alignment with the gravity line and to determine if there is any twisting of the head and neck. Finally, the total body should be viewed in terms of whether it is being held in good alignment and balance and to see if any lateral tilts of the total body exist (Fig. 9-38).

Posterior view. The student is instructed to assume the same position in relation to the posture screen as in the anterior examination, except that his back is now turned to the screen, that is, with the inner ankle bones over the marker on the floor. The posterior examination should give the instructor an opportunity to double-check many of the conditions noted from the anterior view and will also allow the instructor to make an evaluation of certain other conditions that cannot be checked during the anterior view examination. Foot alignment can again be checked, with special emphasis this time being placed on whether the forepart of the foot is abducted, the top part of the calcaneous bone is rotated medialward, the heel cords are bowed in, and the inner and outer malleoli are of approximately equal prominence. It should also be checked to see if the inner sides of the malleoli and the inner sides of the femoral condyles are about the same distance apart and whether the legs are in good, straight alignment. Previous judgments about bowlegs and knock-knees can be double-checked in the posterior view. The level of the hips can also be checked.

The gravity line passes directly up through the cleft of the buttocks and through the center of the spinous processes of each of the vertebrae, bisecting the head through its center. The posterior examination is the best for the instructor to evaluate the student for scoliosis (rotolateral curvature). If a lateral curvature exists, further examinations should be made to see if there is any rotation or torque in the pelvic girdle. The degree of lateral deviation and the amount of rotation that has taken place in the spinal column should also be checked. All the areas where lateral deviation of the spine could be present are indicated on the posture card, along with a place to indicate the degree of severity. The examination of the spinal column can be made more meaningful, if scoliosis is suspected, by marking the posterior surfaces of the spinous processes of the vertebrae with a skin pencil so that the curves can be observed more accurately (Figs. 9-38, *B* and *C*). The sides of the trunk are also checked as they were in the anterior

view for any abnormal unilateral curvatures and for any creases or bulges on one side only, which would indicate the presence of a tilt or of a lateral spinal curve.

From the posterior view, the shoulder blades or scapulae are viewed to determine whether they are flat against the rib cage, whether the medial borders have been pulled laterally in abduction, and whether the medial border and the inferior angle of the scapula project outward from the back of the rib cage. This latter condition is known as a "winged scapula." The distance between the medial borders of the scapulae can be measured with a tape measure and this distance can be compared with measurements taken after corrective exercises have been assigned to pull the scapulae together and flatten them against the rib cage. The head position must also be checked from the posterior view to verify the findings of the anterior examination relative to the presence of a head tilt or head twist.

If differences between the anterior and the posterior examinations occur, they may be a result of the fact that the student is sighting on the gravity line in the anterior view and is standing in a stiff or posed position. If this visual cue is used by the student, it should be removed. One way to do this is to have the individual close the eyes at the conclusion of the posterior examination; keep the feet in exactly the same position; bend over at the waist; and freely swing the arms, shoulders, and upper body back and forth from side to side. Then have the student stand up again, keeping the eyes closed; double-check the posture from the posterior view. This should help to identify the natural standing body alignment (one that *feels* comfortable to the student) and should rule out the factors of posing and using the eyes for correct alignment.

Lateral view. For the lateral or side view, the student stands with his left side to the screen (the side facing the screen is the one shown on the posture examination form). The feet are placed on either side of the + drawn on the floor, with the inner malleolus about 1½ inches behind its center. Deviations in alignment and posture can readily be observed through the screen. Abnormalities in flexion and extension of the toes may be easier to see from the side than they were from the front. The lateral examination is used to verify conditions noted in other phases of the examination. The whole conformation of the foot should also be checked for such things as redness, swelling, heavy calluses, undue rotation, or pressure on the various areas of the feet and ankles.

The center line of the screen should pass about 1 inch anterior to the external malleolus, just behind the patella at the knee, and through the center of the hip at about the center of the greater trochanter of the femur bone. If the student has back knee, the gravity line will fall too far forward in relation to the patella; if he has bent knee, it will fall too far back (toward the center of the knee).

If the student has a total forward or backward lean of the body, his alignment is basically correct at all joints, except the ankle, where he is leaning too far forward or backward. In this case, as the examiner checks the reference points, he will find that they become progressively farther out of alignment with each segment from the foot to the head. If the alignment is correct at the ankle and at the shoulder, but the center of the hip is too far forward, the individual will have a total body sway, whereas if the hips are too far back, he will have a distorted position of the low back and buttocks. If the alignment is correct at the ankle, knee, and hip, but the shoulder and the head are positioned too far posteriorly, the student will have what is called a posterior overhang. It is quite easy to identify these various conditions when the body landmarks are viewed in relation to the gravity line of the posture screen (Fig. 9-39). The amount of deviation is ascertained by judging the distance the affected body parts are out of alignment in relation to the grids of the posture screen. Correc-

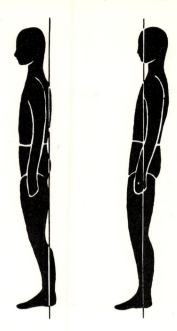

Fig. 9-39. Total body forward and backward leans (plumb line test).

tive procedures for leans and sways are presented in Chapter 5.

Forward or backward pelvic tilt can be quickly checked in the examination through the posture screen by marking either the anterior and posterior superior iliac spines and checking them against the horizontal lines of the screen or by marking the anterior spine of the ilium and the symphysis pubis and checking this alignment against one of the vertical lines. It is usually easier to evaluate these landmarks if the student places a finger on each of them so that they can be seen more easily by the examiner.

The vertebral spine should then be checked throughout its length for what would be termed its normal curvatures. In the region of the lower back, the two conditions that are noted are (1) excessive hyperextension in the lumbar spine, a condition called *lordosis*, and (2) too little curve in the lumbar spine, known as *flat low back*. When the lumbar spine goes into a flexion curve, it is called *lumbar kyphosis*. This is not observed frequently, however. Usually associated with these lower back conditions are a pelvic tilt forward (with lordosis) and a pelvic tilt backward (with a flat low back). Often associated with these conditions, especially with lordosis, is abdominal *ptosis*. Ptosis refers to a relaxation of the lower abdominal muscles with a sagging of the abdomen forward, often accompanied by misplacement of the pelvic organs. The degree of severity of this deviation must be judged subjectively (Fig. 9-14).

In the region of the chest and shoulders, the normal curvature of the spine is one of mild flexion. The abnormal condition that would be looked for in the thoracic spine is an excessive amount of flexion in this region, which, in its severest form, is called

humpback. Any abnormal increase in flexion is known as *kyphosis*. Kyphosis is often associated with a flattening of the chest and rib cage and, frequently, with deviations in the alignment of the shoulder girdle, called *forward shoulders* and *winged scapula*. Although these four conditions are often found in the same individual, they do not necessarily occur together. The winged scapula, mentioned in the posterior examination, should be checked again from the lateral position to see whether the inner border projects to the rear and whether the inferior angle projects outward from the rib cage. The degree of deviation in

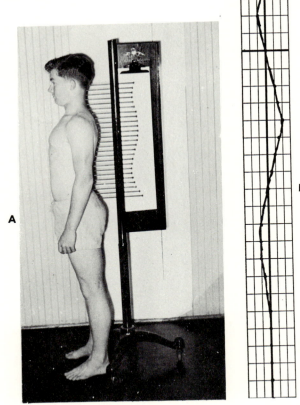

Fig. 9-40. Conformator examination. **A,** Instructor ready to chart life-size spinal curves on attached sheet of paper. **B,** Conformator examination charted to scale on the posture examination card or graph paper by viewing conformator through the grids of a posture screen. (See Fig. 20-24.)

forward (round) shoulders is judged subjectively and is related to how far forward of the gravity line the center of the shoulder falls.

In the region of the neck, the most common condition found is a forward position of the cervical vertebrae accompanying a forward head. An abnormal amount of hyperextension in the cervical or neck vertebrae exists when the individual has attempted to correct a faulty head position by bringing the head back and the chin up. All the anteroposterior curves of the spine (discussed previously) can be judged subjectively as to the degree of severity or can be measured more objectively through the use of a conformator (Fig. 9-40).

If the instructor believes that students are posing for the examination, the technique described at the last part of the posterior examination can be used to disorient them.

In all the examinations described previously, the instructor must be alert to the possibility that one postural deviation often leads to, causes, or is the result of another. It is a pattern of the human body to attempt to keep itself in some semblance of a state of balance (homeostasis). Therefore when one segment or various segments of the body become malaligned, it is customary (sooner or later) for the body to attempt to compensate for this by throwing other segments out of alignment, thus obtaining a balanced position. An example of this would be the individual with lordosis who compensates with kyphosis and forward head. The individual with a simple C scoliosis curve in the spine may compensate for this with a complex S curve (an effort to return the spine, and thus the body, to a state of balance).

Tests for functional-structural conditions
Description

Several tests may be used to determine whether spinal curvatures are functional (involving the muscles and soft tissue) or structural (involving the bones). Postural deviations that are the result of

muscle and soft tissue imbalance are considered functional and will often disappear when the force of gravity is removed. Structural posture deviations have gone beyond the soft tissue stage, with involvement of the supportive bones and connective tissue, and are not eliminated by the removal of gravitational influences.

Instructions for use

Prone lying test. The prone lying test is designed to check anteroposterior or lateral curves of the spine. Functional curves will disappear or will be decreased when the student assumes the prone position on a bench, a table, or the floor.

Hanging test. The hanging test has the same uses as the prone lying test. The individual hangs by his hands from a horizontal support. Functional curves disappear or are decreased in this position (Fig. 9-41, B).

Adam's test. The Adam's test is used to determine whether a lateral deviation of the spine (scoliosis) is functional or structural. The student assumes his normal standing position, then gradually bends his head forward, continuing with the trunk until the hands approximate the toes. The instructor stands a short distance behind the student and observes the student's spine and the sides of the back as the student *slowly* bends forward. If the spine straightens and if the sides of the back are symmetrical in shape and height, the scoliosis is considered functional. Corrective procedures should be started under the direction of a physician (Fig. 9-41, C).

If the spine does not straighten and if one side of the back (especially in the thoracic region) is more prominent (sticks up higher) than the other as the student bends forward, the scoliosis is judged to be structural. In structural cases, the rotation of the vertebrae accompanying the lateral bend of the spine causes the attached ribs to assume a greater posterior prominence on the convex side of the curve. This curve does not disappear in the Adam's test after bony changes occur in the spinal column.

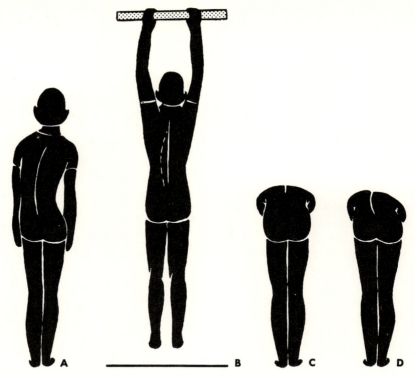

Fig. 9-41. Test for functional-structural scoliosis. **A,** Left C curve scoliosis. **B,** Hanging test for scoliosis. Note straight line indicates spinal position during hanging test. **C,** Adam's test showing functional scoliosis. **D,** Adam's test showing structural scoliosis.

Structural cases must be cared for by an orthopedist (Fig. 9-41, *D*).

Uses and limitations. The Adam's test is used by physicians, therapists, and physical educators to analyze lateral spinal curves. It provides an evaluation of scoliosis, which can be verified through the use of x-ray examination, if desired.

Photography

Photography can be used in many aspects of the adapted physical education program, especially in all types of posture examinations. It can be used successfully in photographing the individual behind the posture screen. This has some advantages over other kinds of examinations, since it provides a permanent record of how the student actually looked at the time of the examination. It also serves as a motivating device for the student, since he can then see deviations and the instructor can point out what can be done to correct them. The posture picture also may be evaluated by the instructor to determine the severity of various conditions, especially when a posture screen is used, since deviations can then be evaluated in relation to the grids of the screen. In doing posture photography through a posture screen, it is necessary to standardize procedures completely so that photographs can be taken quickly and accurately when the need arises. This can be done by determining the proper distance, the proper settings for the camera, and the proper lighting to be used. It is also important to provide a proper backdrop behind the subject so that a clear, well-defined picture is obtained each time a student is photographed (Figs. 9-38 and 20-24). The use of videotape is also an excellent way to record and study posture.

The teacher and student can immediately evaluate the static and moving posture pictures thus recorded.

Moving posture examinations

Description. Many persons have been critical of static posture evaluations, indicating the following:

1. Students are likely to pose in this type of examination.
2. When a plumb line or posture screen is used, the student may use it to obtain visual cues to correct faulty posture.
3. The posture examination does not indicate the student's habitual standing posture.
4. No attention is given to posture and alignment as they would relate to students' movements in activities.

For these reasons, it is wise to include, as a part of the total posture examination, certain phases in which the student is actually in motion and during which he may or may not know that he is being examined. This may be accomplished in several different ways. One is to deploy the class for exercises, observing them as they perform during the exercise program and when they remain in a standing or sitting position between exercises. To enable the examining teacher to identify those students with major deviations and to record this properly on the student's examination form, students must either be organized in a fashion in which the instructor knows all the students by name or by a number or students may be removed from the group as posture deviations are noted. Their names should then be taken so that the posture deviations noted are recorded for the proper student.

Another technique that can be used to evaluate posture and body mechanics during movement is to have the students arranged in a large circle around the teacher, or with the teacher standing at the periphery of the circle, and then have the students walk, run, or do various kinds of activities as they move continuously around the circle. The teacher or therapist identifies those children who are in special need of posture correction and removes them from the circle. Their names are then recorded, along with the appropriate information regarding their posture deviations. As a part of each of these two types of examinations, especially if they are given in lieu of any type of static examination, the students should also assume a normal standing position with the teacher evaluating posture from the front, lateral, and rear views.[3, 9]

REFERENCES

1. Adams, W. C., et al.: Foundations of physical activity, Champaign, Ill., 1968, Stipes Publishing Co.
2. Clarke, H. H.: Application of measurement to health and physical education, Englewood Cliffs, N.J., 1967, Prentice-Hall, Inc.
3. Corrective physical education, Los Angeles, 1958, Los Angeles City Schools.
4. deVries, H. A.: Physiology of exercise for physical education and athletics, Dubuque, Iowa, 1973, William C. Brown Co., Publishers.
5. Hansson, K. G.: Body mechanics and posture, J.A.M.A. **128:**947-953, 1945.
6. Jorris, T. R.: The relationship between abdominal muscle shortening and anterior-posterior pelvic tilt. Unpublished doctoral dissertation, University of California at Los Angeles, Los Angeles, 1960.
7. Kelly, E. D.: Adapted and corrective physical education, New York, 1965, The Ronald Press Co.
8. Logan, G., and Dunkelberg, J.: Adaptations of muscular activity, Belmont, Calif., 1964, Wadsworth Publishing Co., Inc.
9. Lowman, C. L., Colestock, C., and Cooper, H.: Corrective physical education for groups, Cranberry, N.J., 1928, A. S. Barnes & Co., Inc.
10. Lowman, C. L., and Young, C. H.: Posture fitness significance and variances, Philadelphia, 1960, Lea & Febiger.
11. Morrison, W. R., and Chenoweth, L. B.: Normal and elementary physical diagnosis, Philadelphia, 1955, Lea & Febiger.
12. Rasch, P. J., and Burke, R. K.: Kinesiology and applied anatomy, Philadelphia, 1975, Lea & Febiger.

RECOMMENDED READINGS

Barrett, M., et al.: Foundations for movement, Dubuque, Iowa, 1968, William C. Brown Co., Publishers.

Billig, H. E., Jr., and Lowendahl, E.: Mobilization of the human body, Stanford, Calif., 1949, Stanford University Press.

Broer, M. R.: An introduction to kinesiology, Englewood Cliffs, N.J., 1968, Prentice-Hall, Inc.

Crowe, W. C.: The use of audio-visual materials in developmental (corrective) physical education. Unpublished master's thesis, University of California at Los Angeles, Los Angeles, 1950.

Crowe, W. C., Arnheim, D. D., and Auxter, D.: Laboratory manual in adapted physical education and recreation, St. Louis, 1977, The C. V. Mosby Co.

Davis, E. C., Logan, G., and McKinney, W.: Biophysical values of muscular activity, Dubuque, Iowa, 1965, William C. Brown Co., Publishers.

Drury, B. J.: Posture and figure control through physical education, Palo Alto, Calif., 1966, National Press Books.

Kendall, H. O., and Kendall, F. P.: Developing and maintaining good posture, Phys. Ther. **48**: 319-336, 1968.

Krusen, F. H., editor: Handbook of physical medicine and rehabilitation, Philadelphia, 1971, W. B. Saunders Co.

Lilly, L. J.: An overview of body mechanics, Palo Alto, Calif., 1967, Peek Publications.

Metheny, E.: Body dynamics, New York, 1952, McGraw-Hill Book Co.

Mueller, G. W., and Christaldi, J.: A practical program of remedial physical education, Philadelphia, 1966, Lea & Febiger.

Rusk, H. A.: Rehabilitation medicine, ed. 3, St. Louis, 1971, The C. V. Mosby Co.

Williams, M., and Lissner, H. R.: Biomechanics of human motion, Philadelphia, 1977, W. B. Saunders Co.

Williams, M., and Worthingham, C.: Therapeutic exercises for body alignment and function, Philadelphia, 1957, W. B. Saunders Co.

10

MUSCULOSKELETAL DISORDERS

ACUTE

■ The National Safety Council in their 1974 report, which surveyed the number of accidents occurring during the years 1971 through 1973, indicated that there were annually over 62 million accidents causing activity restriction. Of that number, there were over 14 million disabilities so serious as to result in confinement in bed.[1] A significant number of accidents also occur as the result of sports activities. The young person is subject to many physical hazards that may be attributed to living an active life. There are hundreds of thousands of sports injuries sustained each year, with well over 41,000 serious enough to require hospitalization.[5]

By their very nature, many sports activities invite injury. The "all out" exertion required, the numerous situations requiring body contact, and the play that involves the striking and throwing of missiles establish hazards that are either directly or indirectly responsible for the many and varied injuries suffered by those engaged in sports.[2] The highest incidence of sports injuries is in the category of sprains and strains, with the greatest number occurring to the lower limbs.

Often, the physical educator is called on to assist individuals, both young and old, who have received some acute musculoskeletal condition. It is not uncommon that the adapted physical educator must help in managing a sports injury or must establish a reconditioning program for a student after an auto accident. The acute traumatic injury is characterized as being *sharp, intense, having rapid onset,* and *usually being of short duration.* Trauma to the musculoskeletal system causes tissue to be either compressed or elongated. Classification of injuries falls into two broad categories: exposed and unexposed. Exposed injuries refer to wounds that expose external tissue, whereas unexposed conditions occur to underlying tissue.[5]

The reaction of the body to those traumatic forces that tear, crush, overstretch, or shear tissue produces the classic inflammatory quintet: *local heat, swelling, redness, pain,* and *loss of function.* Immediately after injury, there occurs, first, constriction of blood vessels and, then, capillary dilation. After capillary dilation, an osmotic fluid imbalance causes blood and exudation of serum to extravasate into the surrounding tissue areas. Pain is produced by swelling and resultant pressure on sensory nerves as well as hormones that destroy tissue. Associated with inflammation is the removal of debris by phagocytosis and repair. Contained within the serum exudate are the ingredients for repair that, eventually, form a granulation tissue and, finally, a fibrous connective tissue scar.[2]

UNEXPOSED INJURIES

Unexposed or internal injuries affecting the musculoskeletal system, in general, fall into two categories: trauma by compression and trauma by stretching.

Trauma by tissue compression

Injuries to the body that occur by compression of tissue are separated into (1) contusions resulting from sudden and direct blows to the body or other forces that compress and crush tissue and (2) the chronic pressure conditions produced by a constant abnormal external force on the body.

An acute injury to the body can produce varying degrees of muscle spasm and vascular hemorrhage with associated pain. Repeated contusions to a single area under constant abnormal pressure can cause chronic inflammatory conditions. However, chronic compression problems are most apparent with persons who have worn poorly fitting shoes over a long period of time. Shoes that are too long, too short, too narrow, or too pointed cause toes to become deformed (Chapter 9).

Trauma by tissue stretching

Those injuries that occur primarily by the mechanism of stretch are described as strains, sprains, dislocations, and fractures.

Strains

A strain is described as a pulled muscle, with trauma being attributed to an excessive stretch or forcible muscular contraction. The extent of injury is characterized as first, second, or third degree and, additionally, as slight, moderate, or severe. The pathological condition ranges from little or no hemorrhage and low-grade inflammation to the severe rupture of the musculotendinous unit or complete evulsion of a tendon from its bony attachment.

Sprains

Direct or indirect trauma to a joint, affecting its stabilizing connective tissue, results in a sprain. An articulation forced beyond its anatomical limitations can result in pathology in ligamentous, capsular, and synovial membranous tissue as well as tendons crossing or contiguous to the joint. As in strains, sprain severity is depicted by first, second, and third degrees and ranges from a very minor tearing to complete separation of supporting structures. The recipient of a sprain may have symptoms ranging from minimal discomfort to severe joint tenderness, loss of function, and swelling.

Dislocations

The traumatic displacement of a bone from its usual position within a joint is generally termed a dislocation. More specifically, a complete articular disunion is called a *luxation*, whereas a partial separation is considered a *subluxation*. Many severe sprains have, in reality, been dislocations that have spontaneously reduced themselves into proper alignment. The pathological condition that occurs as a result of a dislocation is extensive, with stretching and tearing of articular tissue as well as those tendons associated with movement of the part. Besides affecting the structure of stabilization, avulsion chip fractures may occur from the force of trauma. Once an articulation has been disrupted by such force as to cause severe sprain, subluxation, or luxation, the chances of recurrence are very possible. A chronic recurring dislocation often requires surgical intervention to reestablish stabilization.

Fractures

Fractures represent interruptions in the continuity of a bone and are classified as either closed or open. A closed fracture is one in which there is no external wound; conversely, an open fracture displays external tissue damage. Although fractures are commonly caused by shearing forces, they can occur as a result of direct external forces that crush the bone.

After a fracture, there is damage to the periosteum and adjacent soft tissue structures, primarily blood vessels, nerves, connective tissue, and muscles. There is hemorrhaging and noticeable inflammation. The repair and healing of the bone ends involve a number of processes, namely, formation of a granulation tissue mass, fibrous connective tissue junction, or hard callus and the final development of new rigid bone.

BASIC CONCEPTS IN PHYSICAL RECONDITIONING

The major concern of the adapted physical educator with individuals who have experienced serious acute traumatic impairments is one of reconditioning. The term "reconditioning" implies that through an exercise program, an individual will be returned to the same degree of conditioning as before the injury. In cooperation with the physician, the teacher establishes an individually designed exercise program for the student.

Prolonged bed rest or inactivity after trauma to the musculoskeletal system results in delayed recovery. Physicians and reconditioning specialists generally agree that an exercise program is needed for all muscular and skeletal involvements, whether preoperative preparation, postoperative recovery, or general rehabilitation of acute conditions. It is important that the affected person engage in a general physical fitness program as well as rehabilitation of the injured part.

A relatively healthy individual who has incurred an acute musculoskeletal impairment should *avoid inactivity* as a means to restoration. Lack of activity results in muscular atrophy and the loss of joint flexibility and general coordination. Prolonged bed rest may lead to a generalized debilitation that may extend the recuperation period. Authorities generally agree that a carefully guided program of activity encourages healing and shortens the time of recovery, particularly in cases of acute musculoskeletal conditions.

The traumatic conditions discussed in this chapter are commonly found to occur to active persons, those involved in accidents, the weak, and the infirm. Each is described in terms of its *anatomical implications, mechanism of injury,* and *pathological condition* and a *rationale for reconditioning* is presented. There is no intent here to give a complete discussion of all traumas, but only to discuss those injuries that have a high incidence among the school-aged population.

THE FOOT, ANKLE, AND LEG

The 26 bones composing the skeleton of the foot are primarily structured for strong, flexible, coordinated movement. Architecturally, the foot forms an anterior metatarsal arch, an outer longitudinal arch,

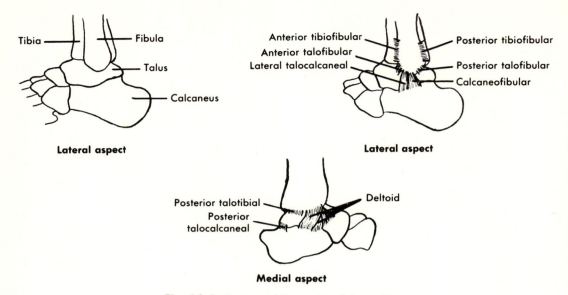

Fig. 10-1. Bones and ligaments of the ankle.

and the high inner longitudinal arch on its medial aspect. The main function of the arch is to absorb the shock of weight bearing and to allow space for plantar muscles, nerves, and blood vessels. Body weight is conducted to the foot via the leg bone of the tibia through the supporting bone, the talus. A mortise is formed by the malleoli of the fibula and the tibia and, with the aid of collateral ligaments, it stabilizes the talus. Below the talus is the calcaneus. The foot makes surface contact with the calcaneus and the metatarsal heads. An intricate system of plantar muscles and elastic and inelastic connective tissue serves to uphold the shape and arches of the foot. Additional support is afforded by a suspension of muscles stemming from the leg and ending within the longitudinal arch. Dorsiflexion, together with plantar ankle flexion, is permitted at the talotibial articulation, whereas inversion and eversion of the foot take place at the talocalcaneal joint.

Structurally, the ankle joint is relatively strong as a result of its bony and ligamentous arrangements. Because of the direction of weight bearing, the medial collateral, as compared to the lateral collateral, ligament offers the greatest ankle stability. Bony strength is added to the medial collateral ligament by the arrangement of the talus over the calcaneus. Laterally, the ankle is architecturally weaker and more subject to sprains than on the medial side (Fig. 10-1).

The leg is composed of the tibia and fibula and the soft tissues surrounding them. Three fascial chambers contain the muscles, blood vessels, and nerves. The anterior compartment contains those constituents that control the action of dorsiflexion, namely, the tibialis anterior, the extensor hallucis longus, the extensor digitorum longus, the anterior vessels, and the anterior tibial nerves; a lateral compartment houses the muscles of the peroneus longus and the peroneus brevis; and a posterior compartment confines the motor mechanisms of plantar flexion and inversion, primarily the soleus, posterior tibialis, long flexors of the toes, and gastrocnemius muscles. The main weight-bearing bone of the leg is the tibia. It is triangularly formed at its upper two thirds and changes to a more oval shape in the lower one third. The fibula's primary function is serving

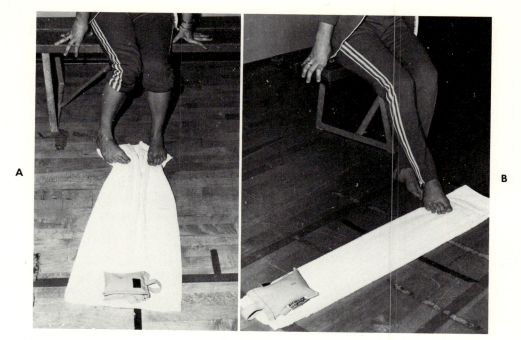

Fig. 10-2. Foot exercises. **A,** No. 13 (p. 109), building mounds. **B,** No. 14 (p. 110), foot curling. (Courtesy California State University, Audio Visual Center, Long Beach, Calif.)

as a point for muscle attachment. Connecting the fibula and tibia is the strong tissue sheet of the interosseous membrane.

Foot injuries

The foot is extremely vulnerable to trauma. Serious injury may occur as a result of the following:

1. An individual's falling from a height and landing on the feet
2. Objects falling on the foot
3. Striking toes against an immovable object
4. Twisting and wrenching forces

Fractures to the phalanges are most common consequent to a stubbing action; to the talus and calcaneus consequent to falling; and to the metatarsals consequent to objects falling on them, although fractures at the base of the fifth metatarsal are associated with severely sprained ankle and violent foot inversion. Spontaneous fractures can arise from prolonged use of feet, as occurs in walking or running. Tendon and connective tissue injuries have the highest incidence in the plantar and lateral aspects of the foot. However, sprains and strains may arise at almost any site. The sprained foot commonly affects ligaments that stabilize the intertarsal or tarsometatarsal joints. A traumatic arch sprain can occur as a result of a sudden overstretching of the plantar aspect of the foot.

Reconditioning

Reconditioning the foot after injury involves the prevention of edema and fluid stasis; immobilization, when applicable; mobilization; and graded exercises. The tendency toward swelling after injury requires the physical therapy of immediate elevation, pressure, and cold application. Uncontrolled edema may result in eventual fibrosis and chronic irritation.

Physical restoration is implemented during the convalescent period by active movements of the toes within the margins of pain and safety (Fig. 10-2). The physical educator must give consideration to the main foot functions and redevelopment of the injured muscles (see Chapter 5 and Figs. 5-13 and 5-14).

Ankle injuries

Most ankle injuries occur as a result of the foot being forcibly turned inward or outward on the leg while supporting the body weight. The primary cause of ankle injuries is stepping on uneven surfaces. The highest incidence of trauma to the ankle occurs when the foot is violently inverted; however, the most serious pathological condition results from eversion, which affects the main supporting tissues of the

ankle and longitudinal arch. The scope of ankle injuries ranges from the mild stretching of stabilizing ligamentous tissue to fractures of both malleoli, or even ankle dislocation.

An ankle sprain results in stretched or torn ligamentous fibers and muscle tendons. The inversion sprain affects the anterior tibiofibular ligament, the anterior talofibular ligament, the calcaneofibular ligament, and the posterior talofibular ligament in varying degrees, not to mention the straining of the peroneal tendons (Fig. 10-3, A). Eversion sprains primarily affect the medial collateral deltoid ligament, with an associated pathological condition in the plantar ligaments and tendons. Severe abnormal twisting of the foot, inwardly or outwardly, can result in fractures of the lateral or medial malleolus such as are incurred in skiing injuries.

Serious ankle damage is manifested in loss of movement and inability to bear weight. Marked swelling, pain, and discoloration (ecchymosis) often are displayed. Severe ankle joint derangement often requires immobilization by cast or strapping and the prevention of weight bearing for a varied length of time.

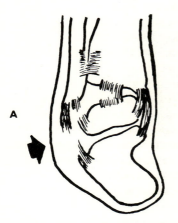

A

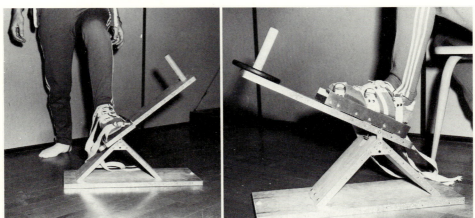

B

C

Fig. 10-3. A, Lateral ankle sprain. **B,** Ankle exercise machine; foot eversion. **C,** Foot dorsiflexion. (**B** and **C** Courtesy California State University, Audio Visual Center, Long Beach, Calif.)

Reconditioning

Care of severe acute ankle affections demands control of edema by means of cold pressure, elevation, support by adhesive strapping, or casting. Weight bearing may be restricted and crutches required or a plaster walking cast may be applied for immobilization in the care of fractures or severe sprains.

The primary objective of ankle reconditioning is to restore normal joint function. Movement at the tibiofibular-talar articulation approximates 20 degrees of dorsiflexion and 45 to 60 degrees of plantar flexion. Normal movement may be encouraged immediately after injury, once fracture has been ruled out. Early exercise often aids in venous and lymphatic drainage. When initial soreness decreases, the physician may allow the patient to engage in modified activity and limited weight bearing.

The saying, "Once a sprain, always a sprain," points up the fact that stretched or torn ligaments do not repair themselves. Exercise cannot be expected to restore injured ligaments nor can it be expected to fully strengthen strained tendons crossing the ankle joint. Therefore full ankle stability after severe derangement is doubtful and should not be expected.

With the permission of the physician, the student may begin a graded program of inversion, eversion, plantar flexion and dorsiflexion, and exercises against resistance. To provide normal mechanical continuity between ankle and foot, an exercise program should also include toe and arch routines. A number of choices of ankle resistance devices are available to the individual with a sprained ankle. Specialized resistance machines, weighted iron boots, sandbags, and manual resistance may afford an overload program to the injured ankle (Fig. 10-3 and Chapter 5).

The criterion for resumption of normal activity should be whether the student can pass a variety of ankle stress tests, such as the following:

1. Walking without a limp

2. Balancing on the toes of the affected ankle without pain
3. Jumping up and down with ease while bearing full weight on the affected ankle
4. Running at full speed in a zigzag pattern

Shin splints

Shin splints is a condition associated with pain in the area of the anterior or posterior aspect of the tibia. It most often occurs to athletes or active individuals who engage in repetitive walking or running on a nonresisting surface. Although shin splints may occur suddenly and transitorily, it may also appear gradually and become a chronic disability. Many factors have been attributed to causing shin splints; the primary causes are the following:

1. Running or walking on nonresistant and uneven surfaces
2. Poor running or walking form
3. Running on the balls of the feet too early in the training program
4. Postural and structural foot anomalies[9]

Most authorities agree that shin splints is a chronic inflammation of the muscles and connecting tissue in the shin region, primarily resulting from irritation to the calf muscles and plantar flexors; however, it occasionally occurs from irritation to the extensor muscles of the lower leg.

Nontraumatic problems of the shin region, such as stress fractures, anterior tibial syndrome, and leg overuse, may, in their early stages, closely resemble shin splints. The stress fracture occurs spontaneously in the tibia or fibula from overuse, whereby the synergistic muscle coordination is overcome by fatigue. Acute anterior tibial compartment syndrome is considered a very serious condition leading to ischemic necrosis from hemorrhage within the fascial boundaries.[9]

Reconditioning

Physical therapy of shin splints requires heat, rest, supportive strapping, and static stretching in positions of plantar and dorsi-

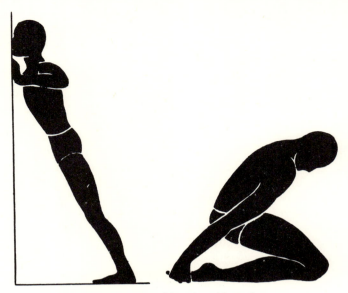

Fig. 10-4. Stretching for shin splints.

flexion (Fig. 10-4). deVries[4] determined that muscle spasm is an important cause of the shin splint symptoms and could be relieved by a daily routine of static stretching of both the anterior and posterior aspects of the lower leg.

THE KNEE AND THIGH

The knee has an extremely high incidence of injury among active young persons, particularly those engaged in football and skiing. As an articulation, the knee is considered to be an unstable ginglymus, or hinge type, joint. Having an extremely shallow bony structure, the knee's functional stability is based mainly on the support of its muscles and ligamentous arrangement. Structurally, the knee joint is the largest and one of the most complicated joints in the body. It is formed by the lateral and medial femoral condyles, the tibia, and the patella. Two semioval cartilages (menisci) serve to deepen the shallow depression of the tibia. Ligamentous stability is afforded the knee, laterally and medially, by collateral ligaments and anteriorly and posteriorly, by internal cruciate ligaments (Fig. 10-5, *A* and *B*). The primary move-

ments of the knee consist of flexion and extension, with some secondary internal and external rotation. Although the ligaments prevent abnormal movements, the primary knee joint stability is acquired through the gastrocnemius, the hamstring, and the quadriceps muscles (Fig. 10-5, *C* and *D*).

The thigh consists of the femur and associated musculature, blood vessels, and nerves. There are four groups of thigh muscles, based on their primary action: flexors, extensors, abductors, and adductors.

The patella is the largest sesamoid bone in the body; it lies within the quadriceps muscle tendon. Its primary function is to provide protection to the anterior aspect of the knee joint and to increase the mechanical advantage during extension. The two most prevalent injuries of the patella in the active young person are dislocation and fracture.

Acute patellar dislocations may result from a direct blow or sudden twist when the knee is flexed. Dislocations of this type happen most often to individuals who have poor quadriceps tone or a shallow patellar groove. *Genu valgum*, or knock-knee, is

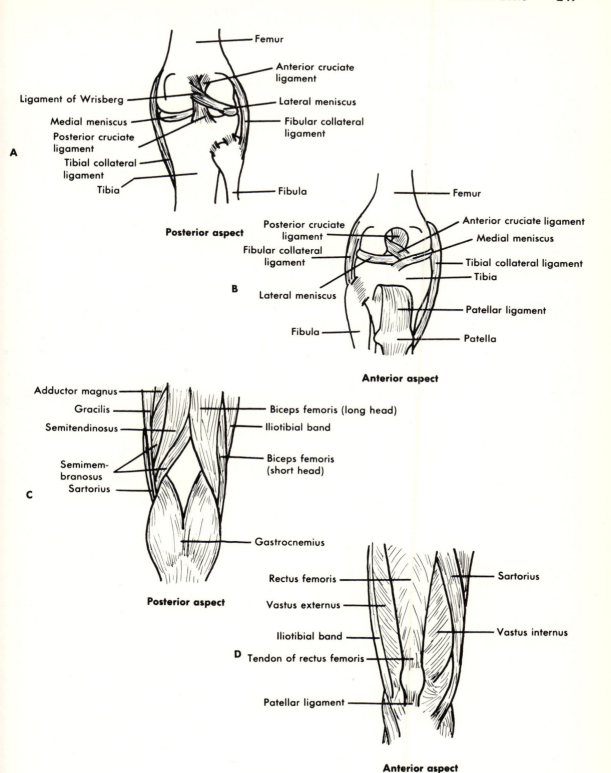

Fig. 10-5. Knee anatomy.

also a contributing factor, along with the increased tibial femoral angle that is common in the physically mature female. O'Donoghue[7] described the mature female as being more prone to patellar dislocations because of her broader pelvis, resulting in an increased angle at the patella, therefore pulling laterally on full knee extension. Treatment of the dislocated patella often requires corrective surgery and immobilization. Activity is then increased through a graded quadriceps exercise program.

Fractures of the patella are not as prevalent as dislocations. They result from a direct blow or from a sudden severe pull that fragments some portion of the patella. Because of the possibility of developing a roughened articular surface, surgery may be required to remove a portion of, or the entire, patella.

Repeated trauma to the kneecap can lead to the condition known as chondromalacia, which is a softening of the articular surface. Chondromalacia eventually develops into degenerative changes and a state of chronic inflammation. Other articular surfaces that commonly develop chondromalacia in the rapidly growing adolescent are the knee and hip (Chapter 11).

Knee sprains

Because of the structural shallowness of the knee joint, it is very vulnerable to abduction, adduction, and torsion injuries. Violent activity, as in football or skiing, places great stress on the knee joint. Injury often follows when the foot is planted firmly and the knee is either struck from the outside inward or rotated on its long axis.

The *medial collateral ligament* has the highest incidence of sprain, occurring most often when the knee receives a direct blow, which causes the foot to evert and the knee to be forced inward in an unlocked position. Although not usually as serious as the medial, the lateral collateral knee sprain results from a forced adduction of the leg and an internally rotated knee. In both

instances, there is an instability of the affected side besides a tendency toward effusion, hemarthrosis (blood in the joint), and pain.

The *anterior cruciate ligament* can be abnormally stretched or torn by a violent internal rotation of the femur while the foot is planted with the knee adducted and flexed or by hyperextension while the knee is internally rotated on the femur. Conversely, the posterior cruciate ligament can be injured when the femur is externally rotated and the foot is fixed with the knee in a flexed and adducted position. A fall on a flexed knee can also result in a posterior cruciate sprain. Anterior cruciate injury results in forward displacement of the tibia in relationship to the femur, whereas the posterior cruciate sprain results in backward displacement and instability. In each case of injury, there is usually swelling and effusion of blood into the joint.

The mechanism *hyperextension knee sprain* can result from a direct force to the planted foot, causing the knee to move backward abnormally. Depending on the severity of trauma, the hyperextension injury can result in sprain to the medial collateral and anterior cruciate ligaments, besides straining tissue in the popliteal region.

Reconditioning

Very often, the physical educator wll be charged with helping a student who is about to have, or who is recovering from, knee surgery. There has been a recent trend toward early knee surgery when symptoms reveal definite joint derangement, especially in the "unhappy triad," indicating trauma to the medial collateral ligament, medial meniscus, and anterior cruciate ligament.

Profound atrophy and weakness are common to the quadriceps extensor mechanism after knee injury or surgery. Weak quadriceps muscles, in general, mean a defective and unstable knee joint. Physical restoration of the knee requires a concentrated exercise regime for strength and flexibility of the gastrocnemius and both the quadri-

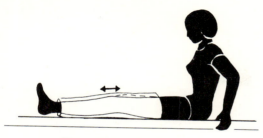

Fig. 10-6. Quad setting.

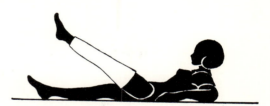

Fig. 10-7. Straight leg raises with hip flexion.

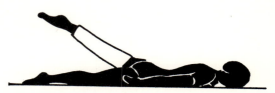

Fig. 10-8. Straight leg raises with hip extension.

ceps and hamstring muscle groups. Eliminating the hamstring and gastrocnemius muscles from the reconditioning program results in failure to provide a balance of knee strength and leaves the student vulnerable to additional trauma.[7]

A graduated exercise program of reconditioning will, in most instances, consist of the following seven procedures:

1. Quad setting
2. Straight leg raises with hip flexion
3. Hip extension
4. Toe raises
5. Leg swings
6. Hamstring conditioning
7. Progressive resistance exercises

Quad setting (Fig. 10-6), or muscle tensing, is a procedure whereby the student performs an isometric or static contraction of the quadriceps muscles for a period of between 6 and 10 seconds, without knee movement and until some fatigue is sensed. Many athletic trainers start this exercise immediately after injury to prevent muscle wasting or after knee surgery in an attempt to restore normal muscle strength as soon as possible.

Straight leg raises with hip flexion (Fig. 10-7) is executed against gravity, first in a sitting position, which emphasizes the three single joint muscles of the quadriceps group and then, gradually, in the supine position, which brings into action all four muscles. The effectiveness of the exercise is increased by the individual leaning back on the hands to a final position of long lying. The second and third exercise positions increase the stress placed on the rectus femoris muscle. The student at-

tempts to maintain the knee in a locked position while raising the leg about 6 inches above the level of the hip. When 15 to 20 repetitions can be accomplished for two or three bouts during the day without undue discomfort, the physician may allow graduation to leg swings. Gradual resistance can also be applied to the straight leg raising exercise by progressively adding sandbags to the extended leg.

Straight leg raises with hip extension (Fig. 10-8) should be executed to exercise the gluteus maximus and hamstring muscles. The student takes a prone position and lifts the affected leg approximately 6 inches above the hip level. Like the straight leg raise with hip flexion, this exercise is conducted 15 to 20 times, with two to three bouts daily. Sandbag weights can also be applied for progressive resistance exercise (Fig. 10-9).

Because the gastrocnemius (Fig. 10-10) assists in flexion at the knee as well as in plantar flexion at the ankle and because it provides posterior stability, it should be included in the reconditioning exercise regimen. Exercise of the gastrocnemius can best be accomplished by the progression

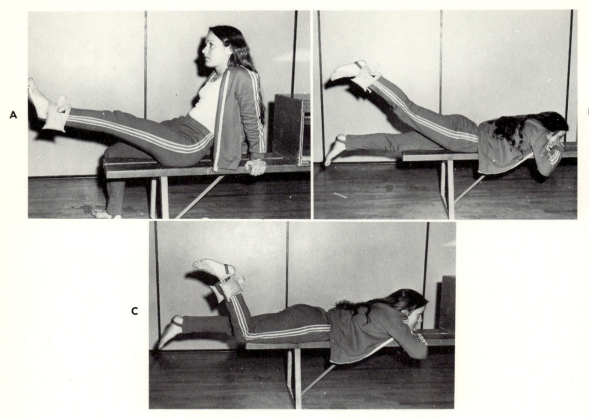

Fig. 10-9. Using sandbag weights in a progressive resistance exercise program for the knee. (Courtesy California State University, Audio Visual Center, Long Beach, Calif.)

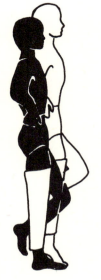

Fig. 10-10. Toe raises.

of toe pointing without weight bearing, weight bearing and *toe raises,* and weight bearing plus resistance, for example, carrying a weight in the hands or on the shoulder and initiating toe raising. From 15 to 20 repetitions should be initiated in each set of exercises. A full stretch of the Achilles tendon should be attempted after each toe raise, which is accomplished by standing with the ball of the foot on a raised block.

Leg swings (Fig. 10-11) may be incorporated with the straight leg raises or may be reserved as a progressive movement, depending on the extent of knee damage and the wishes of the physician. The patient executes them by sitting on a table or bench and freely swinging the lower leg in flexion and extension and gradually increasing the arc of the swing.

The primary purpose of leg swings is to aid in muscle redevelopment, restore joint flexibility, and increase normal circulation for the resolution of effusion or joint swelling. Resumption of normal knee movement

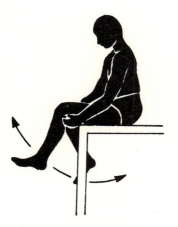

Fig. 10-11. Leg swings.

should be encouraged as soon as possible without hindering the healing process.

Hamstring strength is essentially for the posterior support of the knee. Too often, this muscle group is neglected in the total knee reconditioning program. Lying in the prone position, the athlete, first without resistance, curls the affected leg. Gradually, resistance is added until the strength of the hamgstring group has been developed to the extent of being 50% to 60% that of the quadriceps group.

Isotonic progressive resistance exercises usually represent the final exercise stage for the reconditioning of the knee. By the use of resistance applied to the ankle or foot of the affected side, the patient extends the leg through a full range of movement against gravity (Fig. 10-12). The quadriceps and hamstring groups and the gastrocnemius must be given equal attention for the restoration of full joint function.

Weight bearing parallels the return of muscle function and joint stability. As the student becomes reconditioned, he gradually progresses from inability to bear weight to crutch walking and full mobility.

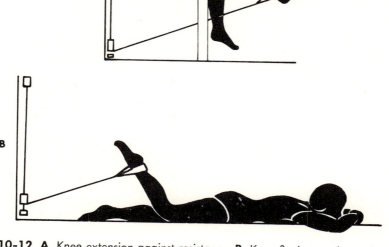

Fig. 10-12. A, Knee extension against resistance. **B,** Knee flexion against resistance.

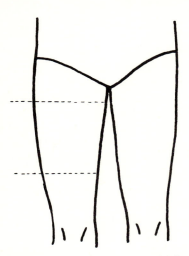

Fig. 10-13. Sites for measuring thigh circumference.

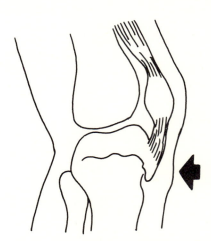

Fig. 10-14. Osgood-Schlatter condition of the knee.

The criterion often used to determine recovery from knee derangement is the return of strength and flexibility equal to or exceeding that of the unaffected side, restoration of normal circumference (Fig. 10-13), and the ability to move easily without favoring the part.

Osgood-Schlatter condition

Many terms have been applied to the Osgood-Schlatter condition; the most prevalent are "apophysitis," "osteochondritis," and, most common, "epiphysitis of the tibial tubercle." It is not considered a disease entity, but the result of a separation of the tibial tubercle at the epiphyseal junction (Fig. 10-14).[10] The cause of this condition is idiopathic, with direct injury thought to be the main inciting factor. Direct trauma as in a blow, osteochondritis, or an excessive strain of the patellar tendon as it attaches to the tibial tubercle may result in evulsion at the epiphyseal cartilage junction. Disruption of the blood supply to the epiphysis results in enlargement of the tibial tubercle, joint tenderness, and pain on contraction of the quadriceps. It usually occurs in active adolescent boys and girls between the ages of 10 and 15 years who are in a rapid growth period. If not

properly cared for, deformity and a defective extensor mechanism may result; however, it may not necessarily be associated with pain or discomfort. In most cases, Osgood-Schlatter condition is acute, is self-limiting, and does not exceed a few months' duration.

Local inflammation is accentuated by leg activity and ameliorated by rest. The individual may be unable to kneel or engage in flexion and extension movements without pain. Even after arrest of symptoms, Osgood-Schlatter condition tends to recur after irritation.

The physical educator may, from the complaints of the student, be the one to detect this condition, in which immediate physician referral should be made. Early detection may reveal a slight condition whereby the individual can continue a normal activity routine, excluding overexposure to strenuous running, jumping, and falling on the affected leg. All physical education activities must be modified to avoid quadriceps strain, while, at the same time, preparing for general physical fitness.

Complete abstinence of all knee joint movement must be maintained when the inflammatory state persists. Forced inactivity, provided by a plaster cast, may be the only answer to keeping the overactive adolescent from using the affected leg. While immobilized in the cast, the individual is greatly restricted; weight bearing may be held to a minimum, with signs of pain at the affected part closely watched by the physician.

Reconditioning

Although Osgood-Schlatter condition is self-limiting and temporary, exercise is an important factor in the full recovery of the individual. Physical education activities should emphasize the capabilities of the upper body and nonaffected leg to prevent their deconditioning.

After arrest of the condition and removal from immobilization, the individual is given a graduated reconditioning program. The major objectives at this time are reeducation in proper walking patterns and restoration of normal strength and flexibility of the knee joint. Strenuous knee movement is avoided for at least 5 weeks and the demanding requirements of regular physical education classes may be postponed for 6 months or longer, depending on the physician's recommendations. Although the period of rehabilitation places emphasis on the affected leg, it must also include a program for the entire body.

The criteria for the individual to return to regular physical education would be as follows:

1. Normal range of movement of the knee
2. Quadriceps strength equal to that of the unaffected leg
3. Asymptomatic evidence of the Osgood-Schlatter condition
4. The ability to move freely without favoring the affected part

Following recovery, the student should avoid all activities that would tend to contuse, or in any way irritate again, the tibial tuberosity.

THE HIP AND PELVIS

The hip is an extremely powerful joint with great bony, ligamentous, and muscular strength. It serves as the main supporting structure of the body in the upright position. Without proper integrity of the hip joint and its associated structures, ambulation becomes difficult or even impossible. Although designed to withstand great and repeated stress, the hip is vulnerable to epiphyseal separations in the early growth stages and to fractures in old age. Dislocations of the hip are more prevalent than fractures in young active individuals because they have more viable and elastic tissue about the joint, compared to the porous and degenerative hip of elderly persons. Sprains, dislocations, and fractures will be considered in this section, whereas congenital and degenerative conditions are discussed in Chapter 11.

Sprains and dislocations

Any movement that exceeds the hip's normal range can result in injury. A torsion force with the foot planted and the body twisting on its long axis can result in sprain or dislocation. A direct force to the knee while the thigh is flexed and adducted, such as striking the dashboard in an auto accident, can result in fracture and dislocation of the femoral head. A common complication of the hip dislocation or fracture, particularly in older individuals, is injury to the sciatic nerve or disruption of the ligamentum teres carrying the main nutrient artery to the head of the humerus.

INGUINAL HERNIA

A hernia is a protrusion of an organ through an abnormal opening. The most prevalent site is in the abdominal region. Millions of persons in the United States suffer from some type of hernia, the majority of which are of the inguinal type. However, along with inguinal hernia, there is a high incidence of femoral and umbilical hernia. Generally, the inguinal hernia is more prevalent in men and occurs most often in childhood, whereas the femoral hernia is most prevalent in women.

The inguinal canal is found in the lower abdomen just above Poupart's ligament and serves as a passageway for the spermatic vessels and the vas deferens in the male and the round ligament in the female. It extends about 1½ inches in length, with a downward and inward direction. The canal's internal and external openings are termed the internal and external abdominal rings.

There are two types of inguinal hernias: congenital and acquired. The congenital or direct hernia is primarily associated with the descent of the testes before birth and is often discovered soon after birth. Many of these types close spontaneously with a truss, which is a mechanical device that aids in reducing the hernia by placing external pressure at the site; however, surgery for the congenital inguinal hernia is the choice of many physicians.[8]

The second highest incidence of inguinal hernia occurs between the ages of 16 and 20 years[8] and is categorized as acquired or indirect. This is best described as a sac protruding through the internal inguinal abdominal ring. An incomplete hernia would still be in the inguinal canal, whereas a complete hernia extends past the subcutaneous external ring and descends into the scrotum.

The femoral hernia, unlike the inguinal hernia, is associated with the female sex. A portion of the lower intestine protrudes through the femoral ring that is provided for the femoral vessels leading to the upper thigh.

There are many reasons attributed to the occurrence of hernia. Some common congenital causes may be inherited weakness of the lower abdomen, faulty descent of the testes, or abnormal enlargement of the internal inguinal ring. An acquired hernia can stem from trauma, as from a blow or lifting a heavy object; from pregnancy; or from degeneration. In general, the anatomy of a hernia may be divided into three parts: the mouth, the hernial ring, and the body. The body of the hernia consists of a sac that protrudes outside the abdominal cavity, often containing a portion of the abdominal viscera.[5]

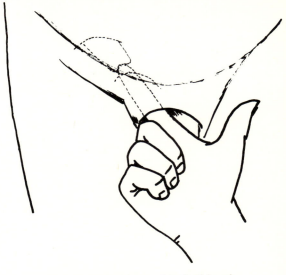

Fig. 10-15. Palpating an inguinal hernia.

Early symptoms of the hernia are indicated by a swelling in the area of the internal inguinal ring that expands while the abdomen is under strain and contracts under slight pressure (Fig. 10-15). Pain on exertion may also be elicited in the region of the groin.

The inguinal hernia, besides causing discomfort and aggravation, can also be a serious threat to health. A number of complications may aggravate hernial conditions; these include infection, incarceration, and strangulation. The incarcerated hernia is an irreducible hernial sac. An incarcerated hernia, if not treated promptly, may become strangulated and result in tissue damage, severe pain, and shock.

The student with a hernial condition should be aware of the inherent dangers and should be encouraged to obtain corrective surgery as soon as feasible. While in the preoperative situation, a restrictive physical education program must be afforded. Activities that produce extreme fatigue or intra-abdominal strain, such as weight lifting, gymnastics, track and field and breath-holding activities, must be avoided. Programming emphasis should be placed on proper body mechanics, mild to moderate exercises, voluntary deep breathing, and lower limb movement while in a seated or lying position.

THE SPINE

The spine is composed of individual vertebral segments consisting of 7 cervical, 12 thoracic, and 5 lumbar vertebrae; a sacrum; and a coccyx. Although each vertebral region has individual features, in general, they are designed for weight bearing, protection of the spinal cord, muscle attachment, and trunk and head mobility. Vertebrae become increasingly large as they progress downward to accommodate for the upright posture. Adding to the complexities of the spinal column are the cervical, dorsal, and lumbar curves that accommodate gravity while the individual is in the erect position.

Many authorities consider the vertebral column as still being in an evolutionary stage of adaptation. This assumption is reached because of the inadequate way the individual adjusts to the various forces applied to the spine. In essence, the spine must function as both stationary support and a dynamic unit.[3]

Gross movement of the spine consists of the combined articulations of each vertebra. Between two vertebrae are articular facets that form joints. Each articular facet has a synovial membrane and is joined together by ligamentous tissue. Between the bodies of each vertebra are fibrocartilaginous discs composed of a hard outer fibrocartilage and a gelatinous center, the *nucleus pulposus,* which provides shock-absorbing qualities to the entire spine. Gross movement of the spine is initiated by a gliding action of the individual joints, combined with the adaption of the intervertebral cartilages. The cervical region is permitted free flexion and extension, whereas head tilting takes place with the combined movement of rotation and torsion. The thoracic spine moves laterally more easily than it flexes and extends because of its bony limitations. Although lateral bending and rotary movement are limited

in the lumbar spine, flexion and extension are permitted.

Spine injuries

Back disorders, primarily of the lower back and neck, are becoming increasingly more prevalent in today's population. Cailliet[3] estimates that 80% of the human race will complain of back pain, particularly in the low back region. Lack of exercise and poor muscle tone, combined with the hazards of modern living, serve to predispose individuals to acute back problems. Pathological problems of the back fall mainly into three categories: congenital, mechanical, and traumatic. Congenital and mechanical affections are considered in Chapters 9 and 11, respectively.

The back regions that are most susceptible to musculotendinous ligamentous injury are the cervical and low back regions, each being unique in its potential to injury. The neck, as the result of its flexibility, is able to withstand a great deal of traumatic force applied to it. However, sudden twists, forced hyperextension, or a quick snap of the head can produce varying degrees of damage. The primary muscles involved are the upper trapezius and the sternocleidomastoid. A strain of the neck musculature may appear as wryneck or acute torticollis. Deeper injury may affect ligamentous supporting structures or may result in herniation of the cervical intervertebral disc. Automobile accidents involving rear-end collisions are producing increasingly great numbers of *whiplash* injuries, whereby the recipient's head is snapped forcefully forward and back, tearing and stretching supporting tissue.

The individual with various anatomical weaknesses, congenital or acquired, in the low back region is prone to acute conditions. The individual with poor abdominal muscle tone or faulty vertebral alignment, with its concomitant muscular imbalance, has the stage set for future injury and chronic low back pain. Whether it is acute or of gradual onset, trauma plays a primary role in low back affections. The sequence

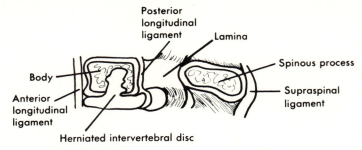

Fig. 10-16. Sagittal section showing herniated disc.

of injury usually occurs after a sudden trunk twist or bending from the waist that places acute stress on inflexible atonic musculature or structurally deformed low back vertebrae. The low back injury may be reflected in a dull ache, pain radiating down a leg, muscle spasm, or restricted movement. Occurring from the same mechanisms as the lumbosacral sprain is the herniated lumbar disc (intervertebral disc syndrome). Often, the herniated disc is a product of gradual degeneration over a period of time. A sudden strain to the lumbar region increases the internal pressure of the intervertebral disc, forcing the nucleus pulposus to push outward, usually posteriorly (Fig. 10-16). The protruding nucleus pulposus may cause pressure on adjacent nerves, resulting in pain and incapacitation.

Dislocations of the vertebral column have the highest incidence in the cervical region. A hyperextension or severe torsion force can result in dislocation or cervical fracture. Torque of the head or neck places most stress on the cervical atlas and axis and, if of great enough intensity, can lead to spinal cord damage, paralysis, or even death.

Violent hyperflexion of the trunk, or falling from a height and landing on the feet or buttocks, can produce a vertebral fracture, particularly in the lumbar or dorsal region. Bony fragments may lacerate spinal nerves or even the cord, causing partial or complete paralysis of the lower limbs.

Reconditioning

Severe acute neck conditions, such as are incurred in dislocations or fractures, are immobilized by a cast or skeletal traction. This procedure may be carried on for weeks or even months. In lesser injuries such as whiplash the neck may be immobilized by a cervical collar. The period of neck splinting allows healing to take place without aggravation by neck movement. During this period of immobilization, general conditioning exercises should be carried out for the entire unaffected parts of the body. Emphasis particularly should be placed on the upper extremities to avoid contractures and a loss of shoulder joint range of movement. If the student is required to be in a recumbent position, muscle tensing and range of movement exercise must be carried out to all the major joints several times a day. When the student is permitted active neck movement, mobility in all directions is the first concern and then a graded strength program is initiated.

Reconditioning of acute low back problems requires an understanding of the anatomical complexities involved. Rest is often prescribed through the acute stages. If corrective surgery has been given, a muscle setting program should be executed several times a day while the patient is in the recumbent position. When active exercises are allowed, a program of stretching, strength development, and reeducation is initiated. Postural control and good body alignment are of the utmost importance. Abdominal strength must be developed and lumbosacral flexibility must be acquired in order that proper pelvic alignment is re-established. *Because of the pull placed on the lumbar curve by the iliopsoas muscle, double straight leg raising exercises while the student is in the supine position are contraindicated.* Along with the graded exercise program, the student should be taught how to carry on normal daily activities such as sitting, standing, walking, or running without undue stress and tension in the low back region.[6]

The following exercises, divided into seven basic categories, are often given to persons with low back problems associated with faulty lumbar pelvic alignment, muscle imbalance, and inflexibility:

1. Low back stretching
2. Abdominal strengthening
3. Pelvic rolling
4. Quadriceps stretching
5. Hip flexor stretching
6. Hamstring and heel cord stretching
7. Postural reeducation

Specific exercises for hamstring stretching, heel cord stretching, and postural reeducation are discussed in detail in Chapter 5.

Low back stretching is employed because a tight low back prevents normal trunk flexion. Individuals with an accentuated lordotic curve often are unable to fully round their backs. A safe exercise for sufferers of a pathological low back condition is executed from a supine position (Fig. 10-17). Knees are first pulled alternately to the chest and then, if without pain, are brought together to the chest. Each stretch should be statically held for at least 30 seconds and then gradually released. Variations of this stretch are sitting in a chair and touching the heels with the fingertips and allowing the head to slowly move between the legs.

Abdominal strengthening is necessary because, as discussed in Chapters 5 and 9, weak abdominal muscles are often associated with pain and disorder of the low back

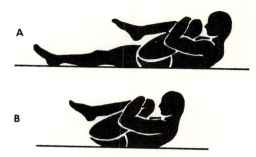

Fig. 10-17. Stretching the low back.

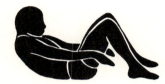

Fig. 10-18. Abdominal strengthening using an abdominal curl.

region. Strengthening should be executed without strain being placed on the lumbar spine and, specifically, the iliopsoas muscle. An effective exercise is the abdominal curl (Fig. 10-18). The subject assumes a hook lying position with one arm extended forward. Maintaining the hips and knees in a flexed position, the person slowly curls the trunk, starting with the chin on the chest and executing 5 to 10 repetitions of the exercise.

The *pelvic rolling* exercise is designed to strengthen the lower abdominal muscles, stretch the lumbosacral muscles, and educate the subject to proper pelvic positioning, as discussed in Chapters 5 and 9. The subject assumes a hook lying position with hands folded behind the head (Fig. 10-19). The lordotic curve is flattened by rolling the pelvis backward. Holding the flattened position, the subject contracts the gluteal muscles (pinches the buttocks together) and raises the tailbone from the mat approximately 3 inches, holding the position for 10 seconds, executing 5 to 10 repetitions of the exercise.

Quadriceps and hip flexor stretching is

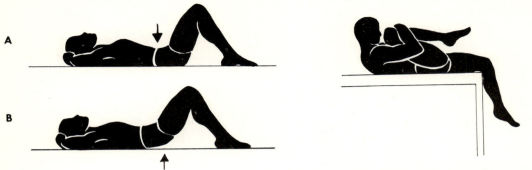

A

B

Fig. 10-19. Pelvic rolling.

Fig. 10-20. Quadriceps and hip flexor stretching.

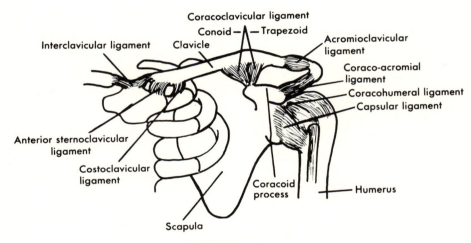

Coracoclavicular ligament

Conoid — — Trapezoid

Interclavicular ligament   Clavicle   Acromioclavicular ligament

Coraco-acromial ligament

Coracohumeral ligament

Capsular ligament

Anterior sternoclavicular ligament

Costoclavicular ligament

Coracoid process   Humerus

Scapula

Anterior aspect

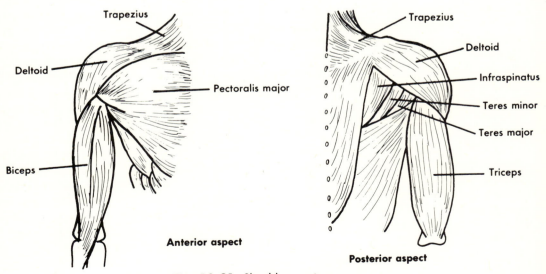

Trapezius

Deltoid

Pectoralis major

Biceps

Anterior aspect

Trapezius

Deltoid

Infraspinatus

Teres minor

Teres major

Triceps

Posterior aspect

Fig. 10-21. Shoulder anatomy.

important because tight quadriceps, primarily the rectus femoris, and hip flexors (iliopsoas muscles) are often associated with lordosis and low back pain. Stretching of these areas is difficult and requires very exact positioning. Two stretches are suggested. The first stretch is conducted from a supine position. The subject pulls the knee of one leg to the chest while the other leg is maintained in an extended position (Fig. 10-20). Caution must be taken that the extended leg does not rise from the floor. A longer stretch can be achieved if the extended leg's knee is allowed to bend over the end of a table or bed. The stretch position should be held for 30 seconds and then the legs should be alternated. The subject must be advised to keep his low back flat while stretching. A second stretch can be conducted with a bench or chair. Placing one foot on a chair with the lower leg and thigh at approximately a 90-degree angle, the subject extends the other leg backward, with the knee slightly flexed. Stretching takes place when the person leans forward, rounds his back, and lowers the pelvic level. Positions of the legs are alternated, with each stretch being held for 30 seconds.

THE SHOULDER COMPLEX

The shoulder complex or girdle, in contrast to the stable pelvis, is designed to provide free mobility. It is formed by the clavicle, scapula, humerus, and associated ligaments and muscles (Fig. 10-21). The clavicle, as it joins the sternum, forms the only skeletal contact the shoulder complex has with the thorax. It forms a strut or bridge to the scapula, which, in turn, holds the head of the humerus. The shoulder complex is composed of four separate articulations that allow for a scapulohumeral rhythm to take place: the glenohumeral, coracoclavicular, acromioclavicular, and sternoclavicular articulations.

Shoulder articulations

The *glenohumeral articulation* is classified as enarthrodial, or ball and socket, and

is formed by the round head of the humerus joining the shallow concavity of the glenoid fossa. A loose synovial capsule surrounds the joint, which is reinforced by ligaments. Tendons crossing the joint serve to strengthen and reinforce the ligamentous arrangement.

The *coracoclavicular joint* allows for only slight movement of a syndesmotic type. Its prime function is to suspend the scapula and the clavicle, which are held together by the strong coracoclavicular ligaments.

A gliding articulation, the *acromioclavicular joint*, is composed of the lateral end of the clavicle and the acromion process, forming a very weak union. Its primary support is produced by a joint capsule reinforced by superior and inferior ligaments.

The clavicle, at its medial end, articulates with the outer angle of the manubrium called the *sternoclavicular joint*. It is held in place on the sternum by strong ligamentous bands.

The dynamics of the shoulder complex are extremely lengthy and complicated, belonging to a kinesiology text; therefore we intend to provide a description of those motions that are pertinent to specific injuries and their restoration.

Shoulder injuries

Because of the shoulder complex's structural design, which provides mobility with little articular strength, it is extremely vulnerable to trauma. Falls on the outstretched hand, a severe torsion of the humerus, or a direct blow to the shoulder girdle can result in various pathological conditions. The more prevalent injuries to the shoulder complex include strains, sprains and dislocations, and fractures.

Strains to the shoulder complex are primarily in the region of the glenohumeral joint. Overstretching of the musculotendinous unit through throwing activities, as in baseball, or torsional stress, as received in wrestling, are common mechanisms of strain. The small intrinsic muscles of the *rotator cuff* (subscapularis, supraspinatus, infraspinatus, and teres minor) are commonly traumatized through forceful over-stretch of the arm in the abducted position.

Sprains and dislocations can occur at any joint in the shoulder complex. A disruption of the sternoclavicular joint occurs from a fall on the outstretched hand or from a direct inward blow, such as may be received in football. The acromioclavicular sprain or dislocation can arise from forces upward or downward against the acromion process. The partial or complete gleno-humeral dislocation represents one of the most common among active young people. Having the highest incidence, the anterior glenohumeral or subcoracoid dislocation is most often received when the arm is abducted and externally rotated.

Shoulder *fractures* most commonly involve the clavicle; however, the upper humerus is vulnerable to fracture and epiphyseal separation in active youths. Anatomically, the clavicle lacks support at its middle third and, consequently, receives most fractures at that site. Clavicular fractures of the greenstick type are received most often by junior and senior high school students.

Reconditioning

Injuries to the shoulder complex often lead to muscle contractures, with a subsequent lack of range of movement, particularly when immobilization is imposed, as in a sling or cast. Severe damage may require surgical intervention, prolonged immobilization, or both. In such situations,

muscle tone must be maintained by muscle setting exercises of the affected part and full range of movement exercise must be provided for adjacent areas such as the elbow, wrist, and hand. Although each disorder of the shoulder must be considered unique for each person, the majority require some form of graded exercise that will restore maximum mobility and strength within individual limitations. Several exercises are specifically designed for shoulder complex reconditioning, including the Codman's pendulum exercise, the wall finger walking exercise, the shoulder wheel, and active rotation.

The *Codman's pendulum exercise* (Fig. 10-22) is conducted in a stooped position to eliminate the force of gravity. It is designed to mobilize and free the contracted glenohumeral joint capsule. The participant bends from the waist, his affected arm hanging down; in this position, he can perform the shoulder movements of flexion, extension, adduction, abduction, and circumduction in either direction. Within the limits of pain and fatigue, movement arcs are at first made small, gradually being extended along with an increase in executions until 10 have been reached.

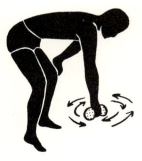

Fig. 10-22. Pendulum exercise for the shoulder.

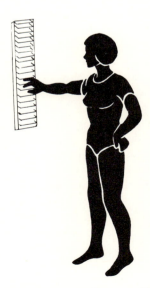

Fig. 10-23. Wall finger walking.

The *wall finger walking exercise* (Fig. 10-23) is designed to provide the participant with an increased range of shoulder movement. In this exercise, the student attempts to walk up the wall with the fingers of the affected arm. Each attempt that is higher than the last is recorded on the wall. Shoulder flexion and/or abduction range of motion can be increased depending on individual requirements.

The *shoulder wheel* (Fig. 10-24) is a machine that is very popular in centers for reconditioning. It is a metal wheel mounted on the wall, with the center axis adjustable to the patient's shoulder level. A wing nut can be tightened in the center to provide the correct resistance for each person. An adjustable handle is affixed to one of the wheel's spokes at a point approximating

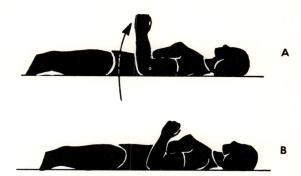

Fig. 10-25. Active shoulder rotation.

the patient's arm length. The shoulder wheel allows the patient to engage in circumduction exercises while facing the wheel and in flexion-extension exercises while standing sideways to the wheel.

Active rotation from a supine position (Fig. 10-25) allows mobilization of the glenohumeral joint without extraneous movements of the other shoulder complex articulations. Rotation is first executed with the arm flexed and the elbow positioned next to the body. External and internal rotation is then attemped. As the patient gains full range of movement, with the elbow held next to the body, the arm is gradually abducted from the body. The rotation movements can be assisted by the physical educator or resisted by pulley or dumbbell weights (Chapter 5).

A number of pieces of equipment are used for developing shoulder function. A length of rope, a towel, or a wand approximately 36 inches long and held at either end provides an excellent means for increasing shoulder girdle function. Such equipment as parallel or horizontal bars and climbing ladders provide the patient with more advanced exercise opportunities (Chapters 5 and 20).

THE ELBOW

The elbow is composed of three articulations, consisting of those between the radius and the humerus, the radius and the ulna, and the ulna and the humerus. The movement of flexion and extension is provided

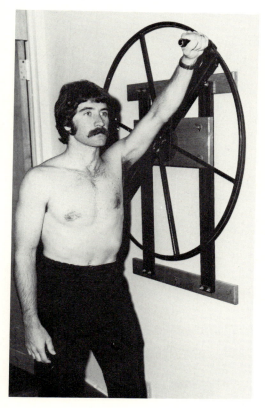

Fig. 10-24. Shoulder wheel. (Courtesy California State University, Audio Visual Center, Long Beach, Calif.)

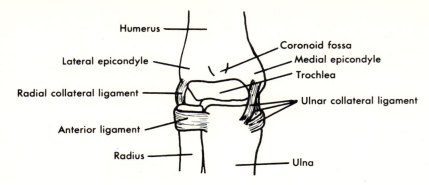

Fig. 10-26. Elbow anatomy.

for in the ulnohumeral joint, whereas forearm rotation takes place at the proximal flat circular head of the radius. Strong collateral ligaments stabilize the elbow laterally and medially, whereas the upper end of the radius is supported by an articular capsule called the angular ring. Adding to the stability of the elbow are the flexors, the biceps, the brachialis, the brachioradialis, and the triceps extensor muscle (Fig. 10-26).

Although basically designed as a strong articulation, the elbow is subject to various acute conditions in active young persons. The mechanism of injury often results from a fall on the outstretched hand, from transmission of an abnormal force to the joint, or from repeated overstretching, as in throwing activities.

A fall on the outstretched hand, a forcing of the elbow joint into a position of hyperextension, or severe torsion while in the flexed position can cause musculotendinous injury, ligamentous stretching, fracture, or dislocation. A dislocation appears as backward, forward, or lateral displacement of the ulna or radius. Repeated acute insults to the tissue of the elbow, as occur in throwing or striking types of activities, often cause an accumulation of inflammation and subsequent scarring. Activities such as pitching, serving in tennis, swinging a golf club, or throwing a javelin commonly cause strain to the elbow joint.

Reconditioning

The elbow, having received injury involving articular structures, has a great propensity for contractures, myositis ossificans, and varying degrees of ankylosis. Therefore a concentrated reconditioning program must be offered in the early stages of injury, while shoulder movements are encouraged, together with active hand and wrist exercises. When free movement is permitted by the physician, active assistive movements of flexion, extension, and rotation are encouraged several times a day within the limits of pain and fatigue. After restrictive tissues have been lengthened satisfactorily, a progressive resistive program may be instituted. The student may be encouraged to carry his books with the affected arm to facilitate stretching. It should be noted, however, that a contracted elbow should never be forced into full extension. Tissue aggravation only encourages the chronic condition of myositis ossificans, often with permanently disabling results.

THE FOREARM, WRIST, AND HAND

The forearm bones consist of the ulna and the radius. The ulna extends directly from the humerus to the carpal region. In contrast, the proximal head of the radius is held by a strong network of ligamentous tissue. Considered an extension of the hand, the radius, compared to the ulna, is much

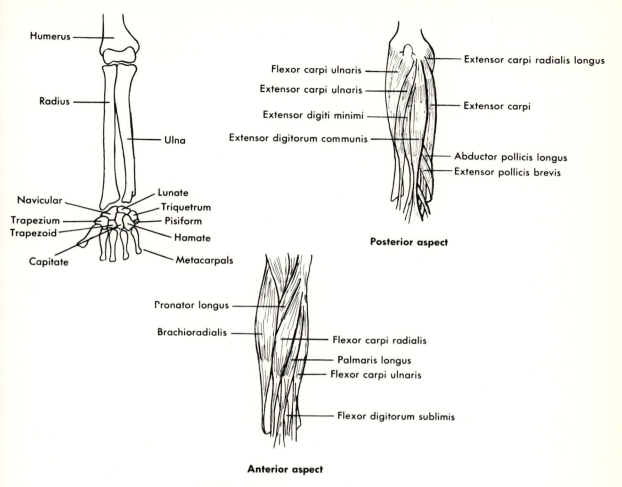

Posterior aspect

Anterior aspect

Fig. 10-27. Forearm and wrist anatomy.

thicker at its distal end than at its proximal end. Architecturally, the wrist is structured to produce great flexibility and to promote hand dexterity. The carpal bones are arranged in two rows and held together by a strong network of ligaments. Although individually the carpal bones move slightly, combined they create great flexibility in the region of the wrist. Anatomically, the hand represents a highly versatile and intricate organ. The 27 bones forming the hand include the 8 carpal bones, the 5 metacarpal bones, and the 14 phalanges (Fig. 10-27).

A complex system of muscles helps carry out the motions of the wrist and hand.

Flexors of the wrist and phalanges consist of superficial and deep muscles. The deep flexor muscles stem from the ulna, the radius, and the interossei and the superficial flexors stem from the internal condyle of the humerus. Wrist and finger extensor muscles originate at the external condyle of the humerus.

Forearm, wrist, and hand injuries

In general, the lower arm is highly susceptible to trauma, with strains, sprains, dislocations, and fractures prevalent among physically active children and young adults.

With the numerous musculotendinous units associated with the lower arm, strains are a common problem. Sudden over-stretching or abnormal and repetitive stress activities, such as throwing a baseball, swinging a golf club, or stroking a tennis racket, may lead to varying degrees of acute, subacute, or chronic lower arm strains.

A joint disruption caused by trauma occurs often to wrist and fingers. The mechanism of wrist injuries is commonly the result of a fall on the outstretched hand or a sudden twist. What is commonly thought to be wrist sprain is often tendon strain. A severe wrist sprain may, in actuality, be a fracture of the navicular bone. A navicular fracture occurs when force is applied, as in sudden hyperextension. The most common dislocation of the wrist is that of the lunate carpal bone. The cause of a lunate dislocation is a forceful hyperextension of the wrist as the radius exerts pressure downward. Stretching of the dorsal carpal ligament allows the lunate to slip forward and out of its bed.

Because of their mobility and the fact that their main support is provided by ligaments, the carpometacarpals are easily subject to sprain. The metacarpophylangeal joint is more mobile than the carpometacarpal joint and more subject to sprain when in an abducted position. Immobilization, up to 3 weeks in duration, is a standard procedure for the thumb sprain or dislocation. The need for a functional and intact thumb demands proper care and rehabilitation procedures.

Sprains and dislocations of fingers are often caused by hyperextension to the extent that ligament and capsular tissues are stretched or torn. Following splinting in a partially flexed position for a period of time with restorative exercises is the usual sequence of care.

The same mechanism that results in sprain and dislocation about the wrist and fingers also causes fractures. The fall on the outstretched hand may produce either the common Colles' fracture or fracture to the navicular bone. A Colles' fracture (Fig. 10-28) can be described as a forward dis-

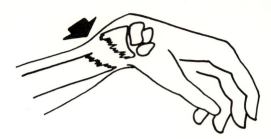

Fig. 10-28. Colles' fracture.

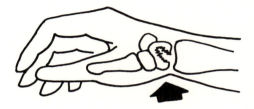

Fig. 10-29. Navicular fracture.

placement of the radius at its distal end. A navicular fracture, as described earlier, is usually a consequence of wrist hyperextension and compression of the radius and second row of carpal bones (Fig. 10-29). Improper diagnosis and inadequate wrist immobilization in the navicular fracture may lead to a condition of aseptic necrosis and bone degeneration, with subsequent permanent wrist damage.

Reconditioning

Fine motor function is of primary importance to the lower arm. Consequently, restoration means forearm rotation, wrist flexibility, and dexterity of fingers. As with the other parts of the body, whenever one part is immobilized, the other parts must be exercised to maintain function. Such activities as squeezing a small ball or a piece of sponge rubber, wringing a towel (Chapter 5), or rolling a piece of paper into a small ball are excellent exercises to reestablish hand strength and facility. Ball squeezing and towel wringing may be added to the exercise routine when range of movement has been reestablished.

REFERENCES

1. Accident facts, 1975, Chicago, 1975, National Safety Council.
2. Anderson, W. A. D., and Scotti, T. M.: Synopsis of pathology, ed. 9, St. Louis, 1976, The C. V. Mosby Co.
3. Cailliet, R.: Low back pain syndrome, ed. 2, Philadelphia, 1968, F. A. Davis Co.
4. deVries, H. A.: Physiology of exercise for physical education and athletics, Dubuque, Iowa, 1974, William C. Brown Co., Publishers.
5. Klafs, C. E., and Arnheim, D. D.: Modern principles of athletic training—the science of injury prevention and care, ed. 4, St. Louis, 1977, The C. V. Mosby Co.
6. Licht, S., editor: Therapeutic exercises, ed. 2, New Haven, Conn., 1961, Elizabeth Licht, Publisher.
7. O'Donohue, D. H.: Treatment of injuries to athletes, Philadelphia, 1976, W. B. Saunders Co.
8. Page, A. H.: Inguinal and femoral hernias, Ciba Clin. Symp. **18:**35-61, 1966.
9. Paul, W. D., and Soderberg, G. L.: The shin splints confusion, proceedings of the eighth National Conference on the Medical Aspects of Sports Medicine, Chicago, 1967, American Medical Association.
10. Raney, R. B., Sr., and Brashear, H. R.: Shands' handbook of orthopaedic surgery, ed. 8, St. Louis, 1971, The C. V. Mosby Co.

RECOMMENDED READINGS

Cailliet, R.: Foot and ankle pain, Philadelphia, 1968, F. A. Davis Co.
Cailliet, R.: Neck and arm pain, Philadelphia, 1964, F. A. Davis Co.
Cailliet, R.: Shoulder pain, Philadelphia, 1966, F. A. Davis Co.
Klein, K. K., and Allman, F. L., Jr.: The knee in sports, New York, 1969, The Pemberton Press.
McLaughlin, H. L.: Trauma, Philadelphia, 1959, W. B. Saunders Co.
Olson, O. C.: Prevention of football injuries, Philadelphia, 1971, Lea & Febiger.

11

MUSCULOSKELETAL DISORDERS
CHRONIC AND CONGENITAL

■ Orthopedic impairments constitute a major challenge to physical education, with an estimated 2.4 million orthopedically impaired individuals under 21 years of age in the United States.[23] It also has been determined that children with congenital malformations constitute about 30% of all the crippled children in the United States.[23]

The term "chronic" is defined in this text as a condition having a very gradual onset and a duration longer than 3 months, whereas "congenital" affections refer to those disorders that are present at birth. This chapter is concerned with the most prevalent of those conditions commonly found in children and young adults. They consist of amputations, arthritis, developmental hip dislocation, epiphyseal hip affections, muscular dystrophy, spina bifida, talipes, and torticollis.

AMPUTATIONS

An amputation refers to the removal of some member, part, or body organ through surgery, trauma, or some congenital malformations. Adams[2] points out that there are over 300,000 amputees in the United States; 32% of their amputations involve the upper extremities and 68% the lower limbs. Of this number, there are approximately 7% under the age of 21 years, 58% between the ages of 21 and 65 years and 35% over the age of 65 years. Amputations may be categorized as congenital, traumatic, or elective. The *congenital amputation* is one in which a body part fails to develop properly during the prenatal period. A *traumatic amputation* occurs as the result of some violence to the body, whereas the *elective amputation* is one in which surgery is performed to ameliorate a disease condition or to correct a congenital or traumatic condition. Commonly, elective surgery is conducted for vascular impairments, infection, or, more often, for malignant tumors in children.[1]

Wherever there is an amputation, a prosthetic appliance must be considered. To employ a prosthesis, a stump must be both free from irritation and functional. Therefore sites of amputations become extremely important. An optimum site for lower extremity amputation is based on the location and extent of normal tissue, type of function required, placement of prosthesis, and stump appearance.[4] Besides these factors, the child's future needs and individual personality must be taken into consideration by the physician.

Lower extremity amputations

The successful surgical amputation requires good circulation to ensure proper healing; it also requires enough remaining stump that a prosthesis may fit properly. The main requirement for a lower limb stump is that it is able to bear weight with an artificial limb and have maximum function. A scar that is improperly positioned by the surgeon may evoke constant irritation by the prosthesis. Abnormal irritation and pressure points by the artificial limb while weight bearing will develop into skin lesions and additional incapacitation.

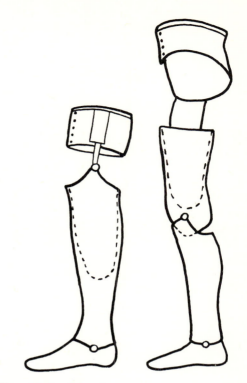

Fig. 11-1. Below-knee prosthesis and above-knee prosthesis.

The lower limb prosthesis consists of a socket for the stump and, depending on the level of amputation, an artificial knee joint, ankle joint, and segmented foot (Fig. 11-1). A conventional artificial foot allows for plantar flexion and dorsiflexion, with rubber bumpers to simulate the action of the gastrocnemius and anterior tibialis muscles. After the fitting of the artificial leg, gait training is performed. The type of prosthesis to be used is determined by the level of the amputated part. Lower limb amputations are categorized primarily into below-knee (BK) and above-knee (AK) types. The most common BK prosthesis used today is the patellar tendon bearing (PTB) with a sack foot. This prosthesis provides the wearer with a closed socket by which the stump fits snugly at its distal end to provide good proprioception.[21] AK amputees who are young and have good stump musculature will generally be fitted with a quadrilateral suction socket prosthesis. The individual with a hip disarticulation requires a prosthesis that is controlled by the action of the pelvis. The Canadian type of hip disarticulation prosthesis provides the user with maximum stabilization and mobility.

Upper extremity amputations

The loss of any part of an upper extremity is often accompanied by severe functional and emotional consequences. Prehension, tactile sense, and balance are affected.

Because of the great variance in upper extremity amputations, classification is extremely difficult. With some exceptions in the hand amputation, a long stump is desirable in order to provide for adaptability in fitting a prosthetic appliance. No single artificial arm can fill all the requirements of the amputee. A choice must be made as to which need will be satisfied: cosmetic, heavy labor, or skilled dexterous work. Every effort is made by the surgeon to reconstruct hand function and to maintain prehension and sense of touch. In an effort to replace some semblance of hand function, various terminal devices have been made for the amputee. The two most common devices are the cosmetic prosthetic hand, having some prehension, and the more useful and adjustable split hooks (Fig. 11-2). Control of the artificial upper limb is frequently provided by steel cables and a shoulder harness.

Children with amputations

Children with amputations, whether acquired or congenital, should be provided with a prosthesis according to their particular growth and development demand.[17] Some authorities have indicated that the sooner a child is provided with an appliance, the sooner he can acquire proper habits of locomotion or dexterity. As the child grows, constant attention should be paid to the fit of the prosthesis. An improper fit may mean the acquisition of poor movement patterns.[6]

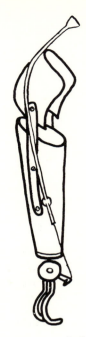

Fig. 11-2. Upper limb prosthesis.

Therapeutic management

After surgery, the patient's stump is usually placed in good alignment. Since the leg stump tends to go into abduction, flexion, and external rotation, it is positioned parallel to the mattress. General postural alignment and good body mechanics are disrupted with the loss of a major extremity, a factor to be considered in the total rehabilitative process.

An elastic bandage is applied early after surgery to control hemorrhage and shrink, toughen, and shape the stump in its preparation for the prosthesis. Swelling caused by edema is prevented by the compression of the elastic bandage and elevation of the part. Stump hygiene becomes the utmost importance in preventing skin problems. A daily routine of cleansing the stump, the elastic bandage, the stump sock, and the socket of the prosthesis must be carried out.

Phantom pain is a normal phenomenon that occurs after the loss of an extremity. Sensations such as numbness and "pins and needles" in the lost limb are common complaints. The reasons for such a phenomenon are various and obscure.

Exercise plays an important part in the management of amputees. Gullickson[7] described the therapeutic exercise needs of the amputee as follows:

1. To increase joint range of movement
2. To correct or prevent contractures
3. To establish proper body alignment and mechanics
4. To provide proper stump circulation
5. To maintain a balance of muscle power, endurance, and coordination
6. To prevent atrophy
7. To toughen the stump for use in a prosthesis
8. To improve the general physical fitness of the amputee

Maximum physical fitness must be established by amputees if they are to be able to withstand prolonged recumbency and the effect the amputation will have on their body mechanics. Ideally, a general program of conditioning should be started in the preoperative stage; however, in most cases this is not feasible unless the amputation is elective and planned well in advance of surgery. Immediately after amputation, a bed exercise regimen should be started, which includes muscle setting of the affected limb and isotonic movement of all other major joints to prevent atrophy and contractures.

Implications for physical education

The amputee poses a real challenge to the physical educator. Because of the varied types and sites of amputation as well as the different personalities involved, physical education programs must be individualized. The pupil should be encouraged to engage in and learn as many different activities as his condition will permit. Of major concern to the pupil is the maintenance of proper postural alignment, good general body balance, proficient use of a prosthesis, a high level of physical fitness, and personal confidence.

Physical education offers the amputee opportunities for development toward independence. The amputee should be encouraged to engage in all physical education activities. Swimming and gymnastics are particularly important in developing the full potential of the amputee. A physical education class is an excellent place for the amputee to acquire a positive self-concept. Embarrassment by the student about the missing body part can be lessened by an understanding teacher and the student's acceptance as an equal participant in physical activities by his peers.

ARTHRITIS

The term "arthritis" is derived from the two Greek roots "*arthro-*," meaning joint and "*-itis*," meaning inflammation. It has been estimated that over 12 million individuals in the United States are afflicted with some form of rheumatic disease. It is difficult to agree on a classification of the many arthritides, primarily because of the lack of accurate knowledge of their etiology. The American Rheumatism Association indicates that the three forms of arthritis most prevalent are arthritis from infection, arthritis from rheumatic fever, and rheumatoid arthritis. Arthritis after trauma and osteoarthritis or degenerative joint disease of the aging also have a high incidence among the general population.

Infectious arthritis

The occurrence and extent of infectious arthritis has been greatly reduced with the advent of antibiotics. Various pyogenic microorganisms, for example, streptococci, staphylococci, gonococci, pneumococci, and meningococci, have been identified as causative agents of infectious arthritis. The disease appears as an acute inflammatory condition of the synovial membrane and hyaline cartilage, with joints becoming swollen, hot, red, and painful. Associated muscle tendons may also become inflamed, resulting in contractures, inactivity, and, subsequently, muscle atrophy. Uncontrolled infection will eventually result in bony deterioration.

Rheumatic fever and arthritis present an involvement of many joints, but without the chronic effect of degeneration of articular tissue. Having its highest incidence in childhood, rheumatic fever is associated with the group A beta-hemolytic streptococcus of the upper respiratory tract. After a general systemic reaction of sore throat and fever, a transitory polyarthritis travels from one joint to another. Carditis may later be detected by the appearance of murmurs, tachycardia, and chest pain.

Rheumatoid arthritis

Rheumatoid arthritis represents the nation's number one crippler, afflicting over 3 million persons. It is a systemic disease of unknown cause. Seventy-five percent of the cases occur between the ages of 25 and 50 years and in a ratio of 3:1, women to men. A type of rheumatoid arthritis called *Still's disease,* or juvenile arthritis, attacks children before the age of 7 years. An infection theory postulates that a microorganism may play an important role. However, there is a great variance in expert opinion as to the exact cause of the disease. Hughes[9] indicated that a great many factors may predispose acquisition. Major contributors could be infection, heredity, environmental stress, dietary deficiencies, trauma, and organic or emotional disturbance.

The disease progresses in the patient, gradually resulting in general fatigue, weight loss, and muscular stiffness. Articular involvement is symmetrical and characteristically found, in its earliest stages, in the small joints of the hand and feet. Tenderness and pain may occur in tendons and muscular tissue near inflamed joints. As the inflammation in the joints becomes progressively chronic, degenerative and proliferative changes occur to the synovial tendons, ligaments, and articular cartilages. If not arrested in its early stages, joints become ankylosed and muscles atrophy and contract, eventually causing a twisted and deformed limb.

The majority of persons afflicted with rheumatoid arthritis recover almost totally with only minor residual effects. However, it has been estimated that about 10% to 15% of cases become crippled to the point of invalid status. The course of the disease, for the most part, is unpredictable, with spontaneous remissions and exacerbations.

Treatment

Medical treatment of the rheumatoid arthritic involves proper diet, rest, drug therapy, and physical therapy. Because of its debilitating effect, prolonged bed rest is discouraged, although daily rest sessions are required to avoid undue fatigue. A number of drugs may be given to the patient by the physician, depending on individual needs, for example, salicylates such as aspirin relieve pain, gold compounds may be used for arresting the acute inflammatory stage, and adrenocortical steroids may be employed for the control of the degenerative process.[18] Physical therapy is primarily concerned with preventing contracture deformities and muscle atrophy by the use of heat, massage, and graded exercise.

Accompanying chronic rheumatoid arthritis are psychological, social, and economic problems. Psychosocial problems can be as difficult to resolve as those manifested by the disease. The arthritic may feel sensitive about his condition, particularly when deformity is apparent. The theory has been advanced that the rheumatoid arthritic often displays extreme dependence, insecurity, feelings of inadequacy, and an inability to cope successfully with the demands of the environment. The following eight personality characteristics of rheumatoid arthritics have been proposed[15]:
1. Leading quiet lives
2. Being shy and feeling inadequate
3. Having marked feelings of inferiority
4. Being self-sacrificing
5. Being overconscientious
6. Having a strong need to serve others
7. Being obsessive-compulsive
8. Having a tendency toward depression

Peer adjustment may pose a serious problem for the afflicted adolescent. However, as with any reaction to a disease entity, adjustment is personal and individual.

Exercise requirements

The exercise requirements for the arthritic fall into three major categories: those that prevent deformity, those that prevent muscle atrophy, and those that maintain joint amplitude and basic function. The physical educator can use gradual or static stretching, isometric muscle contraction, and graded isotonic exercises to advantage.

Preventing deformity is a major concern of the arthritic. In the acute stage, when muscle contractures are prevalent, splinting is a common practice. While lying in bed and splinted, the patient is encouraged to engage in muscle tensing exercises numerous times during the day. Such a program tends to prevent general weakness and maintains a balance of strength.

Preventing muscle weakness from inactivity is very important if the arthritic is to maintain joint function. Muscle setting exercises, isometrics, and isotonic exercises must be employed throughout the convalescence of the patient. Particular emphasis is paid to the gluteus and knee extensor muscles, which are extensively used in ambulation.

Maintenance of normal joint range of movement is of prime importance for establishing a functional joint. Stretching is employed, first, passively by the therapist and, then, is gradually undertaken by the patient.

Implications for physical education

A pupil with arthritis may need rest periods during the school day. These should be combined with a well-planned exercise program. Activity should never increase pain or so tire an individual that normal recovery is not obtained by the next day.

Because of the nature of arthritis, an activity program must be based on the particular requirements of the individual. If the disease has been arrested from the acute stage, a variety of sports and game activities may be initiated; however, abnormal physical stress or injury must be avoided

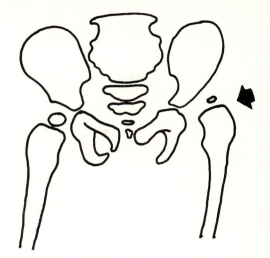

Fig. 11-3. Developmental hip dislocation.

at all costs. Swimming is an excellent activity for the arthritic; however, the water must not be chilling. Additional individual sports might include archery, golf, badminton, tennis, or weight training. Exercises that improve joint range of movement should be conducted daily by the patient. Posture training and good body alignment must be stressed in all aspects of the arthritic's daily living.

HIP AFFECTIONS
Developmental hip dislocation

The developmental hip dislocation, commonly called the "congenital hip," refers to a partially or completely displaced femoral head in relation to the acetabulum (Fig. 11-3). Haas[8] estimated that it occurs six times more often in females than in males; it may be bilateral or unilateral, occurring most often in the left hip.

The cause of the congenital hip dislocation is idiopathic or unknown, with various reasons proposed. Heredity seems to be a primary causative factor in faulty hip development and subsequent dysplasia. Faulty prenatal development as the result of an abnormal in utero position or injury from the birth process is a possible additional cause. The practice of a physician holding a newborn child by its feet or binding the

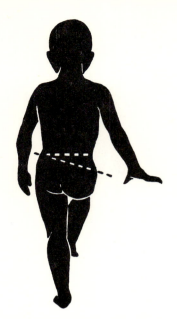

Fig. 11-4. Trendelenburg test.

infant in swaddling clothes, with thighs adducted or internally rotated, may force the hip to become dislocated. Michele[11] cited that only about 2% of developmental hip dislocations are, in actuality, congenital and therefore produced by a defective germ cell.

Generally, the acetabulum is shallower than the nonaffected side and the femoral head is displaced upward and backward in relation to the ilium. Ligaments and muscles become deranged, resulting in a shortening of the rectus femoris, hamstring, and adductor thigh muscles and affecting the small intrinsic muscles of the hip. Prolonged malpositioning of the femoral head produces a chronic weakness of the gluteus medius and minimus.[11] A primary factor in stabilizing the hip in the upright posture in the iliopsoas muscle. In the developmental dislocated hip, the iliopsoas muscle serves to displace the femoral head upward; this will eventually cause the lumbar vertebrae to become lordotic and scoliotic.

Detection of the hip dislocation may not occur until the child begins to bear weight or walk. Early recognition of this condition may be accomplished by observing asymmetrical fat folds on the infant's legs and by restricted hip abduction on the affected side. A positive *Trendelenburg test* (Fig. 11-4) reveals that the child is unable to maintain the pelvis level while standing on the affected leg. In such cases, weak abductor muscles allow the pelvis to tilt downward on the nonaffected side. The child walks with a decided limp in unilateral cases and with a waddle in bilateral cases. No discomfort or pain is normally experienced by the child, but fatigue tolerance to physical activity is very low. Pain and discomfort become more apparent as the individual becomes older and as postural deformities become more structural. Medical treatment of the developmental hip dislocation depends on the age of the child and the extent of displacement. Young babies with a mild involvement may have the condition remedied through gradual abduction of the femur by a pillow splint, whereas more complicated cases may require traction, casting, or surgery to restore proper hip continuity.

Exercise therapy is given as soon as the splint for fixation of the femur in the adducted position is removed. Slowly, the thigh is returned to a normal position. Heat and massage are given to encourage circulation. Active exercise is permitted, along with passive stretching to contracted tissue. Primary concern is paid to reconditioning the movement of hip extension and abduction. When adequate muscle strength has been gained in the hip region, a program of ambulation is conducted, with particular attention paid to walking without a lateral pelvic tilt.[11]

Implications for physical education

A child in the adapted physical education program with a history of developmental hip dislocation will, in most instances, require specific postural training, conditioning of the hip region, continual gait training, and general body mechanics. Swimming is an excellent activity for general conditioning for the hip and it is highly recommended. Activities should not be en-

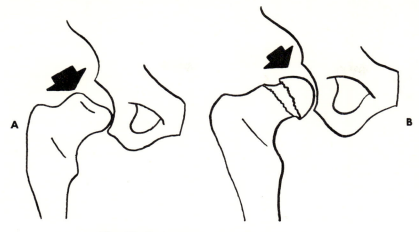

Fig. 11-5. A, Coxa plana. **B,** Coxa vara.

gaged in to the point of discomfort or fatigue.

Coxa plana

Coxa plana is the result of chondromalacia or osteochondritis dissecans, an abnormal softening, of the femoral head. It is a condition identified early in the twentieth century independently by Legg of Boston, Calvé of France, and Perthes of Germany. Its gross signs reflect a flattening of the head of the femur (Fig. 11-5, *A*) and it is found predominantly in heavily built boys between the ages of 4 and 12 years. It has been variously termed *osteochondritis deformans juvenilis, pseudocoxalgia,* and *Legg-Calvé-Perthes disease.* The exact cause is not known; trauma, infection, and endocrine imbalance have been suggested as possible causes.

This condition is characterized by necrosis and degeneration of the capital epiphysis of the femoral head. Osteoporosis, or bone rarefaction, results in a flattened and deformed femoral head. Later development may also reveal a widening femoral head and a thickened femoral neck. The last stage of coxa plana may be reflected by a self-limiting course in which there is a regeneration and an almost complete return of the normal epiphysis within 3 to 4 years. However, recovery is not always

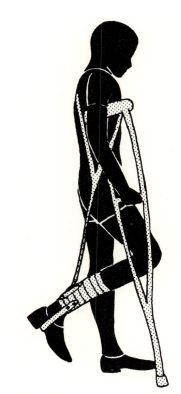

Fig. 11-6. Sling and crutch for hip conditions.

complete and there is often some residual deformity present. The younger child with coxa plana has the best outlook for complete recovery.

The first outward sign of this condition is often a limp favoring the affected leg, with a pain referred to the knee region. Further investigation by the physician may show pain on passive movement and restricted motion in internal rotation and abduction. X-ray examination will provide the definitive signs of degeneration. The physical educator may be the first person to observe the gross signs of coxa plana and bring it to the attention of parents or physician.

Treatment of coxa plana primarily entails the removal of stress placed on the femoral head by weight bearing. Bed rest is often employed in the acute stages, with ambulation and nonweight-bearing devices used for the remaining period of incapacitation. The sling and crutch method for nonweight bearing is widely used for this condition (Fig. 11-6).

Coxa vara and coxa valga

The adult femoral head or neck of the femur is at a normal angle of inclination of about 128 degrees. An abnormal increase in this angle is termed *coxa valga* and a decrease is called *coxa vara* (Fig. 11-5, *B*). Coxa vara and coxa valga are disturbances in the proximal cartilage or epiphyseal plate of the femur that result in alteration in the angle of the shaft as it relates to the neck of the femur. Steindler[19] describes the pathomechanics of coxa vara and coxa valga as resulting from the combined stresses of an abnormal increase or decrease in weight bearing. A variation of more than 10 to 15 degrees can produce a significantly shortened or lengthened extremity.[19]

Coxa valga and coxa vara can result from many etiological factors, for example, hip injury, paralysis, nonweight bearing, or congenital malformation. Coxa vara and coxa valga are described according to where the structural changes have oc-

curred in the femur, that is, neck (cervical), head (epiphyseal), or combined head and neck (cervicoepiphyseal). Two types of conditions have been recognized: the congenital and the acquired. The congenital type may be associated with the developmental hip. However, of the two, the acquired coxa vara is, by far, the most prevalent and occurs most often in adolescent boys between 10 and 16 years of age. It is commonly termed *adolescent coxa vara*.

Adolescent coxa vara is found in boys who have received a displacement of the upper femoral epiphysis. Boys who are most prone to adolescent coxa vara have been found to be obese and sexually immature or tall and lanky, having experienced a rapid growing phase. Trauma, such as is incurred in a hip fracture or dislocation, may result in an acute coxa vara or, more often, through constant stress, a gradual displacement may take place. Whatever the mechanism of injury, the individual experiences progressive fatigue and pain on weight bearing and progressive stiffness, combined with a limited range of movement. As in coxa plana, a limp is apparent, which reflects weakness in the hip abductor muscles and pain referred to the region of the knee. With displacement of the epiphyseal plate, the affected limb tends to rotate externally and to abduct when placed in flexion.

Management in the early stages of coxa vara involves crutch walking and the prevention of weight bearing to allow revascularization of the epiphyseal plate. Where deformity, displacement, and limb shortening are apparent, corrective surgery may be elected by the physician.

Implications for physical education

The individual with an epiphyseal affection of the hip presents a problem of muscular and skeletal stability and joint range of movement. Stability of the hip region requires skeletal continuity and a balance of muscle strength, primarily in the muscles of hip extension and abduction. Prolonged limited motion and non-weight bearing may result in contractures of tissues surrounding the hip joint and an inability to walk or run with ease. Abnormal weakness of the hip extensors and abductors causes the individual to display a positive Trendelenburg sign.

A program of exercise must be carried on by the child if he is to prevent muscle atrophy and general deconditioning caused by lack of activity. Muscle-tensing exercises for muscles of the hip region when movement is prohibited are conducted, together with isotonic exercises for the upper extremities, trunk, ankles, and feet.

When the hip becomes asymptomatic, a progressive isotonic nonweight-bearing program is first initiated for the hip region. Active movement emphasizing hip extension and abduction is recommended. Swimming is an excellent adjunct to the regular exercise program. When the physician considers the patient free from a pathological joint condition, weight-bearing exercises can commence. Program dosage should never exceed the point of pain or fatigue until full recovery is accomplished. A general physical fitness program emphasizing weight control and body mechanics will aid the student in preparing for his return to a full program of physical education activities.

MUSCULAR DYSTROPHY

Muscular dystrophies are chronic, progressive, degenerative, noncontagious diseases of the muscular system, characterized by weakness and atrophy of the muscles of the body. Muscular dystrophy is probably the most serious disabling condition that can occur in childhood. Although not fatal in itself, the disease contributes to premature death in most known cases because of its progressive nature. Late in the disease, connective tissue replaces most of the muscle tissue. In some cases, deposits of fat give the appearance of well-developed muscle. Despite the muscle atrophy, there is no apparent central nervous system involvement in the disease.

Although the exact incidence of muscular dystrophy is unknown, estimates place the number afflicted with the disorder in excess of 200,000 in the United States. It is estimated that more than half those cases known fall within the age range of 3 to 13 years.

The exact cause of muscular dystrophy is not known. Speculation regarding etiology includes faulty metabolism (related to inability to utilize vitamin E), endocrine disorders, and deficiencies in the peripheral nerves. There is some indication that an inherited abnormality causes the body's chemistry to be unable to carry on proper muscle metabolism. Wallace[25] indicated that heredity influences the severity of the disease and that the distribution of the affected muscles in individual patients is determined primarily by the linkage of a faulty gene.

There are numerous classifications of muscular dystrophy, with regard to the muscle groups affected and the age of onset. However, four main clinical types of muscular dystrophy have been identified. They are the pseudohypertrophic type, the facioscapulohumeral type, the juvenile type, and the mixed type.

Pseudohypertrophic type

The pseudohypertrophic type is the most prevalent type of muscular dystrophy and is usually recognized between the ages of 4 and 7 years. It is largely confined to males. Symptoms displayed by the child that give an indication of the disease are the following:

1. Decreased physical activity, compared with children of commensurate age
2. Delay in the age at which the child walks
3. Poor motor development in walking and stair climbing
4. Little muscular endurance
5. A waddling gait with the legs carried far apart
6. Walking on tiptoe
7. Moving to all fours when changing from a prone to a standing position

8. Weakness in anterior abdominal muscles

9. Weakness in neck muscles, which makes it difficult to sit erect

10. Pseudohypertrophy of muscles, particularly in the calves of the leg, which are enlarged and firm on palpation

11. Pronounced lordosis and gradual weakness of lower extremities

As the disease progresses, imbalance of muscle strength in various parts of the body occurs. Deformities develop in flexion at the hip and knees. The spine, pelvis, and shoulder girdle also eventually become atrophied. Contractures and involvement of the heart may develop with the progressive degeneration of the disease. In general, the later the age at which the disease is observed, the slower it progresses. Consequently, persons who are afflicted later may perform functional activities longer.

Facioscapulohumeral type

The facioscapulohumeral type of muscular dystrophy is the second most common. The onset of symptoms or signs of the facioscapulohumeral type is usually recognized between the ages of 3 and 20 years, with the most common age of onset between 3 and 15 years. This form of muscular dystrophy affects the shoulder and upper arm and the person may have trouble in raising his arms above his head. There is also a weakness in the facial muscles and the child may lack the ability to shut his eyes, whistle, close his eyes completely when sleeping, or drink through a straw. A child with this type of disease often appears to have a masklike face that lacks expression. Later, involvements of the muscles that move the humerus and scapula will be noticed. Weakness usually appears later in the abdominal, pelvic, and hip musculature and anomalies such as scoliosis and lordosis develop in the spine. This type of muscular dystrophy is often milder than the pseudohypertrophic type and some persons with it have been able to live useful lives. Facioscapulohumeral muscular dystrophy usually progresses slowly.

Juvenile type

The juvenile type begins in late childhood, adolescence, or early adult life. Muscle atrophy is more general, with the muscles of the shoulder girdle being affected first. The progression is usually slower than in the types mentioned previously and persons afflicted with this type live longer.

Mixed type

The mixed version of muscular dystrophy may occur between the ages of 30 and 50 years. Involvement is most likely to appear in the area of the scapula and pelvis. This type may take on many of the characteristics that appear in the pseudohypertrophic type.

Implications for physical education

The age of onset of muscular dystrophy is of importance to the total development of the child. Those who contract the disease after having had an opportunity to secure an education, or part of an education, and develop social and psychological strengths are better able to cope with their environment than those who are afflicted with the disease prior to the acquisition of basic skills.

Although the characteristics of patients with muscular dystrophy will vary according to the stage that the disease has reached, some general characteristics are as follows:

1. There is a tendency to tire quicky.

2. There may be a tendency to lose fine manual dexterity.

3. Truitt[22] and Ripley and associates[14] concluded that children with muscular dystrophy have normal intelligence, but lack motivation to learn because of isolation from social contacts and limited educational opportunities.

4. Progressive weakness tends to produce adverse postural changes.

5. Emotional disturbance may be prevalent because of the progressive nature of the illness and the resulting restrictions placed on opportunities for socialization.[22]

Nothing currently known will arrest muscular dystrophy once it begins. Because of the negativism prevalent in some cases as a result of the inability of these children to serve a social purpose, this lack of knowledge has been a serious deterrent to expansion of educational plans for patients with muscular dystrophy. However, it is worth noting that scientific research may be close to solving unanswered questions regarding the disease and eventually the progressive deterioration of muscles may be halted.

Inactivity seems to contribute to the progressive weakening of the muscles of those with muscular dystrophy. Exercise of muscles involved in the activities of daily living to increase strength may permit greater functional use of the body. Furthermore, exercise may assist in reducing excessive weight, which is a burden to those who have muscular dystrophy; therefore the diet should be high in protein and low in carbohydrate content for the purpose of weight control.

One must recognize that the dystrophies cannot all be considered the same; therefore the physical and social benefits children can derive from physical education programs are different. Those who have milder forms of muscular dystrophy, which progress slowly, can derive many benefits from well-constructed adapted physical education programs and children should be allowed to play as long as they can.

A great deal can be done to prevent deformities and loss of muscle strength from inactivity. If a specific program is outlined during each stage of the disease, it is possible that the child may extend the ability to care for most of his daily needs for many additional years. In addition to the administration of specific developmental exercises for the involved muscles, exercises should include development of walking patterns, posture control, muscular coordination, and stretching of contractures involved in disuse atrophy. It should be noted, however, that all exercises should be

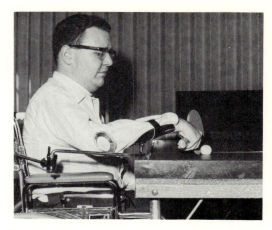

Fig. 11-7. A student with muscular dystrophy finds Ping-Pong enjoyable. (Courtesy The American Association for Health, Physical Education, and Recreation.)

under the direction of a physician. In an attempt to achieve social and emotional progress from activities, it may be desirable to blueprint the activities around the remaining positive strengths so that enjoyment and success can be achieved (Fig. 11-7).

The progressive weakness and muscle deterioration make the child with muscular dystrophy particularly susceptible to respiratory infections. Therefore the physical educator should be particularly alert not to expose these children to damp environments or to situations that are conducive to respiratory infections.

CONGENITAL SPINAL COLUMN MALFORMATIONS
Spina bifida

Of the dysplastic congenital defects occurring to the spine, spina bifida is the most common. Spina bifida implies congenital malformation of the posterior aspect of the spinal column, in which some portion of the vertebral arch fails to form over the spinal cord. It has been estimated that spina bifida occurs in 1 of 1,000 infants born, of which 80% do not survive the first year. Spina bifida might appear as an external herniation of meninges, meningo-

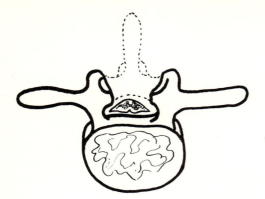

Fig. 11-8. Spina bifida occulta.

cele, or myelomeningocele or, more commonly, as spina bifida occulta without an external sac (Fig. 11-8). In any type, spinal cord involvement may occur, producing varying degrees of neurological impairment. However, neurological disturbances may be completely absent in spina bifida occulta or may not become symptomatic until later in life.[9] "Spina bifida occulta is the unfused condition of vertebral arches without any cystic distension of the meninges. There may or may not be changes in the overlying skin, neurological signs, or pathological changes in the spinal cord."[20]

Children who are paraplegic from spina bifida are often able to move about with the aid of braces and crutches. Of considerable concern is the prevention of contractures and associated foot deformities, for example, equinovarus, through daily passive flexibility exercises.

Implications for physical education

No particular program of physical education can be directly assigned to the student with spina bifida. Some students have no physical reaction and discover the condition only by chance through X-ray examination for another problem. On the other hand, a student may have extensive neuromuscular involvement requiring constant medical care. A program of physical education based on the individual needs of the child should be planned.

Spondylolysis and spondylolisthesis

Spondylolysis and spondylolisthesis result from a congenital malformation of one or both of the neural arches of the fifth lumbar vertebra or, less frequently, of the fourth lumbar vertebra. Spondylolisthesis is contrasted to spondylolysis on account of its anterior displacement of the fifth lumbar on the sacrum. Forward displacement may occur as a result of a sudden trauma to the lumbar region. The vertebrae are moved anteriorly because there is an absence of bony continuity of the neural arch and the main support is derived from its ligamentous arrangement. In such cases, individuals often appear to have a severe lordosis.[19]

Many individuals have spondylolysis, or even spondylolisthesis, without symptoms of any kind, but a mild twist or blow may set off a whole series of low back complaints with localized discomfort or pain radiating down one or both sides. The pathological condition may eventually become so extensive that surgical intervention will be required.

Implications for physical education

Physical education can provide the person with a painful low back because of spondylolysis or spondylolisthesis with a graduated exercise program that may help prevent further aggravation and, in some cases, remove many symptoms characteristic of the condition. A program should be initiated similar to that of ameliorating the postural malalignment of lordosis, with primary concentration on the strengthening of abdominal muscles; the lengthening of low back muscles; and the segmental realignment of legs, pelvis, and spine (Chapters 5 and 9). Games and sports that overextend, fatigue, or severely twist and bend the low back should be avoided. In most cases, the physician will advise against contact sports and heavy weight lifting.

TALIPES (CLUBFOOT)

One of the most common deformities of the lower extremities is talipes or clubfoot.

Talipes is a term derived from the Latin *talus,* meaning ankle, and *pes,* meaning foot. This defect can be acquired or congenital. The acquired clubfoot can develop from a spastic paralysis, as in cerebral palsy or other neuromuscular disease, which eventuates in bone and soft tissue changes. A congenital clubfoot is by far the most prevalent type. However, the pathogenesis is not clearly understood. A defective germ cell, inheritance, arrest of fetal development, muscle imbalance, or faulty in utero position have been advanced as possible causes.

A clubfoot deformity is characterized by the position in which the foot is formed and may be described as *equinus* (plantar flexion), *calcaneus* (dorsiflexion), *varus* (inversion), or *valgus* (eversion). The clubfoot deformity, if not corrected, would force the individual to walk on the ankles rather than on the sole of the foot.

Talipes equinovarus

Talipes equinovarus has the highest incidence, amounting to 70%, among the congenital forms of clubfoot. Adams[1] described talipes equinovarus as being adducted and inverted at the subtalar, midtarsal, and anterior tarsal joints, while contracted tissue pulls the foot into a plantar flexed position (Fig. 11-9). The calcaneus fails to grow, remaining small or underdeveloped. If not corrected early in life,

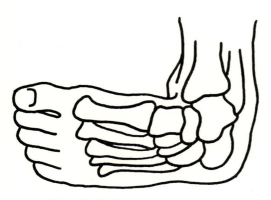

Fig. 11-9. Talipes equinovarus.

the individual with talipes equinovarus develops an awkward gait and walks on the outside of the foot and ankle.

Therapeutic management

Treatment of the clubfoot may be conservative or operative. If the deformity is recognized soon after birth, a plaster cast is employed to retain the foot in an overcorrected position. Special clubfoot shoes with a ridged steel pole may be employed for the prewalker to help maintain the proper position of the foot. Various corrective shoes may be worn and splints applied to continue the development of proper foot alignment until amelioration is achieved.

Implications for physical education

The pupil's limitations and capabilities will depend on the extent of residual derangement and deformity. A handicapped child with a severe malformation may be restricted from standing long periods or may be unable to walk without fatigue. Activities requiring running and jumping must be modified.

Exercise cannot be considered a means for correcting a clubfoot. However, a graded program should be given the pupil that will maintain or improve muscle tone, improve ambulation, and develop good body mechanics (Chapters 7 and 9). Team and individual sports activities are beneficial for the pupil with clubfoot, but they may have to be adapted to prevent the deleterious effects of extensive running, jumping, and kicking (Chapter 8).

TORTICOLLIS

Torticollis, or wryneck, is an acquired or congenital neck deformity characterized, most often, by a shortening of the sternocleidomastoid (Fig. 11-10) and, occasionally, the scalenus, platysma, splenius, and trapezius muscles. It appears as a flexion and tilting of the head, together with rotation toward the affected side.[13]

Acquired torticollis may develop from an acute, subacute, or chronic inflamma-

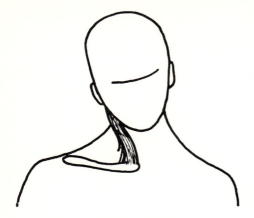

Fig. 11-10. Torticollis.

tory process resulting from strains, sprains, or wounds. Habit patterns such as those developed by defective eyesight or hearing difficulties may tend to produce a postural torticollis. Other acquired conditions may be psychogenic in nature and can be produced by a psychoneurotic tic, which contributes to a chronic torticollis.[5]

Congenital torticollis can result from malposition of the head in utero, defective cervical vertebral development, or disruption of circulation to the neck muscles. Continuous muscle shortening eventually leads to scar development and contractures. As the child grows older, facial deformity may be noted. The face on the contracted side becomes flattened, with the eye and mouth distorted downward.

Therapeutic management

Medical care for the acute wryneck involves rest, traction, heat, massage, mild manipulation, and, in some cases, a Thomas collar for immobilization and support, depending on the patient's requirements.[5] Chronic and congenital torticollis requires more extensive and prolonged medical management than acquired torticollis. In mild cases, stretching exercises or bracing may be employed. However, with the more complicated conditions, surgery with bracing might be the treatment of choice, followed by an extensive physical therapy program. The total psychological, sociological, and

medical implications of the pupil must be kept in mind. Often, grave psychological problems arise from bodily disfigurement.

Implications for physical education

The reaction of the pupil to his condition is individual and depends on his basic psychological makeup. Lack of feelings of personal worth or self-esteem may occur as a result of an unusual appearance and the negative reaction of peers. The physical educator should provide an atmosphere of acceptance and encouragement for the child.

An individual with torticollis is not usually limited in physical activity. When permitted by the physician, a program of graded exercises should be employed to increase the strength of weakened neck musculature and to stretch contracted tissue. In some cases, topical heat applied to the shortened area will aid muscular relaxation and elongation. Wale[24] suggested that active exercises for torticollis should include head side flexion away from the contracted side, with rotation movement in the direction of the affected side.

Because the student is usually capable of a great variety of sports activities, he should be introduced to as many as possible. For students whose torticollis is psychogenic in origin, low-tension activities such as swimming, golf, and tennis are suggested.

REFERENCES

1. Adams, J. C.: Outline of orthopaedics, Baltimore, 1966, The Williams & Wilkins Co.
2. Adams, R. C., et al.: Games, sports, and exercises for the physically handicapped, Philadelphia, 1972, Lea & Febiger.
3. Anderson, W. A. D., and Scotti, T. M.: Synopsis of pathology, ed. 9, St. Louis, 1976, The C. V. Mosby Co.
4. Burnham, P. J.: Amputation of the lower extremity, Ciba Clin. Symp. No. 16, 1964.
5. Cailliet, R.: Neck and arm pain, Philadelphia, 1964, F. A. Davis Co.
6. Daniels, A. S., and Davies, E. A.: Adaptive physical education, New York, 1975, Harper & Row, Publishers.
7. Gullickson, G., Jr.: Exercises for amputee. In Licht, S., editor: Therapeutic exercise, ed. 2,

New Haven, Conn., 1961, Elizabeth Licht, Publisher.

8. Haas, H.: Therapeutic dislocation of the hip, Springfield, Ill., 1963, Charles C Thomas, Publisher.
9. Hughes, J. G.: Synopsis of pediatrics, ed. 4, St. Louis, 1975, The C. V. Mosby Co.
10. Klafs, C. E., and Arnheim, D. D.: Modern principles of athletic training—the science of injury prevention and care, ed. 4, St. Louis, 1977, The C. V. Mosby Co.
11. Michele, A. A.: Iliopsoas, Springfield, Ill., 1962, Charles C Thomas, Publisher.
12. Prior, J. A., and Silberstein, J. S.: Physical diagnosis, ed. 4, St. Louis, 1973, The C. V. Mosby Co.
13. Raney, R. B., Sr., and Brashear, H. R.: Shands' handbook of orthopaedic surgery, ed. 8, St. Louis, 1971, The C. V. Mosby Co.
14. Ripley, H. S., et al.: Personality factors in patients with muscular dystrophy, Am. J. Psychiatry 99:781-787, 1943.
15. Rotstein, J.: Arthritis performance, Philadelphia, 1965, W. B. Saunders Co.
16. Rusk, H. A.: Rehabilitation medicine, ed. 3, St. Louis, 1971, The C. V. Mosby Co.
17. Salter, R. B.: Disorders and injuries of the musculoskeletal system, Baltimore, 1970, The Williams & Wilkins Co.
18. Stecher, P. G., editor: The Merck index, ed. 8, Rahway, N.J., 1968, Merck & Co., Inc.
19. Steindler, A.: Kinesiology of the human body, Springfield, Ill., 1955, Charles C Thomas, Publisher.
20. Swinyard, C. A., editor: Comprehensive care of the child with spina bifida manifesta, New York University, Rehabil. Monogr. No. 31, 1966.
21. Tosberg, W. A.: Upper and lower extremity prosthesis, Springfield, Ill., 1962, Charles C Thomas, Publisher.
22. Truitt, C. J.: Personal and social adjustments of children with muscular dystrophy, Am. J. Phys. Med. 34:124-128, 1955.
23. U.S. Department of Health: Welfare services for crippled children, Public Health Services Publication No. 2137, Washington, D.C., 1971, U.S. Government Printing Office.
24. Wale, J. O., editor: Tidy's massage and remedial exercises, Baltimore, 1961, The Williams & Wilkins Co.
25. Wallace, H. M.: The muscular dystrophies. In Frampton, M. E., editor: The physically handicapped and special health problems, Boston, 1955, Porter Sargent, Publisher.

RECOMMENDED READINGS

Cailliett, R.: Foot and ankle pain, Philadelphia, 1968, F. A. Davis Co.

Cailliett, R.: Low back pain syndrome, ed. 2, Philadelphia, 1968, F. A. Davis Co.

Cailliett, R.: Shoulder pain, Philadelphia, 1966, F. A. Davis Co.

Licht, S., editor: Therapeutic exercise, ed. 2, New Haven, Conn., 1965, Elizabeth Licht, Publisher.

12

CARDIORESPIRATORY
DISORDERS

■ "Cardiovascular" includes all diseases of the heart and the blood vessels throughout the body. This includes rheumatic and congenital heart conditions, coronary heart disease, hypertensive heart disease, and cerebrovascular disease. The rheumatic and congenital heart conditions are the primary heart disorders found in the public schools. Moreover, 25 million Americans live with some type of heart or blood vessel disease.[1] This chapter is concerned with fundamental principles of establishing physical education programs for children with heart disease of the congenital and rheumatic types and physical education programs that may help in delaying the degeneration of the cardiovascular system in regard to coronary heart disease and hypertensive heart disease. Heart disease in children is a major problem and commands the attention of the physical educator whenever this condition confronts him. It is imperative that teachers have a general understanding of the heart and circulatory system (Figs. 12-1 to 12-3) and of the major kinds of deviations in the cardiovascular system and know how to plan programs within the capabilities of children who suffer from these deviations.

Cardiovascular diseases are estimated to cause more than 54.3% of all deaths in the United States.[1] Compared to other disabilities, heart conditions cause the greatest number of restrictions in physical activity. Congenital heart disease and rheumatic fever are the heart disorders that occur most often in children of school age. It is estimated that there are about 500,000 children in this country suffering from rheumatic fever[19] and that rheumatic fever and rheumatic heart disease account for approximately two thirds of all heart disease in children.[35]

CLASSIFICATION OF HEART MURMURS

When the blood flows past the valves of the heart, sounds are made that are easily detected by a stetheoscope. Heart murmurs are of two types. The first is a functional murmur, which is believed to result from a physiological disturbance. In these cases, there is usually no sign of heart disease. The murmur may disappear on another examination.

The second type of murmur is the organic murmur, which is usually a result of some defect of the heart. Organic murmurs may be either acquired (caused by disease) or congenital (present at birth). On many occasions, the mitral and aortic valves are afflicted. Valve affliction may cause either regurgitation (imperfect closure of the valve, permitting a backflow) or stenosis (incomplete opening of a valve, which restricts the flow of blood). The organic murmur usually warrants the close supervision of the physical educator, for this type of murmur generally is associated with some form of cardiac disease.

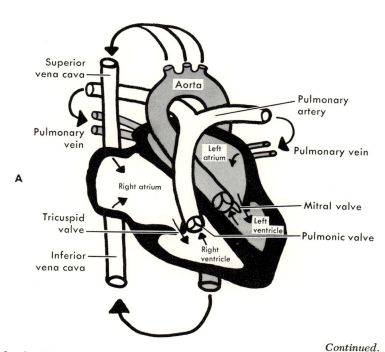

Continued.

Fig. 12-1. A, Blood flow through the normal heart. **B,** Blood flow through the heart. *1,* Blood enters right atrium; *2,* then flows to right ventricle; *3,* goes to the lungs through the pulmonary artery; *4,* returns from the lungs to the left atrium; *5,* then goes to the left ventricle; and *6,* flows through the aorta into the body.

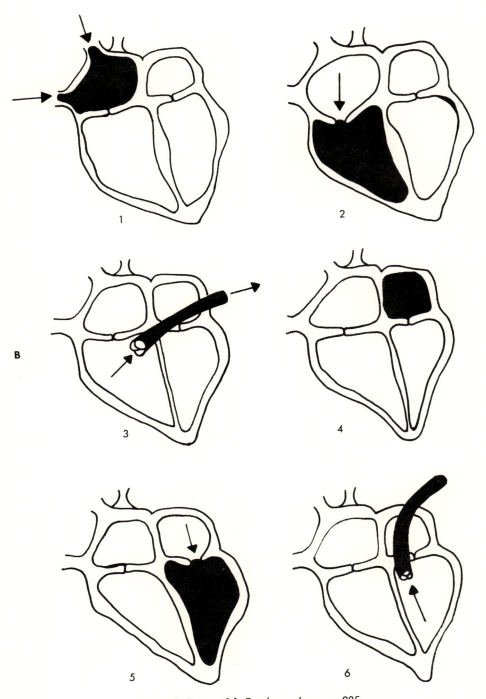

Fig. 12-1, cont'd. For legend see p. 285.

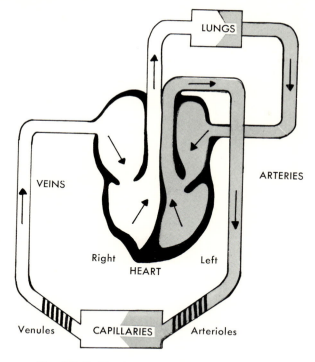

Fig. 12-2. Circulation to the lungs and body.

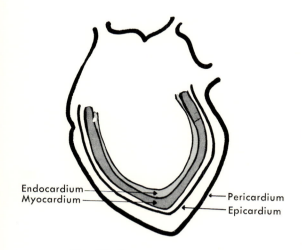

Fig. 12-3. Layers of the heart.

MAJOR TYPES OF CARDIOVASCULAR DISEASE

The American Heart Association[44] listed four major types of cardiovascular disease:

1. Rheumatic heart disease, which damages the heart and its valves, muscles, and blood vessels by scar tissue and is caused by rheumatic fever
2. Congenital heart disease, which is a malfunction of the heart occurring in fetal life
3. Hypertensive heart, commonly known as high blood pressure, which places a prolonged stress on the heart and major arteries
4. Coronary heart disease, or arteriosclerosis of the coronary arteries, a condition in which the coronary arteries become sclerotic, or hardened and narrowed and the passage of blood through the channels becomes more difficult. The chief cause of coronary heart disease is

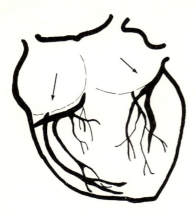

Fig. 12-4. Arrows indicate coronary arteries.

atherosclerosis, that is, the formation of atheromas or fat masses on the lining surface of the coronary arteries (Fig. 12-4).

The first two of these conditions, rheumatic heart disease and congenital heart disease, are commonly found in school-aged children. The latter two are the result of a degenerative cardiovascular system and are prevalent among the aging population, but often have their origins in poor health practices of younger persons.

Rheumatic fever

Rheumatic fever is a disease that school-aged children may contract. Rheumatic fever ranks first in causes of death in children and adolescents from 5 to 19 years of age. Consequently, it presents a great problem to physical education teachers in the public schools.

Although the direct cause of rheumatic fever is not known, the disease is an acute infection related to a hemolytic streptococcus. There are three main phases in the development of rheumatic fever. In the first stage, the youngster has a sore throat caused by a streptococcus infection. He then recovers, in the second phase, for 1 to 4 weeks; the third phase begins when he contracts acute rheumatic fever, which may last for weeks and months. The following are a number of warning signals that may

be of use to the educator, school nurse, or physician:

1. Failure to gain weight
2. Pallor
3. Fatigue
4. Poor appetite
5. Frequent colds and sore throats
6. Tonsil or adenoid problems
7. Scarlet fever or any known streptococcal infection
8. Unexplained nosebleeds
9. Unexplained fever
10. Pains in arms, legs, or joints
11. Unusual restlessness, irritability, twitching, or jerky motions
12. History of previous rheumatic fever
13. Behavior and personality changes
14. Poor schoolwork by a child who has previously done well
15. Breathing difficulties, rapid breathing, exceptionally slow breathing, or arrhythmical breathing

During the acute attack of rheumatic fever, there are usually symptoms that are caused by the localization of inflammation. The inflammation may be in the joints; in the skin, in the form of a rash; in the brain, causing Saint Vitus's dance; and in the heart, causing a faulty closure of the heart valves. There is also marked fever and migration of heat, pain, and swelling from joint to joint. In many instances, the first attack of rheumatic fever is very mild and difficult to diagnose. Consequently, most of the children who have contracted rheumatic fever escape the first time with little or no heart damage. However, there is no immunity built up to rheumatic fever. On the contrary, there is a strong tendency for the disease to recur. Therefore it is extremely vital that the initial attack of rheumatic fever be diagnosed as such so that precautions can be taken to withstand or prevent a second attack.

Through the administration of antibiotics that destroy the streptococcus bacteria, effective prevention of recurring attacks of rheumatic fever can be achieved. Without prophylactic medication, second attacks occur in from 50% to 70% of children who have had one attack.[28] Once the initial attack of rheumatic fever has manifested itself, primary interest is not so much in the heart or in the amount of physical activity in which the child is engaged, unless severe damage has occurred, but in the practice of preventing streptococcal infection. In the event that a child is in a preventive program against rheumatic fever and contracts a streptococcal infection, more often than not, penicillin will eradicate the infection. Therefore the American Heart Association has listed the following guides to assist persons in identifying possible streptococcal infections:

1. Did the sore throat come on suddenly?
2. Does the youngster complain that his throat hurts most when he swallows?
3. Does it hurt him under the angle of his jaw when it is pressed gently with the fingers? Are the lymph glands swollen?
4. Does he have fever? How much? (Streptococcal infections bring on fever between 101° and 104° F.)
5. Does the child complain of headache?
6. Is he nauseated?
7. Has he been in contact with anyone who has had scarlet fever or a sore throat?

When deterrents of the recurring attacks in rheumatic fever are not successful, in many instances, the heart is permanently injured. Injury is usually manifested in one or both of the values on the left side of the heart. The valves heal by means of scars, which leave the heart rough or deformed. This deformity may prevent the valves from functioning properly. The valves may also become narrowed (stenosed). Recurring attacks of rheumatic fever usually subside during adolescence (Fig. 12-5).

Congenital heart disease

The range in the severity of congenital heart disease is great. The defect can be so mild that it in no way affects the child or it can be so severe that the consequence is death. It is a disease that occurs in many combinations as a result of defective fetal development of the heart and vessels of the circulatory system. The incidence of congenital heart disease is estimated at 1% or 2% of all the organic heart diseases. Some of the causes of congenital heart disease have been associated with metabolic and endocrine disturbances, infectious virus, or vitamin deficiencies during the first 3 months of pregnancy. German measles during the first trimester of pregnancy has been believed to contribute to possible congenital heart disease. Great advances in heart surgery during the past few years have made it possible to correct congenital heart defects that would former-

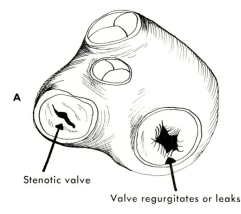
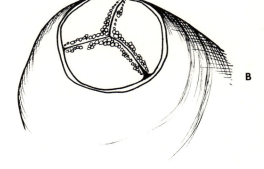

Stenotic valve

Valve regurgitates or leaks

Fig. 12-5. A, Rheumatic disease of heart valves. **B,** Rheumatic disease along cusps of aortic valve.

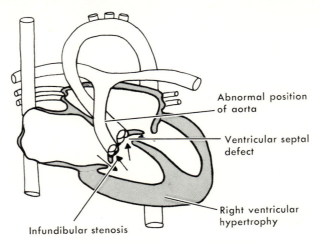

Abnormal position of aorta

Ventricular septal defect

Right ventricular hypertrophy

Infundibular stenosis

Fig. 12-6. Tetralogy of Fallot.

ly have resulted in death so that the child may now live and have the possibility of a satisfying life in the future. However, it should be noted that not all children with congenital heart defects can benefit by operation.

The following are some of the specific disorders of congenital heart disease:
1. Patent ductus arteriosus, in which the passageway between the pulmonary artery and the aorta remains open after birth and some of the blood that should go through the aorta is short-circuited to the lungs. This works to the disadvantage of both the pulmonary and the general circulations.
2. Tetralogy of Fallot ("blue baby"), congenital abnormalities that consist of an opening of the septum between the ventricles and abnormal positioning of the aorta to the right in such a manner that it lies over a defect of the septum of the left ventricle so that some blood leaves the aorta, which results in enlargement of the right ventricle and a decreased amount of the blood going to the lungs for reoxygenation (Fig. 12-6).
3. Coarctation of the aorta, constriction of the aorta; generally after the arteries branch off to the head and arms. This

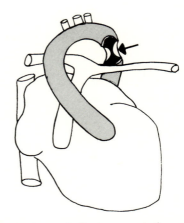

Fig. 12-7. Arrow indicates coarctation of aorta.

causes limitation of blood to the tissues and organs of the body together with high blood pressure in the upper extremities and low blood pressure in the lower extremities, which, if not corrected, lead to later complications (Fig. 12-7).

CLASSIFICATION OF CARDIAC DISEASES

The approval of the activity program for a child with a cardiac disorder must come from the physician. Therefore most diagnostic referral forms that come from medical personnel use the standard classification procedures developed by the American Heart Association. The classification represents an estimate as to what the person can do in response to effort. This classification provides enough information for a teacher so that a child with a cardiac disorder will not be unduly restricted from physical activity. The classification of patients with diseases of the heart is as follows:

Class I: Patients with heart disease, but without resulting limitation of physical activity. Ordinary physical activity does not cause undue fatigue, palpitation, dyspnea, or anginal pain.

Class II: Patients with cardiac disease resulting in slight limitation of physical activity. They are comfortable at rest. Ordinary physical activity results in fatigue, palpitation, dyspnea, or anginal pain.

Class III: Patients with cardiac disease resulting in marked limitation of physical activity. They are comfortable at rest. Less than ordinary activity causes fatigue, palpitation, dyspnea, or anginal pain.

Class IV: Patients with cardiac disease resulting in inability to engage in any physical activity without discomfort. Symptoms of cardiac insufficiency or of the anginal syndrome are present even at rest. If any physical activity is undertaken, discomfort is increased.

The complementary classification is as follows:

Class A: Patients with a cardiac disease whose ordinary physical activity need not be restricted.

Class B: Patients with cardiac disease whose ordinary physical activity needed not be restricted, but who should be advised against severe or competitive physical efforts.

Class C: Patients with cardiac disease whose ordinary physical activity should be moderately restricted and whose more strenuous efforts should be discontinued.

Class D: Patients with cardiac disease whose ordinary physical activity should be considerably restricted.

Class E: Patients with cardiac disease who should be at complete rest, confined to a bed or a chair.

In addition to the classification of a child with a cardiac disorder for the purpose of assisting teachers in the administration of physical activity, the Ohio State Department of Education has stated some general rules for administering activity to the child who has cardiac disease. They are as follows:

1. Children should be observed and reclassified at regular intervals.
2. All children should have their temperatures taken daily.
3. All cardiac children should have rest periods, with frequency depending on the severity of the condition.
4. Perhaps the best guide for determining limitations is the response to exercise and the frequency with which shortness of breath occurs.

MEDICAL DIAGNOSTIC PROBLEMS

Medical personnel assume the responsibility of defining the limits of physical activity for the child with heart disease. Diagnostic difficulties are encountered when attempting to determine the limits of physical activity for the child. The following are some of the problems that face diagnosticians:

1. The physician's experience in cardiac practice. Many advances have been made and are currently being made in heart disease. Consequently, the physician must be aware of the most recent evidence for proper diagnosis.[5]
2. The physician's own personal attitudes toward heart disease. Some physicians are cautious in their diagnoses and wish to protect their patients as well as themselves professionally. As a result, there is a tendency to "overdiagnose."[12] Furthermore, Vodola[13] indicates that, for many years, some physicians have disapproved of physical activity for those exhibiting circulorespiratory problems.

There is a recent trend that indicates that physicians are inclined to include graded activities for cardiac patients after careful evaluation of the limits to be imposed. Improved diagnostic techniques are also available to the physician.

NATURE AND NEEDS OF THE PERSON WITH CARDIAC DISABILITY

The person with cardiovascular disability must not overstep his bounds in either the physical or the emotional dimension of living, for doing so can mean disaster. Consequently, walking this tightrope can cause both emotional disturbance and psychic disorders. Furthermore, cardiovascular impairment in some is a dynamic thing, with the person either deteriorating or being rehabilitated so that he can live a more fully functioning life. This means that a person living under these circumstances must constantly make adjustments to his environment to maintain the balance between his capabilities with respect to his heart. This also confronts the person with psychological and emotional problems. He may withdraw and underestimate his capabilities, thereby unnecessarily placing substantial obstacles in his way to independent living. He may suppress the seriousness of the condition and perform acts that may jeopardize his life.

Cardiovascular disability also stands in the way of fulfillment of optimal vocational experiences, for schoolwork is often missed and experiences may be few, narrow, and distorted. Therefore it is of the utmost importance that education be concerned with the establishment of orderly progression and increasing standards of performance and achievement for these children. Since one cannot deny the fact that the possibility of anxiety increased above the norm is prevalent among children with cardiovascular impairments, it is not surprising that many of these persons manifest characteristic traits such as overstriving, perfectionism; resentfulness; tight restrain, an inability to express aggression; insecurity; conflict avoidance; a passive nature with a great need for the respect of authority; and a noticeable tendency to neglect health, to minimize symptoms, or to reject illness. Although these traits may be prevalent among all handicapped populations, it is nevertheless important that an awareness be developed in physical education teachers to help them better understand possible manifestations of disease in children with cardiovascular impairment.

Psychological and emotional characteristics

Personality function is dependent on the brain and its physical health. If there is a reduction in the cerebral flow as a result of cardiovascular impairment, mental symptoms may frequently be seen in cardiac patients. Therefore it is possible to assume that there is a relationship between the cardiovascular system and personality function.

The physical educator should be interested in the response of the cardiac patient to various forms of physical exercise and various forms of psychological effort and stress. It may be well to point out that the age of onset of the heart disability may be a variable in the emotional problems facing the cardiac patient. The child who has had a heart disability from birth and one who has acquired a heart disability have different adjustment problems. A child with a congenital cardiac condition, for instance, may be restricted in active play throughout the process of development. Consequently, emotional immaturity may result. On the other hand, the child who is in adolescence or has had some years of uninterrupted growth may have progressed further in social, psychological, and physical development.

When a physical handicap such as cardiovascular impairment causes emotional complications and when the two conditions exist simultaneously, each condition increases the problems presented by the other.

The child with cardiac disability in physical education

Because heart disease is so complicated and not well understood among professionals dealing with the child who has cardiac disease, fears and apprehensions have long interfered with their educational management. The role of the physical educator in dealing with the child who has cardiac disease is to create a protective environment and yet to provide activities that keep the child from feeling different. Children with cardiovascular impairment require the same educational opportunities and have the same needs as typical children. Therefore it is important to look at the physiological bounds and develop the best life within them.

There is no doubt that the needs of children with heart disease are great. Therefore there are two alternatives for educational placement of these children in the public schools: a regular class or a special class. The present tendency is to integrate the child with cardiac difficulties with peers in regular classes, for every child wants to be like other children. However, the possibility is still recognized that a child might profit less from being in a regular class, where he cannot possibly compete satisfactorily, than he would in a special class for the physically handicapped, where the program is geared to his limitations. Regardless of whether the physical educator finds the child with cardiac disability in regular or adapted classes for the physically handicapped, the teacher is obligated to meet the needs of that particular child. Some suggestions for teachers of these children are as follows:

1. Provide opportunities in physical activities for biological and sociological development of the child.
2. Take special precautions to counter ill health, for example, colds and streptococcal infections.
3. Appraise the physical status of the child.
4. Correct remediable defects.
5. Develop in each child a positive attitude toward body care.
6. Base educational practices on precepts of child growth and development.
7. Provide opportunity for a balanced program of activities and recreation in an atmosphere free from tension and strain.
8. Take an interest in planning to meet the recreational needs for the child in the community.
9. Maintain a positive attitude toward a child's disability and try to create this attitude in the rest of the students.

Children's feelings about themselves and their physical condition are often more important than the condition itself. The class period should be modified to fit the needs of the child with cardiac impairment.

When a child or adolescent has been separated from a normal environment as a result of restricted experience because of cardiovascular deficiency, a lower academic level and general immaturity and dependency may be found. Unnecessary restriction of physical activities for such a child gradually gives way to the individualization of treatment to suit the needs of the child and his disease. Individualization is the keynote for physical activity for such a child because there are vast differences between types of heart disease.

There is impressive evidence that, in many cases, physical training can enhance some elements of cardiovascular functioning in some heart patients, when approved by the physician. Examples of physical training for persons with heart conditions have been reported by Trap-Jensen and Clausen,[41] who state that physical training causes striking improvements in exercise tolerance of patients with angina pectoris. In addition, Frick, Katila, and Sjögren[15] indicate a trend toward larger stroke volume of physically trained heart patients compared to controls. Other examples are a reduction of blood pressure and serum lipids and a lower heart rate. All these factors may reduce the demands on the heart. Thus it appears that physical training under proper guidance can be of value to the cardiac patient. The rehabilitation movement has demonstrated that the traditional practice of permanent bed rest for most of these patients was not only unnecessary, but a mistake from both psychological and physiological standpoints. Kraus and Raab[26] stated that the courage to take a calculated risk has already been proved fully justified and, today, physicians who recommend carefully graded exercise practices for their cardiac patients no longer expose themselves to the dangers of being condemned by their clientele and their colleagues.

IMPLICATIONS FOR PHYSICAL EDUCATION

There is great variability among children who have cardiac disorders. Therefore the amount and kind of exercise to be prescribed for a child with a cardiovascular disability must take into account the individual and his particular disability. Once the program has been prescribed for a child, with the consent of the doctor, the teacher must be a keen observer and impress on the cardiac patient the importance of staying within the prescribed limits of exercise. Activities should be discontinued immediately in the event that the child shows stress. Perhaps the best indicators of a stressful situation involving physical activity are heart rate and blood pressure.

The following are some of the controls that should be used as a guide to keep the child with cardiac disability within the limits of his capabilities:
1. Reduce the cadence of the exercise.
2. When using progressive exercises, start in a lying position, then a sitting position, and finally a standing position.
3. Keep the number of repetitions low.
4. Be sure to check for cardiac stress; check heart rate and blood pressure and watch for shortness of breath.
5. Make the dosage congruent with the reaction of the student to the exercise.
6. Aerobic exercise, within the established physical bounds of the child, should provide for maximum improvement.

Types of formal exercise, in most cases, can be adapted to the individual's condition. However, it is suggested that competitive games that are of a highly emotional nature and reach considerable intensity in participation, for example, football, basketball, baseball, or soccer, should be carefully evaluated before including them in the program for the child with cardiovascular impairment. Situations that involve high intensity with regard to physical activity and highly charged emotional situations should be avoided. Activities that involve hill or rope climbing should be closely evaluated in regard to the capabilities of such a child; the energy expenditure involved in these activities is considerably more than the energy expenditure of activities on level ground. Greater stress may be placed on the heart as a result of such activities.

A physical education program should be designed to meet the needs of children with cardiac conditions on all school levels. The cost of oxygen to the heart is the real key to a choice of activities or exercises. An aerobic program can thus be planned within the bounds of the person with cardiac involvement. There are many games that are a part of the elementary school physical education curriculum that are acceptable with regard to physical dosage for children of moderate cardiac disability. Games that do not require sustained activity and that allow for rest between activities are permissible for the child with moderate disability. At the outset, the activities of the physical education program should be modified with respect to distance traveled, duration of the exercise, and dosage of exercise until both the instructor and the student are aware of the capacities of the student. It is best to abstain from activity that is severe or of long duration. The student should not swim or run for distances or at high speeds unless he has proved that this intensity of activity is within his capabilities.

Progressive exercise is an important feature of a rehabilitation program for a person with cardiovascular disability. The following basic progressive procedures are suggested:
1. All exercise should be short and slow in the beginning of the program, with increasing rhythm and longer duration as the program progresses.
2. The first phase of activity should in-

volve the exercise of individual limbs from a lying position only.

3. Later, the student may exercise from a sitting position, then standing, and then progress to walking exercises or exercises that involve mild mobility, followed by light gymnastics or developmental activities.

4. Breathing exercises and relaxation training may be indicated by the physician.

An example of a progressive exercise program is the system of progressive walking and hill climbing developed by Oertel.[11] The system involves progressive walking and hill climbing in which the work load is extended by the distance walked or the height of the hill climbed.

EXERCISE PROGRAMS FOR CARDIAC PATIENTS
Prerequisites

There are several prerequisites needed for the effective utilization of exercise treatment programs for persons who have heart conditions. Some of them are as follows:

1. A classification sequence in which diagnosed patients can be placed
2. Evaluation procedures to determine the level of the individual's functioning and activity capability
3. Activity loads for specifically identified individuals
4. Individual prescriptions of activity for each person
5. Objectives and goals for each person

Prior to entering an activity program, the participants should be medically screened and then informed of the benefits and risks of such a program. Information should be provided both on the effects of training and fitness on cardiovascular function and on potential risks. It may be wise to make a brochure that answers some of the questions individuals may have about the program.

Cardiovascular assessment

Cardiovascular assessment is an essential feature of the total exercise program. It is important that cardiac contraindications be identified. These may be ascertained through medical physical examinations, chest x-ray films, biochemical assays, metabolic tests, and electrocardiograms. As a rule, the administration of these tests will detect cardiac murmurs, arrhythmias, hypertrophy, intraventricular blocking, hypertension, congenital anomalies, diabetes, hypercholesterolemia, heavy smoking, signs of myocardial insufficiency, and other risk factors. In addition, it is advisable to test, under dynamic conditions, the physiological competence of the individual in relationship to physiological parameters that indicate the presence of current functioning of the individual. Steady state of the heart rate during bicycle ergometer exercise or recovery rate from step or treadmill tests are not enough, in and of themselves, to furnish an adequate index of initial level of physical conditioning for the patient.

It is important that goals be set prior to the initiation of the activity program in order to facilitate measuring the progress of the learner. The goals to which the programmer may project are increases in the parameters of measurable laboratory functioning (oxygen uptake) and the behavioral capability to produce greater amounts of activity as a result of progression through the program. When objectives are set for an exercise program, it should be possible to measure progress toward attaining the preformulated objectives.

Physical training and coronary heart disease

The goal of physical training is to attain physical fitness conducive to good cardiovascular function and good health. The attainment of the desired level of fitness should occur in orderly fashion, usually at a restrained rate of progress. This is necessary if programming is to be beneficial for persons who possess great variability in cardiovascular functioning.

Recently, a number of deaths have been reported in subjects undergoing currently popular "do-it-yourself" jogging programs.[20] The high incidence of death in the natural course of programming, regardless of the level of physical activity, makes it impossible to exclude all deaths from any regimen. It would therefore be unreasonable to discontinue programs where the occurrence of death and myocardial infarction are not increased. Instead, specific steps must be taken to educate subjects and professional staffs in the proper use of this modality. The statement made by the American Heart Association's Committee on Exercise emphasizes this by stating:

> For the sedentary individual there is serious risk in the sudden unregulated and injudicious use of strenuous exercise. But it is a risk that can be minimized and perhaps even eliminated through proper preliminary testing and the individualized prescribing of exercise programs.[2]

To clarify the term "risk," the following definitions are suggested:

1. Persons *at risk* or *at high risk* are those who have a few, a majority, or all of the established risk factors pointing toward the potential development of coronary heart disease. An exercise testing and conditioning program, properly supervised, should prove useful in reducing these risks.
2. If used freely, the term *"risk"* or *"high risk"* is synonymous with *"hazard,"* indicating an existing potential danger of unhealthy occurrences when individuals are physically stressed.

Before a sedentary person begins unrestricted exercise, he should have a thorough medical examination to exclude contraindications. This should include orthopedic, respiratory, and cardiovascular evaluation. It should also include an assessment of physical fitness. Other sources[2] offer details of contraindications to exercise testing.

TESTS OF PHYSICAL CONDITION

Most exercise tests for an evaluation of physical work capacity or, more specifically, maximal oxygen uptake, are based on a linear increase in heart rate with increasing oxygen uptake or work load. However, all predictions from submaximal tests should be done with caution. When persons of different age groups are included, some sort of correction factor must be included, since the maximal heart rate declines with age.[3] Even when the tests are carried out during strictly standardized conditions, the methodological error in a prediction of the maximal aerobic power is considerable (standard deviation = 10% to 15%). They can, however, be applied as a valuable screening test for the evaluation of the functional capacity of the oxygen-transporting system; they may provide a useful method for selecting out the best, the worst, and the average persons from a group.

Objective tests to determine the effect of training on different functions are both important and desirable. Such tests may be an aid in the development of the program and they encourage the individual to continue training. The submaximal bicycle ergometer test is a simple, inexpensive, and reliable test. In longitudinal studies, it is an advantage to apply a test where variations in body weight do not complicate the choice of work load and, in this connection, the bicycle ergometer is superior to treadmill or step tests. At the very least, indirect measurements (or prediction) can give an indication of the person's physiological fitness for endurance-type work and periodic retesting can give an indication of improvement. Such evaluation also constitutes a strong motivational tool for the participants.

A maximum heart rate can be determined from standard tables and then exercise prescriptions can be started somewhere below the 60% level and then gradually increased. The prescription of exercise follows certain basic guidelines that are applicable to all individuals, regardless of their age, state of health, or functional capacity. To be meaningful, the exercise prescription must include the type(s) of physical activity, the *intensity*, the *duration*, and the *frequency*. The task of exercise prescription is much more difficult for sedentary persons, for older persons, for those who have risk factors, and particularly for those who are symptomatic. Thus for each individual, the degree of risk associated with exercise involves the following:

1. The severity of the exercise relative to the habitual intensity of exercise performed
2. Age
3. Functional capacity
4. Health
5. Risk factors
6. Symptomatology

The target level for training is defined as that level at which or below which progressive abnormalities occur. Target levels for training should be used only as guidelines. These levels must be adjusted for each subject individually, with the aid of clinical observations and response to the initial effort test to arrive at an "actual" target level. This actual target level may vary somewhat from day to day, depending on daily fluctuations in the subject's other activities.

One *met* is the equivalent of a resting oxygen consumption, which is approximately 3.5 ml/kg/minutes. Mets during exercise are determined by dividing work metabolic rate by resting metabolic rate. The met cost of treadmill work is dependent on body weight, but the met cost of bicycle ergometry is independent of body weight.

The intensity of the exercise may be prescribed by mets or by heart rate.

Exercise prescription by mets

The peak and average intensity of exercise may be estimated by determining 90% and 70% of the individual's functional capacity. Thus for a person with a maximum functional capacity of 8 mets, intensity would be calculated as follows:

Peak conditioning intensity =
$$0.9 \times 8 = 7.2 \text{ mets}$$
Average conditioning intensity =
$$0.7 \times 8 = 5.6 \text{ mets}$$

There is an alternative method that sets a sliding scale for estimating the average conditioning intensity.[2] The sliding scale allows for the variability resulting from known differences in the intensity that can be tolerated by persons with different functional capacities. The baseline intensity is set at less than 60% of the functional capacity in mets.

Mets may be estimated from the work load performed (Table 12-1) or by calculating oxygen intake from measurements of minute ventilation and expired gas composition. Either estimate of mets may be used effectively in exercise prescription.

In supervised exercise programs, it would appear that the greatest hazard might like-

Table 12-1. Energy expenditure in mets during stepping at different rates on steps of different heights*

Step height		Steps/minute			
Centimeters	Inches	12	18	24	30
0	0	1.2	1.8	2.0	2.4
4	1.6	2.1	2.5	2.9	3.7
8	3.2	2.4	3.0	3.5	4.5
12	4.7	2.8	3.5	4.1	5.3
16	6.3	3.1	4.0	4.7	6.1
20	7.9	3.4	4.5	5.4	7.0
24	9.4	3.8	5.0	6.0	7.8
28	11.0	4.1	5.5	6.7	8.6
32	12.6	4.4	6.0	7.3	9.4
36	14.2	4.8	6.5	8.0	10.3
40	15.8	5.1	7.0	8.7	11.7

*From American College of Sports Medicine: Guidelines for graded exercise testing and prescription, Philadelphia, 1975, Lea & Febiger.

wise lie in the subject's overactivity, above and beyond that which is appropriate for him at any given time. Associated with this hazard are potential errors in the exercise prescription, which call for levels of activity that are inappropriately excessive. This factor is controllable with proper supervision of the training sessions.

In the untrained, progressively greater restrictions need to be placed on exercise regimens. This frequently means that, in the beginning, subjects are trained at paces that are less demanding than those they themselves might choose. The initial workout should not exceed 2 or 3 mets for a sedentary person, with 1 met as the increment of step size.

Intensity of exercise

The most difficult problem in designing exercise programs is the prescription of the appropriate exercise intensity. The percentage of functional capacity a given individual is able to sustain for a given conditioning period is quite variable. Consideration must be given to the fact that the capacity for performing routine or conditioning work is relatively less in persons with low functional capacities (6 mets or less) than it is in those with high functional capacities. One group indicates that reasonable estimates for exercise prescription are that during conditioning sessions, *peak efforts* should not exceed 90% of functional capacity and *average intensity* should approximate 70% of functional capacity. The duration can then be set empirically on the basis that the participant recovers fully.[2]

In the early stages of a conditioning program, precise control of effort is necessary to ensure that participants do not create difficulty by expending too much effort and peak efforts may need to be lowered to less than 60% of functional capacity and then gradually increased. These controls continue to be useful at all stages of a conditioning program because they enable the participant to expend the most energy per unit time. Furthermore,

improvements, plateaus, or regressions in performance can be evaluated quickly and efficiently.

Target levels for training

Exercise prescriptions are determined largely by the heart rate and electrocardiogram (ECG) response to the initial effort test. The purpose of the initial exercise test is to determine the target level for training and to provide a basis for future comparative fitness measurements.

Patterns of exercise in the symptomatic subject do not differ greatly from those used in nonsymptomatic subjects, except for the factors that determine peak severity. For nonsymptomatic subjects with normal response to exercise tests, these would include a predetermined heart rate; for those who respond abnormally, these would include the level at which progressive abnormality occurs, for example, some untoward event occurs and thus places an upper limit on exercise. As work capacity increases, exercise programs are changed to challenge the individual and thus the target range is increased.

PRINCIPLES AND TRAINING

An adaptation to a given load takes place gradually; in order to achieve further improvement, the training intensity has to be increased. There is, however, no linear relationship between the amount of training and the training effect. For instance, 2 hours of training each week may cause an increase in maximal oxygen uptake by 0.4 liter/minute. The rate and magnitude of the increase varies from one individual to the next. It is important to ascertain what amount of training may produce a satisfactory result. Less effort is demanded to maintain a reasonable degree of physical condition than to attain it after a period of prolonged activity. Since maximal oxygen uptake and cardiac output can be attained at a submaximal speed, this lower speed is probably optimal as a training stimulus. As pointed out, even work loads demanding only a submaximal oxygen uptake do improve the physical condition for *very* untrained individuals.

Potential hazards in prescriptions for cardiac patients

Some factors or practices frequently associated with physical training sessions of normals should be specifically prohibited or extreme caution used with the cardiac patient. Close supervision is essential until the subject and the physician have been educated as to the pattern, progression, and regression of abnormalities and a study has been made of the coronary arterial circulation.

Improvements in work tolerance may be associated with gross changes in the anatomy of the coronary arterial system, as characterized by coronary arteriograms.

Features that constitute additional stresses to the cardiovascular systems, and that therefore should be avoided, are as follows:

1. It is well known that thermal stress (extremes of heat and cold) can evoke considerable strain in man.
2. Sudden death when snow shovelling is caused by a combination of the effects of cold exposure and sudden severe effort in an unconditioned subject. Care should be taken to be preconditioned, enter the cold gradually, keep the chest covered, and intersperse work with rest periods.
3. The ingestion of fluids at extreme temperatures is known to produce cardiac arrhythmias, but fluids are needed to prevent dehydration.
4. Large meals tend to divert a greater portion of the cardiac output to mesenteric vascular beds.

Guidelines for exercise testing and prescription for cardiac patients

1. When properly prescribed, physical activity is beneficial, since it maintains or increases functional capacity and may modify some risk factors associated with atherosclerotic disease.
2. Initial prescription, including upper limits of exertion, and subsequent modifications can be safely determined from knowledge generated from repeated graded exercise tests given under medical supervision.
3. The attainment and maintenance of functional capacity and work loads commensurate with ability is a concern of professionals, particularly for those individuals considered *at risk* from an injudicious increase in their physical activity level.
4. Fitness is relative and must be individualized.
5. Subject's symptoms can be useful in assessing limitations in physical training.

In summary, the minimal amount and type of exercise required to achieve optimal physical fitness and to protect against lethal coronary attacks need to be better delineated. There is also a need to demonstrate whether or not physical reconditioning after a coronary attack actually reduces the propensity to recurrence and prolongs life. The hazards as well as the benefits of carefully supervised exercise programs need to be ascertained, but there is much to suggest that the potential benefits far exceed the hazards. More discrete guidelines and criteria are needed to delineate the indications and contraindications and to ensure safety and efficacy.

RESPIRATORY DISORDERS

Respiratory disorders (particularly asthma), like cardiovascular disorders, often impair the opportunity for individuals to participate in self-fulfilling physical activity. The research attempting to determine the relationship between physiological parameters and specific individually planned instruction on respiratory function is not as well documented as in the cardiovascular area. However, there are many authorities who do affirm the positive benefits of physical activity for the individual with asthma.[6, 7, 21, 31] Until there is further substantiation of the therapeutic value of physical activity for those suffering from respiratory disorders, caution must be taken.

Allergies and asthma

Allergy is a term used to designate the hypersensitive reactions of some persons when exposed to certain foreign substances called "allergens," which are harmless in similar amounts to most other persons. Allergies are estimated to affect about 16 million persons in the United States.[22] Persons may be allergic to many different substances that affect them in varying degrees; among these substances are the following:

1. Foods (strawberries, eggs, chocolate, wheat, pork, nuts, citrus fruits, etc.)
2. Inhalants that attack the respiratory tract (pollens, tobacco smoke, vapors, dust, perfumes, etc.)
3. Substances that come in contact with the skin (dyes, poison ivy, poison sumac, fur, leather, animal hair, etc.)
4. Infectious agents (bacteria, viruses, fungi)
5. Drugs (vaccines, antibiotics, serums)

The forms of allergy that are of greatest consequence to the physical educator are probably those caused by inhalants such as pollens and dust particles that affect the respiratory tract. In the United States, there are 13.5 million victims of hay fever, the most common indication of allergy. Hay fever and asthma are of particular consequence to the physical educator since, because of them, endurance in physical activity is seriously curtailed. Inhalation of certain pollens, grasses, dust, or particles in the environment or in the gymnasium is a common cause of allergy.

Treatment

The treatment of allergies is a medical problem. In some instances, physical educators may be able to identify such cases. In the event that allergies are identified among their students, referrals should be made to the physician. There are four possible approaches in treating conditions of allergies:

1. *Avoiding the substance causing the allergy.* It may be possible to avoid the allergen that is causing the problem. This, of course, is dependent on locating the cause of the allergy. Possible adjustments made for children who are allergic to pollens in the fall might be prescribed, for example, indoor activity that would free them from the pollens present on the athletic field. Precautions that might be taken to assist in deterring the effects of allergens are avoidance of certain mat coverings that might contribute to allergic conditions, reduction of the dust in the gymnasium, a change in diet, or the withdrawal of a drug.
2. *Desensitization.* The desensitization process is carried out by injecting, in progressively increasing doses, an extract of the causative antigen. This procedure is followed in the cases of pollens, dust, vaccines, and serums.
3. *Antihistamines.* Antihistamines counter or reduce the symptoms produced by excessive release of histamine into the blood.
4. *Hormone therapy.* Adrenal or pituitary hormones often are instrumental in bringing relief to the person with an allergy.

Implications for physical education

In many cases, children with allergies must make adjustments to the activities of their physical education classes. However, it must be realized that the necessary adjustments vary greatly with the intensity, frequency, and duration of the allergy attack. Allergies often reduce the ability of the child to withstand the onset of physical fatigue and he may need to withdraw from an activity while his classmates continue. This affects him emotionally and socially because he is thus made different from his peers. Asthmatic children often fall into this category. However, these children may be helped in several ways. Some of the ways are as follows:

1. Adapt the activity to provide an oppor-

tunity to play with peers and develop social characteristics desired for all children in physical education programs.

2. Improve the physical fitness of the child through progressive developmental activities.

3. Teach and improve neuromuscular skills commensurate with the child's ability. This will enable him to participate in wholesome leisure activities in the form of carry over sports. There is evidence that programmed exercise for children with asthma is beneficial and that progressive activity increases lung capacity, which, in turn, may reduce the number and severity of asthmatic attacks. Children with asthma in the elementary grades may participate in games of low organization and movement exploration activities. As a rule, these activities enable a child to perform at his own rate. However, at the junior high and high school levels, in which competitive play is part of the program, adaptations for children with severe allergies must be taken into consideration. Activities such as dancing, specific developmental exercises, badminton, softball, shuffleboard, tennis, bowling, and golf are acceptable games for children with severe allergies. However, the fundamental rule to consider when placing children with allergies in physical activity is to let each child participate in activities commensurate with current abilities.

Bronchial asthma

Bronchial asthma usually results from allergic states in which there is an obstruction of the bronchial tubes or the lungs or a combination of both. Usually the bronchial tubes are attacked by spasms of the bronchial musculature and excess mucus, which causes an insufficient amount of air to flow into the lungs. When attacks occur, mucus fills the bronchial tubes and makes it difficult for the person to breathe when he exhales. The asthmatic attacks vary in length and intensity; some last only a matter of minutes, whereas others may persist for days. Asthmatic attacks may come about as the result of many circumstances, for example, exposure to cold air, smoke, irritating gases, pollen, and other allergy-producing substances. Asthma accounts for 11.4% of all chronic conditions in children under the age of 1 year and for 22% of all days lost from school, because of chronic conditions, by children between the ages of 6 and 16 years.

Physical activity can play an important part in enhancing the physical functioning of children with asthma. Macman and Itkin[28] point out that physical conditioning may be indicated for a large number of patients suffering from asthma as a means of increasing the usefulness of their lives. Worthy of note is that duration and level of activity are relevant variables to consider when asthmatics are engaged in physical activity. Jones, Wharton, and Buston[24] and Taub[40] indicated that intermittent exercise, for example, ball games, may be suitable experimentation within the framework of individual capability and should be the guide in selection of activity for the asthmatic.

The physical educator can assist the child with asthma in the following ways:

1. Take care not to precipitate an attack through vigorous activity.

2. Attempt to develop physical fitness through physical activity within the student's capacity.

3. Teach motor skills that will enable the child to participate in the team games of his peer culture and carry over activities for later life.

4. Instruct in relaxation skills, correct posture, and breathing exercises.

5. Provide opportunities for social growth by involving the student in adapted activities with his peers.

Exercises for the asthmatic child should be concerned with full chest excursion, including the stretching of restricted musculature and the strengthening of weakened trunk muscles. Because complete expiration is difficult as a result of bronchial spasm, the student is encouraged to breathe diaphragmatically. Instructions are given to expand the abdomen with inhalation and to force exhalation as completely as possible. To emphasize the breathing-out phase, the student is told to make a sound with the mouth as in blowing out a candle. Students who find it difficult to completely empty the lungs of air may aid themselves by applying hand pressure to both sides of the chest. Breathing should be taught from all positions: reclining, sitting, and standing. Many games can be activities to aid the asthmatic child in learning to breathe properly, for example, short-distance jogging with the student breathing rhythmically by inhaling and exhaling on each step or blowing a Ping-Pong ball across a table to an opponent, emphasizing short inhalation and long, forceful exhalation. (Points may be scored by blowing the Ping-Pong ball off the other side of the table.) To increase the force and time of the exhalation, the table can be raised so the ball must be blown up an incline. Balls can also be suspended from strings and the student then tries to blow the ball as high as possible with long, controlled exhalations.

The asthmatic child's condition should be reassessed periodically, for as the attacks become less frequent and exercise tolerance becomes greater, increased exercise dosage should be added to the program of physical activity. Conversely, if a child has recurring and more severe attacks, then further adaptive measures should be taken to ensure participation at optimal levels in the program.

Asthma and physical activity

Experimental programs have indicated that active participation in carefully planned physical education activity may have value to many children having asthma or some other respiratory disorder.[39] In the past, the social environment of the child with a respiratory disorder, as compared to the capable child, has encouraged physical inactivity. In many cases, this pattern of suppressed physical activity leads to a life-style that prevents participation in physical activity, even when the person is free from attacks of asthmatic symptoms. As the result of this attitude, less than optimal physical and social development occurs. Because of this factor, Stein[39] considers that there should be a reexamination of the values of physical activity for the asthmatic child.

There is impressive evidence that high levels of activity can be undertaken with the condition of asthma.[37] Stein uses the illustration of Rick Demontan, Olympic gold medal winner in swimming, and Jim Ryan, who set the world record in the mile run, both of whom achieved these feats despite asthma.[39] Many doctors now recommend that restrictions on physical activities for children with asthma be lessened and that, between attacks, they should be provided with movement opportunities commensurate with their abilities. This concept of developmental physical education expresses the belief that there is an activity level at which all children can perform to further their physical and motor development. Social involvement is an important concomitant.

Asthmatic children can gain strength, endurance, coordination of movement, and, possibly, more efficient pulmonary function as a result of engaging in physical activities. Swimming may be of particular value for persons with asthma.[9] Stein also indicates that swimming seems to provoke less exercise-induced asthma than comparable activities.[39]

There is a great need for physical educators and medical professionals to engage in cooperative efforts so the child with a respiratory disorder may attain the full benefits of participation in physical activities. It is essential that there be dialogue between these professionals so that research can be conducted and programming can be implemented, based on the best information available concerning the nature of the activity program that should be prescribed for those with respiratory problems.

REFERENCES

1. Adams, R. C., Daniel, A. N., and Rullman, L.: Games, sports, and exercises for the physically handicapped, Philadelphia, 1972, Lea & Febiger.
2. American College of Sports Medicine: Guidelines for graded exercise testing and prescription, Philadelphia, 1975, Lea & Febiger.
3. Astrand, I., and Rodahl, K.: Textbook of work physiology, New York, 1970, McGraw-Hill Book Co.
4. Barry, A. J., et al.: Effects of physical training on patients who have had myocardial infarction, Am. J. Cardiol. **17**:1-8, 1966.
5. Becker, M. C., Vasey, C., and Kaufman, J. G.: Social aspects of cardiovascular rehabilitation, Circulation **21**:546-557, 1960.
6. Blumenthal, M. N., and Pederson, E.: Physical conditioning program for asthmatic children, J. Assoc. Phys. Ment. Rehabil. **21**:1, 1967.
7. Blumenthal, M. N., et al.: Controlling asthma through sports and counseling, The Physician and Sportsmedicine **2**:51-54, 1974.
8. Cardiovascular diseases in the U.S.: facts and figures, New York, 1958, American Heart Association.
9. Claverie, E. D.: Changes in pulmonary efficiency and aerobic capacity of asthmatic and non-asthmatic children in a swimming program, Master's thesis, Denton, Texas, Texas Woman's University, 1971.
10. Cureton, T. K.: Physical fitness with normal aging adults, J. Assoc. Phys. Ment. Rehabil. **11**:145-149, 1957.
11. Daniels, A. S., and Davies, E. A.: Adapted physical education, New York, 1975, Harper & Row, Publishers.
12. Durbin, E., and Goldwater, L. J.: Rehabilitation of the cardiac patient, Circulation **13**:410-418, 1956.
13. Ecstein, R. W.: Effect of exercise and coronary artery narrowing the coronary collateral circulation, Circulation Res. **5**:230, 1967.
14. Fisher, P.: Painless myocardial infarction, Northwest Med. **57**:315-318, 1958.
15. Frick, M. H., Katila, M., and Sjogren, A. L.: Cardiac function and physical training after myocardial infarction. In Larsen, A. O., and Malmborg, R. O., editors: Coronary heart disease and physical fitness, Baltimore, 1972, University Park Press.
16. Gardberg, M.: Remarks on the rehabilitation of the cardiac patient, J. Lawson Med. Soc. **109**:335-338, 1957.
17. Hanson, J. S., et al.: Long-term physical training and cardiovascular dynamics in middle-aged men, Circulation **38**:783-799, 1968.
18. Hayden, H., Suggs, A. W., and Beaty, H. W.: B is for breathing, Outlook **1**:3, 1969.
19. Heart disease in children, New York, 1956, American Heart Association.
20. Hirsch, E. Z., Hellerstein, H. K., and Macleod, C. A.: Physical training and coronary heart disease. In Mohler, I. C., editor: Exercise and the heart, New York, 1973, Academic Press, Inc.
21. Hyde, J. S., and Swarts, C. L.: Effects of an exercise program on the perennially asthmatic child, Am. J. Dis. Child. **CSVI**:383-396, 1968.
22. Johnson, W., et al.: Health concepts for college students, New York, 1962, The Ronald Press Co.
23. Jokl, E.: Safe participation in sports, J.A.M.A. **169**:97-167, 1959.
24. Jones, R. S., Wharton, M. J., and Buston, M. H.: The place of physical exercise and bronchodilator drugs in the assessment of the asthmatic child, Arch. Dis. Child. **38**:539-545, 1963.
25. Kovrigina, M.: In Carter, C., and Carter, D., editors: Cancer, smoking, heart disease, drinking in our two world system today, Toronto, 1958, Northern Book House. 1958, Northern Book House.
26. Kraus, H., and Raab, W.: Hypokinetic disease, Springfield, Ill., 1961, Charles C Thomas, Publisher.
27. Macman, M., and Itkin, I. H.: Four-way study of asthma, Rehabil. Rec. **7**:14-17, 1966.
28. Marienfeld, C. J.: The cardiologist looks at the school child. In Margary, J. J., and Eichorn, J. R., editors: The exceptional child, New York, 1960, Holt, Rinehart & Winston, Inc.
29. McGlynn, D.: Exercise gets to the heart of the matter, Outlook **3**:4, 1969.
30. Naughton, J., et al.: Cardiovascular responses to exercise following myocardial infarction, Arch. Intern. Med. **117**:541-545, 1966.
31. Peterson, K. H., and McElhenny, T. R.: Effects of a physical fitness program upon asthmatic boys, Pediatrics **35**:295-299, 1965.
32. Puthoff, M.: Corrective, developmental, and recreational activities (chronic respiratory conditions), proceedings of the first Statewide Conference on Physical Education for Handicapped Children and Youth, Brockport, N.Y., October, 1972, State University of New York at Brockport.
33. Puthoff, M.: New dimensions in physical activity for children with asthma and other respiratory conditions, Health Phys. Educ. Rec. **43**:75-80, 1972.
34. Rechnitzer, P. A.: Effects of a 24-week exercise program on normal adults and patients with previous myocardial infarction, Br. Med. J. **1**:734, 1967.
35. Rosenson, L., and DeRegniers, S.: The cardiopathic-rheumatic fever. In Frampton,

M. E., and Gall, E. D., editors: Special education for the exceptional, Boston, 1960, Porter Sargent, Publisher.

36. Rowell, L.: Human cardiovascular responses to exercise. In Mohler, I. C., editor: Exercise and the heart, New York, 1973, Academic Press, Inc.

37. Sinclair, W. A.: Physical education and asthma are compatible, Calif. Assoc. Health Phys. Educ. Rec. J. 36:19, 1973.

38. Sloman, G., et al.: Effect of a graded physical training program on the working capacity of patients with heart disease, Med. J. Aust. 1: 4, 1965.

39. Stein, J.: Effects of physical activity and exercise upon asthmatic children, report to U.S. Office of Education, Information Resource Utilization Center. In Physical education and recreation for the handicapped, programs for the handicapped, Washington, D.C., 1975, American Association for Health, Physical Education, and Recreation.

40. Taub, S. J.: Effects of physical therapy evaluated in chronically asthmatic children, Eye Ear Nose Throat Mon. 41:105-106, 1968.

41. Trap-Jensen, J., and Clausen, J. P.: Effect of training on the relation of heart rate and blood pressure on the onset of pain in effort angina pectoris. In Larsen, L. A., and Malmbor, R. O., editors: Coronary heart disease and physical fitness, Baltimore, 1970, University Park Press.

42. Turner, R. W. D.: Diagnosis and treatment of essential hypertension, Lancet 1:897-903, 953-958, 1959.

43. Vodola, T. M.: Individualized physical education program for handicapped children, Englewood Cliffs, N.J., 1973, Prentice-Hall, Inc.

44. Whitehouse, F. A.: Cardiovascular disability. In Garrett, J. F., and Levine, E. S., editors: Psychological practices with the physically disabled, New York, 1962, Columbia University Press.

13

NEUROLOGICAL DYSFUNCTIONS

■ This chapter is dedicated to bringing to the reader a discussion of some of the major dysfunctions within the central nervous system and their implications for adapted physical education. Because of the complex nature of the central nervous system, a brief overview of its anatomy and selected functions will be given.

ORGANIZATION OF THE NERVOUS SYSTEM

The nervous system is "a system of extremely delicate nerve cells, elaborately interlaced with each other, collectively consisting of the brain, cranial nerves, spinal cord, spinal nerves, autonomic ganglion, ganglionated trunks and nerves, maintaining the vital function of reception and response to stimuli."[19] It governs and coordinates all activities of the body, providing a means by which changes in the body's internal and external environment can be accomplished. Those changes are the result of stimuli that cause impulses to occur in specific receptor organs such as are found in the skin, joints, muscles, eyes, ears, and organs of taste and smell. Generally speaking, the nervous system is categorized into the central nervous system (CNS), which is composed of the spinal cord and brain; the peripheral nervous system, which is made up of the cranial and spinal nerves and the organs of the special

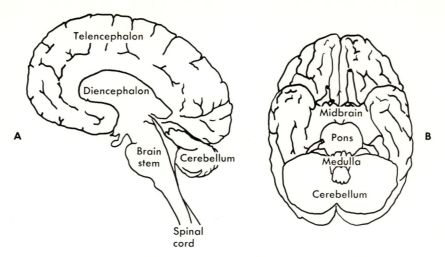

Fig. 13-1. Major regions of the central nervous system.

senses; and the autonomic nervous system, which is concerned with the involuntary control of the body's internal functions.[15]

The major centers of the CNS (Fig. 13-1, *A*), ranging from the less to the more complex, are the following: (1) spinal cord, (2) brain stem, (3) cerebellum, (4) diencephalon, and (5) telencephalon. The functioning of the CNS follows a hierarchy of complexity beginning in the spinal cord and ending at the uppermost aspect of the telencephalon, or cerebral cortex. Reflex responses and servomechanisms (feedback loops) also become progressively more complex as growth, development, and maturation take place. As maturation and development occur within the normal nervous system, inhibition of neutral responses takes precedence over those responses concerned with excitation.[19]

The *spinal cord* is divided into the cervical, thoracic, lumbar, and sacral levels and receives all the bodily sensations below the face. It contains centers that deal with sensorimotor integration, autonomic responses, ascending and descending nerve pathways, receptive and expressive neurons for receiving and responding to both visceral and somatic stimuli, and inter- and intraspinal nerve pathways. It is also a center for the less complicated primitive reflexes.

The *brain stem* is subdivided into the medulla, the pons, and the midbrain (Fig. 13-1, *B*). In general, the brain stem contains ascending and descending nerve pathway centers that are mainly concerned with the degree of an individual's alertness and the ability to stay awake for a prolonged period of time. This arousal system is known as the reticular system and can be found throughout the CNS, but is concentrated in the brain stem. The brain stem also regulates sensory and motor neurons, integrates muscle tone, and controls the reflex functions of breathing and heart action. Emanating from the brain stem are 10 of the 12 cranial nerves concerned with facial functions.

The *cerebellum* is considered by many to both directly and indirectly receive impulses from all the senses of the body, integrating and coordinating their function, for example, in the maintenance of muscle tone and the control of synchronous muscle action. The cerebellum is concerned with the functions of the vestibular system, especially with the functions of body balance and those reflexes that maintain the body's major segments in proper relationship. Moore[19] describes the cerebellum as "the monitor and integrater for past, present, and future neuromuscular behavior."

The *diencephalon,* or interbrain, lies between the brain stem and the telencephalon. It is made up of the thalamus, hypothalamus, epithalamus, metathalamus, and other structures. Basically, the diencephalon is a complex for sensory integration and serves as a relay nerve center leading to and from the major senses, with the exception of the sense of smell. On the other hand, the hypothalamus is the master controller of the endocrine and autonomic nervous systems.

The *telencephalon* is the uppermost aspect of the CNS and is composed of three important regions: the basal ganglion, the limbic system, and the cerebral cortex. The basal ganglion provides integration of the sensorimotor centers concerned with unconscious stereotyped behavior such as the maintenance of muscle tone that is required for the upright posture. It also facilitates and inhibits automatic reflex behavior that is exhibited in the cross pattern arm swing during walking. The basal ganglion is the major storage center for "learned," or semiautomatic, reflexes commonly seen in games and sports activities or in the routine activities of typing, writing, dressing, and eating. On the other hand, the limbic region seems to be primarily concerned with controlling the emotions and personality as well as memory storage. It should be noted, however, that memory and reflex behavior are not confined to any one area of the nervous system. The highest level of sensorimotor behavior is found in the cerebral cortex, which is a main center for learning communication. It has receptive and expressive areas as well as centers that are primarily concerned with association, perception, memory, and personality. In general, the cerebral cortex makes it possible for humans to recognize a stimulus, associate it to some past events, and create new patterns of behavior that may be used immediately or stored for future use.

Sensory and motor are terms commonly referred to in the movement sciences. They, in all probability, should not be separated

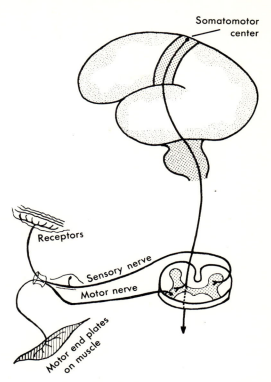

Fig. 13-2. Upper and lower motor neuron. From the motor area of the cerebrum, an impulse is conveyed by an upper motor neuron that is essential for voluntary movement. The lower motor neuron originates from the anterior gray column of the brain stem or spinal cord with its axon penetrating motor end plates of a muscle by a peripheral nerve, allowing for muscular activity.

into two words, but should be referred to as *sensorimotor* because sensation is usually followed by a response (Fig. 13-2). The body receives sensation from three primary sources, namely, exteroceptors, interoceptors, and proprioceptors.[18] The *exteroceptors* receive sensations, for example, pain, temperature, and feel, from the periphery or outside of the body and through the special senses of seeing, hearing, smelling, tasting, and maintaining equilibrium. The *interoceptors* receive sensations, for example, hunger, pain, and abnormal muscle stretching and cramping, from the interior of the body. The receptors that deal with movement and body posture are the *pro-prioceptors* found in muscles, tendons, joints, fasciae, and the vestibular labyrinth organ. It should be noted that the proprioceptors also provide the human organism with a body position sense known as kinesthesia. A fourth set of receptors might be added to this list of sensory sources; they would be called the *exteroproprioceptors*. They are concerned with vibratory sense and fine tactile discrimination necessary for object identification through manipulation (stereognosis).

NERVOUS SYSTEM LESIONS AND DYSFUNCTIONS

Because of the complexity of the nervous system, complete understanding of all the factors that adversely affect it is impossible at this time. However, this section will be mainly concerned with those conditions with which the adapted physical educator or therapist may come in direct contact. The term "lesion" here refers to a specific pathological site that can be identified on examination. Dysfunction does not necessarily refer to a lesion, but, more generally, to the absence of complete or normal functioning.

Nerve and spinal cord disorders

An injury to a peripheral nerve is followed by varying degrees of functional loss, up to and including a complete paralysis. Proprioception, skin sensation, and various tendon reflexes may be partially or completely disrupted. Pathology in the spinal cord also can produce a variety of problems involving both the sensory and motor systems. For example, acute poliomyelitis is a viral disease that attacks the anterior horn cells of the spinal cord, preventing nerve impulses from reaching a muscle via a peripheral nerve. Destruction or disruption of the anterior horn cell can result in a flaccid type of paralysis, followed by atrophy of that muscle. Degenerative conditions occur in the spinal cord, creating varying degrees of dysfunctions, for example, in muscular dystrophy. Trauma to the spinal cord can also create numerous adverse conditions, including partial or complete paralysis, depending on the extent of nerve cell damage. Paralysis is usually named for the number of parts of the body affected, for example, monoplegia refers to paralysis of one limb; diplegia, two limbs; triplegia, three limbs; and quadiplegia, four limbs. Hemiplegia refers to paralysis of one half of the body. The reader should also note that peripheral nerves have the capacity to regenerate about 1 to 2 mm/day, whereas nerve fibers and cells within the CNS do not effectively regenerate.

Brain stem disorders

Disorders that emanate from the brain stem region can produce many different abnormal symptoms, depending on the sensory or motor pathways affected. Generally speaking, lesions in the brain stem can result in muscle spasticity or hypotonicity and deficits in tactile discrimination such as pain or temperature alterations. Postural and/or survival reflexes such as swallowing, breathing, and heart function may also be adversely affected.

Cerebellar disorders

Dysfunctions within the cerebellum can create severe problems in the motor system, five of which predominate, namely, ataxia, hypotonia, asthenia, tremor, and nystagmus. *Ataxia* may be manifested in a number of ways, for example, disturbance in balance, posture, and locomotion; inability to synchronize movement patterns that may involve several joints; *dysmetria*, or inability to stop a movement at a certain desired spot; and *dysdiadochokinesia*, or inability to make rapid or opposite movements such as finger tapping or fast alteration of the forearm in pronation and supination. *Hypotonia*, as a result of a cerebellar disorder, may be reflected by a decrease in tendon reflexes as well as *asthenia* or paresis in which skeletal muscles may tire readily after only minor activity. *Tremor* may also be present in cerebellar dysfunction. This is especially evident when the in-

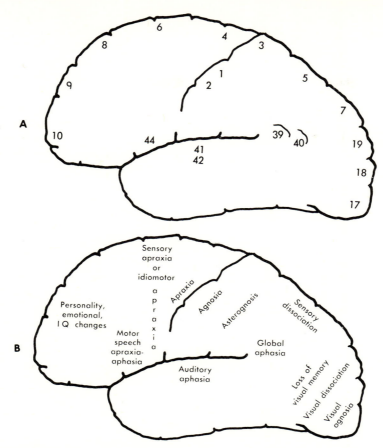

Fig. 13-3. Brodmann's areas. **A,** Areas located on the left cerebral hemisphere. **B,** Dysfunction in relation to Brodmann's disease.

dividual attempts to execute a purposeful movement. *Nystagmus* implies a constant involuntary movement of the eyeball when it is moved away from the center resting position. Besides these impairments, cerebellar dysfunction can also produce *dysarthria*, in which there occurs speech that is slurred and, often, difficult to understand.

Cerebral disorders

The cerebral cortex is considered by many authorities as the final center for the integration of neural function.[15] Although there are specific areas within the cerebrum that can be pinpointed as having specialized functions, there are many other functions that cannot be clearly delineated.

However, Brodmann's cortex areas are presented here for descriptive purposes (Fig. 13-3).[15] For example, Brodmann's motor strip (area 4), which is located in the frontal lobe of the brain, provides fine and gross motor control. Dysfunction within this area can result in alternating involuntary muscle contraction and relaxation (clonic contraction) or in the persistent and sometimes violent muscular contraction that characterizes the grand mal epileptic seizure. On the other hand, area 6, lying just in front of area 4, is commonly known as the premotor area and provides supplementary gross motor control and ability in learning new movement skills. Lesions in the premotor area alone may produce muscle spasticity, whereas lesions in area 4 alone may result in a flaccid paralysis or a floppy muscle. The remaining portions of the prefrontal lobe are considered by many to be essential for abstract thinking and judgment. Dysfunction in this region often produces bizarre, and sometimes unpredictable, personality behaviors.

Dysfunctions within the primary sensory and associative regions of the cortex may create a variety of symptoms, for example, a lesion in Brodmann's area 17 may prevent stimuli from coming to the cortex via the eyes, whereas, on the other hand, dysfunction in area 18 may prevent a visual stimulus from being analyzed by an individual. The process of "knowing," or gnosis, involves the comparison of a stimulus with some past experience. Inability to recognize or associate sensory data is known as agnosia. Therefore a dysfunction in the region of the parietal lobe of the cerebral cortex may result in a condition in which the individual is unable to identify common objects through the combined senses for feel and manipulation (astereognosis). The person with dysfunction in the sensory and associative regions of the cortex may find it extremely difficult to identify the sides of the body (laterality), revealing subsequent disturbances in body image. Of great importance to all movement therapists is the general condition of apraxia, or the inability to initiate purposive motor acts. In this condition, the sensory and motor systems could be functioning normally; however, dysfunction in associative fibers going to the motor cortex makes effective motor planning difficult or impossible.

Abnormal reflex behavior

Reflexes are bodily responses that are mechanical and automatic in nature and are essential for human development. The normal infant brings with it, at birth, critical reflexes necessary for survival such as breathing and digestion, in addition to the reflexes of sneezing, coughing, sucking, and rooting.[21] The foundations for adaptive and postural reactions are also present, together with those reflexes that direct visual, auditory, skin, and deep tendon responses. The newborn displays gross muscular reactions when startled or placed in body positions that require postural adjustments. Fiorentino[14] states:

> From birth onward, we are activated by powerful afferents. These come from the outside world through exteroceptors such as eyes, ears, skin; internally, from interoceptors and proprioceptors.
> [Although] the entire nervous system is involved in all reflexes to a greater or lesser degree, reflexes in the infant, for the most part, are dominated by the spinal cord and brain stem.*

Gradually, as maturation takes place, the primitive reflexes diminish in strength, becoming inhibitive or superimposed by a higher order of reflex behavior. Higher level motor skills are made possible only when the primitive reflex behavior has satisfactorily been overcome and maturation of the higher CNS has taken place.[14]

Dysfunction within the CNS can delay the inhibitory control of higher centers over primitive reflexes, preventing the integration of more complex motor behavior. Brain injury at birth may prevent the individual from ever fully overcoming primitive reflexes. On the other hand, a brain injury in later life might cause a loss of the once acquired inhibitory responses, reverting back to a more primitive reflex behavior. The brain-injured person often displays immature postures and movement patterns that may be further disrupted by abnormal muscle tonus in various parts of the body.

Spinal reflexes predominate during the first 2 months of life. They are considered phasic, coordinating the muscles of the extremities in patterns of total extension or flexion.[13,14] Reflexes at the brain stem level are usually present in the infant from the first 4 to 6 months of life and have mainly to do with postural changes that the infant negotiates while in a reclining position. The midbrain reflexes, on the other hand, assist the infant up to about 12 months

---

*From Fiorentino, M. R.: Reflex testing, methods of evaluating C.N.S. development, Springfield, Ill., 1963, Charles C Thomas, Publisher.

of age, helping to establish head-body relationships and the beginning locomotor skills of rolling over, sitting up, and raising the body up to an all-fours position on the hands and knees. Final reflex control is accomplished at the cortical level, gradually emerging after 6 months of age and continuing throughout life. Cortical level reflexes are primarily concerned with the dynamics of equilibrium in the upright bipedal position.

SEVERE NEUROMOTOR DISORDERS

The term "cerebral palsy" has been used since the beginning of this century to denote those conditions that stem from brain injury. More descriptive terms are "cerebral dysfunction" and "neuromotor disorders," which include a wide variety of conditions, including mental deficiency, convulsive disorders, and impulse disorders, including hyperkinetic behavior; minimal cerebral system dysfunction; and visual, auditory, and perceptual problems.[11]

Cerebral palsy is a condition, rather than a disease. It denotes a number of types of neuromuscular disabilities, characterized by disturbances of voluntary motor function. The degree of motor involvement of children with cerebral palsy may range from those who have serious physically disabling effects to those who have little physical disability.

Statistical estimates indicate that approximately 1 in 14,000 births in the United States results in severe brain injury.[1] This points to a need for continuing emphasis on a search for programs and techniques in education that will provide for optimal living potential in the adult years.

Conditions that give rise to neuromotor disorders may be operative during the prenatal, natal, or postnatal periods. Authorities believe that approximately 30% of the cases occur during the prenatal period, 60% during the natal period, and the remaining 10% from postnatal causes. Prenatal causes may be material infection such as rubella, syphilis, and toxoplasma; metabolic malfunctioning; toxemia; diabetes;

placental abnormalities such as fetal anoxia; and excessive radiation.

Natal causes fall into two basic categories: compression of the head with unusual pressures and trauma and inadequate air exchange in the newborn. Conditions that may give rise to neuromotor disorders from unusual pressure may be the following: breech extraction, contracted pelvis of mother, difficult forceps delivery, prolonged labor, precipitate delivery, placenta praevia, and separation of the placenta.

Postnatal causes may be trauma; infection such as encephalitis, meningitis, and brain abscesses; anoxia; neoplasms; toxic poisons; hyperpyrexia; vascular accidents; and blood group incompatibility.

Since the extent of the brain damage that results in neuromotor dysfunction varies greatly, diagnosis is related to the amount of dysfunction and associated motor involvement that has occurred. Severe brain injury may be evident shortly after birth. However, children with cerebral dysfunction who have slight brain damage and little motor involvement may be difficult to diagnose. In the milder cases, developmental lag in the motor and intellectual tasks required to meet environmental demands may not be detected until the child is 3 or 4 years old. As a rule, the clinical signs and symptoms of cerebral palsy reach their maximum degree of severity at the age of 2 to 4 years. In some cases, children with cerebral dysfunction who have a minor motor involvement and who are not severely handicapped have the greatest difficulties adjusting to their environment. They deviate from normative behavior to the extent that they are different and set apart from their peers. However, the impairments are mild enough that special services for adjustments are not solicited.

"Hard signs" of neuromotor disorders

The different clinical types of cerebral dysfunction display various obvious motor patterns, commonly known as "hard signs." Therefore it is important that the physical educator know the classifications and their characteristic motor patterns in order to implement physical education programs for those with cerebral palsy. In 1954, the Nomenclature Committee of the American Academy for Cerebral Palsy adopted a classification that was derived from observable symptoms. There were six clinical classifications: spastic, athetoid, rigid, ataxic, tremor, and atonic. Of those with cerebral palsy, 50% are clinically classified as spastic, 25% athetoid, 13% rigid, and the remaining 12% are divided among ataxic, atonic, tremor, and mixed and undiagnosed cerebral palsy conditions.[2]

Spastic

The child with muscular spasticity is greatest in prevalence among the cerebral palsied population. One of the physical characteristics of the spastic type is that muscle contractures that restrict muscular movement give the appearance of stiffness to affected limbs. This makes muscle movement jerky and uncertain. The spastic individual has exaggerated stretch reflexes that cause him to respond to rapid passive stimulation with vigorous muscular contractions. Tendon reflexes are also hyperactive in the part involved. In the event the spastic condition involves the lower extremities, the legs may be rotated inward and flexed at the hips, knees may be adducted, and a contracted gastrocnemius holds the heel off the ground. Lower leg deficiency contributes to a scissors gait that is common among persons with this type of cerebral palsy. When the upper extremities are involved, the characteristic forms of physical deviation in the person with spastic cerebral palsy include flexion at the elbows, forearm pronation, and wrist and finger flexion.

Spasticity is most common in the antigravity muscles of the body. In the child with spastic cerebral palsy, contractures are more common than in any of the other types of cerebral palsy. In the event contractures are not remedied or programmed for, permanent contractures may result. Consequently, the maintenance of good posture is extremely difficult. Because of poor balance among reciprocal muscle groups, innervation of muscles for functional motor patterns is often difficult. Mental impairment is associated with spasticity more than with any other clinical type of cerebral palsy, so the incidence of mental retardation among this group is high.

Athetoid

The athetoid is the second most prevalent clinical type of severe cerebral dysfunction. The distinguishing characteristic of the athetoid individual is recognizable incoordinate movements of voluntary muscles. These movements take the form of wormlike motions that involve trunk, arms, legs, tongue, or muscle twitches of the face. The unrhythmical, uncontrollable, involuntary movements seem to increase with voluntary motion and emotional or environmental stimulus. Because of the athetoid individual's inability to control muscles voluntarily, his posture is unpredictable and poses a problem to him. Involvement in the muscular control of hands, speech, and swallowing often accompanies athetosis.

Rigidity

A central feature of the rigid type is the functional incoordination of reciprocal muscle groups. There is great resistance to slow motion among persons with this type and their stretch reflex is impaired. Mental retardation often accompanies this clinical type of cerebral palsy.

Ataxia

The outstanding characteristic of the ataxic type is a disturbance of equilibrium, which impairs the ability to maintain balance. This impairment in balance becomes evident in the walking gait. The gait of the person with ataxic cerebral palsy is unstable, which causes weaving about during locomotion. Standing is often a problem. Kinesthetic awareness seems to be lacking in the ataxic individual, for the ability to locate objects in three-dimensional space is often impaired. Muscle tone, as a rule, is poor in persons with ataxic cerebral palsy.

Tremor

The tremor clinical type of neuromotor disorder is evidenced by a rhythmic movement that is usually caused by alternating contractions between flexor and extensor muscles. Tremors appear as uncontrollable pendular movements.

Atonia (flaccidity)

Atonia is characterized by a lack of muscle tone. The muscles of the atonic person are often so weak that the activities of daily living are severely hampered.

• • •

Another means of classifying those with cerebral palsy is in regard to the limbs that are affected. The classifications are as follows:

1. Paraplegia—legs only
2. Diplegia—legs mainly, arms slightly
3. Quadriplegia—all four extremities
4. Hemiplegia—one half of the body or the limbs on one side of the body
5. Triplegia—both legs and one arm, or both arms and one leg
6. Monoplegia—one extremity

A third way in which individuals with cerebral palsy are classified is based on the anatomical part that contributes to the palsy. There are three primary classifications, including the following:

1. Pyramidal—usually resulting in spasticity
2. Extrapyramidal or basonuclear—when this part of the nervous system is affected, athetosis, tremors, and rigidity are manifested
3. Cerebellar—resulting in ataxia

General characteristics

Although those with cerebral palsy are usually classified on the basis of motor involvement, damage to the brain generally involves other sensory and psychological impairments. Some of the secondary impairments that may accompany motor involvement are mental retardation, hearing and vision loss, emotional disturbance, loss of perceptual ability, and inability to make psychological adjustments.

Studies also have shown that a substantial number of those with brain injury are visually handicapped. According to Denhoff and Robinault,[11] "various authors agree that over 50% of the cerebral palsied children have ocular-motor defects." In other words, brain-injured children often have difficulty in coordinating their eye movements. The implications of this condition for physical activities that are highly loaded with oculomotor tracking of projectiles point to a need for programs that train for ocular control.[11] A program should be adapted that circumvents this difficulty if it is not remediable.

Loss of hearing is often concomitant with cerebral palsy; however, there is disagreement among investigators as to the incidence of hearing loss among individuals with cerebral palsy. Fish[14a] found that 20% of children with brain injury had hearing losses. When clinical types were compared, children with the athetoid type had the greatest incidence of hearing loss. Although it is apparent that there is greater hearing loss among individuals with cerebral palsy than among a comparable normative population, it is still worth noting that the hearing impairments do not occur with as much frequency as do visual problems.

Those with cerebral palsy are also affected with perceptual handicaps to a greater extent than the typical population. Many gross perceptual distortions have been recorded among the cerebral palsied population that are associated with loss of the sense modes, especially vision and hearing.

Emotional disturbances are another concomitant to cerebral palsy. Children with cerebral dysfunction are often afflicted with significant physical impairment that may deprive them of opportunities for ordinary social experience and thus impair their normal social maturation.[5] Interrelated with maldevelopment in the physical and social spheres may be retarded emotional development. The basic needs of the child with cerebral palsy require fulfillment. These basic needs are recognition, esteem, and independence, all of which are an integral part of participation in the experiences of childhood.[2] Block[6] listed traits that thwart the underlying drives toward approval, acceptance, and self-actualization and that cause or give rise to major psychological problems. They are as follows:

1. Unresolved dependency feelings and excessive need for affection
2. Excessive submissiveness and compliance, which hide underlying hostility
3. Egocentricity with emphasis on expansive self-concepts
4. Compensation for feelings of inferiority and inadequacy by fantasy
5. Resignation, rather than recognition of limitations imposed by the disability
6. Superficial conscious recognition of the handicap and unconscious rejection of the self

Treatment of severe neuromotor disorders

There is no treatment for the repair of a damaged brain. However, the portion of the nervous system that remains intact can be made functional through a well-managed training program. Intervention is needed by the physical educator and other liaison personnel to build functional developmental motor patterns with the operative parts of the body that remain. Each child should be evaluated closely and programs should be formulated utilizing those functional abilities of the child that remedy the disabilities that can be corrected and that circumvent those disabilities that are nonremediable. The clinical type should be considered when determining the dosage of exercise. The athetoid type, because of numerous involuntary muscular activities, is much more active than are the spastic, ataxic, and rigid types, who are inhibited regarding physical activity.

The four prevalent procedures in medical treatment are bracing, drugs, surgery, and rehabilitation. Braces are important as an aid in teaching joint function as well as in assisting in the locomotion of patients who are severely handicapped. Another use for bracing is the prevention of deforming contractures. Drug administration usually serves two functions: (1) aiding in exercise therapy by assisting with relaxation of muscle groups when neuromuscular education is attempted and (2) controlling epileptic seizures through the use of anticonvulsant drugs.

There are differing opinions as to the value of orthopedic surgery for those with cerebral palsy. Certain types of operative procedures have met with considerable success, especially with particular types of cerebral palsy. Physical growth of children affects the efficiency of muscle and tendon surgery; however, surgery, for the most part, is not curative, but, rather, gives assistance in the functional activities of daily living. Tenotomies (or tendon surgery) of the adductor and hamstring muscles seem to be the most valuable surgical procedures for adults.

Implications for education

One of the great problems that has interfered in the successful education of children with cerebral palsy is the lack of acceptance by general educators of the emotional, intellectual, and physical disabilities in learning areas. The multitude of behavioral differences displayed by these children indicates a need for various educational approaches and programs.

A number of educational facilities are designed to cope with educational problems of children with brain injury. Some of these sources of education are the following:

1. Home instruction for severely physically disabled children with cerebral palsy who cannot attend school and who are not suitable for schools
2. Hospital schools that serve children with the more severe handicaps
3. Institutions for the mentally retarded, for those children with cerebral palsy who have subaverage intelligence
4. Sheltered care facilities for near-normal children with cerebral palsy who have severe physical handicaps
5. Special schools, or classes in public schools, that are organized for crippled children

6. Mainstreaming into regular school classes for children who will benefit

In many instances, the teacher has more opportunity to meet the total needs of the child with cerebral palsy than do other professional personnel. There are often various adjunct therapies that also work in behalf of the the child. The educator should be aware of these therapies and should make an effort to coordinate the physical education program with other therapeutic endeavors in a rehabilitation program. Although the educator may be only a part of the total rehabilitation program, the educator and the parents will carry on the greater portion of the work with the child, for they often have greater opportunity to put the needs of the child into the total perspective of present and future living.

One of the main responsibilities of the teacher of the child with severe brain injury is to provide an environment that will afford opportunities for maximal personal adjustment and the development of mental health. A prerequisite for creating this type of environment is for such teachers to be well-adjusted themselves, for there are many instances in which problems that the child encounters will be reflected in behavioral problems for the teacher. Therefore it is critical that teachers be warm and understanding and have a genuine interest in each child, regardless of the problems the child may present. Rejection of the child by the teacher does not provide an atmosphere conducive to personal adjustment.

Even though a child may differ physically, he wants to be socially equal to his peers.

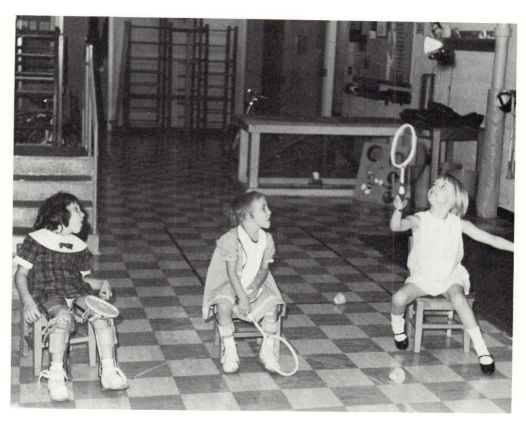

Fig. 13-4. Cerebral palsied children with different abilities playing together. They may differ physically, but they want to engage in activities with their peers. (Courtesy Dr. Julian Stein, American Association for Health, Physical Education, and Recreation.)

Therefore the teacher should attempt to provide opportunities for the brain-injured child to learn in an environment in which he can enjoy normal experiences, as do his nonhandicapped classmates. This requires highly specialized and individualized techniques and demands ingenuity, inventiveness, and patience on the part of the teacher.

Children with brain injury, in addition to motor involvement, often have perceptual problems that necessitate instructional adjustment (Fig. 13-4). There are many areas of perceptual disturbance; therefore it is necessary to identify particular perceptual dimensions that are not functioning properly for a child. Cruickshank[8] identified specific areas of perceptual disability: (1) distinguishing form and color, (2) recognizing spatial relationships, (3) differentiating between high and low or loud and soft sounds, (4) seeing the whole, and (5) following simple directions. There is growing evidence that some of the perceptual characteristics mentioned can be improved through training.[17] Perceptual training techniques are developed primarily through visuomotor and sensorimotor training programs. The aspects of such a program include developing locomotor patterns, balancing, bouncing, performing actively to rhythm, developing ocular control, and using devices that detect form perception. All these perceptual activities are inherent in most physical education programs. However, the quality of physical education programs could be improved by identifying and implementing programs of activities that might enhance these particular perceptual characteristics (Chapter 3).

Typical children bring with them to school a broad experiential history of activities that have accrued during their preschool years. This experiential history lays the background for later, more complex skills. However, in the case of the child with severe brain injury who has been handicapped in the acquisition of motor experience, a program of readiness for the more complex skills should be implemented by going further back in the stages of motor development. The purposes of such a readiness program may be to provide developmental experiences that are meaningful, to stimulate interest and curiosity, to develop satisfactory motor perception, and to build toward greater proficiency and specificity in motor skills. The readiness period may take considerable time in order to prepare the child with cerebral palsy socially, emotionally, and physically for the more complex learnings that will give meaning to his leisure time, vocational pursuits, and adult living. The prerequisites to administering physical activity or teaching physical skills are psychological, sociological, and physiological readiness for the activity.

Physical education for the severely neurologically impaired

Physical educators disagree as to the primary objectives of a physical education program for those who are severely neurologically impaired. Some authorities think that the major purpose is to enhance physical development and muscular control, whereas others place greater emphasis on psychosocial effects, rather than on remedial work adjunctive to physical and occupational therapy. If a child receives regular occupational and physical therapy, the need for this type of activity in physical education classes is less than if he were not in such a program. The psychosocial effects of a physical education program must be determined within the perspective of adjunctive therapy that takes place outside the school. In some cases, physical therapy and occupational therapy are so minimal that the child needs the assistance of the physical educator in developing and restoring neuromuscular function. Regardless of whether restoration of developmental motor patterns and the overcoming of contractures are administered by the physical therapist, occupational therapist, or physical educator, the program should be under the supervision of medical personnel.[10]

Because the needs of each child are different, the program should be different for each child and carefully guided by a physician. A number of techniques are needed to cope adequately with the physical habilitation of the child with cerebral palsy. These therapeutic techniques include the following:

1. Muscle stretching to relieve muscle contractures, prevent deformities, and permit fuller range of active motion
2. Gravity exercises that involve lifting the weight of the body or body part against gravity
3. Muscle awareness exercises to control specific muscles or muscle groups in movement
4. Neuromuscular reeducation exercises, that is, movements performed through their current range to stimulate the proprioceptors and return the muscles to greater functional use
5. Reciprocal exercises to stimulate and strengthen the action of the protagonist
6. Tonic exercises to prevent atrophy or to maintain organic efficiency
7. Relaxation training to assist in the remediation of muscle contractures, rigidity, and spasms
8. Postural alignment to maintain proper alignment of musculature
9. Gait training to educate or reeducate walking patterns
10. Body mechanics and lifting techniques to obtain maximum use of the large muscle groups of the body
11. Proprioceptive facilitation exercises to bring about maximal excitation of motor units of a muscle with each voluntary effort to overcome motor functioning paralysis
12. Ramp climbing techniques to improve ambulation and increase balance, a form of progressive, resistive exercise for the purpose of developing strength

There is impressive evidence that motor skills, muscular endurance, and strength can be developed in these children through progressive exercise and activity in an adapted physical education program. In many instances, the environment of enforced inactivity in which brain-injured children have developed has left them short of their potential development. The opportunities for adapted physical education to enhance maximum physical development of these children are great. Furthermore, children with cerebral palsy frequently do not develop adequate basic motor skills because of their limited play experiences.

When the child participates in a group activity, it may be necessary to adapt the activity to the child's abilities or to modify the rules of the game. An example of rule adaptation for the handicapped child in soccer would be narrowing the goal area that he must defend. Another strategy of activity adaptation might be to require the child with cerebral palsy to play in a position that requires a slower pace or demands less activity than some other position in the game. An example of this might be the goalkeeper in a soccer game. This position is usually less active than the other positions on the team. Positions in many sports vary in the degree of mobility needed by the child to play them.

In addition to using rule modification and adaptation of activity, the program must consider the capabilities of each individual child. Children with spasticity, athetosis, and ataxia differ greatly in function. For instance, the spastic child finds it easier to engage in activities in which motion is continuous. However, in the case of the athetoid child, relaxation between movements is extremely important to prevent involuntary muscular contractions that may thwart the development of skills. Ataxic children have a different motor problem: they are usually severely handicapped in all activities that require balance. The motor composition of the basic types of cerebral palsy, as well as of each individual child, is an important variable in the selection of activities. Rest periods should be frequent for children with cerebral palsy. The length and frequency of the rest periods should vary with the nature of the activity and the severity of the handicap. The development of a sequence of activities varying in degree of difficulty is important. This provides an opportunity to place each child in an activity that is commensurate with his ability and proposes a subsequent goal to work for.

Certain physical activities are appropriate at each of the developmental levels in the physical education curriculum. By and large, the classwork in adapted physical education for those with cerebral palsy at the elementary school level should be taken from general program materials and should be directed toward developing fundamental movements such as walking, running, jumping, throwing, skipping, hopping, and kicking. These movement patterns serve as a foundation for the later learning of more complex motor skills. In addition, music, rhythmic activities, and story plays, accompanied by games of low organization, should be an integral part of the elementary school physical education program. The junior high school level curriculum should be in keeping with the activities of the peer group of the child with cerebral palsy. Such activities may include developmental exercises, the development of body mechanics, and games that lead up to highly organized sports activities. In the high school program, games of our culture that have carryover activities such as bowling, archery, badminton, rhythms, swimming, shuffleboard, and golf are important activities for the child with cerebral palsy to learn, for they provide the media of social interaction and worthy fulfillment of leisure time in postschool years.

For optimal development in motor skills, physical education should be extended to the individual with cerebral palsy beyond formal education because it usually takes such children longer to acquire skills than it does typical children. Furthermore, recreational services that are commensurate with their abilities should be provided for these persons in the postschool years. To date, the greater emphasis has been placed on recreational services for young children with cerebral palsy rather than on the adult population.

MINIMAL NEUROMOTOR DISORDERS
"Soft signs" of neuromotor disorders

As discussed earlier, brain injury and its resultant dysfunction appear to be on a continuum, with symptoms ranging from the more obvious "hard signs" to the less obvious, and sometimes subtle, "soft signs." Another expression commonly given to the large area of minor neurological problems is "minimal nervous system dysfunction." The individual coming under this heading, besides displaying some coordination difficulties, may have problems in perception, conception, memory, speech, language, emotional behavior, and the cognitive skills required in reading, writing, and arithmetic.[4] Those individuals deemed to have minimal gross and fine motor control may be considered physically awkward or clumsy. Touwen and Prechtl[22] have identified seven factors that can be found in children classified as having a minimal nervous system dysfunction, namely, hemisyndrome, dyskinesia, synkinetic or associated movement, balance disturbances, auditory perceptual disturbances, problems in emotional behavior, and the inability to perform a fast sequential or rhythmical movement.

A hemisyndrome refers to a weakness and a decrease in muscle tone on one side of the body, making gross motor activities difficult. Dyskinesia is reflected by movements that are jerky, slow, or irregular, usually when attempting fine or small muscle skills. Synkinetic movements become apparent when a movement is attempted on one side of the body and mirrored on the other. The ability to effectively perform static or dynamic balance such as standing on one foot or walking heel-to-toe on a balance beam may also be disrupted. Auditory-perceptual problems such as difficulty in responding to verbal commands or inability to understand or remember directions may also be associated with minimal cerebral dysfunction. Other characteristics are problems in performing rhythmical movements, such as marching or dancing. Children may also display an inability to make quick repeated movement changes such as are required in tapping a finger or foot. Emotional problems may stem directly from the cerebral dysfunction or may result from difficulty in coping with the demands of the environment.

The physical educator and therapist should note that a child having a number of neuromotor soft signs may be considered a "klutz" in our society.[4] Unable to play effectively with other children, ridiculed by adults for being careless, the clumsy child is often an unfulfilled and unhappy person. Programs of physical education and recreational activities should be more sensitive to individuals with minimal motor deficits, providing them with greater opportunities to overcome their specific problems and find success in developing a variety of movement skills.

Problems in arousal

Managing the level of arousal when confronted with a given stimulus has been primarily assigned to the reticular system found throughout the CNS. Dysfunction in this system can result in two major problem areas: hyperactivity and hypoactivity.

Hyperkinetic impulse disorders may be caused by some organic cerebral dysfunction, may have a genetic antecedent, or may reflect a lag in the maturation and development of the nervous system. As a result of the problem, the child may display a number of behavioral characteristics such as impulsivity, distractibility, disorganization, explosiveness, or an inability to delay gratification. Often, the hyperactive child is described as behaving as a child much younger than would be expected or as one that is "driven" and out of control. It has been suggested that hyperkinetic activity is the result of an inability to properly filter out and monitor stimuli; the individual is therefore bombarded by unselected stimulation from the environment.[11]

There have been many strategies and methods suggested for treatment of the hyperactive child. These have met with varying success. In general, these approaches can be classified into the following: medications, behavior modifications, environmental engineering, and movement methods.

Since as early as 1937, CNS stimulants have been used to benefit the hyperkinetic child. In more recent years, amphetamines such as methylphenidate (Ritalin) have been used increasingly with countless children deemed hyperactive. Under a competent physician trained in the area of learning and behavioral problems, appropriate medications may be a useful tool. However, abuse of these drugs may create problems that have yet to be determined.

The use of positive reinforcement techniques in the home and school environments has found some success in helping the hyperactive child gain self-control. In contrast to punishment, reinforcement by reward has been found to be more successful, especially in keeping to a minimum the child's feelings of degradation and worthlessness, often associated with hyperactivity.[7]

Engineering the environment has been found to be successful with some children. By eliminating distracting influences from the environment and helping the child focus on one type of stimulus at a time, concentration may be improved.

Assisting the hyperactive child through selected movement methods has also been found to be beneficial by many educators and movement therapists, for example, it has been found that neural inhibition occurs following the application of slow, repetitive activities. Inhibition and relaxation are produced by sending inhibitory impulses to the bulbar section of the brain, which contains a large grouping of reticular nerve fibers. Slow stroking of the skin; neutral warmth, such as that in a tepid bath; gentle rhythmical rocking; and soft sounds in a slow rhythmical pattern will inhibit the arousal system.[20] Relaxation training such as the Jacobson technique (Chapter 6) assists in reducing the aroused state. Other movement methods that have been found very successful in helping the hyperactive child gain self-control are games requiring rhythm, a well-defined and structured motor response, and gross and fine muscle coordination.[7]

Hypokinesis, or hypoactivity, implies less than average activity. The hypoactive child is one in whom there is too little arousal, lethargy, and, sometimes, sleepiness. Unlike the child with hyperkinetic impulse disorders, the child who is hypokinetic is often in the background, causing no problems for the parent or teacher. Other characteristics might be having poor coordination, being disliked by peers, being a poor player, having poor muscle tone, and being sloppy about his person and things. Once medical implications such as endocrine dysfunction or disease have been discounted, a program for the underaroused individual can be instituted. Mainly, those activities that stimulate the nervous system should be used, for example, in fast and irregular rhythms or activities that stimulate the child's vestibular system: bouncing, fast rolling, spinning, tilting, and swinging. Exercising against a resistance should also be considered a major body stimulator and activities that involve quick muscle stretching will produce a stimulation to those muscles being stretched.

CONVULSIVE DISORDERS

Convulsive disorders, or epilepsy, refers to a clinical syndrome in which the central features, seizures or convulsions, are a result, in part, of a disturbance in the electrochemical activity of the brain. There are recurrent disturbances of consciousness that may or may not be accompanied by muscular involvement. There is a relatively high incidence of convulsions in children; however, convulsions are not necessarily indicative of epilepsy. Convulsive disorders are grossly misunderstood by the lay public in that associations are often made between epilepsy and mental defect and emotional disturbance. Consequently, the lay public may often view the disorder with fear and prejudice. Although these fears are unfounded, it cannot be denied that epilepsy

can affect the alertness, vitality, and social and emotional adjustment of a child; this may make him less effective in an educational setting.[23]

A physical education teacher may have occasion to serve an epileptic child and it is important that the teacher be familiar with the disorder. However, it must be remembered that children with epilepsy are children first and may differ from other children only in that they have the potential for occasional seizures. More often than not, if there is maldevelopment in personality variables, it is the result of psychosocial conditions, rather than epilepsy itself.

It is difficult to arrive at an accurate reporting procedure to determine the prevalence of epilepsy because of the fear some persons have about letting others know of the disorder. However, there are an estimated 1,860,000 persons with epilepsy in the United States.[17]

Although epilepsy is widespread, drugs have been developed that can control epileptic seizures in approximately 80% of the cases. Unfortunately, less than 50% of all epilepsy patients receive effective treatment.

There is speculation concerning the cause of epilepsy; however, there is no thorough understanding regarding the cause. Although epilepsy may not be said to be inherited, the predisposition to the disorder appears to be inherited, for there is a tendency for epilepsy to run in families. Epileptics are classified into two main categories, according to cause: unknown causes (idiopathic) and known causes (symptomatic).

Idiopathic epilepsy includes all those cases in which no structural damage in the nervous system can be found. Approximately 60% to 70% of the cases of epilepsy fall within this group.

Symptomatic convulsive disorders may be caused by a host of factors, among which may be acute infection to the brain; trauma; allergies; abnormality of prenatal conditions; emotional instability; malnutrition; birth injuries; and infections such as encephalitis, meningitis, and cardiovascular disorders.

Classification of seizures

Many classifications of seizures have been suggested in the literature regarding epilepsy. Perhaps the classification most beneficial to the physical educator is that of six groupings that have been proposed, based on the physical appearance of the child during the seizure, electroencephalographic findings, and the effects of drugs in controlling the seizures. The classifications are as follows:

1. Jacksonian seizures
2. Convulsive seizures
3. Grand mal seizures
4. Psychomotor seizures
5. Petit mal seizures
6. Autonomic seizures

The principal features of these six types of seizures can be summarized as follows: in the first type, symptoms are localized; in the second, excessive movements are the main feature; in the third, transient loss of consciousness is the main characteristic; in the fourth, the central feature is amnesia; in the fifth, there is a brief loss of consciousness; and the last type is manifested by functionally independent, spontaneous symptoms.

Jacksonian seizures

Jacksonian seizure patterns are characterized by an upward march from an extremity such as an arm or a foot. The attack may start at the finger and spread progressively to the wrist, arm, and shoulder, where it is maintained unless it spreads to other body parts. This seizure may then become a grand mal and is often associated with organic lesions of the brain. It may be accompanied by a feeling of numbness and there may be alternate contraction and relaxation of muscles.

Convulsive seizures

Convulsive seizures usually localize on one side of the body or a single extremity, but do not march. The attack is often initiated by alternate contraction and relaxation movements of the face or of an extremity. It is also common for the hands and eyes to turn to one side.

Grand mal seizures

The grand mal seizure is the most common type of attack. It is estimated that approximately 50% of those who have grand mal seizures experience a warning period in which dizziness and numbness occur; this is called an "aura." This warning allows the person to lie down and prepare for the seizure. In some instances, an epileptic child may go through the aura period without going into a full seizure. The physical educator should be aware of the aura so as to prepare to assist during the attack.

A person who has never witnessed a grand mal seizure may find the first attack traumatic. When persons undergo a seizure of the grand mal type, they may drop to the floor; convulse with body stiffening, writhing, and twisting; experience alternating contractions and relaxations; drool; lose bladder and bowel control; fall into unconsciousness; and then usually enter a deep sleep.

Psychomotor seizures

It is important that the physical education teacher have knowledge of the psychomotor seizure because it takes the form of abnormal behavior patterns and might be misinterpreted as warranting punishment. This seizure is characterized by a period of amnesia and tonic spasm may or may not be present. When muscular hyperactivity is present, it may be accompanied by a bluish coloring of the skin and drooling. The child may lose partial contact with reality or may be completely out of contact with his surroundings. The child may be inactive or hyperactive during the seizure. Other characteristics of the psychomotor seizure might be the child's making unconscious sucking noises with the mouth or aimless movements with the hands, striking another child, tearing up paper, moving about the room in a daze, or performing other bizarre psychic behaviors. Consciousness is not lost during this attack; however, the child has no memory of these happenings. This type of seizure, because of the different forms that it takes, often leads to mistaken psychological diagnoses.

Petit mal seizures

There are no overt convulsions during the petit mal seizure; however, consciousness is lost for a few seconds. A child may continue an ongoing activity, but motor activity is minimal and there may be a few flickering movements of the eyelids and face or mild rhythmical jerkings of the hands and arms. The seizure begins abruptly and, after it is over, the trend of conversation or the activity is resumed by the child as if nothing had happened. Petit mal seizures are more frequent in children than in adults and attacks range in frequency from 1 to 200 a day. During the seizure, the child is inattentive and displays a blank look on the face. This type of seizure is difficult for the educators to diagnose, for the unknowing teacher may consider the child a daydreamer or inattentive. The seizure may be accompanied by myoclonic jerks in which a single jerk of an arm or trunk muscle occurs without apparent loss of consciousness. It may also be accompanied by a sudden postural collapse of muscles with consequent nodding of the head; if the collapse is generalized, the child may even fall down.

Autonomic seizures

The autonomic seizure is rare. This seizure consists of periods of flushing, sweating, fast heartbeat, gagging, heightened blood pressure, or fear that occurs without obvious cause. Unconsciousness is absent.

Psychosocial adjustment

Many persons regard epilepsy with fear because they do not understand the nature of the disorder. Consequently, there is great social and economic prejudice expressed toward epileptics by the nonhandicapped majority. As a result, the social handicap manifested by the disorder is often more important than the physical deficiency itself. Much of the prejudice displayed toward epilepsy is caused by inadequate information about the disorder. Many misinformed lay persons often develop a stereotyped concept of the epileptic personality. Attitudes unconsciously reflect ancient beliefs that were attributed to the seizures and that led to the social degradation of persons with epilepsy. These views of the nonhandicapped majority have great implications for the social, psychological, educational, and vocational problems of the epileptic's adjustment.

Convulsive disorders in childhood must be considered as having psychological significance in the development and formation of personality. It is assumed that fear of social embarrassment through a seizure, in the case of the more obvious seizure types, and concern over the etiology of the illness are great deterrents to the healthful personality development of epileptic children.

Inasmuch as public misconceptions regarding epilepsy still prevail in many communities, the educational opportunities for epileptic children, in many cases, are lacking. Usually, epileptic children can attend school and participate in regular physical education activities with their peers, but they are often confronted with prejudice that may adversely affect their schooling. Hopefully, in the ensuing years, this prejudice against epilepsy will be twarted to the extent that the deprivation of opportunity in education will not still prevail. The physical educator is assisting in breaking down stereotyped concepts that lead to prejudice toward children having this disorder. If gains can be made in reducing public prejudice, personality development among epileptics will possibly be enhanced.

Characteristics of epileptics

Considerable research has been done on the intellectual abilities of children with epilepsy. A summary of the literature on the characteristics of epileptics would suggest the following:
1. Categorically, epilepsy does not significantly affect intelligence. There are epileptics who are in the upper ranges of intellectual functioning and epileptics who are mentally retarded. Epileptics who are mentally retarded may be retarded for the same reasons that non-

epileptics are retarded and epileptics of higher levels of intelligence may function as such for the same reasons non-epileptics do so.

2. Epileptics, as a group, appear to be within the normal range of intelligence, but are slightly below the mean.
3. There is an apparent lack of data that indicate progressive mental deterioration of epileptics.
4. Mental impairment in epileptics may be caused by adverse social and psychological factors associated with the disorder and these factors may deter cognitive development.
5. The development of anticonvulsant medication provides opportunities for increased socialization and development of sound mental health in the epileptic.
6. It is unlikely that anticonvulsant medication results in significantly impaired psychological functioning.
7. It is unlikely that anticonvulsant medication results in significantly impaired intellectual functioning.

The prejudiced views of the nonhandicapped majority of persons often precipitate stresses, which, in turn, can be responsible for emotional conflict within an epileptic person. Therefore it is not uncommon to find those with convulsive disorders who encounter emotional problems exceeding those of the typical population. The physical and motor characteristics of epileptic children are as variable as with so-called typical children. However, it may be hypothesized that variability among this population in motor and physical characteristics is great. It would be anticipated that there are epileptics highly skilled and highly developed in the motor and physical areas as well as epileptics who are poorly skilled and poorly developed in the same areas.

Treatment of convulsive disorders
Drug therapy

Medical advances, through the development of anticonvulsant drugs, have made it possible for most children with epilepsy to attend regular classes. It is estimated that approximately 80% of epileptics can, with guidance, secure an education in regular classes and engage in vocations with success. Drugs reduce both the frequency and the severity of the seizures to socially acceptable levels. Drugs are usually administered under the direction of a physician on the basis of the type and nature of the seizure. Some of the common anticonvulsant drugs that are used to control seizures are phenobarbital, diphenylhydantoin (Dilantin), trimethadione (Tridione), paramethadione (Paradione), methylphenylethyl hydantoin (Mesantoin), and phenacemide (Phenurone). Drug administration must be supervised carefully because of side effects that might occur. Anticonvulsant drugs apparently work in one of two ways: either they depress the function of nervous tissue or they replace a chemical substance that is lacking and thus raise the convulsive threshold to above its normal level. Dosages are usually reduced for patients who have been free of seizures for a given period of time.

Surgical treatment

Surgical techniques for the removal of defective areas of the brain can be beneficial in controlling seizures. Conditions that may indicate surgery are brain tumors, abscesses, scar tissue, or depressed fracture of the skull. There are, however, relatively few convulsive disorders requiring neurosurgery.

Psychological treatment

Some form of psychological treatment is often indicated for children suffering from epilepsy. The form of such treatment varies from one individual to another. Lack of treatment often results in perpetuation of the handicap, for it usually affects social and emotional behaviors. Such treatment seems warranted because there is impressive evidence showing a relationship between seizures and psychological variants such as fear, frustration, and unacceptable interpersonal relationships.

An environment conducive to optimal growth of physical and mental health is most helpful. To achieve this end, good personal hygiene and regular meals with a balanced diet are essential. Regular periods of physical activity, conducted in an atmosphere that exposes the child to a minimum of emotional stress and promotes productivity and normal behavior, are of great benefit. Also, there should be a structured life-style, with regular times for sleeping, eating, and physical activity.

Teacher's role during a seizure

The poise of the teacher during a student's seizure is of tremendous importance, for the teacher can properly manage the situation so that there is maximum understanding on the part of the other students and minimum disruption of the class.

If the teacher conveys the idea that a seizure may possibly occur during the day, the children will be assured that the one seizure will be survived with ease and they can go on about their own work. It is important that the teacher know the kind of seizure to expect from a given child, the medication the child is receiving, and the restrictions that the physician has ordered. Some persons experience a warning period called the aura. If the aura can be detected, it will give the teacher the opportunity to place the student in a safe place and prepare the class for the ensuing experience. This will also give the teacher time to lower the student to the floor and thus prevent possible injury from falling when the seizure hits. The teacher should loosen any apparel that may constrict the student's movement and should not try to restrain the student from the convulsive stage of the seizure. A soft object such as a folded handkerchief should be placed between the back teeth when student's mouth opens to prevent the student from biting his tongue or cheek. After the attack, the child should be moved to a quiet room until full consciousness is regained. In the event that sleep follows the seizure, the child should not be awakened.

Implications for physical education

It is now accepted that general physical activity is beneficial to children with epilepsy (Fig. 13-5). This is a result partly of the psychological therapy that play and activity have for children and partly of the physiological benefits of such activity. Vigorous activity seems to enhance drug therapy and resistance to seizures. Physical activity is also instrumental in the development of cardiovascular fitness. The capacities for physical activity and the nature of seizures among the epileptic population vary considerably. Therefore the physical education program should be planned on an individual basis.

Like any other child, handicapped or nonhandicapped, an assessment of needs must be made and then subsequent programs implemented to meet these needs. However, in the case of epileptic children who have controlled seizures and who are enrolled in regular classes, there is little reason why they cannot participate in the same physical education program as their classmates. Epilepsy itself does not necessarily contraindicate competitive and contact sports or the use of gymnastic apparatus.[3] In addition, in some cases of epilepsy, it may be necessary to limit activity on pieces of apparatus that are of considerable

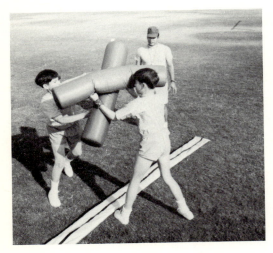

Fig. 13-5. Children with epilepsy need programs of vigorous physical exercise.

height because of the possibility of injury to the child if he were to fall.

Swimming does not seem to be an activity that is contraindicated in even the most severe cases of epilepsy. However, a buddy system employed in the case of the child with epilepsy enhances the safety factor. There is consensus that epileptics should not perform physical activities where a fall would result if a seizure were experienced without warning. Such activities would include rope climbing and gymnastics that involves parallel bars, trampolines, and so forth. However, individual consideration remains the basic determinant. Body contact sports for children with epilepsy should be considered on the basis of individual evaluation. It cannot be denied that there is some risk associated with some of these activities. If the physical, social, and emotional objectives of a physical education program can become a reality to a child, then a small risk may be warranted. To fulfill the needs of an epileptic child in the physical education program, it is imperative that the instructor know the nature, limits, and implications of the epilepsy of a particular child and obtain a recommendation from the child's physician.

THE MULTIHANDICAPPED CHILD

The multihandicapped child is one who is afflicted with several handicapping conditions. Combinations of sensory, emotional, mental, perceptual, neurological, physical, and motor handicaps may be present. Athough it is important for the physical educator to attend to the individual's total development, this section is primarily concerned with those aspects of programming over which the instructor has the greatest control: the physical and the motor. The aspects of growth and development are purported to be interrelated. Thus it may be possible through physical and motor improvement of the multihandicapped to effect positively concomitant aspects of development.

If muscles are weak, progressive techniques in the development of strength should be applied. These techniques in progression are passive exercise, active-assistive exercise, active exercise, and progressive-resistive exercise. The increments of a progressive-resistive exercise should be small and gradual and, since there may be spasticity in the strength of muscles within a group, attention should be given to see that a particular movement is coordinated. All remaining neuromuscular units should be integrated into the movement pattern.

In the case of severe damage to motor cells, it may be necessary to design programs that enhance the activities of daily living so that the individual may function independently in the environment. These training programs might include the development of basic skills such as standing, walking, stair climbing, feeding, grooming, and other self-help activities. In the case of persons who are severely impaired, functional training is a long process requiring a great deal of patience. The medical profession and special instructional staff are usually required to plan and implement functional training programs for the multihandicapped child who is afflicted with severe motor involvement.

Activity programs that will enhance the development of strength, endurance, and coordination will be of invaluable aid to the child. It is necessary to remember that each multihandicapped child is different. Therefore there can be no one program for all children. The assessment of individual ability must be made with a particular program in mind to meet the needs of each particular child. However, certain considerations common to all multihandicapped children who participate in the physical education program should be taken into account. In general, activities should be selected that represent the widest range of activities appropriate to the child's age group and the program constructed should fit each pupil's individual needs. When the program is being constructed, it should be determined whether the activities might create muscular imbalance by strengthening one group of muscles at a faster rate than the antagonistic group. Selection of activities also involves finding the game or activity that can circumvent the disability. For instance, if there is involvement in the legs, it is possible to select activities that can be accomplished through proficiency with the arms.

The multihandicapped pupil may be afflicted with paralysis, weak antigravity muscles, and tight reciprocal muscles. The consequences of these atypical aspects of physical deterrents may contribute to the development of abnormal patterns of motion and faulty body alignment. Therefore the restoration and the maintenance of correct body alignment and movement patterns are of great importance to the prevention of malalignment. Particular attention should be paid to weakened antigravity muscles such as the abdominal muscles, the extensors of the spine, the hip extensors, the trapezius, and the gastrosoleus muscles. If these muscles are weak, it is of the utmost importance that developmental programs be implemented to strengthen these areas. There are cases in which the antigravity muscle groups are beyond repair for functional use. In such cases, it may be necessary for the physician to prescribe supporting appliances such as braces.

More often than not, because multihandicapped youngsters are handicapped physically, they have had little opportunity to participate in recreational activities. Consequently, they have not had enough play during the developmental process and are likely to be left short of desirable experiences of a recreational nature. It is necessary to remember that recreation is derived from the meaning that the child himself attaches to the activity. It must be fulfilling and it must bring fun, self-expression, and socialization into the life of the child. Recreation for the multihandicapped child, in general, should be an activity from which he obtains pleasure or diversion from the routine of the day's activities. Usually, it will be some activity in which he has developed a competency, for recreation, by definition, means to re-

create some activity that has been performed in the past and to recreate it for the sheer pleasure that the activity brings to the child.

Water activity is of special value to the multihandicapped child, for the water provides buoyancy that facilitates the movement of affected limbs. It also has value in that it tends to relax tensed muscles so that movement may eventually become more efficient through greater reciprocal innervation between muscle groups. It is in the water that the physically handicapped child can most closely approximate the movement ability of typical children.

In summary, physical education has a vital role in the physical restoration of the multihandicapped child. The activities in which he engages should be broad in scope so that they contribute to physical, social, and recreational needs. Each child's needs must be met with respect to program implementation.

REFERENCES

1. Adams, R. C., et al.: Games, sports, and exercises for the physically handicapped, Philadelphia, 1972, Lea & Febiger.
2. Allen, R. M.: Cerebral palsy. In Garrett, J. F., and Levine, E. S., editors: Psychological practices with the physically disabled, New York, 1962, Columbia University Press.
3. American Academy of Pediatrics: The epileptic child and competitive school athletics, Pediatrics 42:700-702, 1968.
4. Arnheim, D. D., and Sinclair, W. A.: The clumsy child: a program of motor therapy, St. Louis, 1975, The C. V. Mosby Co.
5. Bice, H. V.: Some factors that contribute to the concept of self in the child with cerebral palsy, Ment. Hyg. 38:120-131, 1954.
6. Block, W. E.: Personality of the brain injured child, J. Exceptional Child. 21:91-100, 1955.
7. Cratty, B. J.: Remedial motor activity for children, Philadelphia, 1975, Lea & Febiger.
8. Cruickshank, W. M., editor: Cerebral palsy, its individual and community problems, Syracuse, N.Y., 1966, Syracuse University Press.
9. Cruickshank, W. M., Bice, H. V., and Wallen, N. E.: Perception and cerebral palsy, Syracuse, N.Y., 1957, Syracuse University Press.
10. Daniels, L., Williams, M., and Worthingham, C.: Muscle testing techniques of manual ex-

amination, Philadelphia, 1957, W. B. Saunders Co.

11. Denhoff, E.: Cerebral palsy: the preschool years, Springfield, Ill., 1967, Charles C Thomas, Publisher.
12. Denhoff, E., and Robinault, I.: Cerebral palsy and related disorders, New York, 1960, McGraw-Hill Book Co.
13. Fiorentino, M. R.: Normal and abnormal development, Springfield, Ill., 1972, Charles C Thomas, Publisher.
14. Fiorentino, M. R.: Reflex testing, methods of evaluating C.N.S. development, Springfield, Ill., 1963, Charles C Thomas, Publisher.
14a. Fish, L.: Deafness in cerebral-palsied school children, Lancet 2:370-371, 1955.
15. Gatz, A. J.: Manter's essential of clinical neuroanatomy and neurophysiology, ed. 3, Philadelphia, 1966, F. A. Davis Co.
16. Hoffly, J. E., and Angers, W. P.: Understanding the child with epilepsy, Catholic School J. 67:27-29, 1967.
17. Kephart, N. C.: The slow learner in the classroom, Columbus, Ohio, 1960, Charles E. Merrill Books, Inc.
18. Layshon, G. A.: Programmed functional anatomy, St. Louis, 1974, The C. V. Mosby Co.
19. Moore, J. C.: Neuroanatomy simplified, Dubuque, Iowa, 1969, Kendall/Hunt Publishing Co.
20. Moore, J. C.: The nervous system, proceedings of the third national workshop for rehabilitation personnel in sensorimotor treatment techniques, St. Louis, Dec. 10-14, 1974, University of Missouri, St. Louis.
21. Olson, W. C.: Child development, ed. 2, Boston, 1959, D. C. Heath & Co.
22. Touwen, B. C. L., and Prechtl, H. F. R.: The neurological examination of the child with minor nervous dysfunction, Philadelphia, 1970, J. B. Lippincott Co.

RECOMMENDED READINGS

Clarke, H. H., and Clarke, D. H.: Developmental and adapted physical education, Englewood Cliffs, N.J., 1963, Prentice-Hall, Inc.
Daniels, A. S., and Davies, E. A.: Adapted physical education, ed. 3, New York, 1975, Harper & Row, Publishers, Inc.
Denhoff, E., and Robinault, I. P.: Cerebral palsy and related disorders, New York, 1960, McGraw-Hill Book Co., Inc.
Fait, H. F.: Special physical education: adapted, corrective, developmental, ed. 2, Philadelphia, 1966, W. B. Saunders Co.
Wolf, J. M., editor: The multiply handicapped child, Springfield, Ill., 1969, Charles C Thomas, Publisher.

14

SENSORY DISORDERS

BLINDNESS AND PARTIAL SIGHT

■ Visual impairments may have varying adverse effects on children, creating a special challenge to adapted physical educators. Attention to visual problems should not be so great that concern for the development of the whole child is lost. The development of the whole child in his normal environment with concurrent awareness of individual differences is of paramount importance. Children with visual impairments must be approached with regard to their own unique characteristics. This means that each child should be evaluated regarding such factors as motor abilities, physical development, psychological adjustment and personality organization, nature and extent of handicap, abilities, interests, and limitations.

The child who has a loss of vision may also be impaired in the function of mobility and may be less able than typical children in motor abilities. Therefore there is a great need for blind children to be provided with opportunities, through adapted physical education, that will compensate for their movement deficiencies.

Children with loss of vision are, for educational purposes, classified as blind (*those who are educated through channels other than vision)* or partially sighted *(those who are able to be educated, with special aids, through the medium of vision, with consideration given to the useful vision they retain).*

For legal purposes, blindness is determined by visual acuity and is expressed in a ratio with normal vision in the numerator and comparison in the denominator, for example, 20/30 vision means that the eye can see at the distance of 20 feet what a normal eye can see at 30 feet. The legally blind are described as those who have a visual acuity of 20/200 or less in the better eye after maximum correction or who have a visual field that subtends an angle of 20 degrees or less in the widest diameter.

There are varying degrees of blindness. If a person is not completely and totally blind, it is still possible to make functional use of whatever vision remains. Some blind persons have little residual vision and are unable to perceive motion and discriminate light. These individuals lie at the upper end of the continuum of blindness. Some blind persons, however, are capable of perceiving distance and motion, whereas others possess these capabilities and are also able to travel with the use of residual vision.

Students who are educationally blind in that they received their education through means other than vision have been known to play a highly skilled game of handball. In the event the ball is black on a light ground, the motion of the handball may be perceived well enough by two blind persons to engage in the participation of this activity. In handball doubles, a sighted person may be paired with a blind partner. The sighted player then indicates to the blind partner the direction of the ball, which can subsequently be differentiated from the light-colored wall.

The point that is to be stressed is that when a person carries the label of blind, it does not necessarily mean that the majority of the activities in a typical physical education program are out of bounds. Rather, a person's capacity for specific ac-

tivity depends on the degree of blindness that a person possesses.

The term "partially sighted" refers to persons who have less than 20/70 visual acuity in the better eye after correction, have a progressive eye disorder that will probably reduce vision below 20/70, or have peripheral vision that subtends an angle less than 20 degrees. Hathaway[10] referred to partially sighted children as those who have undergone eye operations and require physical and psychological adjustment to such conditions as *enucleation* (removal of an eye) or those who have muscle anomalies and conditions that necessitate reeducation of the abnormal eye. Each child must be considered according to his ability to function, regardless of the nature or degree of his visual handicap. In some instances, a child may fall within the range of normal vision, but may have progressive eye difficulties or a disease of the eye or body that seriously affects vision. In cases such as this, children may be placed in an educational environment with those who are partially sighted. Children of this nature also warrant close scrutiny in the physical education program.

Visual defects

There are several defects in vision that may cause loss of vision. Some of these visual defects are the following:
1. Refractive errors such as myopia, hyperopia, and astigmatism
2. Structural anomalies such as cataracts
3. Infectious diseases of the eyes
4. Impaired muscle function of the eye such as strabismus and nystagmus

Kerby[13, 14] reported that 49% of the visual defects found among partially seeing children are caused by errors in refraction, the most prevalent of which are hyperopia, myopia, and astigmatism. These abnormalities of vision are concerned with the internal ciliary muscles of accommodation, which increase the curvature of the lens. *Hyperopia,* or farsightedness, is a condition in which the light rays focus behind the retina, causing an unclear image of objects closer than 20 feet from the eye. The term implies that distant objects can be seen with less strain than can near objects. *Myopia*, or nearsightedness, is a refractive error in which the rays of light focus in front of the retina when viewing an object 20 feet or more from a person. *Astigmatism* is a refractive error caused by an irregularity in the curvature of the cornea of the lens, causing parts of the light rays from a given object to fall behind or in front of the retina. As a result, vision may become blurred.

In addition to the internal muscles of the eye mentioned previously, there are external ocular muscles that control the movement of the entire eyeball. The two most prevalent defects of external muscle function of the eye are strabismus and heterophoria. Strabismus, or cross-eye, results from the inability of the eye muscles to coordinate; consequently, they do not focus simultaneously on an object and the eye turns in or out. When the eye turns inward, the condition is called *internal strabismus;* when the eye turns outward, it is called *external strabismus.* In the event the eye turns inward and then outward, the condition is called *alternating strabismus.*

Efficient vision involves the coordination of two separate images coming into each eye, which become fused into a single image within the brain. *Heterophoria* is a defect in the muscular balance of the eyes, causing the eyes to deviate from the normal position for efficient binocular fixation. Simultaneous fixation is attempted through forced muscular effort. *Esophoria* is a condition in which the eyes pull inward and *exophoria* is a condition in which they pull outward. If the eyes pull upward or downward, the condition is described as *hyperphoria.*

Eye specialists

There is a need for teamwork between educational, medical, and other personnel who serve children who have limited vision. Therefore the educator should un-

derstand the roles of professionals who are involved with eye care and should know who is responsible for rendering each service. Eye specialists include the following:

1. The ophthalmologist, a licensed physician who specializes in the treatment of eye diseases and optical defects
2. The optometrist, a nonmedical practitioner licensed to prescribe and fit glasses and deal with optical defects of the eyes without the use of drugs or surgery
3. The optician, a skilled technician who grinds lenses and makes up glasses
4. The orthoptist, an assistant who provides eye exercises and orthoptic training as prescribed by medical personnel

Identification of visual impairments

Vision tests are extremely important in order to identify and remedy vision disorders and to facilitate the education of handicapped persons. The most important single test of vision is the Snellen test, which is a measure of visual acuity. This test is the most widely used because of the expediency with which it can be administered to a child by nonprofessional personnel and also because it can be used with young children. The Snellen chart can detect such conditions as myopia, astigmatism, higher degrees of hyperopia, and other eye conditions that cause imperfect visual images. However, it must be remembered that the chart primarily measures central distance visual acuity. It does not give indications of near-point vision, peripheral vision, convergence ability, binocular fusion ability, or muscular imbalance. It is easy to see that a thorough vision screening program must include tests supplementary to the Snellen test. Other visual screening tests suitable for educational purposes are the Massachusetts vision test, the Keystone Telebinocular test, and the Orthorator test. Hathaway[11] recommended the Massachusetts vision test as a reliable procedure for acquiring more data about visual disorders. This test battery consists of the illuminated Snellen E chart, a plus lens test for hyperopia, and a test for horizontal and vertical muscle balance at 20 feet as well as for horizontal muscle balance at reading distance.

Limitations in peripheral vision constitute a visual handicap, particularly in activities involving motor skills. Consequently, knowledge of this aspect of vision may assist the physical educator in determining methods of teaching and types of activities for the impaired child. Peripheral vision is usually assessed in terms of degrees of visual arc and is measured by the extent to which a standard visual stimulus can be seen on a black background viewed from a distance of about 39 inches when the eye is fixed on a central point.

It is difficult to evaluate the results found on a given test of vision, for two persons with similar vision characteristics on a screening test may display different visual behavior physically, socially, and psychologically.

Although objective tests of vision are of paramount importance in screening procedures, it should be emphasized that, regardless of specific tests that have been used, it is always wise to supplement this screening with daily observations. Daily observation for symptoms of eye trouble is of particular importance in the early primary years so that visual handicaps may be remedied or circumvented early in the learning process. Symptoms that may indicate eye disorders and that may be observed by the physical educator are the following:

1. Eyelids that are crusted and red, in which stys or swelling appear
2. Discharges from the eyes
3. Lack of coordination in directing vision of both eyes
4. Frequent rubbing of the eyes
5. Inattention when sustained visual activity is required or when looking at distant objects
6. Tenseness of the body
7. Squinting
8. Forward thrust of head
9. Walking overcautiously
10. Faltering or stumbling
11. Running into objects not directly in the line of vision
12. Failure to see objects readily visible to others
13. Sensitivity to normal light levels
14. Inability to distinguish colors
15. Difficulty in estimating distances
16. Bloodshot eyes

Incidence

It is difficult to assess the incidence of blindness and partial vision because of the differing definitions of blindness and the problems that exist in identification. Consequently, dependable statistics on the incidence of blindness in the United States are seriously lacking, although there is a growing awareness that a greater incidence of blindness and vision impairment exists than had been believed previously. It is estimated that there are 85,000 partially sighted children of school age in the United States. There are a considerable number of children with visual defects who are not categorized as either blind or partially sighted. Estimates indicate that approximately 20% of elementary school children and 30% of high school students have some visual defect.

Classification

There are many ways of classifying persons with loss of vision. They may be classified according to cause, topography, degree of vision loss, time of onset, or collateral effects. The underlying causes of vision loss include infectious diseases, accidents and injuries, poisoning, tumors, and prenatal influences. Prenatal causes account for 41.8% of blindness, poisoning for 19.3%, heredity for 14.3%, tumors for 5.1%, injuries for 4.9%, and infectious diseases for 7.4%.[13]

Classification by topography refers to the part of the eye affected, the nature, and the location of the eye defect. These classifications include defects of the retina, the crystalline lens, and the optic nerve.

Perception of vision falls on a continuum.

It is important for the physical educator to be aware of the amount of residual vision that a partially sighted person has. The residual vision can fall on a continuum extending from slight impairment (20/70) to total blindness.

Factors that may enhance the functioning of the more severely handicapped person in his environment may occur in the perception of light, motion, and form at varying distances from the individual. Still another factor related to degree of impairment of total vision is the amount of residual peripheral vision. These factors must be interrelated in order for the individual with loss of vision to adapt successfully to his environment.

Lowenfeld[16] suggested that it is necessary to consider the time of onset of the vision loss as well as the amount of vision one possesses. In the event that blindness was acquired after the preschool years of life, the child has had opportunities to acquire perceptual experiences that will better enable him to cope with his environment at a later time. The early developmental period in which the child explores both his environment and his own physical abilities is of critical importance.

Knowledge of the degree of vision loss and the time of onset is significant to the physical educator because these considerations have a bearing on the development of physical and motor characteristics and the acquisition of motor skills.

Developmental factors

Vision loss has serious implications for the general development of motor, academic, intellectual, psychological, and social characteristics at various age levels. In many instances, intervention with training programs and guidance is necessary to meet the developmental needs of the maturing child with a loss of vision. It is important to have some knowledge of how the child with vision loss may develop physically, socially, and psychologically so that the educator can be alert to cope with needs that may arise.

Evidence indicates that blind pupils in the public schools are educationally retarded when compared to their sighted peers of the same chronological age.[1, 10] Some of the reasons why this may be true are that (1) the blind enter school later, causing an educational lag, which usually persists throughout the school career; (2) they may have a maladjustment at the onset of blindness, making it difficult to stay abreast of sighted peers; and (3) they need to master new tools such as braille reading and writing. The physical educator must be alert to detect educationally retarded blind children. He must not be misguided by grade placement, but must assess and meet the physical, motor, and social needs of each child.

Physical activity is essential for optimum child growth and development. Through movement experiences, the child with a vision loss gains a better understanding of himself, others, and the world around him. However, limited vision restricts physical and motor activity, which, in turn, limits the range and variety of experiences the child may encounter. He then becomes less effective in meeting the demands of his environment. Opportunities for manipulating toys and objects are extremely important in the early life of the blind child because it is through touch and feeling, rather than through vision, that he learns about the physical world.

Providing an environment in which the child with a vision impairment can develop optimally is a great challenge. Because of the limitation in vision, the blind child is often slower in learning such skills as walking, talking, prehension, feeding, and socialization unless he is given special help that will assist in developing these traits.

Norris and Brody[22] found that blind children showed delayed mastery of motor responses in tasks requiring fine motor coordination. There is impressive evidence that fine motor coordination develops with fluency only after the child has had experiences in gross motor activity. This would point to a need to provide environmental experiences for both gross and fine motor activities. Norris and Brody[22] also stressed the importance of opportunities for physical activity and expressed the opinion that the physical development of blind children is usually normal, although the rate may be slower than for children with normal vision.

Research available regarding the social maturity of blind children reveals that, in general, they receive significantly lower social maturity scores than children who see.[17, 18, 21] Whether the cause of the retarded development in social maturity is blindness or an aspect of the manner in which the blind person relates to his environment is not known. Physical education programs may well be an important medium for enhancing the social maturity of blind children.

Mannerisms

Some mannerisms that blind persons may display include rocking backward and forward, rubbing the eyes with the fists, turning around and around, waving the hands in front of the face, and bending the head forward and backward. There is speculation that through training and guiding the visually limited to learn to do things for themselves and through involvement in physical activity, these mannerisms may be overcome.

Perception
Obstacle perception

When a blind person stops walking before coming to a wall or a large object that obstructs his intended path, this is called obstacle perception. Some authorities have indicated that obstacle perception can be learned.[27] It appears to be a function of audition, in which the person responds to an environmental need. Blind persons are capable of avoiding obstacles by detecting changes in pitch as they move about in their environment and develop an awareness of objects.

Sensory perception

It was once a prevalent notion that visually limited children compensated for defective vision with supersensitive hearing, touch, taste, and smell. However, it is now accepted that the visually limited do not possess natural compensation.[25] It is possible that blind children utilize their other sensory abilities better through increased attention to them and through practice and opportunities for learning. A sighted person may be unaware of auditory stimuli in his environment, whereas a blind person would attach great significance to the stimuli; however, there may be little difference between the actual hearing abilities of the blind person and the seeing person.

Psychological and social adjustment

The emotional and social characteristics of the visually limited have not, as yet, been conclusively defined. However, Cowan, Underburg, and Verrillo[6] found that, regarding the relationship between the degree of disability and psychological and social adjustment, better adjustment was associated with greater visual disability. These findings indicate that degree of visual disability does not necessarily lead to proportionate maladjustment. Conclusions drawn from this study were that social and emotional maladjustment, as typically defined and measured, are not necessary consequences of limitations in vision and that such maladjustment that does occur is not directly proportional in severity to, or necessarily directly related to, visual limitation.

Psychological and social adjustment of the blind cannot be separated from the attitudes with which the nondisabled view them. The lack of respect of one's peers may create a need for a disproportionate amount of social and emotional adjustment by comparison with that found among a nondisabled population. The adjustment of blind persons is not blindness itself and, more than likely, does not produce maladjustment. The correlates of maladjustment are to be found in deficiencies of respect accorded the individual, rather than a lack of visual experience.

The uphill battle and social adjustment of the blind requires special attention; sighted persons gain social habits through imitation, but the blind need direct instruction in everyday social adjustment. The emotional and social climate of the physical education class can be structured so that the blind child will be able to function comfortably at his own level and assist in establishing wholesome social relationships or it can contribute to his frustration by creating situations that accentuate, rather than minimize, his differences.

The ultimate goal of the class atmosphere for the child with vision loss is to provide experiences that will assist him in adjusting to the seeing society in which he must ultimately live. The selection and method of experiences in the physical education program are critical. These experiences should not be of such a nature that the blind child is overprotected to the extent that growth is inhibited; rather they should provide challenge, yet remain within the range of the child's capabilities for achieving physical and social success.

The problems that confront the teacher regarding successful emotional and psychological adjustment of the visually limited involve both the visually limited child and the nondisabled child. Guidelines for achieving the goal of adjustment for teachers of visually handicapped children are as follows:

1. Provide opportunities for participation and enjoyment in new experiences
2. Find ways in which they are free to grow and develop at their own rate
3. Find ways in which they can best contribute to the groups that are satisfying to them
4. Help them become acquainted with their physical surroundings

Equally important in the social and psychological adjustment of visually handicapped children is the attitude of nondisabled persons toward them. Physical education teachers working with children who are visually handicapped should attempt to minimize the stereotyped manner in which the visually limited child receives an education and should encourage children to help blind children with some techniques that will clarify situations for them.

Mobility

One of the greatest problems caused by blindness is the difficulty in moving about in one's environment, for success in school and at work in later years depends on mobility. Certainly, the importance of moving about cannot be underestimated, for it tends to force independence in the blind individual, which, in turn, leads to opportunities for social and psychological development.

A program of training in mobility for the blind in the gymnasium or playing areas will greatly increase the degree of independent functioning a person with vision loss may attain in a physical education program. The orientation and training program should help the individual cope with his physical surroundings effectively with regard to his developmental level. The training program should also assist in successful interaction with peers as well as with the physical facilities and equipment. It must be remembered that some blind persons have enough vision to travel about. This vision may be called "travel vision." The individual capabilities of each child should be assessed to determine the extent of the training program.

Educational placement

The physical education teacher may be requested either to instruct a class in which visually limited children are integrated with the regular class or to instruct a class composed solely of visually limited children.

There is a growing awareness that similarities are greater than differences when visually limited children are compared with seeing children. Therefore integration of the visually limited child is becoming more prevalent because it places emphasis on positive aspects of the child and minimizes his differences. It is also generally believed that educational methods can be adapted to meet individual needs.

Although integration is desirable, if possible, for the child who is visually limited, educational placement is an individual matter and dependent on a number of factors. Consequently, integration with the regular class may not be the best educational placement for all children who are visually limited. Some of the factors that should be considered in the placement of the visually limited child are the following:

1. Visual acuity
2. Interests, capacities, and abilities
3. Size of the class
4. Amount of attention the teacher must provide for the child
5. Social, emotional, and intellectual level of development
6. Available equipment and facilities for adequate functioning with the regular class
7. The physical educator's competency to initiate an adapted physical education program for the visually limited child

Implications for physical education

The teacher must be able to respect individuals who are atypical in vision. It is of extreme importance that educators focus their attention on what abilities the visually limited child has, rather than on what he has not, for the purpose of creating an environment conducive to optimal growth. An assessment of the needs, abilities, and limitations of the visually limited child is necessary, with subsequent program development according to defined needs. This is a challenging task for a teacher; however, it has been pointed out by many good teachers that instructing the visually limited has enabled them to do a better job with typical children because it was necessary to plan more carefully when working with the visually limited group.

Some of the basic considerations prerequisite to effective education of the visually limited child are as follows:

1. Skilled observation of motor performance and behavioral characteristics as individuals and as group participants
2. Recognition of differences in the manner in which the child who is visually limited learns (as compared to the typical child), followed by appropriate adaptive methodology
3. Understanding of the growth and development of physical and social competency
4. Knowledge of appropriate curricula and methods in physical education for the visually limited

High quality physical education programs can enhance the visually limited child socially, emotionally, and physically. Loss of vision, by itself, is not a limiting condition for physical exercise. There is apparently no limit to the amount of developmental exercises of muscular strength and endurance that can be administered to this group of children. Through developmental exercise, it is hoped that the visually limited child will develop esthetic qualities such as good posture, graceful body movement, and good walking and sitting positions. It is also hoped that he will develop and maintain a healthy, vigorous body with physical vitality and good neuromuscular coordination. In addition to physical benefits, it is hoped that the physical education program will contribute to such social-emotional outcomes as security and confidence on the part of the visually limited and will promote acceptance of the handicapped by their sighted peers (Fig. 14-1).

Adapting methods and activities

Children with limited vision are capable of participating in numerous activities; however, the degree to which participation is possible is dependent on factors already mentioned. Therefore it is recommended that there be available broad curriculum areas at appropriate levels of development to accommodate each child. It must be remembered that children with limited vision may represent a cross section of any school population with regard to motor abilities, physical fitness characteristics, and social and emotional traits. The purpose of adapting methods and activities for the visually

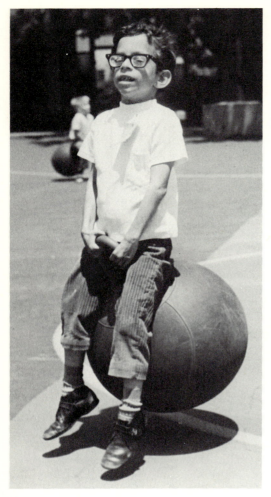

Fig. 14-1. Blind children can participate in numerous physical activities. However, they must know their constraints in space. (Courtesy Dr. Julian Stein, American Association for Health, Physical Education, and Recreation.)

should provide confidence for them to cope with their environment through increasing their physical and motor abilities. It should also produce in them a feeling of acceptance as individuals in their own right. To achieve these goals, the program should include adaptation of the general program of activities, when needed; additional or specialized activities, depending on the needs of the child; and special equipment, if needed.

The physical educator who is administering activities to children with limited vision should take special safety precautions. Some considerations that may enhance the safety factor in physical education programs for the visually limited are the following:

1. Secure knowledge through medical records and observation of the visually limited child's limitations and capabilities
2. Orientation of the child to facilities and equipment
3. Special equipment giving direction, such as guidelines in swimming and running events, deflated softballs, etc.

Adaptation of teaching methods

The visually limited child must depend on receiving information through sensory media other than vision. Audition is a very important sensory medium of instruction. Another sensory medium that can be used is kinesthesis through manual guidance and movement of the body parts administered by an instructor or another student. This gives assistance in comprehension of body position and body action of the visually limited student. The blind child has little understanding of spatial concepts such as location, position, direction, and distance; therefore skin and muscular sensations give meaning to body position and postural change in motor activity. The manual guidance method (accompanied by verbal corrections) is often effective in the correction of faulty motor skills, for two senses are utilized for instruction. A technique used with some success in the integrated class is

limited is to provide for blind children many of the experiences that sighted children learn primarily through visual observation. The goal of group activity in which a child with limited vision participates is to assign a role that the child can carry out successfully. It is undesirable for him to be placed in the position of a bystander.

Adaptation of the physical education program for visually limited individuals for the teacher to use the blind child in presenting a demonstration to the rest of the class by manually manipulating the child through the desired movements. This enables the visually limited child to get the tactual feel of the move being performed on him and instruction to the sighted class members is not deterred.

Providing information, rules, and tests in braille for the visually limited to study in advance of a presentation in class may be helpful. Advance study enables the visually limited child to receive a greater understanding of the presentation of the materials.

Instructional aids that may be applicable for the physical education teacher are the following:

1. Teachers should be alert to the behavioral signs and physical symptoms of visual difficulties in all children.
2. Teachers should not let visually limited children exploit their visual limitations to the extent that they withdraw from participation or underachieve in motor performance.
3. Teachers should arrange seating with regard to the child's range of vision. Glare should be reduced and accommodations made for appropriate light contrasts between figure and ground when presenting materials.
4. Teachers should develop a respect for the particular way in which the child learns, such as tactual-kinesthetic methods and use of auditory cues for direction in space.
5. Teachers must learn respect for individual differences and take time and effort to accept these differences and cope with them (Chapter 8).

Adaptation of skill activities

Because of the great visual content included in the components of certain games, some skill activities are more difficult to adapt to the visually limited than are others. In the case of the more severely handicapped, participation in the more complex activities may be extremely difficult to modify. However, the skills comprising a game may be taught and lead-up games with appropriate modifications will usually be within the grasp of the child. Some adaptations to basic sports skills are discussed in this section.

Basketball

1. *Passing—additional use of audition*
   a. A sighted person should call the visually limited child's name when the ball is to be passed to the visually limited child.
   b. Sighted classmates may snap their fingers with their hands raised to guide the height of a pass executed by visually limited children.
   c. When a ball is passed to a visually limited person, it should be done so with a bounce pass so that the speed and direction of the ball can be detected.
2. *Dribbling—additional use of kinesthesis*
   a. Teaching progression in the dribble is important. The child should first bounce the ball with two hands in a stationary position, then bounce it with one hand in a stationary position, and then move forward and backward while bouncing the ball.
   b. The child should take short steps when dribbling on the move. This will enable the student to push the ball downward instead of outward to achieve greater control of the ball.
3. *Shooting—additional use of kinesthesis and audition*
   a. The teacher should use verbal instruction and manual guidance. Manual guidance is an efficient method when a gradient response is needed by the participant.
   b. Direction and distance of a shot can be aided if a classmate stands under the basket and talks or calls to the visually limited child.
4. *Guarding—increased space*
   a. The visually limited child should be provided with greater space in which to move when executing guarding drills.

5. *Game participation—increased tactility*
   a. The teacher should have the visually limited child play with a sighted player in each position during the early teaching of the game.
   b. A scoreboard that can be read tactually can be constructed from fiberboard to inform blind persons of the score of the game, fouls, time remaining, etc.

Baseball
1. *Decreased space*
   a. The baselines should be shortened; the more severe the handicap, the shorter the baselines should be.
   b. For a totally blind batter, the ball containing a noisemaker can be pitched by rolling it on the ground. The batter should swing the bat parallel to the ground. The more severe the handicap, the larger the ball should be.
2. *Tactile aid*
   a. In the case of an integrated class, sighted children can guide the runners in the base paths. An additional aid to the runner is to station sighted class members at each base for further guidance of the visually limited runners.
3. *Adaptation of the rules of the game*
   a. If a totally blind person picks up a grounder, the runner is automatically out if between bases.

Football
1. *Adaptation of position*
   a. Children who have the greatest visual handicaps should be placed in the line. End positions and backfield positions are more difficult for the visually limited child because of visual factors inherent in the positions.
2. *Adaptation of the rules of the game*
   a. When playing touch football, modify the game so that potential violent contact is minimized, perhaps requiring only one hand touch anywhere on the runner for the more severely handicapped. More difficult tags can be required for the less handicapped.

3. *Adaptation of space per pupil*
   a. The number of contestants on each team should be reduced so that collisions will be less likely to occur.

Soccer
1. *Adaptation of position in accord with ability*
   a. Persons with greater loss of vision are more able to play the defense and goal positions than the front line.
2. *Modify equipment*
   a. The ball should be modified so that it is softer in order to minimize the danger of the blind child's being struck by a hard object. Deflate the ball slightly to retard the rolling progress of the ball when teaching special classes for the blind.
   b. Skills should be emphasized in the form of lead-up games.

Track and field
1. *Participation*
   a. All events are feasible for participation by the blind, with the exception of hurdling.
2. *Additional use of kinesthesis*
   a. Cables should be strung between track lanes to guide runners with severe vision loss.
3. *Adaptation of position*
   a. The child with a visual limitation should be given the outside lane when running against a sighted child. In the special class, those with greatest vision loss should be placed in the outside running lanes to avoid their being in proximity to two persons.
4. *Auditory aid*
   a. In the integrated class, sighted students can run ahead of the visually limited child and call his name in the longer races.
   b. In endurance running in the integrated class, a sighted student may run beside the visually limited child and use his voice as an orientation device for the visually limited child. The position of the visually limited child should be maintained without his touching his partner.

c. The more severely handicapped children may use the standing high jump instead of the running high pump. However, if the running high jump is attempted, a square piece of tin may be taped to the floor of the take-off point, which, on contact, will convey to the jumper that he is taking off at the right distance from the bar.

d. The visually limited child can perform the running broad jump with the assistance of one sighted child at the far end of the broad jump pit to give an auditory signal for direction and a second child to run with him to inform the visually limited child when it is time to jump.

5. *Tactile aid*
   a. In relay racing, the child with severe vision loss can run first to avoid receiving the baton. A sighted student should run as a guide with the child when the exchange of the baton is made to the next person.

Field hockey

1. *Kinesthetic aid*
   a. Dribble: The visually limited child should tap the ball a short distance and in a straight line. If the ball is lost on the dribble, small circular movements that become progressively larger should be made with the stick until the ball is located. When the ball is too far away, the visually limited child should be notified.
   b. Bullies: The player keeps the stick in contact with the ball and takes the bully in the same manner as do sighted children.

2. *Auditory aid*
   a. Passing: Teammates should give auditory sounds when they wish to receive a pass.

Bowling

1. *Kinesthetic aid*
   a. A guide rail should be placed beside the approach so that the visually limited person may receive aid in direction when delivering the ball.

Gymnastics

1. *Participation*
   a. Gymnastics and work on the apparatus are activities that can be performed by totally blind children.

2. *Adaptation of position*
   a. Provisions should be made for adequate space for performance for the visually limited child.

3. *Tactual orientation:* Each piece of apparatus should be tactually observed before participation.

4. *Tactual observation:* Tactual observation of the stunts to be performed is desirable.

Trampoline

1. *Auditory aid*
   a. Removal of the center cables from the mat of the trampoline will assist in centering the bounce of the child. The voice of the instructor should be used to center the bounce. Verbal direction can be given with respect to the position of the person bouncing.

2. *Kinesthetic aid*
   a. The teacher should jump with the child and then inform him of the correct time to execute the seat drop.
   b. The child should first assume a position of landing, then begin a drop from the hands and knees, progress to the feet, and, finally, execute the front drop.

Locomotor skills

1. *Aid by increase of space*
   a. Adequate room should be provided for performance. The child should be assured that there are no obstacles.

2. *Kinesthetic aid*
   a. Hopping and jumping may be taught by having the visually limited child feel the upward and downward movements of a classmate.
   b. The visually limited child should link arms with two classmates who skip forward until the rhythm of the movement is developed and it becomes possible for him to skip alone.

Swimming
1. *Kinesthetic aid*
   a. As in land skills, kinesthetic orientation is a good instructional tool for achieving proficiency in most of the swimming skills.
   b. Manual guidance of the participant's body and limbs and tactual observation of a sighted swimmer's skills are valuable instructional tools. When teaching swimming to the visually limited, adaptive and lead-up techniques are useful.
   c. Walking in the water is a lead-up to the "flutter kick."
   d. The "dog paddle," as a lead-up to the "American crawl," provides tactual stimulation of both arms and legs throughout the entire stroke.
   e. Kickboards and flotation devices are of great value, for they give support to the body and make it possible for the child with a vision loss to explore his environment in the water.
   f. The child should be supported under the shoulder blades to assist floating on the back.
   g. A slide provides assistance for entry into the water.
   h. Guide ropes assist swimmers in staying in their lanes and prevent them from bumping the edge of the pool.
   i. Handrails are useful for orientation when mounted near the sidewalls.
   j. The diving board should be covered with nonslippery material.
2. *Auditory aid*
   a. Auditory cues should be used to inform the visually limited child when he is to make a turn while swimming.
   b. Belt flotation devices or support around the waist gives confidence to the child when treading water.
   c. In water entries, the visual limitation of a student requires that the progression necessary for achievement of a successful dive be in small increments. The first step should be an attempted entry from the steps of the pool, followed by a jump from the deck, and then a headfirst entry with the instructor holding both hands of the diver with one hand and holding correct head position with the other hand. This should be followed by the unassisted headfirst entry.

• • •

One of the chief problems to be confronted in the social and psychological adjustment of the visually limited person is the lack of opportunity for social participation with sighted persons. Recreational opportunities provide a possible outlet for making social contact with the sighted population and also provide self-expression for the visually limited individual (Chapter 8).

DEAFNESS AND IMPAIRED HEARING

Hearing represents one of the strongest lines of communication between persons and the world in which they live. Children who have permanent hearing impairment are afflicted with a handicap that often has an impact on their total development, adjustment, and personality. The responsibility of meeting the special needs of such children requires the cooperation and skills of many disciplines. The purpose of this section is to afford a background into the nature and needs of those who are deaf and hard-of-hearing and to discuss the role of physical education in meeting these needs as part of the total educational process.

Hearing is subjective in that two persons experiencing the same sound will attach different meanings to the sound. Similarly, the meanings attached to impaired hearing by scientists and by educators who work with deaf and hard-of-hearing individuals are different. Therefore it seems desirable to examine the implications of hearing loss as viewed by these two disciplines.

Science's concern for hearing loss is with regard to two objective measures that can be recorded by the audiometer. These measures are *pitch* (or tone) and *intensity* as measured by the decibel (dB).

Hearing loss plotted in decibels on a linear scale does not represent the limits of human audition. However, quantitative degrees of hearing loss may be of some value to the physical educator.

The degree of hearing impairment, in many cases, is associated with quantitative hearing loss as measured by the decibel. The following is an example of what might be expected from persons placed on various points of a hearing-loss continuum:

Loss not in excess of 15 dB does not represent any severe impairment. However, if the hearing loss is in the range of 30 dB, some impairment in communication may be evident. In the event the deficit is in the range of 50 dB, serious impairment in communication may be expected. Speech can be heard only through amplification if the decibel measurement is in the range of 75 dB loss. When the decibel range reaches 90 dB loss in the better ear, the individual is close to total deafness.

Threshold acuity is of limited interest to educators, for their primary concern is with the effects of the hearing loss as it relates to the learning process. The acquisition of speech and language development is basic to the subsequent development of the individual. Therefore the time of onset of deafness is a critical factor in determining the effects that it may have on the learning situation. A child who is afflicted with a hearing loss early in development progresses more slowly than one who is afflicted with a loss later in the developmental process.

Relevant to the education of children with auditory handicaps is the classification of hearing losses established by the Conference of Executives of American Schools for the Deaf.[5] These groupings, which have been made primarily to lay a foundation for education, are listed as follows:

1. *The deaf:* Those in whom the sense of hearing is nonfunctional for the ordinary purposes of life. This general group is made up of two distinct classes, based entirely on the time the loss of hearing occurred.
   a. *The congenitally deaf:* Those who were born deaf.
   b. *The adventitious deaf:* Those who were born with normal hearing but in whom

the sense of hearing became nonfunctional later through illness or accident.
2. *The hard-of-hearing:* Those in whom the sense of hearing, although deficient, is functional with, or without, a hearing aid.*

Worthy of note is the fact that this definition does not take into account other types of hearing loss that may also have educational implications. The proper diagnosis of a hearing defect is very important, for the educational program may be dependent on it. Categories of deafness that should be known and considered in the educational planning of the student are the following:

1. *Psychogenic deafness:* A condition in which the receptive organs function adequately and there is no damage to the nervous system, but, for emotional reasons, the person does not respond to sound.
2. *Central deafness:* A condition in which the receiving mechanism of hearing is functioning properly, but an abnormality in the CNS prevents the person from hearing. This disorder is often referred to as auditory or sensory aphasia, or word deafness.
3. *Perceptive or sensorineural deafness:* A condition caused by a defect of the inner ear or of the auditory nerve in transmitting the impulse to the brain.
4. *Conductive loss:* A condition in which the intensity of sound is reduced before reaching the inner ear, where the auditory nerve begins. Since hearing loss is a problem that is multidimensional in nature, it is important that the educator form no generalized concept regarding the deaf or hard-of-hearing child without considering such relevant factors as degree of hearing loss, age of onset, and type of hearing loss.

Incidence

In the United States, there are approximately 18 million hearing-impaired in-

*From Committee on Nomenclature, Conference of Executives of American Schools for the Deaf, Am. Ann. Deaf 83:1-3, 1938.

dividuals, 3 million of which are children. Also, it has been estimated that 5% of school-aged children have some hearing deficiency with 1 or 2 out of 10 of this group requiring special educational attention.[25] This means that adaptive procedures must be considered in cases of hearing loss, but only a few hearing loss cases will require completely altered educational methods.

There is evidence that hearing loss is on the increase. Reasons for this increase may be the following:

1. The lengthening of the life span, accompanied by deterioration of the sensory processes among the aged
2. An increase of hearing loss among infants whose lives have been saved by modern medicine, but who were born with a defective hearing mechanism
3. The impairment of the hearing mechanism by the loud noises of modern technology
4. The use of more thorough identification and screening procedures to detect hearing loss among the population at large

Causes

Deafness may occur before birth, at birth, or after birth. Some hearing defects are acquired, whereas other hearing defects are hereditary in nature. Myklebust[20] found 39.1% of the incidence of deafness to be acquired, 22.6% to be hereditary, and 38.8% to be of unknown origin.

Various types of hearing impairment may result from particular causes, which may be listed as follows:

1. *Psychogenic deafness:* Personality inadequacies generally associated with neuroses or psychoses.
2. *Central deafness* (affecting the auditory pathways within the CNS): Diseases of the brain affecting the auditory pathways, such as cerebral tumor or abscess, arteriosclerosis, cerebral hemorrhage, and multiple sclerosis. Another form of central deafness is auditory aphasia, which is caused by a lesion in the cortex and association paths of the brain, preventing comprehension, concept formation, and symbolization through audition.
3. *Sensorineural impairment:* Sensorineural impairment may be a result of prenatal, natal, or postnatal causes.

Hearing tests

There are two purposes in the assessment of hearing loss. One purpose is to determine how well the person's hearing serves the process of communication; the other is to see what can be done in terms of auditory rehabilitation. The educator is mainly concerned with hearing tests for the first reason. It is desirable to have children diagnosed at the earliest possible age so that correctable defects may be cared for adequately. If this is done, the impairment will not interfere greatly with the development of the child. Gesell and Amatruda[8] have suggested the following list of signs of hearing loss:

1. *Hearing and comprehension of speech:* (a) General indifference to sound; (b) lack of response to the spoken word; (c) response to noises as opposed to words.
2. *Vocalization and sound production:* (a) Monotonal quality; (b) indistinct speech; (c) lessened laughter; (d) meager experimental sound play; (e) vocal play for vibratory sensation; (f) head banging, foot stamping for vibratory sensation; (g) yelling, screeching to express pleasure or need.
3. *Visual attention:* (a) Augmented visual vigilance and attentiveness; (b) alertness to gesture and movement; (c) marked imitativeness in play; (d) vehemence of gestures.
4. *Social rapport and adaptation:* (a) Subnormal rapport in vocal games; (b) intensified preoccupation with things rather than persons; (c) puzzled and unhappy episodes in social situations; (d) suspiciousness and alertness, alternating with cooperation; (e) marked reaction to praise and affection.
5. *Emotional behavior:* (a) Tantrums to call attention to self or need; (b) tensions, tantrums, resistance, due to lack of comprehension; (c) frequent obstinacies, irritability at not making self understood.*

---

*From Gesell, A., and Amatruda, C. S.: Developmental diagnosis, New York, 1974, Harper & Row, Publishers.

Informal methods

The electric audiometer is the most refined instrument for the detection of hearing loss. However, informal methods may still be of use for the rough appraisal of a child's hearing. Some of the tests are as follows:

1. *The watch tick test:* A watch is brought progressively closer to the child's ear until he acknowledges the sound of the watch.
2. *The coin click test:* This test is administered in relatively the same manner as the watch tick test. It is for the purpose of detecting high-frequency losses.
3. *The conversational test:* The child is placed 20 feet from the teacher and is spoken to in a regular conversational tone. In the event the child cannot hear the examiner, the examiner moves closer and closer. If the child has difficulty hearing at 10 to 20 feet, he should be referred for a more thorough examination.
4. *The whisper test:* This test is administered in a manner similar to the conversational test except that the examiner uses a whisper.

The electric audiometer

Thorough assessment of auditory acuity requires the investigation of a number of different aspects of hearing. Some of the aspects of hearing evaluation are the following:

1. Testing the ability to discriminate pitch and loudness
2. Determining the ability to hear and understand speech
3. Checking the sensitivity to increases in loudness
4. Determining the ability to tolerate loudness
5. Considering the possibility of functional or sensory impairment

The assessment of all these hearing characteristics is beyond the training of the educator. However, the "sweep check" test, a screening test using a standard pure tone audiometer, can be administered by a nonspecialist examiner. Six pitches (300; 500; 1,000; 2,000; 4,000; 8,000 cycles/second) are presented to the subject at an intensity of 10 to 15 dB. Failure to hear at least five of the six tones indicates a need for referral. It is possible to examine 15 to 20 persons an hour by administering this test.

Characteristics

Even though Meyerson[20] stated that most samplings of deaf children revealed considerably lower scores on measures of intelligence, educational achievement, and personality than did the groups with which they were compared, he cautioned that this should not be interpreted as convincing evidence that hearing impairment is directly or necessarily related to intelligence, educational achievement, or personality. It also has been stated that deaf children are generally from 2 to 4 years retarded educationally and that the large majority of them do not complete the eighth grade. This is supported by Fusfeld,[6] who found that of 134 applicants to Gallaudet College (a college for the deaf), the median grade achievement on the Stanford achievement test was grade 9.2. It is difficult to assign meaning to much research in the education of the deaf because of the inability to control such variables as experiential and social deprivations, institutionalization, and methods of instruction. The sensory deficit of hearing often creates a deprived environment that gives rise to unequal opportunities to explore the environment and develop and pursue interests. These inequalities probably place the child with hearing impairment in a disadvantageous position compared with a typical child.

Developmental factors

Hearing loss that afflicts the youngster in the early phases of development impairs the total developmental process. One of the effects of deafness is to limit the child's play experience with other children. Play in the preschool years is important in learning social skills and in the development of motor skills. In play situations, the deaf child is often uncertain as to the part he should play in the game and therefore he often withdraws from participation. Thus the role of play, which is so important to the social, psychological, and motor aspects of development in typical children, is usually limited in the deaf child.

The socializing effects of play that are experienced by typical children are not experienced to the same degree by deaf children. Consequently, slower social development occurs in deaf children. It is in social maturation that the handicap of deafness is most apparent.[21] Studies have indicated that the average deaf child is retarded in social maturity as compared with the average hearing child of his age. This retardation is probably partially caused by language inadequacy that results from the hearing loss.

The deaf child, because of his impaired ability to function socially with his peers and because of the limitations imposed on him by his restricted developmental experiences, is most likely to be subjected to more strain than the hearing child. Therefore the young deaf child may be less emotionally mature than a hearing child of the same age because of the greater number of frustrations he has experienced. Heider and Heider[12] reported a study in which deaf and hearing children were compared in a game situation. It was observed that in situations in which pairs of typical children and pairs of deaf children interacted, there was more tendency for the hearing child to dominate the activity than for a deaf child to dominate. The games played were also classified with respect to structuralization. Again, it was shown that those of the hearing group were more highly organized and showed greater continuity of structure. These findings were explained by the fact that the hearing children had more effective means of communication to control the social situations. This study is indicative of the effects of the inability to communicate in a play situation and the resulting effect on some aspects of personality.

The age of onset of the hearing deficiency is definitely important to the effect the disorder has on the total developmental processes. If the child does not lose his hearing until after speech has developed, he has some concept of the process of communication. However, if a child is born with a severe hearing impairment, he is lacking a valuable tool for learning and his developmental progress is usually retarded.

Case history

Case histories often provide valuable information about children with limited hearing. The following information may be of relevance to the educational process:

1. Type, amount of loss, cause, and age of onset involved in impairment
2. Psychological impact of the onset on the student and the family
3. Student's major modes of communication and problems arising from communicative limitations
4. Effects of the disability in the social, educational, recreational, and domestic spheres
5. Behavior, attitudes, achievements, and aspiration of the student
6. History of diagnostic experiences and rehabilitative measures, including special education
7. Attitudes, motivations, and problems concerning education
8. Presence of other disabilities (visual defects and organic brain damage)
9. Health and medical problems

These data, if obtainable, should provide comprehensive information on which the future educational and rehabilitative program can be built.

Parent education

Parent participation in the education of a child who has a hearing loss is very important. Many parents who face rearing a child with severe hearing impairment have little knowledge of what they can and should do. It is important that the parents of the deaf child do not delay the child's social and educational life, pending enrollment in a school. After the child is in school, it is important for the parents to have a general idea of how the child's hearing is developing, how his basic education is progressing, and how certain aspects of the school program can be extended to the home. The purpose of parent education is to assist the parent in gaining a more realistic outlook regarding the child's future. There is general agreement that parent educational programs are necessary and that orientation is an essential part of any program for the child with impaired hearing.

Rehabilitation

Great individual differences exist among those who are deaf and hard-of-hearing regarding their response to various stimuli. The educational limitations caused by these individual differences must be taken into consideration. For example, persons with tinnitus (a ringing in the ears) are highly sensitive to noise and vibration and may not perform well in a noisy educational facility such as the gymnasium. Deaf children with impaired semicircular canals, which affect balance, should not climb to high places to perform. Also, some children with hearing loss cannot participate in activity where there is excessive change in temperature, dampness, or dust.

Methods of training

There are two prevalent methods of educating deaf persons. They are known as *oralism* and *manualism*. The oral method involves the media of lip reading and facial gestures for communication, with no associated use of hand signs. The manual method makes use of hand signals (signing) to express thoughts. Recently, educators of those who are deaf and/or hard-of-hearing have stressed the importance of *total communication*, whereby the child is taught to use the avenues of communication: lip reading; facial and body gestures;

and hand signs, along with verbalization, whenever possible.

Children with a hearing loss should be taught to make as much use of their residual hearing as possible. Teaching the child with a hearing loss to use what hearing he has is called "auditory training" and consists of improving the child's listening skill. This type of training systematically develops the child's discrimination of gross sounds and rhythm patterns of speech sounds in words, the consonants. In addition to auditory training, which is designed to enhance the communicative process, lip reading and speech training are also used. Worthy of mention is the fact that special skills training, as a rule, takes up little of the program time. However, some authorities believe that this form of compensatory education is the most important part of the plan to prepare the hard-of-hearing child for life in a hearing world and that more time should be devoted to such programs.

A number of hard-of-hearing children are enrolled in regular physical education classes and adaptation in instructional techniques should be made for optimal learning. Many hard-of-hearing children wear hearing aids. If this is the case, it may be best to remove the aids when vigorous physical activity is scheduled. However, once the hearing aid is removed, the student is handicapped in audition and learning, particularly through the verbal medium, so that instructional adjustments are necessary. One adjustment that can be made easily is to place the child close to the instructor so that greater amplification of speech is received. A second adjustment that may help is for the instructor to keep his face in view of the hard-of-hearing child.

When one sensory avenue to gathering information is impaired, it is necessary to rely more on other senses. In the case of children with hearing loss, visual aids have a great significance in instruction. Visual demonstrations, blackboard work, films, and slides are important instructional aids for the deaf. To get the attention of the class, waving the hands or turning off and on lights has proved effective in some instances.

Implications for physical education

The objectives in a physical education program for hard-of-hearing children are the same as those for typical children. However, loss of hearing, which impairs the ability to communicate effectively with others, is a great social handicap. Therefore an objective that should be given priority is the provision of opportunity for social interaction through games with other students. Also, deaf children tend to have poor body mechanics and poor patterns of locomotion. Although the activities in physical education for deaf and hard-of-hearing persons are similar to those in the regular program and although deaf and hard-of-hearing persons may function well in regular programs, there is an obvious need for special and compensatory attention to those who are deaf to fulfill the objectives of the physical education program (Chapters 4 and 8).

In the preschool and early elementary school levels, suggested activities for the deaf are those that develop basic motor skills and rhythm activities. Valuable instruments for such rhythmical activities are percussion instruments such as cymbals, triangles, drums, and tambourines, for these instruments are capable of producing vibrations to which the deaf child can respond.

Deaf and hard-of-hearing children do not, as a rule, need a different set of activities from typical children. However, in many instances, because of the limitations imposed by the hearing disorder, development is retarded. Therefore it is wise to be aware of possible physical underdevelopment and poor motor coordination among deaf and hard-of-hearing persons. If some children have these deficiencies, the program should try to remedy or ameliorate them. Physical characteristics that should be provided for in the physical education program for those who are deaf

and hard-of-hearing include muscular strength and endurance, cardiovascular endurance, flexibility, and body coordination. In addition to these physical and motor characteristics, the sense of balance should be assessed carefully because, in some instances, the function of the vestibular mechanism, which is responsible for balance, may be damaged. A balance program should be designed for such students and their progress assessed. If a child is unable to progress in overcoming this difficulty, it may be necessary to plan a program that would partially circumvent the impairment of balance. These children are often unable to hear auditory signals that give them warnings of impending danger. It is necessary to use visual signals of warning in this instance (Chapter 3).

APHASIA (SEVERE ORAL LANGUAGE HANDICAP)

Aphasia refers to a disturbance in language behavior having an organic base. It is a defect or loss of the power of expression by speech, writing, or signs or of the power of comprehension of speech or written language. Since language behavior involves visual, perceptual, and symbolic processes, interference with any of these processes may have an effect on language. The central focus of this discussion will be on the visuomotor aspects of human development and its effects on the acquisition of language.

Aphasia can occur in both children and adults. It may be incurred (1) through trauma as the result of a direct blow to the head; (2) by a cerebral vascular accident (CVA), commonly called a "stroke"; (3) by a tumor; or (4) from a disease. In addition, severe emotional or physical traumas, excessive rejection, or total isolation can become the basis of an emotional withdrawal and can cause aphasia.

It should be noted that aphasia may be reflected in perceptual disorganization, disturbance in learning, problems in secondary motor functioning, and limitations in abstracting with respect to specific language symbols.

Characteristics

Aphasic children often have difficulty in the discrimination of sound that is to be organized into words. In addition to the problems of converting auditory informa- tion into meaningful symbols, other symp- toms such as impaired laterality, rest- lessness, inattention, emotional outbursts, distractibility, hyperactivity, hypoactivity, short attention span, aggressiveness, unusual

Table 14-1. Maturational milestones, motor correlates, and language development*

Age	Language stage	Motor development
12 to 16 weeks	Coos and chuckles	Supports head in prone position. Responds to human sounds by turning head in direction of sound source.
6 months	Exhibits babbling, resembling one-syllable utterance. Makes identifiable combinations such as "ma," "da," "di," "du."	Sits without props, uses hands for support.
8 months	Exhibits lalling and some echolalia.	Stands by holding onto object. Grasps with thumb opposition.
10 months	Exhibits distinct echolalia, which approximates sounds heard. Responds differentially to verbal sounds.	Creeps efficiently. Pulls to standing position. May take a side step while holding onto a fixed object.
12 months	Reduplicates sounds in echolalia, possibly first words for identification. Responds appropriately to simple sounds.	Walks on hands and feet. May stand alone. May walk when held by one hand or may even take first step alone.
18 months	Possesses repertoire of 3 to 50 words, some 2-word phrases. Reveals intonational patterns through vocalizations. Experiences great increase in understanding of language.	Walks with ease. Runs. Can build two-block tower. Begins to show hand preference.
24 months	Possesses vocabulary of 50 or more words for naming and for bringing about events. Utilizes 2-word phrases of own formulation.	Can walk up or down stairs. Plants both feet on each step.
30 months	Experiences vocabulary growth proportionately greater than at any other period of life. Speaks with clear communicative intent. Makes conventional sentences (syntax) of three, four, and five words. Still includes many infantilisms in articulation. Exhibits good comprehension of speakers in surroundings.	Can jump. Can stand on one foot. Exhibits good hand and finger coordination. Can build six-block tower.
36 months	Possesses vocabulary that may exceed 1,000 words. Demonstrates syntax much like that of older person in surroundings.	Runs proficiently. Walks stairs with alternating feet. Has established hand preference.
48 months	Demonstrates linguistic system essentially like that of adults in environment, except for articulation (phenomic production). May begin to develop own "rhetorical" style of favorite words and phrases.	Can hop on one foot (usually right). Can throw a ball to an intended receiver. Can catch a ball in his arms.

*Modified from Lenneberg, E. H.: Biological foundations of language, New York, 1966, John Wiley & Sons, Inc.

fears, excessive gregariousness, severe to mild emotional problems, catastrophic reactions, unpredictable behavior, and unusual compulsions may be present. However, it is not uncommon for the aphasic child to demonstrate a considerable number of motor competencies.

Although in a great many severely aphasic persons, extremely poor motor coordination may be present, motor difficulties often manifest themselves in poor eye-hand coordination, a failure to perform specific complex movement tasks, and awkwardness in the fundamental motor skills.

Behavioral disorders often thwart the development of language and those abilities that are prerequisite to language. Some children with aphasia show signs of distractibility and perseveration. This disintegrated behavior must be dealt with before either language or the prerequisites of language can be effectively developed. For the aphasic child, it is important that the environment be constructed so that effective perception and language behaviors can be developed. These procedures are discussed in Chapter 13.

The physical educator can make a contribution to the child with aphasia through a motor development program that has the capability of assisting in the correction of perceptual distortions and motor retardation.

Maturational milestones and motor correlates

Lenneberg[15] has drawn a parallel in graphic form between language stages and motor development (Table 14-1). Motor correlates with an increase in speech capability may be associated with greater movement potential of the child. The parallel is most interesting. However, there is little scientific information on causal relationships of speech development as a function of development of motor capability.

Implications for physical education

Children with any disorder should be permitted to participate in physical ac-

tivity that is commensurate with their ability. In the case of aphasic children, on many occasions, the physical prerequisites for participation in activity are present. If this is the case, then vigorous activity to enhance the physical motor and perceptual capabilities should be employed by the physical educator.

The nature of the handicapping condition of aphasia is one that primarily involves communicative skills. An important part of the teaching process utilized by the teacher to aid the aphasic learner involves the use of precise symbols for communication. The following teaching suggestions are made to the instructor of the aphasic child:

1. Use a few simple words with gestures to communicate objectives.
2. Specify what the child is to do with precision.
3. Use a multisensory approach to communicate with the child.
4. Be consistent with the signaling system. In the event that this is not done, there may be a discrepancy between inputs that require the same behavior on different occasions.
5. Repeat the instruction of tasks to be learned, if necessary.
6. Provide opportunity and time for the child to process information and do not expect quick responses to instructions.

Programming

The physical education program for the aphasic child should be designed for perceptual-motor development and the development of language through physical activity or movement. The child should also learn the concepts and ideas that stand for the word or words relating to a specific activity or movement.

The perceptual-motor evaluation can be of assistance for an educational therapist in the remediation of language disorders. Many assessment tools may overlap in their design. Some tests that may be of value are the following:

1. *Goodenough Draw-A-Man Test*[9]: The child is scored on the details of drawing a man.

2. *The Purdue Perceptual Motor Survey*[24]: The child performs gross motor activities that assess the body schema, copy-of-design tests, and oculomotor ability.
3. *The Oseretsky tests*[23]: This scale is composed of six separate items with chronological age norms. The scale measures general static coordination, dynamic coordination of the hands, general dynamic coordination, motor speed, simultaneous voluntary movements, and asynkinesia (inability to perform without overflow or superfluous movements).
4. Luria's[17] dynamic organization of movements, which include (a) motor tests of the ability to reproduce rhythm, (b) tests of the ability to shift from one motor pattern to another, (c) bimanual tasks of simultaneous relationships of two hands, and (d) body image tasks.

Selected activities

There are several types of physical activity that may be used to assist postulated prerequisites of speech development. These include gross motor and fine motor skills that involve auditory, visual, and tactile stimulation. The training activities listed here may provide a base for sequential programming. For a program to become effective, it must possess a sequence of activities capable of reaching the learner. Instructional programming techniques may be applied to most of the activities discussed in this section.

Gross motor activities. Gross motor activities may include any of the following:
1. Running, skipping, hopping, or leaping to auditory inputs
2. Jumping over obstacles or on patterns with a specific command
3. Executing locomotor tasks with the eyes closed
4. Executing balancing tasks with the eyes closed
5. Starting and stopping on command
6. Climbing stairs to an auditory beat
7. Throwing and catching on command
8. Kicking and throwing for accuracy

Visual memory tasks. Visual memory tasks may include either of the following:

1. Superimpose cut-out body parts with a corresponding outline and drawing them in on a blank circle
2. Reassembling an outlined figure that has been cut apart

Identification of body parts. Identification of body parts may include any of the following:
1. Kicking a ball with the foot
2. Slapping a ball with the hand
3. Rolling a ball up the arm
4. Tapping a ball with the fingers
5. Dropping a ball on the toes

Training children with impaired perceptions

For the majority of children with aphasia, activities should involve small groups of children and simple motor patterns that will initiate conversation before, during, and after the actual activity or movement.

It has been suggested that a basic or fundamental list of words (minimum of 35 words to be sufficient) be developed or worked on with the aphasic child. This basic list consists of words such as "over," "under," "across," "top," "bottom," "right," "left," "up," "down," "forward," "backward," "front," "back," "side," "through," "around," "slow," and "fast." It is also recommended that these words be posted on a bulletin board or written on the blackboard so certain words may be assigned on a particular day.

Using this basic word list, the child can then be requested to do simple things such as "Show me 'up,'" "Tell me how many," "How are you moving?" "Who is moving?" Once the aphasic child can understand and demonstrate these fundamental words and clearly understand their meaning, it is time to build on this basic list of words. Additional words can then be added to the list or the same list can be used by progressively increasing the complexity of the words, for example, (1) rub hands, (2) rub hands fast, (3) rub hands very fast, (4) John, rub your hands very fast, and (5) John, I want you to rub your hands very fast. A child might be asked to (1) stand up, (2) walk to the door, (3) jump up and down three times, (4) come back to the chair, and (5) sit down.

Visual perceptual training. The aphasic child must be able (1) to form visual relationships by changing direction in motor performance, (2) to organize and synthesize the peripheral and focal visual fields, and (3) to translate into movement that which is perceived. Some suggested activities to achieve these goals are stacking blocks, stringing beads, performing pegboard activities, stacking rings on pegs, turning the pages of a book, pulling off socks, and lacing a shoe.

Tactile perceptual training. The inability to recognize objects through the sense of touch impairs comprehension of the environment through another sensory avenue. Some children need training in identifying objects by touch. Education in this modality to develop its fullest capacity will further the total learning process. Some suggested activities might involve identifying blocks of different shapes by having the child look at and feel each of several differently shaped blocks and, with closed eyes, identifying objects by touch. This may be done by using a ball, a doll, a top, a toy train, a piece of fruit, etc. Other activities involve the child's tracing with his finger (guided by the teacher) around a form and then pointing to the matching space in a form board. This may be done first with the eyes open and then with the eyes closed.

Auditory perception and memory training

The motor-aphasic child may find it difficult to execute the movements indicated by spoken words because of a loss of memory in recalling the motor patterns described by speech. In such cases, there is a need to relearn word-motor patterns.

Training children with impaired auditory perception in listening and interpreting sound or speech is important. It is necessary to train first in awareness and then in discrimination of gross sounds. If the child has no difficulty, the teacher should proceed first to awareness and discrimination of finer sounds and then to awareness and discrimination of voice and speech. These children usually need "alerting" in responding to auditory stimuli; they must understand thoroughly what is expected of them and they need intensive practice. Some specific techniques are discribed here. The educator should place the child in front of a mirror so he may watch himself and others practice words being formed. Learning may take place by watching and imitating others. The mirror provides visual feedback that may assist in establishing relationships between the motor and auditory aspects of speech behavior. Some children may also need the assistance of a mirror or manual manipulation to learn how it feels to say the words.

The following are a few of the types of questions that might be asked of a group:

1. The children may be asked to "run and touch the fence." While the children are participating, questions may be asked such as "What are we doing?" "How are we moving?" "Show me touch," and "Touch me."
2. One or two children may be picked to lead exercises and said to or asked, "Do your favorite exercise," "What exercise are we doing?" "Are we moving fast or slow?"
3. Hoops may be used and children may be asked, "Jump through the hoop," "Jump in the hoop," "What color is the hoop?"
4. Awareness of persons in a group should be encouraged by asking, "What is next to you?" "How many are in the group?"
5. Perceptual questions may be asked, such as "Show me 'in,'" "Show me 'out,'" "Are you hopping on one foot or two?" "Tell me what you are doing," "Show me 'forward' and 'backward.'"

These activities offer specific examples and demonstrate actual teaching techniques now used to help the aphasic child. A well-balanced program for the aphasic child cannot and should not be overlooked. The program should not only include activities involving language training and retraining but also activities that build and improve on the child's physical conditioning and fitness.[4]

REFERENCES

1. Adair, M.: Working with the slow-learning blind child, Int. J. Educ. Blind **17**:37-39, 1951.
2. American Foundation for the Blind: Am. Foundation Blind Bull. Legislation ser. **13**: 5, 1959.
3. Bradway, K. V.: Social competence of exceptional children. III. The deaf, the blind and the crippled, J. Exceptional Child. **4**: 69, 1937.
4. Carpenter, R. D.: Why can't I learn, Glendale, Calif., 1972, Regal Books.
5. Committee on Nomenclature, Conference of Executives of American Schools for the Deaf, Am. Ann. Deaf **83**:1-3, 1938.
6. Cowan, E. L., Underburg, R., and Verrillo, F. G.: Adjustment to visual disability in adolescence, New York, 1961, American Foundation for the Blind.
6a. Facts on the major killing and crippling diseases in the United States, New York, 1971, National Health Education Committee.
7. Fusfeld, I.: The academic programs of schools for the deaf, Volta Rev. **57**:63-70, 1955.
8. Gesell, A., and Amatruda, C. S.: Developmental diagnosis, New York, 1957, Harper & Row, Publishers.
9. Goodenough, F. L.: Draw-A-Man Test, Chicago, 1934, World Book Encyclopedia Co.
10. Greaves, J. R.: Helping the retarded blind, Int. J. Blind **23**:163-164, 1953.
11. Hathaway, W.: Education and health of the partially seeing child, ed. 4, New York, 1950, Columbia University Press.
12. Heider, F., and Heider, G.: Studies in the psychology of the deaf, Psychol. Monogr. **53**:158-169, 1941.
13. Kerby, C. E.: Causes and prevention of blindness in children of school age, New York, 1952, National Society for the Prevention of Blindness.
14. Kerby, C. E.: Causes of blindness in children of school age, Sightsaver Rev. **28**:10-21, 1958.
15. Lenneberg, E. H.: Biological foundations of language, New York, 1966, John Wiley & Sons, Inc.
16. Lowenfeld, V.: Creative and mental growth, New York, 1952, Macmillan Publishing Co., Inc.
17. Luria, A.: Higher cortical functions in man, New York, 1966, Basic Books, Inc., Publishers.
18. Maxfield, K. E., and Field, H.: The social maturity of the visually handicapped preschool child, Child Dev. **13**:1-27, 1942.
19. Menninger, C. A.: Mental effects of deafness, Psycholanal. Rev. **11**:144-155, 1924.
20. Myerson, L.: A psychology of impaired hearing. In Cruickshank, W. M., editor: Psychology of exceptional children in youth, Englewood Cliffs, N.J., 1955, Prentice-Hall, Inc.
21. Myklebust, H. R.: The psychology of deafness, New York, 1960, Grune & Stratton, Inc.
22. Norris, M. S., and Brody, R. H.: Blindness in children, Chicago, 1957, University of Chicago Press.
23. Oseretsky, N. A.: Metric scale for studying the motor capacity of children. In Lassner, R.: Annotated bibliography of the Oseretsky test of motor proficiency, J. Consult. Clin. Psychol. **12**:37-47, 1948.
24. Roach, C., and Kephart, N. E.: The Purdue Perceptual Motor Survey, Columbus, Ohio, 1965, Charles E. Merrill Publishing Co.
25. Seashore, C. E., and Ling, T. L.: The comparative sensitiveness of blind and seeing persons, Psychol. Monogr. **25**:148-149, 1918.
26. Silverman, S. R.: Hard of hearing children. In Davies, H., and Silverman, S. R., editors: Hearing and deafness, New York, 1960, Holt, Rinehart & Winston, Inc.
27. Werchel, P., Mauney, J., and Andrew, J. G.: The perception of obstacles by the blind, J. Exp. Psychol. **40**:746-751, 1950.

RECOMMENDED READINGS

Agranowitz, A., and McKeown, M. R.: Aphasic handbook for adults and children, Springfield, Ill., 1964, Charles C Thomas, Publisher.

Bauman, M. K., and Yoder, N. M.: Adjustment to blindness re-viewed, Springfield, Ill., 1966, Charles C Thomas, Publisher.

Buell, C. E.: Physical education for blind children, Springfield, Ill., 1966, Charles C Thomas, Publisher.

Cruickshank, W. M., and Johnson, G. O.: Education of exceptional children and youth, Englewood Cliffs, N.J., 1971, Prentice-Hall, Inc.

Daniels, A. S., and Davies, E. A.: Adapted physical education, New York, 1975, Harper & Row, Publishers.

Haring, N. G., and Schiefelbusch, R. L., editors: Methods in special education, New York, 1975, McGraw-Hill Book Co.

Hirst, C. C., and Michaelis, E.: Developmental activities for children in special education, Springfield, Ill., 1972, Charles C Thomas, Publisher.

Kesster, J. W.: Psychopathology of childhood, Englewood Cliffs, N.J., 1966, Prentice-Hall, Inc.

Myklebust, H. R., editor: Progress in learning disabilities, New York, 1975, Grune & Stratton, Inc.

Roberts, A. C.: The aphasic child: a neurological basis for his education and rehabilitation, Springfield, Ill., 1966, Charles C Thomas, Publisher.

15

MENTAL RETARDATION

■ It is now recognized that mental retardation is not an absolute concept. It is not fixed, immutable, or static, but is a dynamic concept that can be changed in varying ways. Years ago, psychologists were engrossed with the idea that intelligence was fixed and could be measured in some absolute manner. Early concepts of mental retardation viewed the disorder as being one that was inherited and essentially incurable. This notion gave rise to hopelessness on the part of professionals and resulted in a social and biological separation of those who were mentally retarded. It is now recognized that this was a fallacious notion, for intelligence is dependent on the measures used, the readiness and experience of the child, and many other variables. Mental retardation also changes with societies. Thirty years ago, society was more agrarian than today. The advances in modern technology make it much more difficult for those who are mentally retarded to cope with contemporary society. It is becoming evident that mentally retarded children are in need of ever increasing added educational assistance in order to function optimally in contemporary society.

DEFINITION OF MENTAL RETARDATION

In 1973, The American Association on Mental Deficiency (AAMD)[13] redefined mental retardation as follows: "Mental retardation refers to subaverage general intellectual functioning existing concurrently with deficits in adaptive behavior, and manifested during the developmental period."

It is important that physical educators be aware of this concept so that they may coordinate their efforts with other professional areas and develop an awareness of how physical education may best serve the mentally retarded.

Explanation of terms

Terms used in defining and discussing mental retardation are explained as follows:

Mental retardation: Incorporation of all the meanings used historically to such concepts describing mental retardation as amentia, feeblemindedness, mental deficiency, mental subnormality, idiocy, imbecility, moronity, etc.

Subaverage: Performance that is greater than one standard deviation below the population mean of the age group involved on measures of a standard IQ test.

General intellectual functioning: An assessment of performance on one or more of the various objective tests developed for that purpose.

Developmental period: For practical purposes, approximately 16 years.

Adaptive behavior: Primarily, the effectiveness of the individual in adapting to the natural and social demands of his environment; impaired adaptive behavior may be reflected in maturation, learning, and social adjustment. These three aspects of adaption are of different importance as qualifying conditions of mental retardation for different age groups.

Maturation: The rate of sequential development of self-help skills of infancy and early childhood such as sitting, crawling, standing, walking, talking, habit training, and interaction with age peers. In the first few years of life, adaptive behavior is assessed almost completely in terms of these and other manifestations of sensorimotor development. Consequently, delay in acquisition of early developmental skills is of prime importance as a criterion of mental retardation during the preschool years.

Learning ability: The facility with which knowledge is acquired as a function of experience. Learning difficulties are usually most manifest in the academic situation and, if mild in degree, may not even become apparent until the child enters school. Impaired learning ability is particularly important as a qualifying condition of mental retardation during the school years.

Social adjustment: Particularly important as a qualifying condition of mental retardation at the adult level, where it is assessed in terms of the degree to which the individual is able to maintain himself independently in the community and in gainful employment as well as in terms of his ability to meet and conform to other personal and social responsibilities and standards set by the community. During the preschool and school years, social adjustment is reflected in the level and manner in which the child relates to parents, other adults, and age peers.

IMPLICATIONS OF THE NEW DEFINITION OF MENTAL RETARDATION FOR PHYSICAL EDUCATION

Within the framework of the definition mentioned, mental retardation is a term descriptive of the current status of an individual with respect to the two basic criteria of adaptive behavior and intellectual functioning of IQ. It can be seen that a person may meet these criteria of mental retardation at one time in life and not at another. This is often the case with many of the higher grade mentally retarded persons. In many instances, they are not known to be retarded before they enter school and are assimilated into society after school. It is only after they have failed to meet the academic standards set by the public schools that they are placed in special education classes and labeled retarded. On leaving school, they are often employed in the community and become relatively indistinguishable from the normative population. Under the new definition, a sharp rise in the incidence of mental retardation occurs during the school years, with a regression of incidence in the adult years, when these persons are functioning in society. The incidence is great at grade six because many children are unable to achieve an academic level beyond this point.

It is important to note that this definition requires the association of two basic criteria, adapted behavior and subaverage IQ, before a person is termed mentally retarded. The components contributing to mental retardation must be examined by the physical educator in an attempt to plan to remediate or ameliorate these contributing factors. The physical educator can assist the adaptive behavior of the mentally retarded individual by the development and implementation of perceptual-motor training programs through programming of motor activity. This is reported to enhance the utilization of the senses for better cognitive learning (Chapter 3).

Impairment of maturation

In the preschool years, the adaptive behavior criterion for mental retardation rests heavily on sensorimotor development. There is impressive evidence that motor development is central to the ability of the child to cope with his environment. (Indeed, it seems central to the whole developmental process.) Kephart[17] expressed concern with modern technology's decreasing the opportunity for random motor experimentation to assist in developing the senses. Apparently, the impact of physical education programs directed toward sensorimotor development for those children who lag behind developmental norms in

the preschool years is critical in remedying the adaptive behavior criterion for mental retardation. There appear to be trends developing that afford opportunity for the development of programs for preschool children, particularly in culturally deprived areas, where the incidence of mental retardation is relatively high. The identification of potential retarded persons who are behind developmental norms in the motor sphere and subsequent programming appear to be areas that must be given attention in the future. There is evidence, albeit scanty, that learning early generalized motor skills through random motor experimentation is the forerunner of the development of spatial relationships and the abstraction of symbolic content that may lay the foundations for elementary school skills. If this is the case, physical education in the preschool years for those who encounter problems in the development of motor skills is most critical in prevention of the adaptive behavior criterion of learning, which is the qualifying condition for mental retardation in the school years.

Implications of physical education
Implications for learning

Learning difficulties are the important qualifying conditions for mental retardation in the school years. Inasmuch as IQ tests were validated against academic achievement, it is not surprising that IQ scores and ability to achieve academically are closely related. Early educators of mentally retarded persons approached education for those who are mentally retarded through the development of the senses. It was believed that through bombarding the peripheral nervous system with sensory stimuli, pathways leading to the central nervous system (where perception takes place) would be opened. There is some evidence in the literature that physical education programs raise the IQ of the mentally retarded. This would indicate amelioration of the impairment of the learning criteria involved in mental retardation. There is a need for the effects of physical activity on intellectual functioning in retarded groups to be explored further.

Implications for social adjustment

Social adjustment as a qualifying condition of mental retardation refers to the individual's ability to maintain himself independently in the community, with reference to gainful employment and meeting personal and social responsibilities set by the community.

Because the mentally retarded will most likely use motor skills, rather than intellectual skills, in the pursuit of a vocation and because gains have been reported in the development of motor skills among the mentally retarded, motor proficiency has vocational implications for the mentally retarded. Increased motor proficiency may lead to such job possibilities as simple crafts or manual labor, domestic work, routine industrial work such as assembly and production line operations, and agricultural work. There is a need for identifying common psychomotor functions present in many vocations. Programs for the development of motor abilities that have vocational implications and would lead to a higher level of employability for those who are mentally retarded are greatly needed.

Motor proficiency also has implications for the social and recreational activities of mentally retarded persons. The physical educator is a primary source for the development of leisure skills in those who are mentally retarded. Typical persons have intellectual resources from which to draw for recreational experiences. These recreational experiences may include reading, opera, lectures, and social gatherings that have a high component of verbalization. On the other hand, mentally retarded persons are limited in the intellectual sphere and must draw heavily on motor activity for recreational experiences. For this reason, programs of physical education that carry over to recreational motor skills applicable to adult living are of the utmost importance for the mentally retarded. It must be remembered that recreational activity can contribute to the physical, social, and psychological aspects of self-satisfying living for mentally retarded individuals.

Implications for personal-social factors

The definition of mental retardation proposed by AAMD lists three personal-social factors that may contribute to the adaptive behavior criterion of mental retardation. They are (1) impairment in interpersonal relations, (2) responsiveness, and (3) cultural conformity. It is well accepted among physical educators that one of the basic objectives of a physical education program is the development of personal-social aspects of living. Therefore conscientious programs of physical education that fulfill this objective appear to be tools for ameliorating the adaptive behavior criterion of mental retardation.

Impairment in interpersonal relations reflects deficiencies in the individual's ability to relate adequately to peers or authority figures. It may also demonstrate an inability to recognize the needs of other persons in interpersonal interactions. The activities of physical education programs afford great opportunities for the development of interpersonal relations through participation in the games of our culture. It is accepted that many of the team games of current physical education programs require an individual to give up his own personal feelings for the good of the group and to play cooperatively in order to reach common goals. It is often necessary that the individual relate to authority figures to achieve the ends of an activity. The authority figure may be the official of the contest or the teacher. Development of these personal-social traits lies at the heart of the physical education program.

Deficient responsiveness is characterized by an inability to delay gratification of needs and a lack of long-range goal striving; it is also marked by responses of only biological and physical stimuli of comfort or discomfort. In physical activity, it is often necessary to withstand some discomfort to achieve a skill that a person has never before been able to do or to perform an act that has never before been done. This might be the case in the discomforts of learning to swim, tumble, catch a ball, or maintain any type of activity relating to endurance. Inability of mentally retarded children to persist at a physical task was illustrated by Auxter.[2] When mentally retarded children were to sustain a maximum muscular contraction on a hand dynamometer, it was found that they were significantly less capable than the typical children with whom they were being compared. Since psychological limits are reached more quickly than physiological limits, it may well be that the will to sustain activity contributes more to fatigue in a task than physiological endurance. Physical education programs for mentally retarded individuals may well provide the media for reducing lack of responsiveness on their part and contribute to the amelioration of the adaptive behavior criterion.

Deficiencies in cultural conformity reflect behavior that does not conform to social mores or meet standards of dependency, reliability, and trustworthiness. They also refer to behavior persistently asocial, antisocial, or excessively hostile. Physical education programs, as well as all other programs of education, attempt to transmit the desirable characteristics of our culture through their programs.

Implications for sensorimotor factors

In addition to personal-social factors contributing to the maladaptive behavior of those who are mentally retarded, impairment of sensorimotor factors contributes to the inability of persons to adapt their behavior. Reference to impairment in sensorimotor skills is made by the AAMD to disabilities, either gross or fine, in motor coordination. The development of sensorimotor skills of the mentally retarded individual lies within the domain of the physical educator. Indeed, this is one of the primary objectives of the physical education program. In the preschool years, motor activity plays a part in developing the senses. The development of motor skills has implications for the educational, vocational, social, and recreational activities of those who are mentally retarded and is certainly a contributing factor to the criterion of mental retardation of impaired adaptive behavior.

Although the available research reports a discrepancy in scores between retardates and normal individuals on motor tasks, significant improvement has been reported in multiple trial motor learning tasks.[5, 12, 15] This leads to the speculation that physical education programs for the mentally retarded, if conscientiously constructed and implemented, may be of consequence to the amelioration of sensorimotor deficiencies that contribute to the maladaptive behavior criterion of mental retardation.

CLASSIFICATION OF MENTALLY RETARDED PERSONS

Workers in the area of mental retardation recognize that those who are mentally retarded in the generic sense are not homogeneous in nature. Consequently, physicians, psychologists, educators, and sociologists have each evolved their own methods of classification. Mentally retarded persons have been classified according to psychological degree, educational purposes, and etiology; the classification according to etiology will not be discussed here.

Psychological classifications

The psychological classification of the AAMD considers primarily different degrees in mental retardation based on psychological evaluations. These groups are identified in terms of sigma scores on a psychological examination or IQ test. The classification of AAMD using the Stanford-Binet intelligence test as a guide is as follows:

1. Profoundly retarded, IQ under 19—requires complete custodial care.
2. Severely retarded, IQ 20-35—can be trained to care for some of his bodily needs; develops some language; has great difficulty in social and occupational areas.

3. Moderately retarded, IQ 36-51—usually unable to master academic skills; can be trained to perform daily routines; can usually perform in a sheltered workshop.
4. Mildly retarded, IQ 52-68—has some degree of educability in terms of reading and writing; is educable in the area of social and occupational competence.

Educational definitions

The terms "educable" and "trainable" are used to describe mentally retarded children who are found in special classes in the public schools. The educable child compares favorably in characteristics to those described as borderline and mildly retarded in the psychological classification. The IQ range may be anywhere from 50 to 80 or higher, depending on the statutes of the particular legislation of a particular state and the administrational procedures of the particular school. The problem of differentiating between those children who are to be educated in regular classes and those who are to be placed in special classes offered for mentally retarded children is one of paramount importance. The current

trend in legislation in some states is for inclusion of educable mentally retarded children in regular class "mainstreaming." The integrated concept calls for new instructional strategies on the part of physical education teachers because it requires teachers to utilize instructional procedures to accommodate differences in learning styles and performance variability.

The differences between trainable and educable mentally retarded children are that many educable mentally retarded children may be expected to maintain independent living in the community, whereas the trainable child, more than likely, will work within the environment of a sheltered workshop. The educable mentally retarded child is capable of learning some academic skills, but the trainable mentally retarded child usually is severely limited. Furthermore, recent legislation has made it possible for every child, regardless of level of functioning, to have the right to an education. Therefore many children who are profoundly and severely mentally retarded have been enrolled in public schools where

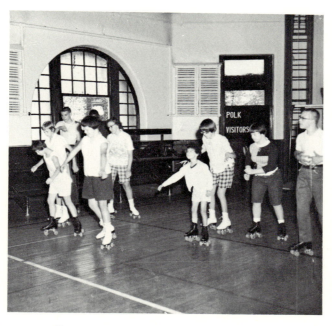

Fig. 15-1. Many mentally retarded children develop leisure skill activity. (Courtesy Neuromotor Therapy Program, Polk State School, Polk, Pa.)

their educational needs must be met. It is worth noting that nearly all the needs of the profoundly mentally retarded are physical and motor. Therefore modification of the physical education curricula and procedures for developing trained personnel are critical needs (Fig. 15-1).

PROGRAMS FOR MENTALLY RETARDED PERSONS

Physical education programs should be based on the nature and need of the learner. As mentioned previously, there is great variability among the mentally retarded population. This is attributable to inherent differences between high-grade and low-grade retardates, causations, and many other disorders that accompany mental retardation.

Associated disorders accompanying mental retardation may be sensory impairments such as blindness, being hard-of-hearing, or deafness; emotional disturbances; and neurological disorders such as cerebral palsy, muscular dystrophy, and problems in perception. It becomes evident that physical education programs for mentally retarded persons must meet a multitude of needs, at all age levels and at all levels of intellectual and physical development.

Differential diagnosis

It is a prevalent practice for the placement of children in special classes to be based on IQ. However, great differences exist among children who have the same IQ. Therefore the physical educator must be more concerned with the individual than with a tag that is designed for educational expediency. To understand the individual, the following suggested areas of diagnosis are listed:

1. *Consideration of associated disorders that accompany mental retardation:* Special educational techniques should be developed for children who are retarded deaf, retarded blind, retarded psychogenic, retarded with cerebral palsy, and slow learners who have partial sensory impairments.

2. *Neurological evaluation:* Electroencephalogram, neurological reflexes should be checked.

3. *Psychomotor examination:* Reaction time, speed of limb movement, aim, hand steadiness, and manual and finger dexterity are evaluated.

4. *Perceptual assessment:* Perceptual disorders may be disruptive in the learning of motor skills. The Frostig developmental scales[9] and the Kephart perceptual motor survey[17] should be employed for evaluation.

5. *Physical fitness test:* AAHPER physical fitness test and Fleishman's physical fitness test may be used.

6. *Motor fitness test:* Measures that include basic motor skills such as running, jumping, and throwing are needed.

7. *Motor developmental scales:* The Gesell developmental scales[10] are recommended.

8. *Etiology:* The individual with an organic case may be more severely retarded in the motor sphere than the cultural-familial retarded person may be.

Retardation in culturally deprived areas

Special programs must be designed for preschool children who show motor or mental retardation. Suggested physical education programs to serve preschool potential retarded persons residing in culturally deprived areas have been described by Kephart.[17] These programs are designed to develop generalized motor patterns, coordinate hand and eye, and develop what is described as body image. For the organic mentally retarded child, a program of motor exploration should be initiated with early training in self-help skills and locomotor development.

Programs for developing preschool motor skills

There are many mentally retarded children who function on motor skills at a preschool level. Mentally retarded children classified as trainable often fall into this group as do young educable mentally retarded children of the primary group. The basic needs of this particular group of mentally retarded children are management and control of the whole body. Therefore the program should be directed toward building a large repertoire of movement skills. These children should be made aware of the body in relation to other parts. There is a need for a great deal of random experimentation and gross body movement, particularly the exploration of gravitational forces. Activities that have proved successful at clinics for preschool mentally retarded children at Slippery Rock State College have been climbing activities on stall bars, tumbling and walking activities on an inclined board, and bouncing activities on a miniature trampoline. Gravitational forces challenge the children and exercise control of these activities. It is important to construct environments so that the child will always achieve some degree of success and still be challenged. Failure or the infliction of pain often makes subsequent participation in the activity undesirable.

One of the basic problems encountered by children in these types of activities is learning to transfer weight from foot to foot without losing balance. One of the primary objectives of the program involving countering gravitational forces is directed toward the enhancement of weight transfer. Another component of a program for preschool children who function at a preschool level on motor skills is the development of basic locomotor and play skills serving as the foundation for more complex skills used in the games of our culture. These skills include running, jumping, throwing, catching, striking, and kicking. This type of training is done by a directive purpose approach where there is a low ratio of instructors to children.

Gains can be made in ocular tracking skills of preschool retarded children by the implementation of catching activities. Objects of varying weights and sizes that travel at different rates of speed are caught by the mentally retarded children. The

speed of the object can be controlled and developmental programs in tracking objects can be implemented for the purpose of hand-eye coordination development. Rhythms also have proved to be popular with these children.

Some teaching suggestions for preschool mentally retarded children are the following:

1. Manipulate body parts manually to achieve desired movement patterns. (Verbal communication is difficult or impossible with some of these children.)
2. Demonstrate the activity. This is of invaluable assistance to these children.
3. Be firm, but accept them and use a positive approach. They often show reluctance to engage in activities; however, if the environment of the activity affords them security and if they have some measure of success as a result of performance, the children usually respond to the initiation of the activity at subsequent times.
4. Use strong auditory and visual cues to focus attention on the task at hand for the more severely retarded. Intensity of the stimulus is important to initiate and sustain activity.
5. Consider individual abilities in attention span.
6. Give encouragement when the children meet with success. However, encouragement should not be indiscriminate.
7. Keep records of progress.
8. Aim for progression in motor and social skills.

Objectives of physical education

The objectives of physical education programs for those who are mentally retarded are the same as the objectives of physical education programs for typical children. An examination of the priority of objectives for typical children, more often than not, reveals that the priority of objectives places intellectual or academic objectives highest on the list. It is in these endeavors that the child spends most of his time. The second priority of objectives favors preparation for a vocation. Typical children are taught skills to enable them to have opportunities to select from a variety of occupational endeavors. The objectives apparently receiving the least attention in the curriculum of the typical child are the social and physical objectives.

When the educational objectives of mentally retarded children are examined carefully, it becomes clear that the priority of these same objectives should be inverted. Inasmuch as trainable mentally retarded children fail in most academic tasks and educable mentally retarded children plateau in achievement of intellectual skills at an elementary level, this objective cannot be held in the same priority as for typical children. Vocationally, mentally retarded persons are usually trained for special occupations falling within their particular capabilities.

Although occupational competency is extremely important to those who are mentally retarded, there is impressive evidence that motor proficiency and social skills are more often the wherewithal of a successful occupation than are intellectual abilities. Therefore because of the extreme importance of physical and social objectives in the education of those who are mentally retarded, it is a necessity that no stone be left unturned in affording mentally retarded persons quality physical education programs. Fulfillment of social and physical development is the substance of physical education programs.

Examination of the subgroups of the mentally retarded with regard to educational objectives shows that it may be that the more severe the retardation, the more significant the physical objective.

Some suggested objectives of physical education for mentally retarded persons are as follows:

1. Development of physical fitness that, hopefully, will afford those who are mentally retarded a better opportunity to cope with their physical environment and give them greater will to live a full life, approaching everyday tasks with vigor.

2. Development of neuromuscular skills to afford opportunities for those who are mentally retarded to participate and enjoy the physical activities of our culture. In the case of the more severely retarded and younger mentally retarded children, development of sensorimotor and self-help skills to enable them to cope better with activities of everyday living is important.

3. Development of social skills through social interaction. Enhancement of both intergroup and interpersonal practices in the school and in the community is important.

4. Emotional development resulting in the ability to accept oneself and others in everyday life situations and the ability to face deterring limitations.

5. Intellectual development resulting in the ability to assemble data, organize information, and remember. In more severely retarded children, ability to discriminate among colors, sizes, shapes, and sounds, as well as to develop perceptual abilities, is worthy of pursuit.

A diagnostic prescriptive approach

The work of Kephart[17] points to the serious consequences of preschool children who lag behind established motor developmental scales. It has been suggested that, in the early years, motor, social, emotional, and psychological development are closely related. Early diagnosis and prognosis for all children who lag behind developmental norms in the motor sphere are recommended. The diagnosis should not be a method to pin a label on a child; it should be a description of the person's needs, characteristics, abilities, and necessary remediation.

Hints for teaching

Those who are mentally retarded are a very heterogeneous group. Many techniques of instruction are necessary to solicit a desired response. Therefore it is difficult to make generalizations that may be helpful in the instruction of all who are mentally retarded in physical education activities. However, as a guide, some teaching hints follow:

1. Consider individual differences when selecting the activities. It is possible to play many games that account for differences in abilities among class members.

2. Select activities according to the needs of those who are mentally retarded.

3. Select activities to meet the children's interest level. However, precautions should be taken against participation in one particular activity to the exclusion of others. Be aware of the development of rigid play behaviors.

4. Do not underestimate the abilities of mentally retarded children to perform skilled movements. There is a tendency to set goals too low for these children. This is particularly true for educable mentally retarded children from cultural-familial backgrounds.

5. Develop recreational skills that make it possible for those who are mentally retarded to integrate socially with members of their family and peers, now and in later life.

6. Select skills primarily on the basis of the development of motor skills. In the past, mental age and chronological age have played too great a part in the selection of physical activities; however, in many instances, they may be irrelevant criteria for the selection of activities.

7. Structure the environment in which the activity takes place so that it challenges the child, yet frees him from the fear of physical hurt and gives him the satisfaction of some degree of success.

8. The lower grade mentally retarded child must be taught to play. This means that physical education is responsible for creating the play environment, developing basic motor skills that are the tools of play, and, occasionally, initiating the activity.

9. The play environment must be one of safety. However, a safe play environment does not necessarily mean that the instructor should provide security to the extent that the child places undue dependency on the instructor for physical safety.

10. Use manual guidance as a method of instruction. The proprioceptors are great teachers of movement. Manual guidance is more important in the younger and more severely mentally retarded children. The less ability the child has to communicate verbally, the greater the consideration manual guidance should have as a tool for instruction.

11. Work for progression in skill development. Use the motor developmental scales for preschool retardates and teaching progression methods used for typical children for those mentally retarded children functioning above the preschool level.

12. Work for active participation on the part of all mentally retarded students.

13. Adapt the activities to the abilities of *each* child. No blanket programs for those who are mentally retarded, as a generic group, should be used.

14. Convey to mentally retarded persons that they are persons of worth, reinforcing their strengths and minimizing their weaknesses.

15. Be patient and content to settle for smaller and slower gains in more severely retarded persons. Often, gains that seem small when compared to typical children are tremendous for the more severely mentally retarded.

16. Use strong visual and auditory stimuli for the more severely retarded children as these often bring the best results.

17. Have many activities at hand from which to draw as attention span is short.

18. Use demonstration as an effective tool for instruction.

19. Keep verbal directions to a minimum. In the cases of more severely retarded children, they are often ineffective.

20. Provide a broad spectrum of activities

having recreational and social significance for later life.

Physical education programs

Because of the heterogeneity of those who are mentally retarded, it is recognized that many types of programs must be developed to meet the needs of all mentally retarded children. The following description of aspects of physical education programs for the mentally retarded children will be broad and generalizations will be made with reference to the generic group called mentally retarded. The aspects of

the physical education program to consider are development of basic skills, development of physical fitness, development of specific skills, and recreation.

Development of basic skills

Basic motor skills refer to the movement patterns that occur in successive stages of development, such as crawling, creeping, walking, running, jumping, hopping, skipping, leaping, and throwing. Knowledge and application of the development of the basic skills may serve as a guide to the physical educator in identify-

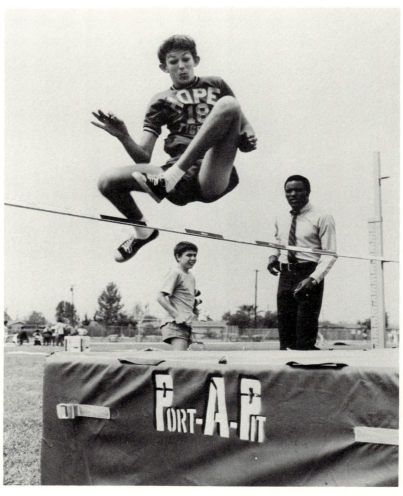

Fig. 15-2. Mentally retarded children may become proficient in sports skills. (Courtesy Western Special Olympics, California, 1971.)

ing the current level of functioning of a particular mentally retarded child and provides information for the subsequent selection of activity.

Attention should also be given to the acquisition of gross motor movements, which, when combined, may form discernible skills. Bending, bouncing, balancing, carrying, and climbing are examples of these gross motor movements.

At the lower levels of mental retardation, the profound, severe, or moderate degree of retardation, in many cases, will determine the ends in motor development that may ultimately be achieved. The more profound the retardation, in general, the lower are the limits of ultimate performance. Profoundly mentally retarded children may develop self-care skills and minimal locomotor skills.

Development of physical fitness

The development of physical fitness must occupy high priority in the objectives of a physical education program for those who are mentally retarded. Research has shown that physical fitness levels of mentally retarded persons can be improved.[20] Basic components of physical fitness that have been identified and that result from vigorous physical exercises are strength, muscular endurance, flexibility, and cardiovascular endurance.

Activities contributing to the development of these characteristics of physical fitness are calisthenics, partner activities that include dual stunts, tumbling, combative games, self-testing activities, relays, games, ladders, jungle gyms, climbing ropes, jump ropes, and gymnasium apparatus.

Development of strength, muscular and cardiovascular endurance, and flexibility are discussed in previous sections of the text (Chapters 5, 10, and 12).

Development of specific skills

Physical education programs for mentally retarded persons should also include opportunities to develop motor skills to enable these persons to participate in the sports activities of our culture. Such activities include gymnastic stunts, trampoline activity, swimming, ice skating, roller skating, bicycling, track events, wrestling, volleyball, hockey, skiing, baseball, soccer, basketball, bowling, golf, and handball. All the lead-up games that serve as forerunners to these more complex activities should be taught in small progressive units (Chapters 4 and 8).

Recreation

Recreational opportunities for those who are mentally retarded (Figs. 15-2 and 15-3) should be provided after the school day terminates, during school vacations, and after formal educational training. There should be adequate provision in the recreation program for vigorous activity such as sports, dancing, active games, swimming, and hiking. Intramural and community sports leagues should be provided for the purpose of using skills developed in the instructional program. In addition, winter outdoor activities such as ice skating, skiing, and snow games should be made available to those who are mentally retarded. It should be remembered that camping and outdoor education programs are other ways of affording expression of skills and interests.

In conjunction with the recreation program, special events scheduled throughout the school year serve to stimulate interests, motivate the children, and inform the community about the progress of the physical education program and the abilities achieved by mentally retarded children. Examples of such events are demonstrations for PTA meetings, track-and-field meets, swimming meets, play days, sports days, pass-punt-kick contests, hikes, and bicycle races.

Volunteers

When working with more severely retarded children, individual attention is often required. Volunteers trained in specific duties can be of assistance to the instructional program as well as to after-

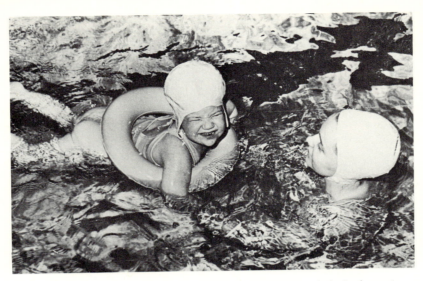

Fig. 15-3. A mentally retarded child learns what she can do in the water.

school and vacation recreation programs. Sources of recruitment for volunteers may be service clubs, women's clubs colleges, high schools, and associations for mentally retarded persons.

SUPPLEMENTAL PHYSICAL EDUCATION PROGRAMS

Mentally retarded children, if at all possible, should be integrated with their peers in regular physical enducation classes. In the event that they cannot participate successfully in regular classes, they should be given special developmental physical education commensurate with their capacity and needs. It is recognized that the regular physical education class may not provide adequate placement for all mentally retarded children. Those who are mentally retarded are behind the norms socially and physically to the extent that they are not motivated to participate with members of the regular class. Consequently, they are often found on the periphery of activity and do not involve themselves in the games and activities of the physical education class. When attempting to integrate, an effort must be made to integrate mentally retarded persons in class activi-

ties. However, if this is not possible, special physical education programs should be adapted to the particular needs of the child.

It is also suggested that any mentally retarded child who can be successfully integrated socially in the unrestricted physical education program, but who has physical or motor deficiencies, receive supplementary physical education to remedy or ameliorate the particular diagnosed motor deficiency. In many instances, erroneous assumptions are made relative to the physical abilities of a person labeled mentally retarded. It is worth noting that, in many instances, mentally retarded boys from special classes are proficient athletes in interscholastic athletics.

EXTENDED OPPORTUNITIES BEYOND FORMAL EDUCATION

Opportunities to learn motor skills and participate in recreation utilizing those skills learned should be available to all beyond the normal years of public-sponsored education. Activities taught during the formal years of schooling must be able to find expression in the form of recreational opportunities at a time subsequent to leaving school. These opportunities should be available to mentally retarded persons of all ages. Physical education for those who are mentally retarded is a relatively recent development. Those who have been deprived of opportunities to participate and learn motor skills should be provided with opportunities to learn these skills and to gain new insights into learning the use of leisure time through physical activity. The desired aspects of physical fitness for the particular age and characteristics of a retarded person should be a part of the extended physical education program.

THE HOME PROGRAM

The amount of time that the physical educator personally will be involved with the mentally retarded child is relatively small. If maximum benefits are to be derived from programs, it is necessary to have a follow-up of activities taught in the form of a home program. Therefore an educational program for parents describing the program to which the children are exposed and the purpose of the program should be provided for implementation in the home. Parents should receive direction and assistance in methods for involving their children in physical activity taking place in the neighborhood and the home.

DEVELOPMENTAL APPROACH AND SEVERELY MENTALLY RETARDED PERSONS

Many profoundly and severely mentally retarded children, in the past, were not included in the process of public education. However, recent legislation and court decisions have made it mandatory that such children receive appropriate education (Chapter 1). As a result, many severely mentally impaired children with limited ability to function in motor skills are now in our public schools. Many of these children are nonambulatory and lack the ability to engage in self-help skills. Therefore motor development is one of their most critical needs. Increased opportunities for physical educators to participate in the motor development of those who are severely handicapped constitute a great challenge.

Many children who are severely handicapped function on motor development scales in the first year of life. It is necessary, through assessment, to determine, with great precision, where these children lie on a motor development continuum, so that purposive programming can be structured for them.

Motor development curriculum

The curriculum for the severely handicapped child who functions on a chronological age scale in the first year of life is rather limited. For the most part, the curriculum is composed of the development of prerequisite abilities that lay the foundation for more complex skills. Often, programming involves motor behaviors that are marks that have been established by researchers in growth and development. However, before these motor landmarks can be achieved, it is necessary for the child to develop several sensorimotor prerequisites. Great precision must be exercised in the implementation of programming according to the principles of learning and development.

Accountability

The financial resources that are necessary to carry out programs for severely mentally handicapped persons are considerable. Low pupil-teacher ratios are usually required to engage these children in the instructional process. There is considerable interest in the accountability of learned behaviors of handicapped children as a result of programming. One way to account for the effects of programming on the development is to calculate as follows:

1. Administer a test to the child that can be translated in terms of rate of development.
2. Compute the rate of development (developmental age [DA] divided by chronological age [CA]).
3. Intervene with the program.
4. Compare the rate of development after

the intervention with the rate at the initial evaluation for changes.

An example of this would be the following:

June, 1976 $\quad \dfrac{\text{DA 1 year}}{\text{CA 8 years}}$ or

$$\dfrac{12 \text{ months}}{96 \text{ months}} = 0.125 \text{ rate of development}$$

June, 1977 $\quad \dfrac{\text{DA 21 months}}{\text{CA 9 years}}$ or

$$\dfrac{21 \text{ months}}{108 \text{ months}} = 0.19 \text{ rate of development}$$

The total rate of development has increased as a result of intervention. Thus there is a need for two types of measurement in the implementation of accountable programming. They are criterion measurement for program activities that have been achieved through programming and changes in developmental rates through intervention.

Communications of program results

Parents and consumer advocates are concerned with the educational progress of handicapped children. Therefore there is a need to translate the program results of their children to parents in behavioral terms. It is desirable to have graphic information that communicates what children have gained as a result of the program. Such graphic procedures require a curriculum from which progress can be measured. This curriculum represents a series of behavioral objectives that are linked together to form a process to which measurement can be ascribed. This is extremely important for personnel working in motor development with severely handicapped children because it enables implementers to measure the instructional results obtained.

Behaviors derived from motor development scales

Bayley,[3] Gesell and Amatruda,[10] and Frankenburg and Dodds[8] have devised motor development scales and assessment tasks that indicate the developmental levels of children. The skills on these scales may be used to assess the developmental levels of severely handicapped children who function at low levels. Although some of the behaviors on the developmental scales are prerequisite to one another, others are not. There is a need to identify those behaviors that are prerequisite to one another on the scales so that orderly progression can be constructed within scales that can be followed in the implementation of programming.

Cephalocaudal development

Children develop from the head to the foot (cephalocaudal development).[20] The application of this principle of development provides guidelines to the implementation of programming for severely handicapped children because it provides the focus for programming developmental purposes. For instance, if a child can lift the head while in the prone position, it may be raised increasingly high. The increased height that the head is raised is indicative of greater development in the cephalocaudal direction because the spinal area closer to the foot is being activated. There is further need of development along this continuum when the child attempts to sit erect. It is then necessary for the child to control the musculature in the lumbar region of the spine so the sitting behavior may be maintained. At a later point in development, control must be gained so the hips, knees, and ankles may move with facility and locomotion may take place. Thus strength and endurance of the musculature along the cephalocaudal continuum must be gained before the prerequisite behaviors of cephalocaudal control can be acquired. In the severely handicapped child, this is often most difficult. The skeleton and the body, which have developed through the process of maturation, often have gained weight incommensurate with the strength and endurance necessary to maintain control of the body. Therefore programs that are designed to develop pre-

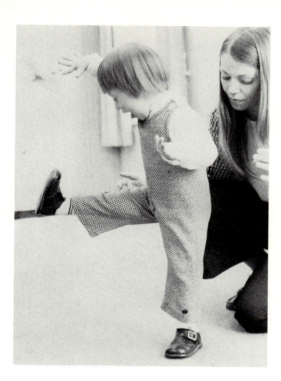

Fig. 15-4. Balancing on one foot is an ability that can be transferred to skills such as stair climbing and many other movement behaviors.

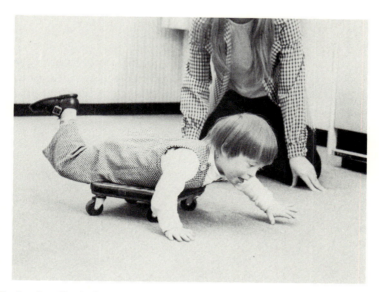

Fig. 15-5. Proximodistal development can be assessed by the movement pattern of the arms as a child moves the scooter. Some children move the scooter from the elbows, using only the shoulder muscles. Others move it with the hand, using the elbow and shoulder muscles. The more highly developed child derives force from the shoulder, elbow, and wrist. This is the higher form of proximodistal development.

requisite strength and endurance are of importance (Fig. 15-4).

Proximodistal development

Another concept of development that provides guidelines for programming is the application of the principle of proximodistal development. This deals with the concept that development proceeds from the midline outward to the extremities. It is possible, through observation of children's movements, to receive information concerning the focus of where most of the programming should be directed, for instance, if most of the movement occurs at the shoulders with little movement at the elbow, the focus of the programming should be directed at the elbow, with activities that integrate the shoulder and the elbow. If the activities involve primarily movement of the elbow and shoulder, movements should be programmed that involve the wrist and require integration of the wrist, elbow, and shoulder. Thus the procedures involve observation of activity at each joint and functional integration with other joints proceeding from the proximal to the distal structures (Fig. 15-5).

Specific and general abilities. It is possible to teach specific skills that incorporate the integration of fingers, wrists, elbows, and shoulders without the application of the principle of proximodistal development. However, there may be a tendency for the skill to be specific and each such skill will have to be learned as distinct and separate. However, the development of proximodistal principles will enable the child to generalize movement patterns to acquire several skills. The facility of learning and a host of other skills will be enhanced. Therefore there is a need to develop both specific skills and movement patterns that facilitate the development of the proximodistal principle (Fig. 15-6).

Types of programs for severely handicapped children

Three categories of motor programming for those who are severely handicapped will be discussed. They are the following:
1. Specific skills that enable social adaptation to the environment
2. Landmark motor behaviors (crawling, creeping, sitting, rolling over, standing, walking, etc.) that serve as guidelines

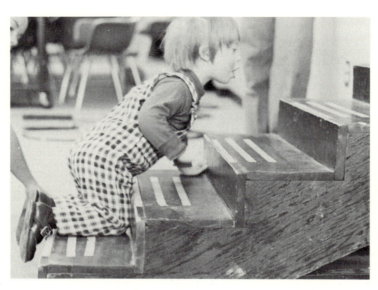

Fig. 15-6. Basic motor skills may be generalized to other movement behaviors. The child has generalized the specific skill of creeping to climbing the staircase.

in development as indicated on developmental scales

3. Ability traits (strength, endurance, flexibility, balance) that serve as prerequisites for skills

Motor diagnosis and prescription (Fig. 15-7)

There must be a direct relationship between the assessment information on a target objective and the programming that will assist in reaching the stated objective. An example of diagnostic and program integrity may involve a child who has been assessed on a developmental scale as not being able to sit erect. This becomes a target behavior and it is then necessary to direct programming that will develop the behavior of sitting. Such programming may include the development of balance from a sitting position and of strength of the musculature that controls the head, including thoracic and lumbar extensors of the spine. Such programming would bear a direct relationship to the assessment of this particular behavior. If a child has been diagnosed as having impaired manipulative

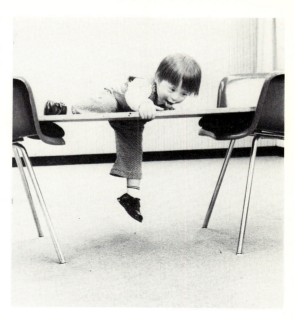

Fig. 15-7. The diagnosis of the ability to climb can be measured by the height of the object over which the body is to move. The programming measures increased efficiency to climb greater heights. The diagnosis and prescription must be in direct relationship to one another.

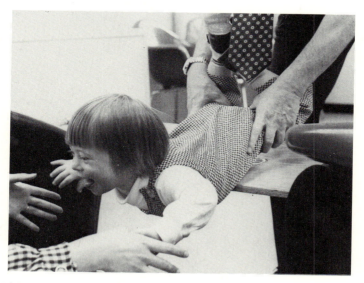

Fig. 15-8. This task is designed to develop the thoracic extensor muscles of the upper back. It is an important activity for appropriate postural development, which is lacking in many severely handicapped children.

skills and cannot execute a pincer grasp, he should be programmed to perform tasks where the pincer grasp is used. The diagnostic test indicates the nature of the programming. The effectiveness of the programming is therefore measured by progress of the child in a positive direction from the base level performance to the target behavior (Fig. 15-8).

Hendricks[14] indicates a relationship between the development of the visual mechanism and the posturing mechanism. The development of control of the posturing mechanism enables the head to right. This affords opportunity for the visual mechanism to be appropriately placed so that it may develop. As the visual mechanism increases in capability, the posturing mechanism rights so that more environmental information may be utilized. Thus there is a need for considering the reciprocal functioning of the posturing and visual mechanism when programming (Figs. 15-9 and 15-10).

As the posturing mechanism is activated, it enables the visual mechanism to develop; head righting also tends to activate the manipulative activity of the child. With increased activity in the manipulation of objects, involving the hand and the eye, perceptual information about objects can be stored through acquiring information by pairing what is felt by the hand and what is seen by the eyes. An essential interrelationship that must be made to facilitate the development of visuomotor abilities of the severely handicapped child is the strength and endurance of the musculature that rights the body. This, in turn, places the visual mechanism where it can more effi-

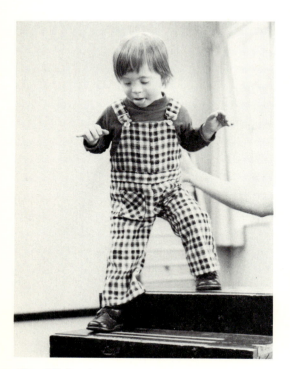

Fig. 15-9. The child's visual mechanism is activated when the eye fixates on foot placement on the stair tread.

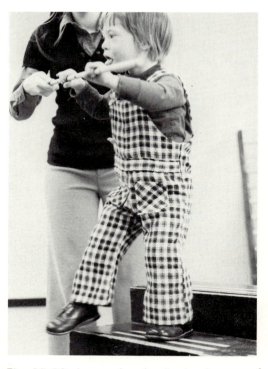

Fig. 15-10. A procedure for the development of kinesthetic awareness of foot placement requires that vision be directed away from the foot. A firm prompt is applied so the child may be successful on the task.

ciently function to interpret environmental objects and events. With the visual mechanism appropriately positioned, greater possibility exists for the eye to inspect the hand and for its manipulation of objects to gain information about the objects, leading to greater hand-eye coordination.

Task analysis

Task analysis is a procedure that can be applied to determine the appropriate selection of activity for a terminal objective for a learner. The analysis can begin at any level, with any stated instructional objective, and asks the question, "To accomplish this behavior, what prerequisites must the learner be able to perform?" For each be-

havior so identified, the same question is asked; thus a hierarchy of objectives based on testable prerequisites is generated. The behavior can begin at any level and always specifies prerequisite components, according to Glaser and Nitko.[11] The task analysis is an essential tool for deriving instructional objectives for severely handicapped children. Task analysis is especially appropriate in the development of self-help skills that involve motor development (Figs. 15-11 and 15-12).

Task analysis of self-help skills

The development of self-help skills that will assist severely handicapped persons in independent self-fulfilling living are of the

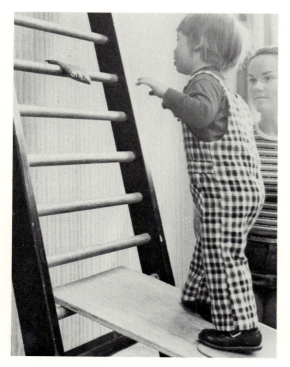

Fig. 15-11. A task analysis of a mature walking skill.

Task analysis	Activity
Walk with vision off of the skill.	A bean bag is placed on the ladder so the visual mechanism focuses on it rather than the feet.
Elaborate the walking pattern.	An inclined walking surface has been designed.

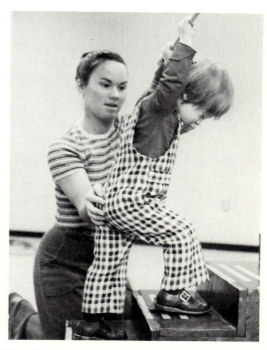

Fig. 15-12. An activity to develop stair climbing skills through task analysis.

Task analysis	Treatment
Keep vision on foot.	The eye must focus on feet.
Maintain dynamic balance.	The stick and implementor's hand prompt the movement of the child up the staircase.

CRITERION PERFORMANCE MEASURE: Demonstrate the ability to feed yourself with a spoon in a socially acceptable manner.

Feeding behavior	Criterion for mastery
1. Sit in chair at table.	Hold the head and trunk erect with no support to the back.
2. Grasp the spoon.	Use a pincer grasp, with the spoon resting on the third finger.
3. Scoop the food.	Scoop from ¾ to 1 teaspoonful.
4. Move the food to the mouth.	Do not spill the food.
5. Accept the food from the spoon.	Move all the food from the spoon into the mouth.
6. Move the food to where it can be mastered.	Keep the tongue in the mouth as the food is moved through the chewing mechanism.
7. Chew the food.	Utilize the teeth and make at least three chews.
8. Swallow the food.	Keep the head in an erect position.
9. Return the spoon to the dish to repeat the process.	Look toward where the next intended bite of food will come from.

---

utmost importance. A task analysis curriculum may be developed through analyzing the prerequisites of various skills. Once the prerequisites have been identified, the child is assessed on each behavior prerequisite to the analyzed skill. From this assessment, a profile of acquired and unacquired behaviors is derived. Subcurricular areas that need development are identified. Thus instruction may proceed from this assessment. The boxed material above presents a task analysis of a feeding skill with prerequisite behaviors of mastery identified for the learner and appropriate programming suggested to facilitate the development of the feeding skill by the learner.

Task analysis of locomotor skills

Severely handicapped persons are often persons who are nonambulatory or who cannot move with efficiency in their environment. Therefore an essential prerequisite for gaining greater independence is the development of a more appropriate means of locomotion. The target objectives of locomotor patterns will vary depending on the developmental level of the child. Basic

movement skills include rolling, crawling, creeping, and walking. Locomotor skills of a higher order, running, hopping, skipping, galloping, and leaping, are often outside the capability of severely handicapped persons (Fig. 15-13).

Task analysis can be applied to locomotor development. If a child cannot grasp with the hands, the diagnostic test must assess his ability along a continuum of behaviors related to the pincer grasp. The effectiveness of the programming is therefore measured by the child's progress in a positive direction, from initially assessed levels of performance to more proficient behaviors along the developmental continuum of pincer grasp behaviors.

If a person cannot walk, a long-range goal often becomes the ability to walk so as to master greater control over the environment. Thus an anatomical analysis might assess movement prerequisites at hip, knee, and ankle joints in relation to the ability areas of flexibility, strength, and endurance. An evaluation of each ability trait is then made at each joint. It is not uncommon for children to possess deficient gaits as a result of loss of range of motion

Table 15-1. Assessment of walking

Anatomi-cal part	Flexibility	Strength	Endurance
Hip	90 degrees	Kneeling or standing	Can stand erect for 7 seconds
Knee	25 degrees	Cannot support weight (stand)	
Ankle	20 degrees	Cannot support weight (stand)	

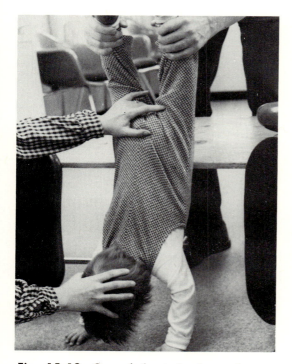

Fig. 15-13. One of the tasks that a learner must perform as a result of a task analysis of the forward roll is to move to a tuck position when the trunk is in an inverted position. A prompting procedure is employed to break up a reflex so the tuck position may be assumed to eventually perform a modified forward roll.

in the ankle, knee, or hip. Table 15-1 presents a sample evaluation of assessment of a walking behavior. This table gives the implementor some indication as to where an anatomical breakdown may result to impair the development of prerequisites for the skills. However, it does not answer the question of deficiencies in patterns of movement involving coordination or movement-balancing prerequisites. These require further analysis. (See Chapter 4 for this type of planning.)

The development of locomotor movement usually requires detailed analysis of all parameters of motor functioning related to the training of the motor patterns with the further isolation and control of the development of each component of the skill. This curriculum procedure is followed by integration of the developed components into functional movement patterns.

Application of learning principles

The curriculum for the severely handicapped child in motor development should be composed of hierarchical, sequential behavioral objectives. With the formulation of behavioral objectives, there is the need to teach new behaviors. Thus it becomes imperative that learning principles be appropriately applied to the learners if they are to progress properly in the developmental continuum. Some aspects of the learning principles that may assist in the development of appropriate behaviors are as follows:

1. *Application of shaping procedures:* Determining the specific sequence of steps that are small enough to enable the child to be successful and yet progress toward the target behavior.
2. *Prompting procedure:* Assisting the child in the response so he may be successful.
3. *Fading the prompt:* Using the minimum amount of prompt necessary.
4. *Reinforcement component building:* Pairing neutral and positive reinforcers, then fading the positive so a transfer to the neutral occurs.
5. *Identification of reinforcers:* Determin-

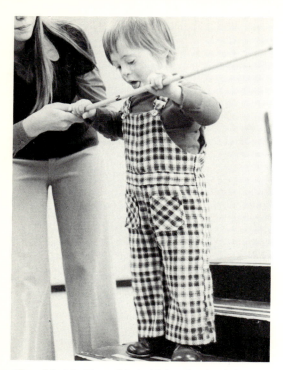

Fig. 15-14. The stick held by the implementor is a prompt that can assist the child to learn to walk up and down the stairs.

ing that a consequence of the performance will strengthen desired behaviors.

6. *Application of learning principles:* Practicing a sequence of (a) reward immediately; (b) reward after, not before; and (c) reinforcement of the correct behavior, being fair, honest, and clear.[16] In addition to these, there are several other principles that can be applied to programming.

It is necessary to apply learning principles to make the instructional processes come alive. The learning process is an essential part of the total delivery system for the severely handicapped child (Figs. 15-14 and 15-15).

Component building

An important instructional technique to apply when working with severely handicapped children is to build the components of the operant learning system. The components of the learning system that need to be built are (1) a greater number of stimulus properties to which the learner may respond and (2) a greater number of

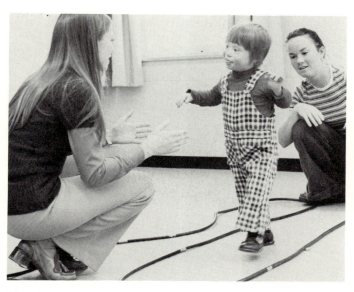

Fig. 15-15. The designed pathway where child is to walk can be narrowed. Thus the walking behavior can be shaped. An implementor waits to apply the learning principle of immediacy of reinforcement when the child walks the pathway without touching the boundaries.

responses that may be used as reinforcers for the child. The procedures for the building of components of the learning process are described in greater detail elsewhere.[18] The procedure of building the components of the learning system involves the pairing of a positive and a neutral stimulus to elicit a response. After repeated pairing, the positive stimulus may be withdrawn; it is hoped that a transfer of the positive to the previously neutral stimulus occurs. The same procedure may be used in building a reinforcer. In the case of building response capability, manual movement of the body can be applied and, through the physical prompting and fading procedure, motoric function that was not possessed before can be given to the child. With the capability of building stimulus, response, and reinforcement capacity for an existing response repertoire, it may then be possible for all children to learn instructional tasks that lie within their grasp. Therefore appropriate programming for the severely handicapped child consists of appropriate selection of objectives through task analysis and the proper application of learning principles to ensure that the objective will be achieved.

Use of the systems approach

There appears to be increased emphasis on the employment of a systems approach to education for the handicapped. Inasmuch as severely mentally impaired children possess limited capability to learn on their own, systematic instruction is a critical need to further their motor development. A systems approach involves a solution to a large problem. The optimal motor development of severely handicapped children is a large problem. To solve this problem, all the components that are brought to bear on the problem need to be identified, isolated, and developed through controls. Some of these components of the instructional process are the following:

1. Developmental curriculum
2. Assessment instruments
3. Programming of the child in the curriculum
4. Application of learning principles
5. Training of personnel
6. Management of personnel with learners
7. Home training programs

When these components have been identified and developed, it is then necessary to establish relationships among the system components, as follows:

1. The diagnostic instrumentation and the program
2. The curriculum and the needs of the learner
3. The program at school and the program in the home
4. The training of implementation personnel for the school and for the home
5. The application of learning principles among personnel
6. The management formats to interforce personnel, pupils, and curriculum
7. The program continuity for the child among teachers (so progress of the child may be continuous)

• • •

Additional information about the developmental approach and the systems approach in dealing with disadvantaged persons in our population is presented in Chapter 4.

REFERENCES

1. Abeson, A., Bolick, H., and Hass, J.: A primer on due process: education decisions for handcapped, Except. Child. 42:68-74, 1975.
2. Auxter, D. M.: Muscular fatigue of mentally retarded children, Train. Sch. Bull. 63:5-10, 1966.
3. Bayley, N.: The development of motor activities during the first three years, Monogr. Soc. Res. Child Dev. 1:1-26, 1935.
4. Blatt, B., editor: Education of handicapped children in Rhode Island, Providence, R.I., 1963, Rhode Island Legislative Commission to Study the Education of Handicapped Youth.
5. Carrier, N., Malpass, N., and Orton, K.: Responses to learning tasks of bright, normal and retarded children, technical bulletin, Project 578, OE-35073, Washington, D.C.,

1961, U.S. Office of Education, Cooperative Research Program.

6. Cratty, B. J.: Perceptual-motor behavior and educational process, Springfield, Ill., 1969, Charles C Thomas, Publisher.

7. Delacato, C. H.: The diagnosis and treatment of speech and reading problems, Springfield, Ill., 1965, Charles C Thomas, Publisher.

8. Frankenburg, W. K., and Dodds, J. B.: The Denver Developmental Scale, Boulder, Colo., 1968, University of Colorado Medical Center.

9. Frostig, M.: Administration and scoring manual for the Marianne Frostig Developmental Test and visual perception, Palo Alto, Calif., 1964, Consulting Psychologists Press.

10. Gesell, A., and Amatruda, C. S.: Developmental diagnosis, New York, 1965, Harper & Row, Publishers.

11. Glaser, R., and Nitko, A. J.: Measurement in learning and instruction. In Thorndike, R. L., editor: Educational measurement, ed. 2, Washington, D.C., 1970, American Council on Education.

12. Gordon, S., O'Connor, N., and Tizzard, J.: Some effects of incentives on the performance of imbeciles, Br. J. Psychol. **45**:277-287, 1955.

13. Grossman, H. J.: Manual on terminology and classification in mental retardation, Baltimore, 1973, Garamond & Pridemarks Press.

14. Hendricks, H.: The vision development process. In Wold, R. M., editor: Visual and perceptual aspects for the achieving and underachieving child, Seattle, 1969, Special Child Publications.

15. Hohman, P.: The relationship between general mental development and manual dexterity, Br. J. Psychol. **23**:279-283, 1933.

16. Homme, L., and Tosti, D.: Behavior technology: motivation and contingency management (units I and II), San Rafael, Calif., 1971, Individual Learning Systems, Inc.

17. Kephart, N. C.: The slow learner in the classroom, Columbus, Ohio, 1961, Charles E. Merrill Publishing Co.

18. Lindsley, O.: Direct measurement and prosthesis for retarded behavior. J. Educ. **148**:57-79, 1965.

19. Oliver, J. H.: The effects of physical conditioning exercises and activities on the mental characteristics of educationally subnormal boys, Br. J. Educ. Psychol. **28**:155-165, 1958.

20. Rarick, G. L.: Motor development during infancy and childhood. (Mimeographed.) Madison, Wis., 1954, University of Wisconsin.

21. Strauss, A. A., and Kephart, N. C.: Psychopathology and education of the brain-injured child, New York, 1955, Grune & Stratton, Inc.

RECOMMENDED READINGS

Bureau of Special Education, Pa.: Challenge to change program guidelines in physical education for the mentally retarded, Harrisburg, Pa., 1972, Pennsylvania Department of Education.

Cratty, B. J.: Developmental sequences of perceptual-motor tasks, Freeport, N.Y., 1967, Educational Activities, Inc.

Cruickshank, W. M., editor: Psychology of exceptional children and youth, Englewood Cliffs, N.J., 1971, Prentice-Hall, Inc.

Drowatsky, J. N.: Physical education for the mentally retarded, Philadelphia, 1971, Lea & Febiger.

Fait, H. F.: Special physical education, Philadelphia, 1972, W. B. Saunders Co.; visual, 59; auditory, 72; orthopedic, 83; cardiopathic, 97, 113-144; mentally retarded, 190; socially maladjusted, 212-225; learning disability, 168-182.

Gallahue, D. L., Werner, P. H., and Luedke, G. C.: A conceptual approach to moving and learning, New York, 1975, John Wiley & Sons, Inc.

Hirst, C. C., and Michaelis, E.: Developmental activities for children in special education, Springfield, Ill., 1972, Charles C Thomas, Publisher.

Kirk, S. A.: Educating exceptional children, Boston, 1972, Houghton Mifflin Co.

Kirk, S. A., and Weiner, B. B.: Behavioral research on exceptional children, Reston, Va., 1963, The Council for Exceptional Children.

Recreation and physical activity for the mentally retarded, Reston, Va., 1966, The Council for Exceptional Children and American Association for Health, Physical Education, and Recreation.

Wedemeyer, A.: Learning games for exceptional children, Denver, 1971, Love Publishing Co.

Zwiren, M. L.: Mental retardation: how can we help? J. Am. Health, Phys. Educ. Rec. **43**:79, 1972.

16

EMOTIONAL DISTURBANCES

■ In recent years, there has been increased awareness by educators of the incidence of emotional disturbance in the public schools. It is estimated that of the 1,300,000 seriously disturbed children in the United States, only 18% are receiving educational service and treatment. Obviously, the need and demand for professional help in the mental health area greatly exceeds the availability of qualified professional personnel and treatment facilities. Therefore it is becoming important that educational personnel learn how to deal with the problems of those who are emotionally disturbed in the normal school setting.

The function of the school is changing from the teaching of academic subjects and stimulating the intellect to meeting the total needs of children. Therefore it is becoming necessary for schools to cope with emotionally disturbed children, whether it is through integration in the regular school setting or placement in a special class for emotionally disturbed children. Children with emotional disturbances often confront physical educators with an impaired ability to learn motor skills and can thus create management problems in the gymnasium. There is an obvious need to employ methods and materials that will provide adequate classroom management and physical education programs that will optimally assist these children to lead self-satisfying, independent lives.

Criteria of disturbance, differences in diagnostic procedures, and inabilities to establish baselines of abnormality make identification of emotionally disturbed children difficult. If children beset with affectional, physical, social, and adult-model deprivations; victims of unrealistic standards; and those resorting to an antisocial code of life were added together, over 20% of the children in the public schools would be considered to have an identifiable learning or emotional disability. Obviously, educators have an opportunity to make great gains in meeting the needs of these children.

There is a trend evolving in which educators are required to provide services that meet the unique needs of emotionally disturbed children. This trend has been apparent with the provision of increased services to more emotionally disturbed children and may be indicative of the following:

1. Increased awareness on the part of educators for establishing special programs to meet the educational needs of emotionally disturbed children
2. Better methods of diagnosis and identification
3. Greater incidence of emotional disturbance among the public school population
4. A combination of these factors

At any rate, this information points to the importance of the development of physical education programs that will meet the needs of emotionally disturbed children.

The term "emotional disturbance" covers a multitude of traits, personality patterns, and behaviors. There is a difference between an "emotionally disturbed" child and a child whose behavior indicates a state of emotional disturbance. Whereas the latter term carries the connotation that a person is confronted with conflict and may be in jeopardy of becoming "emotionally disturbed," a person who is "emotionally disturbed" is considered to possess limited, inflexible, and restricted behavior that impairs adaptation to changing environments. The subsequent results often are accompanied with a reduction of behavioral freedom.

CHARACTERISTICS OF EMOTIONALLY DISTURBED PERSONS

Emotionally disturbed children, as a group, are heterogeneous. This becomes apparent when a person views the behavior of an emotionally disturbed child who is hyperactive and compares this behavior with that of an emotionally disturbed child who is withdrawn. There are many behavioral characteristics that are prevalent among the emotionally disturbed; however, all emotionally disturbed children do not possess all these characteristics. Most emotionally disturbed children will possess deficiencies in at least one of the following categories:

1. Characteristics that impair learning
2. Characteristics that impair interpersonal relationships
3. Characteristics that impair appropriate behavior under normal conditions
4. Characteristics that impair perceptual and motor skill

Learning

Emotionally disturbed children are frequently deficient in abilities contributing to the learning of physical skills. Since the learning process is at the heart of education, it is important that the physical educator be aware of characteristics that emotionally disturbed children often possess. Characteristics that may interfere with the learning of motor skills and the management of physical education classes are the following:

1. Poor work habits in practicing and developing motor skills and aspects of physical fitness
2. Lack of motivation in achieving goals not of an immediate nature
3. Disruptive class behavior on the part of those who are hyperactive
4. Lack of involvement on the part of those who are withdrawn
5. Inability to follow directions or seek help, despite demands for constant attention

6. Short attention span
7. Poor coordination
8. Development of physical symptoms (stomachache, headache, etc.) when confronted with physical activities with which the person is not secure

Interpersonal relationships

Emotionally disturbed children are often impaired in their ability to relate appropriately to their peers. Inability to relate to their peers is often atypical in that those who are emotionally disturbed become easily led by other members of their peer group and become desperate followers. On the other hand, some emotionally disturbed children attempt to express themselves in a desperate effort to become leaders. In play situations, atypical behavior may also be displayed by easy stimulation of others; at the opposite end of the behavioral continuum, the emotionally disturbed child may be antisocial in that he plays alone. There are instances in which emotionally disturbed children want to conform to group patterns but cannot. Physical education programs possess a great opportunity to assist these children in developing appropriate interpersonal relationships.

Emotionally disturbed children are also often impaired in their ability to relate adequately to their teachers. They may demand constant attention by the manifestation of different types of behavior patterns. On the other hand, they may remain inconspicuous and not seek the help necessary to attain physical abilities available for them to learn. Other characteristics that may be displayed by emotionally disturbed children and that may result in impaired interpersonal relationships are little social conscience, easy loss of emotional control, and formation of superficial relationships because of fears of forming close attachments.

Inappropriate behavior under normal conditions

Emotionally disturbed children often display atypical behavior patterns under normal conditions because of difficulty in learning appropriate emotional responses. Some inappropriate behavior patterns that may be displayed under normal conditions are displays of unhappiness or depression; inconsistencies in response; rigidity in expectations of everyday living; displays of such characteristics as carelessness, irresponsibility, and apathy; and low capacity to delay gratification.

Perceptual and motor skill

Deficiencies in perceptual and motor skills make it difficult to perform the more complex activities in which perception and motor control are important. Children impaired in these areas may find it difficult to become proficient in games involving balls or moving objects. Some perceptual and motor difficulties found among those who are emotionally disturbed are difficulty in making space and time assessments (Fig. 16-1), poor motor coordination, development of physical symptoms when activities are presented in which they feel inadequate, and aversion toward sports activities.

Psychological development

Emotionally disturbed children often attain physiological growth without attaining parallel emotional growth. Therefore a need exists for physical educators to be aware of this particular aspect of development and to plan for it just as they plan for the development of the physiological aspects. In many situations, emotionally disturbed children have failed to learn appropriate behaviors because of the environments in which they find themselves. The impaired development of emotional behaviors may often mean that the classroom environment must be altered to accommodate the emotional level of the child. The physical educator must also be aware of the effects of particular classroom settings and relationships with particular emotionally disturbed children. What is of great benefit to one child may be detrimental to another child.

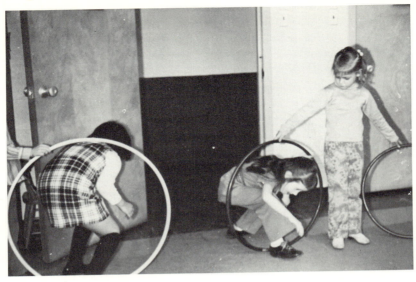

Fig. 16-1. Space-time assessments may be developed by moving the body in space in relationship to objects.

CAUSES OF EMOTIONAL DISTURBANCES

When teaching emotionally disturbed children, teachers sometimes find it helpful to know the cause of emotional disturbance. The knowledge of these causal factors may assist with the prognosis of the emotionally disturbed child and may give cognizance to circumstances that aggravate an already existing condition. There is much speculation as to what causes emotional disturbances. Many clinicians place emphasis on locating a hypothesized environmental source of the disturbance. It is suggested that emotional blocks to learning of environmental nature might be family disorganization, parental ambitiousness, awareness of the impending birth of a sibling, or inability to adapt to a change in environment.

There are differing points of view regarding the predominant cause of the more severe emotional disturbances of childhood. There are many authorities who trace the cause of emotional disturbance to environmental circumstances that occur early in the life of the child. Faulty parental relationships, in particular, are believed by some authorities to account for the cause of a great portion of emotional disturbance in children. On the other hand, there are other authorities who tend to uphold the notion that organic factors that cause a "maturational lag" make an emotional compensation necessary.

Worthy of note are the comments made by Gellhorn and Loofburrow[2] on the basic unity of physiological and psychological action. These authors are of the opinion that psychic events change the function of the nervous system and mental disturbances are caused by a faulty physiological condition of the nervous system. Therefore they conclude that disorders of the mind should be restored through procedures acting on the basic physiological mechanism that determines behavior. If this is the case, it might be speculated that physical activity would be important therapy for the emotionally disturbed. It is known that volitional motor activity induces proprioceptive impulses that, in turn, effectively activate the hypothalamic-cortical system, a powerful determinant of behavior.

IDENTIFICATION

The early identification of children who are emotionally disturbed is extremely important. It is recognized that the earlier educators and mental health specialists can attack this problem, the greater the prospect for ameliorating or remedying it. In many instances, the treatment and education of those who are emotionally disturbed involve the unlearning of behavioral patterns. The sooner identification is made, the less unlearning needs to occur. The physical education teacher can be a key person in the nomination of children for classes consisting of those who are emotionally disturbed because he has an opportunity to view children in many dimensions of behavior.

It is important that teachers have knowledge of their role in screening. The purpose of screening is to determine which children are not functioning properly in a particular behavioral dimension, not to determine what caused the difficulty. The purposes of screening children for emotional disturbance are as follows:

1. To identify children with emotional problems that impair the learning of the child
2. To identify children with emotional problems that disrupt classroom management and prevent others from learning
3. To permit intervention in the disturbance by remedial services (special or adjunctive physical education services)
4. To place children in the educational environment where they can best develop their potentialities

It is not easy to determine which children have problems worthy of intervention with regard to special educational services. Usually, a problem in physical education classes manifests itself by disruption of the work of the student, the desirable cooperation of the group, or the individual's ability to function adequately. A succession of disturbances that may assist educators in identifying the severity of a disturbance are described by Buhler, Smitter, and Richardson,[1] who suggest the following sequence of behavioral patterns that lead to a severe disturbance:

1. Trivial everyday disturbances such as giggling or the lack of concentration that teachers cannot study in detail. Action can be met with counteraction to eliminate this form of disturbance.
2. Repetitious behavior that must be interpreted as a sign of deeper underlying tension.
3. Repetitious behavior accompanied by a serious single disturbance, a tantrum or breaking into tears.
4. A succession of different disturbances: talking when roll is taken, poking the person standing next to the child, staring into space, etc., on different days. This type of behavior is indicative of deep-seated tension and requires the experience of a psychologist or a psychiatrist.

There are other characteristics previously listed that will provide assistance in identifying possibly emotionally disturbed children. More often than not, the teacher is the person making the initial identification of the disturbance, with subsequent referrals to the school psychologist. There is a great need for developing sensitivity to the characteristics of emotionally disturbed children in teacher training programs so that these children may be better served in a public school setting.

Behavioral description

Emotionally disturbed children possess a multitude of traits. Consequently, the label "emotionally disturbed" tells little about a particular person.

It has been traditional to classify emotionally disturbed children with a label describing their behavior. Suggested categories that may be of significance to the physical educator of emotionally disturbed children are the following:

1. *The dimension of personality afflicted:* Personality characteristics associated with emotional disturbance may be immaturity of physical, emotional, social, or psychological traits. Each trait has

implications for physical education programming. Social immaturity limits the child's participation in a hierarchy of social games requiring team play and adherence to discipline with regard to obeying rules. The psychological problems are often perceptual in nature, making it difficult to match perception with motor skills that are associated with many sports activities. In many instances, the emotional instability of the child may have an effect on the physical development.

2. *Overt behavior patterns:* Emotionally disturbed children tend to fall on a continuum from hyperactivity to withdrawal. Children at each end of this continuum pose antithetical problems to the physical educator with regard to program implementation for optimal development.

3. *Degree of emotional disturbance:* Neurosis is a less severe from of emotional disturbance than psychosis. In the latter case, the child loses touch with reality and poses a more difficult problem for the physical educator.

4. *Associated deficiencies:* In some instances, emotional disturbance is accompanied by other disorders such as mental retardation, sensory deterioration, perceptual problems, epilepsy, and obesity.

Learning impairment

Classification according to learning impairment is mentioned to differentiate among the particular types of blocks that may impair a child's ability to learn motor skills and to become developed physically. In the event these particular learning blocks can be remedied or reduced in severity, greater educational domains will open. Some of the fundamental psychological problems that impair the learning of motor skills are problems in relationships with others, impaired communication with others, body image problems, difficulties in both vision and audition or difficulties in one or the other, and language deficiency expressed by difficulty in articulation or syntax.

Well-implemented physical education programs may contribute to the alleviation of problems in relating with others and body image problems. However, more often than not, the other impairments mentioned will have to be circumvented in the process of teaching physical education.

THE TEACHER

The teacher of an emotionally disturbed child is a very important person. The teacher not only teaches physical activities and directs play, but, what is more critical, the child learns patterns of behavior from the teacher. How the teacher reacts in situations occurring in everyday interaction becomes a part of what children expect of themselves and of persons with whom they become involved in daily activity. It is from the teacher that immature children learn how their environment works and how persons cope with themselves.

The teacher of emotionally disturbed children must be stable, flexible, and empathetic toward atypical behavior. However, perhaps the most important ability such a teacher must possess is the ability to perceive what is going on outside himself and what the children are experiencing. Such a teacher provides a medium through which the child may better understand his own behavior and actively change it. This is no easy task. Being in contact with anxiety-provoking persons often stretches the teacher's emotional capacities. It should be recognized that different teachers evoke different responses from different children. A teacher might do well with one emotionally disturbed child and not another. It seems that each teacher responds differently to different types of abnormalities. Some of the behaviors that teachers often must tolerate are implied rejection from the child, conflicting demands made by the child that may range from demanding that immediate needs be met to severe withdrawal, skillful aggressive tactics, and immature behaviors.

Conventional teachers are unaccustomed to these behaviors. However, to succeed in working with these children, teachers must understand and accept their atypical behavior patterns. It may be necessary for teachers to receive special guidance and support to prevent reaching an emotional breaking point.

THE PHYSICAL EDUCATION PROGRAM
Principles of teaching

To conduct a developmental curriculum in physical education for emotionally disturbed children, it is necessary to understand the learning characteristics of emotionally disturbed children in the development of motor skills and to evolve principles taking these characteristics into consideration. The principles of good teaching of emotionally disturbed children in physical education are as follow:

1. *Overstimulation should be provided for emotionally disturbed children, with the exception of the hyperactive disturbed child.* Many emotionally disturbed children need a strong stimulus to focus their attention on the activity at hand. Use tactile stimulation in teaching if the child will cooperate with that particular method. However, avoid overstimulation of the hyperactive emotionally disturbed child.

2. *A variety of methods of teaching and a variety of games that will accommodate children who function at different physical, social, and emotional developmental levels should be used.* The short attention span of these children makes it necessary to have several games on hand so that their interest can be recaptured when an initial activity is no longer productive (Fig. 16-2). Novelty in activities is a great aid in holding their attention.

3. *Distracting objects should be removed.* The attention span can be increased if seductive objects are removed from the immediate environment because the possibilities of involvement in other activity are reduced. Bats, balls, and

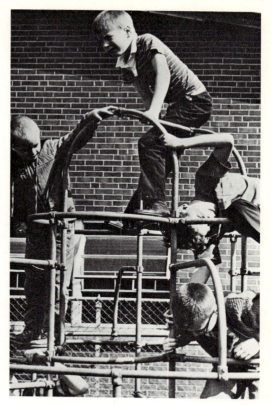

Fig. 16-2. Emotionally disturbed children at play. (Courtesy United States Jaycees, Mental Health–Mental Retardation, Tulsa, Okla.)

other play equipment should be kept out of sight until the time of use, if possible.

4. *Manual guidance has proved to be an excellent method of teaching basic skills to younger emotionally disturbed children.* However, it is not necessarily a good procedure for all disturbed children. A rapport must first be built between the child and the instructor before use of manual guidance or the kinesthetic method of teaching motor skills becomes effective. This method is particularly effective for *autistic* children. Manual guidance is less effective with hyperactive children than with those who are withdrawn.

5. *Limits should be required with regard to use of equipment, facilities, and conduct.* Undue expectations with re-

gard to developmental level of emotions should not be made. However, each child should adhere to behavioral limits within his capabilities. It must be remembered that responsible action toward equipment and facilities involved in play activity affords opportunities for the development of positive behavioral attitudes.

6. *Motor skills and games should be within the child's ability to achieve some degree of success.* Every satisfying experience makes for decreased anxiety and increased self-awareness and confidence.

7. *The instructor should know when to encourage a child to approach, explore, and try a new activity or experience.* A new experience is often met with resistance. In such instances, it is wise to build guarantees of success into the new experience. Subsequent involvement becomes much easier for the emotionally disturbed child. The child who witnesses peers participating successfully in activities sometimes receives impetus to participate with them.

8. *The instructor should discourage stereotyped play activities that develop rigid behavioral patterns.* Emotionally disturbed children often have a tendency to respond to the same objects or activities day after day. After a skill or activity has been well mastered, it may become a deteriorative agent in that it makes the initiation of other activities difficult.

9. *It is not essential to strive for control in all situations.* One of the major goals of education for those who are emotionally disturbed is to effect adequate social adjustment. This does not imply strict obedience to authority but the ability of the individual to adjust to situations independently of supervision. Authoritarian methods can be disastrous in some circumstances. Control should be of such a nature that the preconceived goals of education are being achieved.

10. *Inappropriate interaction among specific children in the class may result in conflicts that disrupt the whole class.* It may be necessary to separate children who interact with one another in a disruptive manner.

11. *The instructor should provide activities within individual abilities and levels of development.* The instructor should know the developmental level of social, emotional, and motor patterns of each child, should be aware of how each child responds to various stimuli and activities, and should plan the program around the child's abilities and disabilities.

It is recognized that the emotionally disturbed population is an extremely heterogeneous group with regard to possessing varying traits. Therefore the guiding principles mentioned are obviously not applicable to all emotionally disturbed children. They are to serve only as a guide to the implementation of programs of physical education for the emotionally disturbed.

Objectives

The objectives of a physical education program for emotionally disturbed children are the same as the objectives held for typical children. The program for those who are emotionally disturbed should stress the development of motor skills and physical fitness, social competence, and personal adequacy. However, it is well to note that these objectives can be pursued through a therapeutic or an educational approach. There have been instances in which physical activity has been used as a therapeutic device for the treatment of emotional disturbance.[11] However, the basic objective of physical education programs is not specifically to eradicate pathological conditions. The objectives of the physical education program should be the development of personal and social competencies that will make the child aware of his own resources and potentialities to optimize the development of self. Physical activities assisting the development of desirable relationships between self and both peers and persons in authority should be provided. Physical activities should also provide constructive and positive new experiences that enhance the concept of self and provide a feeling of worth.

The approach to the education of emotionally disturbed individuals is a central problem needing resolution. The differing approaches have been adequately described by Hobbs[5] for emotionally disturbed children. Hobbs indicates that education places the emphasis on health rather than on illness, on teaching rather than on treatment, on learning rather than on fundamental personality reorganization, on the present and future rather than on the past, and on the operation of the total social system of which the child is a part rather than on the intrapsychic processes exclusively. The primary purpose of the physical educator is to deal with the process of education, not with therapeutic treatment, when implementing programs of physical education for emotionally disturbed children. This does not mean, however, that physical education programs should not and will not have therapeutic effects on emotionally dis-

turbed children. On the contrary, the expectation of well-conceived educational programs should record therapeutic gains with these children. However, the educator's goals must be broader than those of a therapist, who is primarily concerned with the mitigation of a particular disorder.

Although the general objectives for emotionally disturbed children are applicable to typical children, there are specific objectives that may be of higher priority for the emotionally disturbed. These specific objectives of physical education programs for the emotionally disturbed include the following:

1. *The child should generate physical power through the development of the various organic systems of the body.* Emotionally disturbed children need to develop the ability to sustain adaptive effort, to recover from physical exertion, and to resist muscular fatigue. Hopefully, this will enable the child to become more active, demonstrate better motor performance, and become healthier in the organic systems of the body.

2. *The child should develop motor skills that provide opportunities for participa-*

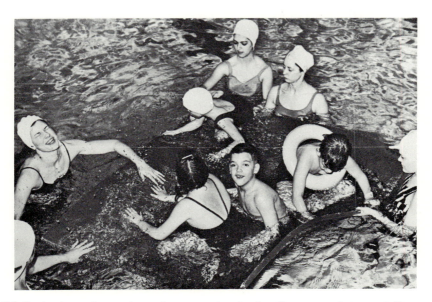

Fig. 16-3. A planned experience in water play in the Slippery Rock State College swimming program for exceptional children.

tion in wholesome leisure-time activity. Motor development is also concerned with making physical movement more useful, proficient, graceful, and esthetic; it is concerned, too, with the contribution to the building of confidence and the enhancement of physical and mental health. Supplementary physical education programs should be provided for children who are deficient in physical fitness and motor development.

3. *The child should be educated to get along with others by developing social competencies through numerous social experiences in games.* Emotionally disturbed children should be helped to unlearn some specific habits causing rejection by adults and peers and to acquire some specific habits making them more acceptable to the important persons in their lives. The physical education program should enhance their self-confidence and add to their joy of living.

Programs of physical education must be of such a nature that each child can accomplish something at his level of ability. Emotionally disturbed children should not be placed in situations in which feelings of insecurity or inadequacy are reinforced by failure to perform the task (Fig. 16-3).

Educational placement

Placement of emotionally disturbed children in an educational setting is a difficult problem. It is becoming obvious that there is no single setting where emotionally disturbed children are best educated. However, it is clear that their education, if possible, should be in the least restrictive environment (mainstream). The possible arrangements in which these children may be educated are as follows:

1. In the regular class with typical children
2. In special classes for emotionally disturbed children
3. In special classes for exceptional children, designed primarily for the mentally retarded
4. In a private institution

The majority of emotionally disturbed children, and particularly the less disturbed, are educated in an integrated fashion in regular classes. There are definite social advantages to integrated placement in that these children are not set apart from their peers and do not carry an educational label that makes them different. However, under such circumstances, the individual needs of emotionally disturbed children may not be met. There may also be a deterring effect on the education of typical children who are in the same class with emotionally disturbed children. When emotionally disturbed children are placed in the regular class, a concerted effort must be made to meet their individual needs through the individualization of instruction.

When emotionally disturbed children cannot be mainstreamed, they may receive an assignment to a special class. Under this type of placement, the physical educator usually teaches the children in the same group in which they are taught throughout the day. Usually, it is necessary to consider physiological differences as well as social and emotional differences because the age range of these groups may extend from early primary to junior high school grade levels. Ordinarily, special classes for the emotionally disturbed are smaller than regular physical education classes. This may provide opportunities for greater attention to individual needs.

The needs and characteristics of all children in a physical education class that contains emotionally disturbed children must be considered in the selection and implementation of physical activities. This is no easy task because of the tremendous variability in characteristics among this group. Hyperactive brain-damaged children may be adversely affected on hearing an overstimulating noise such as one from a drumbeat or the voice of the instructor. On the other hand, a strong stimulus may be greatly needed by other emotionally disturbed children in the same group to focus their attention on the activity at hand.

Behavioral management

The behavioral management of emotionally disturbed children, whether they are in regular or special classes, is a tremendous task. To cope effectively with the behavior of these children in a classroom setting requires that the teacher be an astute observer and a keen psychological tactician. Management demands the analysis of the dynamic interaction of individuals and group forces acting on children during particular activities, together with the skillful application of learning principles.

Certain considerations must be made in managing the behavior of emotionally disturbed children. They must be given the leeway that typical children would be given in a learning situation The teacher should reflect on the developmental level of the child (social, emotional, and physical) and gear expectations accordingly. It should be realized that a problem presented by a child to the teacher is indicative of a problem. It is not reasonable to expect that an emotionally disturbed child will behave in the same manner as a typical child. Therefore the expectations should not be so high that teachers are adversely affected if the emotionally disturbed children do not meet preconceived standards.

It is often difficult to set limits as to when a teacher should intervene to manage atypical behavior displayed in class. The following suggestions* can serve as guidelines of intervention to control classroom behavior:

1. *Reality dangers:* The teacher should intervene if children are involved in physical activity placing them in danger.
2. *Psychological protection:* The teacher should intervene if a group gangs up on a child and uses derogatory remarks that tend to label him as a scapegoat.
3. *Protection of property:* The teacher should intervene when it is evident that school property, equipment, or facilities are in danger of being destroyed or damaged.

---

*From Bulletin of the School of Education, Indiana University, July, 1961.

4. *Protection of the on-going program:* Once the class is motivated in performing a particular activity, intervene if a child who is having difficulty displays disruptive behavior.
5. *Protection against negative contagion:* The teacher should intervene if tension is mounting in an activity and a child with high social power contributes negatively to the activity.
6. *Highlighting a value area:* The teacher may want to intervene to point to an aspect of sportsmanship or rules of the game which may lie slightly below the surface of behavior.
7. *Avoiding conflicts with the outside world:* It is expected that behavior will be controlled when the public or persons other than class members are available to view the class.

Besides knowing when to intervene in the occurrence of inappropriate behaviors in the classroom, the teacher needs to know how to intervene to control such behaviors. The following discussion describes the methods designed to help teachers maintain surface behavior. Redl[9] listed 21 specific influence techniques that he has been able to identify in his work with aggressive boys. The ones most applicable to the management of children in a physical education setting are as follows:

1. *Planned ignoring:* Much of children's behavior is designed to antagonize the teacher. If this behavior is not contagious, it may be wise to ignore the behavior and not gratify the child.
2. *Signal interference:* The teacher may use nonverbal controls such as hand clapping, eye contact, facial frowns and body postures to indicate to the child the feeling of disapproval and control.
3. *Proximity control:* The teacher may stand next to a child who is having difficulty. This is to let the child know of the teacher's concern regarding the behavior.
4. *Interest boosting:* If a child's interest is waning, involve him actively in class activities of the moment and let him demonstrate the skill that is being performed or discussed.
5. *Reduction of tension through humor:* Humor is often able to penetrate a tense situation, with the end result of everyone becoming more comfortable.
6. *Hurdle lesson:* Sometimes a child is frustrated by the immediate task he is requested to perform. Instead of asking for help, he may involve his peers in disruptive activity.

In this event, structure a task in which the child can be successful.

7. *Restructure the classroom program:* If the teacher feels the class is irritable, bored, or excited, a change in program may be needed.

8. *Support from routine:* Some children need more structure than others. Without these guideposts they feel insecure. Structure programs for those that need it.

9. *Direct appeal to value areas:* Appeal to certain values that children have internalized. Some of these values may be relationship between the teacher and child, reality consequences, an awareness of peer reaction, or appeal to the teacher's power of authority.

10. *Remove seductive objects:* It is difficult for the teacher to compete against balls, bats, objects that can be manipulated, or equipment that may be in the vicinity of instruction. Either the objects have to be removed, or the teacher has to accept the disorganized state of the group.

11. *Verbal removal:* When a child's behavior has reached the point where he will not respond to verbal controls, he may have to be asked to leave the room (to get a drink, wash up, or deliver a message—not as punishment).

12. *Physical restraint:* It may be necessary to restrain a child physically if he loses control and becomes violent.

EDUCATIONAL APPROACHES

There are many ways to implement educational programs for emotionally disturbed children. However, only three different educational approaches for emotionally disturbed children will be examined. Although these approaches have been used primarily in academic classroom settings, many techniques are applicable to the implementation of physical education programs. The three approaches are as follows: (1) psychoeducational approach,[7] (2) behavioral modification,[4] and (3) planned experience approach.[10]

Psychoeducational approach

The psychoeducational approach is based on gathering pertinent data about the child and using these data to formulate an educational plan for the child. The teacher is an active member of a team that operates in a framework based on understanding the child. By combining information from educational diagnostic tests and psychological and psychiatric data, the teacher hypothesizes why the child is not learning and plans accordingly. This teaching approach differs from approaches used with normal children in that it has great concern for assessment data. Each child is a school unto himself, with the prescribed activities dictated by speculation from assessment information. Such an individualized method requires a discrete lesson for each child.

If this approach were applied to implementing a physical education program for emotionally disturbed children, it would necessitate the use of a method that Mosston[8] described as individual learning. In this method, learning is the affair of the individual. An individual program is designed and manipulated in a manner that provides for activities that relate to the assessment data. Mosston[8] offered several individual designs that have been used successfully on all levels of physical education. These designs proceed from the simple to the complex; they are individualized on different levels and require different kinds of responsibilities and responses from different individuals. The basis of the individualized programs would come from the results of physical fitness tests and motor ability tests. Strengths and weaknesses of components of the evaluation would be used to formulate the program that would meet the individual's needs. It would appear that this particular method has limited implications for the development of social skills based on social experience. Emotionally disturbed children are capable enough in the performance of the skills but are socially and emotionally immature to the point that the skills cannot be implemented in successful social play in the form of games. One of the great challenges in teaching physical education to emotionally disturbed children is the structuring of environments affording success in social situations. The individualized approach needs to include social learning as well as that of motor skills.

Behavioral modification

Behavior modification in the education of emotionally disturbed children makes practical application of learning theory, operant conditioning, precise objectives, and schedules of reinforcement.[4] The major hypothesis of this approach is that emotionally disturbed children lack order or structure in their environment and in their emotional educational life and tasks to be taught must be specified in detail. To remedy this condition, ways are sought to increase definiteness and the structure of daily classroom experiences. Factors contributing to a structured situation are identified as controlled extraneous stimulation, reduced social activity, and assigned specific educational tasks with constant follow-up. The teacher's purpose is primarily to increase structure, to specify tasks to be learned, and to solidify unclear structure. Good teaching under these conditions means knowing each child well, possessing the ability to persevere, giving specific directions to the child, and having firm expectations and consistent follow-through. The implementation of this approach is expected to bring about behavior that is controlled, constructive, predictive, and orderly. It is of great importance that each moment be planned and that the child engage actively in the task.

The organization of behavior, as a result of behavioral modification, progresses through four stages described as (1) orientation, (2) shaping, (3) cognition, and (4) integration. During the *orientation* period, the children become accustomed to the routines of the classroom environment, the teacher, and the tasks they will be required to perform. All tasks are assigned so that the child will achieve a 95% success experience. The children are introduced to reinforcement procedures.

The next step in the organization of behavior is *shaping*. This refers to presenting a behavioral model repeatedly, obtaining a response, and reinforcing the response. During the shaping period, reinforcement follows each successful task and the success rate should be high.

After shaping has been successful, the child is exposed to the *cognitive* phase of behavioral organization. This phase indicates the child is developing an understanding of the relationship between his behavior and its consequences. During this phase, the child is conditioned to complete projects and to be concerned with quality and efficiency. It is at this stage of behavioral development that reinforcement schedules change from reinforcement of each response to intermittent reinforcement.

From the cognitive stage, the child moves to the most advanced stage of behavioral organization, *integration*. Attaining this stage indicates that the child's behavior is being maintained within the limits of expectation set for him. At this stage, he begins to make his own decisions and realizes the importance of neatness and cooperative work.

Planned experience approach

The planned experience approach recommended by Rhodes[10] is based on the assumption that the forces of growth and the motivational effects of exploration and discovery of emotionally disturbed children are similar to those of typical children.

If children are to recognize their capabilities and resources, it is important that the experiences be planned carefully. Principles that should be applied to the preparation of experiences are as follows:

1. New experiences should be elicited in relationship to old problems. The child's responses will provide the cues to the quality and intensity of the experience and suggestions for additional preparations.
2. The child must be surrounded with opportunities for new experiences that afford chances for adventure, discovery, and exploration (Fig. 16-2).

3. Newly developed abilities should be afforded opportunities for expression.
4. The preparation should involve the engagement of as many sensory channels as possible.
5. The preparation should develop new abilities channeled toward the interests of the child.
6. The preparation should include natural and immediate consequences of the child's activity.
7. The preparation should require only performances in line with the child's present abilities.
8. The teacher should find ways to help the child reflect on the experience and its meaning for him so that it is bound as a permanent record within him.

These guides are most applicable to physical educators in implementing a physical educational program.

The process of *guided discovery* involves establishing an environment that presents a problem and thus awakens the possibility of discovery. In this method, the teacher never gives the child the answer. The student is the focus and must remain so if the process is to continue and succeed. In guided discovery, there is no failure. The student, by himself, evolves the answer. Some of the things students can discover are relationships (similarities and dissimilarities), principles (governing rule), physical movements (intensity and speed), how things are done, and why (Fig. 16-3).

In the process of *problem solving*, the child seeks out the answers independently. In the guided discovery process, the environment is manipulated to guide discovery. In the problem solving style of teaching, the problems have several solutions. The degree of freedom for self-improvement independent of the teacher's control is almost complete. The element of choice, the availability of a variety of solutions, and the climate of encouragement to seek a new response create motivation to participate in activity that may have been lacking in many emotionally disturbed children.

IMPLICATIONS OF PHYSICAL ACTIVITY

Physical activity in the form of play and dance has traditionally been used by mental health specialists both as a tool in diagnosis and as therapy for emotionally disturbed persons. The qualitative aspects of play and the development of motor skills among those who are disturbed have not always received a great deal of attention in the past. However, it is now recognized by educators of emotionally disturbed children that play is not an intermittent freedom from the discipline of academic tasks, but is of educational value and has creative effort in itself.

There is a qualitative aspect to the nature of the physical activity in play that can contribute most to the well-being of the disturbed child. Constructive play of a higher order implies the socialization of children. Usually, emotionally disturbed children must be taught how to play and enjoy physical activity. Once constructive play is learned, it provides a medium through which the child may experiment with self-control and with the control of his environment Play also offers opportunity for social learnings and tension release. Because those who are emotionally disturbed strain the educational program, they are often left out of the extracurricular and intramural activities of a regular school. This is in reverse order of their basic needs for experience in community living (Fig. 16-4).

Play

It has long been known that movement and play have positive effects on the behaviors of emotionally disturbed persons. However, there is a need for research that will answer such questions as: How does a particular game affect a child emotionally? What are the effects of body contact, agility, strength, flexibility, complexity of skill learning undertaken, the rules of the game, the environment, and duration of the game? How do activities limit, provoke, or coerce the expression of children's needs and problems? Research answering these

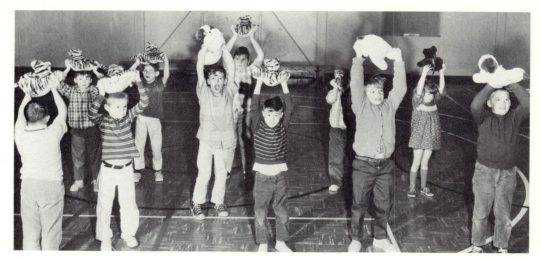

Fig. 16-4. Classroom behavior can be controlled through well-managed activity that gets children involved. (Courtesy Dr. Julian Stein, American Alliance for Health, Physical Education, and Recreation.)

questions would contribute to the systematic evaluation of physical education programs for the emotionally disturbed and their subsequent effects on behavior.

Such research as mentioned has come under experimental conditions. Gump and Sutton-Smith[3] described various types of social interaction among emotionally disturbed children who were participating in swimming. The authors concluded that the activity setting was more important than the activity per se, but the activity was also important because it affects the children's relationships with one another and with the leader. From such data, a person can learn that swimming will put the child in a social climate in which total interaction will be high, whereas crafts will put a child in a milder social climate in which total interaction is low. More research of this nature is necessary to develop programs of physical education that will meet the needs of emotionally disturbed children with particular behavioral problems.

REFERENCES

1. Buhler, C., Smitter, F., and Richardson, S.: What is a problem? In Long, H. J., editor: Conflict in the classroom, Belmont, Calif., 1965, Wadsworth Publishing Co., Inc.

2. Gellhorn, E., and Loofburrow, G.: Emotions and emotional disorders, New York, 1963, Harper & Row, Publishers.

3. Gump, P., and Sutton-Smith, B.: Therapeutic play techniques. In Long, H. J., editor: Conflict in the classroom, Belmont, Calif., 1965, Wadsworth Publishing Co., Inc.

4. Haring, N. G., and Whelan, R. J.: Experimental methods in education and management. In Long, H. J., editor: Conflict in the classroom, Belmont, Calif., 1965, Wadsworth Publishing Co., Inc.

5. Hobbs, N.: How the Re-ED plan developed. In Long, H. J., editor: Conflict in the classroom, Belmont, Calif., 1965, Wadsworth Publishing Co., Inc.

6. Lyons, D. J., and Powers, V.: Study of children exempted from Los Angeles schools. In Long, H. J., editor: Conflict in the classroom, Belmont, Calif., 1965, Wadsworth Publishing Co., Inc.

7. Morse, W. C.: The crisis teacher. In Long, H. J., editor: Conflict in the classroom, Belmont, Calif., 1965, Wadsworth Publishing Co., Inc.

8. Mosston, M.: Teaching physical education, Columbus, Ohio, 1966, Charles E. Merrill Publishing Co.

9. Redl, F.: Managing surface behavior of children in school. In Long, H. J., editor: Conflict in the classroom, Belmont, Calif., 1965, Wadsworth Publishing Co., Inc. (From notes abridged from N. J. Long and R. G. Newman.)

10. Rhodes, W. C.: Curriculum and disordered

behavior. In Long, H. J., editor: Conflict in the classroom, Belmont, Calif., 1965, Wadsworth Publishing Co., Inc.

11. Vaughn, J. E.: The effects of exercises and games activities upon the behavior, body image and self-image of hospitalized male psychotics. Unpublished doctoral dissertation, Springfield College, Springfield, Mass., 1966.

RECOMMENDED READINGS

Altman, L., and Linton, T.: Operant conditioning in the classroom setting: a review of the research, J. Educ. Res. 64:277-286, 1971.

Bateman, B.: Three approaches to diagnosis and educational planning for children with learning disabilities. From proceedings of the international convocation onn children and young adults with learning disabilities, Pittsburgh, Pa., 1967, Crippled Children's Home.

Brown, P., and Presbie, R.: Behavior modification skills, Hicksville, N.Y., 1973, Research Media, Inc.

Cruickshank, W. M., editor: Psychology of exceptional children and youth, Englewood Cliffs, N.J., 1971, Prentice-Hall, Inc.

Hall, R.: Managing behavior: Applications in school and home, Lawrence, Kan., 1971, H. & H. Enterprises.

Haring, N. G., and Schiefelbusch, R. L., editors: Methods in special education, ed. 2, New York, 1975, McGraw-Hill Book Co.

Hewett, F. M.: The emotionally disturbed child in the classroom, Boston, 1968, Allyn & Bacon, Inc.

Long, H. J., and Newman, R. G.: Managing surface behavior of children in school. In Long, H. J., editor: Conflicts in the classroom, Belmont, Calif., 1965, Wadsworth Publishing Co., Inc.

Morse, W. C.: The education of socially maladjusted and emotionally disturbed children. In Cruickshank, W. M., and Johnson, G. O., editors: Education of exceptional children and youth, Englewood Cliffs, N.J., 1958, Prentice-Hall, Inc.

Myklebust, H. R., editor: Progress in learning disabilities, New York, 1975, Grune & Stratton, Inc.

17

OTHER CONDITIONS

MENSTRUATION AND DYSMENORRHEA

Menstruation is a complex process that involves the endocrine glands, uterus, and ovaries. The menstrual cycle, on the average, lasts for 28 days. However, every individual woman has her own rhythmic cycle of menstrual function. The cycle periods usually range from 21 to 35 days, but they may occasionally be longer or shorter and still fall within the range of normality.

Three ounces of blood is the average total amount lost during the normal menstrual period; however a woman may lose from 1½ to 5 ounces.[17] This blood is replaced by the active formation of blood cells in bone marrow and, consequently, does not cause anemia. On occasion, some women may have excessive menstrual flow and, in this event, a physician should be consulted. The average menstrual period is 3 to 5 days, but 2 to 7 days may be considered normal. The average age of onset of menstruation is 12.5 years, although the range of onset may be from 9 to 18 years.

Dysmenorrhea, or painful menstruation, is a common occurrence among some girls and women. The ratio may be as low as 1:4 among college women, indicating that it is the exception rather than the rule. It has been estimated that only 20% to 30% of cases of dysmenorrhea are a result of organic causes such as ovarian cysts, endocrine imbalance, or infections. Most of the causes are of functional origin such as poor posture, insufficient exercise, fatigue, weak abdominal muscles, or improper diet.

Physical activity during the menstrual period

Nolen[15] indicated, in a study of problems in menstruation, that postural deficiency may be responsible for some discomfort, not just during the menstrual period, but also on other days. She found that when posture was improved and good physical condition achieved, the menses did not incapacitate girls for physical education or recreational programs.

Gilman's[10] findings indicate that activity during the menstrual period has proved helpful in the correction of dysmenorrhea. Clow and Sanderson[6] observed that many girls have discovered that if they do not have some form of exercise prior to and on the first day of their period, they may have pain.

A number of studies are concerned with the effect of exercise on menstruation. Runge,[17] who studied 107 college girls who trained 15 hours each week, and Duntzer and Hellendall,[8] who studied 1,561 woman participants in a German athletic festival, found that, in a majority of the cases, training was without effect on the character of the menstrual history. The activities were continued during the menstrual period without impairment to performance ability. In Duntzer's study, it was shown that 55% of the women suffered no decrease in efficiency, while the other 45% showed a decrease in performance either during menstruation or immediately before the onset of flow. The findings of these studies seem to indicate that menstruation has a differential effect on women. It is suggested that menstruation does not necessarily prohibit bodily exercise during flow, but there are exceptions to the rule.

The consensus in the literature would seem to be that excuse from physical education activity because of normal menstruation would be unwarranted.

There has been a question in the minds of some persons as to the feasibility of girls and young women swimming during the menstrual cycles. Phillips, Fox, and Young[16] conducted a survey among gynecologists and other physicians to determine their points of view on this issue. The menstrual period was divided into three phases: (1) the premenstrual period (3 or 4 days prior to the actual onset of the menses), (2) the first half of the menstrual period, and (3) the second half of the menstrual period. The consensus among the doctors and the gynecologists was that restrictions on participation in vigorous physical activity, intensive sports competition, and swimming during all phases of the menstrual period were unwarranted for girls who are free from menstrual disturbances. However, with regard to the first half of the menstrual period, there were some physicians who advised moderation with limited participation in intensive sports competition. The reason for moderation during the first half of the menstrual period is that the flow is heavier during the first 2 or 3 days and some women experience cramps during the first 2 days. Restrictions increase for women with premenstrual discomfort as the severity of the discomfort increases.[16]

Worthy of note is a study performed by Anderson[1] on swimming and exercise during menstruation. This study showed that the incidence of discomfort associated with menstruation was less for an active group of competitive swimmers than for girls who did not participate in swimming activities. Also of interest is the study by Astrand et al.[2] of the training of 30 champions who swam from 6,000 to 6,500 meters each week. They found there was no evidence that the strenuous swimming regimen caused menstrual disturbances.

Exercises for dysmenorrhea

The question has often been asked as to what effects exercise has on dysmenorrhea. Studies have shown that women previously suffering from moderate or severe cases of dysmenorrhea showed a decrease in severity of cramps after performing 8 weeks of prescribed abdominal exercises. These exercises, prescribed for women who had no organic causes for dysmenorrhea, provided relief of congestion in the abdominal cavity caused by gravity, poor posture, poor circulation, or poor abdominal muscle tone. They also provided relief of leg and back pains by stretching lumbar and pelvic ligaments in the fascia to minimize pressure on spinal nerves. Undue muscular tension may also have a bearing on painful menstruation; therefore relaxation techniques and positioning of the body, accompanied by heat from a hot water bottle on the low back area, may relax tensions and consequently lessen the pain. Other relaxation techniques and exercises may also be used to reduce tension in the body.

Women who suffer from dysmenorrhea may benefit by conscientious endeavor in a daily exercise program designed to alleviate this condition. The exercises should provide for improvement of posture (especially lordosis), stimulation of circulation, and stretching of tight fascia and ligaments. The exercises discussed here are suggested to alleviate the symptoms of dysmenorrhea.

Fascial stretch

The purpose of this exercise is to stretch the shortened fascial ligamentous bands that extend between the low back and the anterior aspect of the pelvis and legs. These shortened bands may result in increased pelvic tilt, which may irritate peripheral nerves passing through or near the fascia. The irritation of these nerves may be the cause of the pain. This exercise enhances the stretching effect on the hip flexors and increases mobility of the hip joint[1] (Fig. 17-1).

To perform the exercise, the woman should stand erect, with the left side of her body about the distance of the bent elbow from a wall; the feet should be together, the left forearm and palm against the wall, with the elbow at shoulder height, and the heel of the hand placed against the posterior aspect of the hollow portion of the hip. From this position, abdominal and gluteal muscles should be contracted strongly to tilt the pelvis backward. The hips should slowly be pushed forward and diagonally toward the wall and pressure applied with the hand. This position should be held for a few counts, then slowly a return is made to the starting position. The stretch should be performed three times on each side of the body. The exercise should be continued even after relief has been obtained from dysmenorrhea. It has been suggested that the exercise be performed three times daily. To increase motivation, the girl should record the number of days and times she performs the exercise.

Abdominal pumping

The purpose of abdominal pumping is to increase circulation of the blood throughout the pelvic region. The exercise is performed by assuming a hook-lying position and placing the hands lightly on the abdomen. The exercise is performed by slowly and smoothly distending the abdomen on the count of one, then retracting the abdomen on the count of two, and relaxing. The exercise should be repeated 8 to 10 times[14] (Fig. 17-2).

Pelvic tilt with abdominal pumping

The purpose of this exercise is to increase the tone of the abdominal muscles, which may eventually contribute to relieving dys-

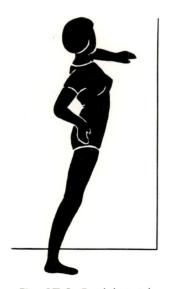

Fig. 17-1. Fascial stretch.

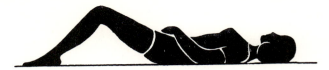

Fig. 17-2. Abdominal pumping.

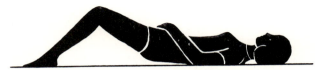

Fig. 17-3. Pelvic tilt with abdominal pumping.

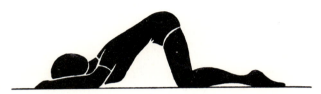

Fig. 17-4. Knee-chest position.

menorrhea.[14] In a hook-lying position, with the feet and knees together, heels 1 inch apart, and hands on the abdomen, the abdominal and gluteal muscles are contracted. The pelvis is rotated so that the tip of the coccyx comes forward and upward and the hips are slightly raised from the floor. The abdomen is distended and retracted. The hips are lowered slowly, vertebra by vertebra, until the original starting position is attained. The exercise is to be repeated 8 to 10 times (Fig. 17-3).

Knee-chest position

The purpose of this exercise is to stretch the extensors of the lumbar spine and strengthen the abdominal muscles. The exercise is performed by bending forward at the hips and placing the hands and arms on a mat. The chest is lowered toward the mat, in a knee-chest position, and held as close to the mat as possible for 3 to 5 minutes.[11] This exercise should be performed once or twice a day (Fig. 17-4).

Implications for physical education

The conclusion that can be reached after viewing the numerous studies on the effects of physical activity and menstruation is that it is not warranted that girls and women be excused from physical education classes because of the menstrual cycle. Social, professional, and athletic schedules cannot be adjusted to each woman's menstrual cycle. It is also realized that many girls and women experience discomfort as a result of menstruation. However, this aspect of femininity must be adjusted, too, so that women can continue normal professional and athletic activities during all phases of the menstrual cycle. The observation has been made that by continuation of activity through the cycle, the impact of menstrual discomfort experienced often decreases.[2]

DIABETES

Diabetes mellitus is a chronic metabolic disorder, the basis of which is the inability of the cells to use glucose. The diabetic's body is unable to burn up its intake of carbohydrates because of a lack of insulin, which is produced by the pancreas. The lack of insulin in the blood prevents the storage of glucose in the cells of the liver. Consequently, blood sugar accumulates in the bloodstream in greater than usual amounts.

There are approximately 1,600,000 known diabetics in the United States and many more unidentified cases. It has been estimated that approximately 65,000 new cases of diabetes develop each year and about 4,750,000 individuals presently residing in the United States, who are now free of diabetic symptoms, will develop diabetes during their lifetime. About 10% of the recorded cases occur among children, according to *Diabetic Fact Book*, published by the United States Public Health Service. However, there is a greater prevalence of diabetes with increasing age; approximately half the people who are afflicted with the disease are over the age of 60 years. Furthermore, there is evidence that the diabetic mother may contribute to greater prevalence of diabetic children.[12] Kogan[12] indicates that diabetic mothers have malformed children 10 times more frequently than nondiabetic mothers.

Teachers should be aware of the symptoms of diabetes in order to help identify the disease if it should appear in any of their students, since early identification and treatment promise the best hope. Symptoms of diabetes include infections that may be slow to heal; fatigue; excessive hunger; itching; impairment in visual acuity; skin infections such as boils, carbuncles, ulcers, and gangrenous sores; and excessive urination and thirst.

The cause of diabetes is, as yet, unknown. There seem to be, however, hereditary predispositions for the acquisition of the disease. Of significance regarding the cause of diabetes is the fact that 70% to 90% of the diagnosed diabetics have a history of obesity as a result of having a high degree of fat and carbohydrate content in their diets. Endocrine imbalances, mental trauma, and sedentary living also appear as precipitating factors in the onset of diabetes.

Although the symptoms mentioned may be important in identifying diabetes, the most reliable method of detecting the disorder is a urinalysis by laboratory examination.

Characteristics

Overweight is one of the best-known characteristics of diabetics, particularly in adults. Reducing to normal weight often brings about definite improvement in a diabetic condition. Another characteristic of the diabetic is susceptibility to infection. Therefore care and prompt treatment must be exercised in the event that abrasions, blisters, cuts, or infections occur in physical education activities. Still another complication the physical educator should be cognizant of is a condition called "insulin shock." This condition occurs when the glycogen stored in the liver is depleted. The patient develops general muscular weakness, mental confusion, vertigo, profuse sweating, trembling, and either a pale or a flushed face. If there is a rapid drop in glycogen, symptoms progress to epileptic-like convulsions. When the warning symptoms appear, the patient should eat or drink something containing sugar.

Treatment

It is important that the physical educator understand diabetes treatment procedures so that cooperative efforts with the medical profession can enhance the total development of the child. Effective control of diabetes solely by diet and oral medication has long been sought. Progress toward this objective has been made in recent years through the development of therapeutic drugs that have the properties of insulin. However, a third factor is important in the control of diabetes. This is participation in exercise, which may help stimulate pancreatic secretions. Insulin injections are usually self-administered by the patient, using hypodermic needles in the upper leg. The injections are generally administered either once or twice daily, depending on the individual's need. Also important in the treatment of diabetes is the psychological adjustment patients themselves must make. In addition, patients must undergo regular health checkups and have periodic urinalyses recorded by medical personnel. They must also realize that the condition still is not curable, although it can be controlled. By adjusting to the disciplines placed on them by the physician, diabetics can expect to live lives as long and productive as nondiabetic persons.

Insulin shock and diabetic coma

In dealing with the diabetic, the physical educator should be aware that a life-and-death situation can arise from too much or too little insulin. In an inadequate dosage of insulin, the early stages produce lassitude, uneasiness, loss of appetite, unquenchable thirst, and excessive urination. As the demand for insulin becomes greater, symptoms of vomiting, dizziness, and even a diabetic coma may result. A coma and shock condition can also occur from the opposite state of too much insulin. Insulin shock or hypoglycemia may cause a loss of consciousness and, unchecked, eventually, a comatose state. In comparing the diabetic coma to insulin shock, certain differences are apparent, namely, insulin shock occurs rapidly, the patient's skin is moist and pale, there is seldom nausea, and the breath does not smell sweet as in cases of diabetic coma.

Exercise and diabetes

Physical exercise is an important aspect in controlling diabetes. Before the discovery of insulin in the late 1920's, diabetes was controlled primarily through diet and mild exercise. Studies conducted before the discovery of insulin, although scanty, show that the number of deaths from diabetes was higher among the group of persons whose occupations were of a sedentary nature than among those with more physically active jobs. From these findings, might be inferred that exercise was a variable in the longevity of the diabetic. Exercise has been considered so valuable to diabetics that it should be looked on as a duty and incorporated into their daily life. Walking and mild exercise were thought to be of sufficient value. Yahraes'[20] findings suggest that there might be a relationship between exercise and efficient control of diabetes.

It must also be emphasized that diabetes does not prevent persons from improving their physical fitness through exercise. Zankle[21] demonstrated that it was possible, through exercise, to increase the Rogers physical fitness index of hospitalized diabetic patients. Furthermore, Engerbretson[9] found that daily insulin dosage in diabetic patients were reduced when accommpanied by exercise. Also, the diabetic control improved during the period of training. In addition, motor fitness of an experimental group subjected to exercise increased during the training period, whereas a nonexercising control group of subjects decreased in motor fitness.

Regular exercise programs are of value to children with diabetes, for exercise may help to stimulate pancreatic secretion as well as contribute to overall body health and assist in maintaining optimal weight, which is a problem for many diabetics. The child with diabetes can participate, in general, in the activities of the unrestricted class. However, in many cases, diabetic patients are more susceptible to fatigue than their nonhandicapped peers. Therefore the physical educator should be understanding in the event the diabetic cannot withstand prolonged bouts of more severe exercise. Adaptations to inabilities on the diabetic's part should be considered.

Implications for physical education

School medical records should be examined in an effort to locate children with diabetes as well as other conditions that may impair the child's education. After the location of such students, programs of exercise should be established, with medical counsel, according to the needs of each student. The limits to the activity each diabetic child can perform vary. Continuous evaluation must be made to determine the capabilities and limitations of each diabetic child in the performance of physical and motor activity. The physical education program for the diabetic child, as all other physical education programs, should follow specific progressive sequences ranging from light to intense and simple to complex with regard to the development of physical characteristics and motor skills. It is of the utmost importance that the initial capability of the child be identified precisely so that no exercise will be prescribed that is more intense or difficult than the child's capabilities permit. Such a situation could be physiologically and psychologically damaging and might retard the child's receptivity to subsequent activity. The setting most suitable for the child with diabetes is in a regular physical education class. In the event his condition warrants adaptation of exercise and games, these adaptations should be made. The social values accrued from participation with the child's peers seem to far outweigh the possible slight stigma that may be placed on him because of the adaptations in his physical education program.

KIDNEY DISORDERS

The kidneys and their related structures are the primary organs for excretion in the body, for they remove nitrogenous wastes and various other substances. In addition, the kidneys also eliminate water and help control the water content and osmotic pressure of the blood; they eliminate excess salts in order to keep proper salt concentration in the blood and they control acid-base balance by secreting an excess of either acid or alkaline residues. Thus it can be seen that the kidneys play an important role in the maintenance of the health of the body.

The rate of kidney secretion is influenced by the pressure of the blood passing through the kidneys. Strenuous and vigorous exercise may cause the blood pressure to increase, thus augmenting the rate of urine excretion. Under the conditions of vigorous exercise or high temperature, there is a loss of water and salts. In the event that the salt loss is great, the water content in the tissues will be decreased and the restoration of normal levels of salt will be difficult to achieve. Therefore it may be that, in the case of kidney disorders, vigorous exercise may be contraindicated. However, the best procedure to follow in the case of a person who has a kidney disorder is to implement the recommendations of the physician with respect to dosage, duration, and intensity of exercise.

Perhaps the most prevalent kidney disorder that occurs in children and young adults is *chronic nephritis*. This disorder often follows acute infections such as scarlet fever, tonsillitis, diphtheria, or even colds. The symptoms for chronic nephritis may be pain in the lumbar region of the spine, fever, frequent and painful urination, and the presence of blood in the urine. If a student has such a disorder, vigorous exercise is usually contraindicated because chronic nephritis usually yields to rest, proper medical care, and, in some instances, antibiotic treatment.

It is interesting to note that Turner[18] indicated that "hollow-back posture" may sometimes interfere with normal kidney function and produce albumen in the urine. Also, severe and prolonged chilling of the body, especially after vigorous exercise, may cause congestion and injury to the kidneys. This is particularly important if the child already has a kidney disorder.

A child who has contracted chronic nephritis should take part in programs of physical education within the current limits of functioning. However, the treatment and activities to be included in the program should be under the direction of the physician.

INFECTIOUS DISEASES

There are several infectious diseases that may be contracted by schoolchildren. In many cases, modification of activity is necessary in order to meet the temporary needs and abilities of these children. Some of the infectious diseases that may require special attention of the physical educator are tuberculosis, pneumonia, streptococcal infections, infectious encephalitis, meningitis, and mononucleosis.

Tuberculosis

Tuberculosis is a disease of the lungs caused by the tubercle bacillus. Predisposing factors are generally conducive for the development of the disease. These factors may include emotional or physical lowering of resistance, alcoholism, a chronic debilitating disease, poor nutrition and hygiene, or a combination of these factors.

No age group is exempt from the disease, but the greatest prevalence of tuberculosis is found among young adults and middle-aged persons.

Tuberculosis is a difficult disease to identify. Perhaps the first indication that such an infection exists may come from a routine radiograph of the chest. However, other minor symptoms that may be associated with the onset of the disorder are symptoms of fatigue, failure to gain weight during growth, low fever, cough, chest pain, or a mild case of influenza.

There is great variability in degree, stage, and type of tuberculosis. Since each case of tuberculosis is different, there are many complex factors that must be resolved by the physician when treating the disease. Usually, complete bed rest is required in active cases until the disease can be brought under control. With the resumption of activities of daily living, general strength and endurance may be developed by the implementation of progressive exercise. Also included in the treatment is a nutritious diet and activities that contribute to both physical and mental health. The child who is returning to school after an attack of tuberculosis is usually unable to engage in the unrestricted physical education program. The activities must be adapted to the child's current level of functioning and frequent periods of rest must be afforded him so that he will not become unduly fatigued. The physical education program for the child recovering from tuberculosis should be under the direction of the physician.

The activity program should be mild at first and contain the element that all good programs contain, which is progression commensurate with the abilities of the afflicted person. Care should be taken to involved the student in activities that do not cause undue fatigue. The milder recreational activities such as swimming, archery, bowling, camping, or golf provide opportunities for the student to participate at the level of his capabilities.

Pneumonia

Pneumonia is an infection of the air spaces of the lung. Usually, the bacteria causing pneumonia gain a foothold through the lowered resistance of a person. There are several types of pneumonia. Some of the most prevalent types are lobar, viral, bronchial, and foreign body.

The lobar type of pneumonia is often manifested with chills, fever, chest pain, coughing, shortness of breath, and inability to withstand the onset of fatigue. The temperature often reaches 104° to 105° F; consequently, bluish discoloration of the lips and skin occurs.

The viral type of pneumonia, which generally occurs in the younger and middle-aged groups, possesses symptoms that are often difficult to identify because of gradual onset. On the other hand, pneumonia may also appear very abruptly after an upper respiratory infection. The most prevalent symptoms indicating the viral type of pneumonia are generalized muscular pains and a slight cough. At times, however, the symptoms may be similar to the more explosive lobar type of pneumonia.

Bronchopneumonia occurs often in children. The lungs are usually inflamed and there is often an inability to withstand the onset of fatigue. A cold is also present.

Foreign bodies may also cause pneumonia, for they often precipitate a cough or low fever. In many instances, through the identification of the specific organism responsible for pneumonia, antibiotic treatment will control the disease effectively. An effort should be made to maintain a balanced nutritious diet. Care should be taken by the physical educator to see that a child who has returned to school after an occurrence of pneumonia is not exposed to environmental conditions that would lower resistance and provoke another attack. Also, progressive exercise, starting with a dosage commensurate with the capacity of the student, should be administered.

Streptococcal infections

The streptococcic bacteria cause a wide variety of diseases. The diseases differ with regard to the portal of entry and the tissues on which the infectious agent acts. Some of the more important conditions caused by the streptococcal bacteria are scarlet fever and streptococcal sore throat such as tonsillitis and pharyngitis. Other diseases include mastoiditis, osteomyelitis, otitis media, impetigo, and other skin and wound infections.

Sources of the streptococcal infection are acutely ill or convalescent patients; discharges from nose, throat, and purulent lesions; or objects contaminated with such discharges. The transmission of the bacteria is by direct contact with the carrier, by indirect contact with objects handled, or by the spreading of droplets whereby the bacteria can be inhaled. Repeated attacks of streptococcal infections of the throat by different types of streptococci are frequent. It appears that neither active nor passive immunization against the streptococcus itself can be accomplished satisfactorily.

When a student is recovering from a streptococcal infection, caution should be exercised with regard to an unwarranted return to an unrestricted physical educa-tion program. The same procedures for implementing exercise for the person recovering from strep throat are applicable to other illnesses: exercise of a progressive nature that is in accordance with the student's current functional capacity. Care must be taken to place the student in an environment that will not cause a lowering of resistance, thereby leaving him vulnerable to recurring streptococcal infections. Streptococcal infections are particularly dangerous to children who have had rheumatic fever. Consequently, the fact cannot be overemphasized that a child who has been afflicted with rheumatic heart disease should be guarded judiciously against streptococcal infections, which could conceivably further impair heart function. Antibiotic injections can be administered periodically to persons who tend to have recurrent streptococcal infections. This constitutes special risks in that the body may build an immunity to the antibiotic; however, for individuals who have had recurring rheumatic fever, antibiotic treatment may be necessary to avoid subsequent streptococcal infections that may prove damaging to the heart.

Infectious encephalitis

Among the many forms of encephalitis, there are two major types: (1) acute nonsuppurative encephalitis that follows or is a part of some infectious disease and (2) the arthropod-borne viral encephalitis.

Nonsuppurative encephalitis

Acute nonsuppurative encephalitis is an acute inflammatory condition of the brain that occurs as a result of complications of various infectious diseases and is characterized by some manifestation of cerebral dysfunction. The condition itself is not contagious, but it may complicate any acute infectious disease, even the common cold. Consequently, the cerebral symptoms may become more prominent than the primary disease. This form of encephalitis may attack all age groups, although children under 10 years of age are more frequently affected than adults.

Symptoms that may give an indication of acute nonsuppurative encephalitis may be headache, visual disturbances (particularly double vision), vertigo nausea, and general weakness. There is usually some change in the sensory media and inattentiveness to ongoing activity may be an observable symptom. It is not uncommon to find such symptoms as convulsions, muscle twitchings or spasms, tremors, ataxias, and aphasia with the disease. Recovery from encephalitis is usually rapid and apparently complete on the surface, but, in many instances, the nervous system is permanently impaired because of degenerative changes that have occurred as a result of the disease.

Arthropod-borne encephalitis

Although there are many forms of the arthropod-borne viral encephalitis, all types produce an almost identical clinical picture. The symptoms that may be present are headache, tight hamstring muscles, stiff neck and back, fever, disorientation, stupor, coma, tremors, and spasticity. The symptoms may occur abruptly or may come about over a period of 1 week or more. When adults contract the disease, tendon and skin reflexes usually remain normal.

Implications for physical education

The physical educator should be aware of changes that may occur in a student who has had infectious encephalitis. In many instances, particularly if there has been degeneration of the nervous system, the mental as well as the physical needs of the individual may be different on his return from such an attack than they were prior to the attack. The physical education teacher should know the limits of activity for each individual case and should be sensitive to adapting the activities so that the child may make a satisfactory adjustment to regular school activities after returning from the ailment. Characteristics that may be manifested after the attack are

inability to withstand the onset of fatigue, impaired motor coordination, and a decrement in measures of strength.

Meningitis

Meningitis is an acute contagious disease characterized by the inflammation of the meninges of the spinal cord. The severity with which persons are attacked by the disease varies greatly. Epidemics of meningitis occur with greater frequency in areas where there are rural communities, as opposed to cities. The disease occurs at any age; however, 40% of the meningitis cases occur in children under 10 years of age. There is also a great prevalence of meningitis among older children and young adults. Epidemics of meningitis are more prevalent in the winter and spring seasons of the year.

The onset of meningitis is, more often than not, abrupt and accompanied by severe headache and chills, followed soon by fever and vomiting. Other characteristics indicating the presence of the disease may be irritability; delirium; stupor; coma; convulsions; constipation or diarrhea; rash; infections of the ear such as mastoiditis, otitis media, difficulty in hearing; or eye conditions such as conjunctivitis, optic neuritis, diplopia, and strabismus. Meningitis is a serious disease because many complications may be associated with it. These complications are pneumonia, otitis media and mastoiditis, arthritis, hydrocephalus, ocular conditions such as conjunctivitis and optic neuritis, cystitis, endocarditis, or pericarditis.

The many forms of meningitis can be classified with regard to four major types with several subheadings under each of the major types. The main classifications are meningococcus meningitis, lymphocytic choriomeningitis, influenzal meningitis, and purulent meningitis. Each form needs to be diagnosed differentially for medical treatment.

Implications for the physical educator

Usually, the convalescent period for meningitis is not as long as for some other communicable diseases. Therefore it may be possible to involve the child more quickly and with greater intensity than is possible in the case of other illnesses.

AUTISM

Autism is a condition in which a person is dominated by subjective, self-centered trends of thought and behavior. The consideration is usually associated with severe disorders of communication and behavior.[5] Furthermore, complications associated with autism may be profound aphasia, psychosis, or other conditions characterized by severe deficits in language ability and interpersonal behavior. Autistic children appear to suffer from a pervasive impairment of their cognitive and/or perceptual functioning, the consequences of which are manifested by limited ability to understand, communicate, learn, and participate in social relationships. The autistic child often possesses characteristics similar to those of the mentally retarded, emotionally disturbed, brain-damaged, and psychotic individual. In general, autistic children are very often multihandicapped in their ability to receive and communicate information, which produces physical and social behaviors that are inappropriate to the demands of their environment. In addition to this, difficulties often arise in the impairment of motor, visual, and auditory perception.

Motor traits of autistic children

There is considerable information concerning the abilities of autistic children. However, the data from the literature conflicts with respect to general aptitude on specific motor traits. There is agreement, however, that, more often than not, autistic children possess limited motor abilities when compared to other children of the same chronological age. There is some evidence, although scanty, that autistic children possess greater variance in profiles of abilities than do normal children. For instance, Carlson[7] reports that autistic children have poor gross motor coordination, yet well-developed fine motor skills. This would indicate that unique patterns of development for gross motor skills are prerequisite to the development of fine motor skills. Autistic children, in many instances, possess uneven profiles of abilities and tend to convert their assets into obvious talents, whereas other aspects of their behavior may become poorly developed.

Gross motor ability

For the most part, autistic children possess abnormalities in gross motor development. They are often clumsy and poorly coordinated. However, there are indications that through proper application of learning principles and developmental curricula, autistic children can be taught to learn gross motor activity. This has been demonstrated by Kozloff,[13] who taught autistic children physical activity through a shaping procedure of increasing the frequency and duration of episodes of self-initiated play.

Perceptual-motor ability

There is information in the literature that autistic children possess distinct limitations in matching perceptual inputs with motor outputs. Some of the limitations are as follows:

1. Inability to clap hands to music, reflecting auditory-motor disability
2. Inability to manipulate objects, the result of visuomotor disability
3. Inability to translate imitation of movement into similar motor patterns, a further example of visuomotor disability
4. Inability to perform self-help skills, the result of impairment in gross and fine motor skills

The autistic child, as a rule, possesses a set of limited motor characteristics. The physical educator thus has a challenge in the development of a most worthy aspect of the functions of everyday living. The application of physical training to autistic children possesses great possibilities of exploration.

Socialization and play

The autistic child often is out of touch with reality and therefore finds it difficult to socialize with other children. It has been hypothesized that stereotyped activity prevents the optimal development of skills. With limitation of skills, it is often difficult for the autistic child to enage in social activities with others. Team or group interaction depends on the severity of the disability. Competitive situations are often frightening and demoralizing to the child and tend to increase his withdrawal.

Instructional activities that enable the autistic child to play effectively are essential. A clear, systematic instructional system is needed in which skills for socialization can be developed with full knowledge of missing prerequisite behaviors and of programming to provide the necessary motor skills that will enable success in social living.

Some characteristics of the autistic child that reduce social opportunities are as follows:

1. *Social withdrawal and unresponsiveness:* These behaviors often make autistic children inaccessible to their peers, their parents, and other adults.
2. *Behavioral inflexibility:* These children appear to function best in highly structured environments in which predictable routines are established. Changes in routine or in the environment tend to upset many autistic children.
3. *Stereotyped behavior:* Many autistic children engage in stereotyped behaviors in which a specific act is repeated over and over. These behaviors often are bizarre and further reduce the children's social acceptance by others.
4. *Self-mutilating behavior:* These behaviors involve acts that injure the child. Some examples of such activity are head banging and biting and hitting oneself. All these behaviors make it more difficult for the child to engage in social activity.

Wing[19] indicates that, in normal play, rules that most children pick up easily cause the autistic child great difficulty.

Many such children possess difficulty in adopting social play behaviors appropriate to the situation, which often results in a withdrawal from the situation. Thus there is a need for a systematic planning of social interaction with others.

Inasmuch as play is a medium in which inabilities of the autistic child can be identified, it may be a medium through which these children may facilitate positive social behavior. There are social sequences of play and prescriptive techniques for facilitation of the social behavior in microsocial environments.[3] The application of these techniques is worthy of trial with autistic children.

There should be concerted efforts made to move autistic children from adult-initiated and side-by-side play to cooperative play with others. This is a formidable challenge. The play of autistic children weakens without the presence of novelty in the environment. Novelty can be introduced in several ways to foster the play behavior of the autistic child; some of these ways are as follows:

1. Skills within the individual can be developed so that he may invent novel ways of manipulating the environment.
2. New playthings may be added to the environment.
3. The child can be introduced to different social settings.
4. Different environmental events may be structured.

Novelty can be added in other ways. To foster play development, it is important to pair the play materials with the skill level of the child. Otherwise, there may be considerable difficulty in motivating the child to interact with the play materials so that skill and social development may occur.

Instructional factors

The literature indicates that if accepted principles of learning are applied to the instruction of children with autism and if target objectives are within their capabilities, progress in learning tasks is feasible. The effective use of shaping procedures in the teaching of a motor skill to autistic children has already been mentioned (Chapter 16). Wing[19] suggests the use of sequential activities for programming the autistic child. The child is then moved at his own rate through the sequence. Another technique that utilizes the principles of learning is the modeling of visual movement to communicate to the child tasks that he is to perform. The use of aversive stimuli, that is, an avoidance type of learning, may be successful, but should be used as a last resort. Therefore with the proper application of learning principles to programming, productive positive learning results are possible with children who are autistic.

The primary dimension that must be considered when teaching autistic children is the nature of the task. This is important in enabling the greatest potential of capability to be developed by the autistic child.

There are indications that tasks that are rather complex and that require complicated processing of information by the learner often are too difficult for the autistic child. Activities that require quick decisions and changing situations are, more often than not, too advanced for the autistic child. Therefore when selecting tasks for the child, it is desirable to perform an analysis of the task according to its complexity in relationship to the ability of the child.

Several instructional techniques can be used with autistic children. It is important that directions be presented in a clear, concise, and simple manner and that a multisensory approach be used to communicate. Also, activities should be presented in such a way that there is not a reversal or mirror image effect, that is, the instructor should plan to present visual information to the group so the children view the behavior from the rear of the instructor.

REFERENCES

1. Anderson, T. W.: Swimming and exercise during menstruation, J. Health Phys. Educ. Rec. **36**:66-68, 1965.
2. Astrand, P. O., et al.: Girl swimmers with special reference to respiratory and circulatory adaptation and gynaecological and psychiatric aspects, Acta Paediatr. (Suppl.) **147**: 1-71, 1963.
3. Auxter, D. M.: Muscular fatigue of mentally retarded children, Train. Sch. Bull. **63**:5-10, 1966.
4. Billig, H. E., Jr., and Lowendahl, E.: Mobilization of the human body, Stanford, Calif., 1949, Stanford University Press.
5. Carpenter, R. D.: Why can't I learn, Glendale, Calif., 1972, Regal Books.
6. Clow, A. E., and Sanderson, M.: Effect of physical exercise on menstruation, Mind Body **30**:19-21, 1923.
7. DesLaurlers, A. M., and Carlson, C. F.: Your child is asleep; early infantile autism: etiology, treatment, parental influences, Homeward, Ill., 1969, Dorsey Press.
8. Duntzer, E., and Hellendall, M.: Munch. Med. Wochenschr. **76**:1835, 1929.
9. Engerbretson, D. L.: The effects of internal training on the insulin dosage, sugar levels and other indexes of physical fitness in three diabetic subjects. Unpublished master's thesis, University of Illinois, Urbana, Ill., 1962.
10. Gilman, E.: Exercise program for correction of dysmenorrhea, J. Health Phys. Educ. Rec. **15**:377-381, 1944.
11. Kelly, E. D.: Adapted and corrective physical education, New York, 1965, The Ronald Press Co.
12. Kogan, B.: Health, New York, 1967, Harcourt Brace Jovanovich, Inc.
13. Kozloff, M.: Reaching the autistic child, Champaign, Ill., 1973, Research Press.
14. Mosher, C. D.: Dysmenorrhea, J.A.M.A. **62**: 1297, 1914.
15. Nolen, J.: Problems of menstruation, J. Health Phys. Educ. Rec. **36**:12, 1965.
16. Phillips, M., Fox, K., and Young, O.: Sports activity for girls, J. Health Phys. Educ. Rec. **30**:23-25, 1959.
17. Runge, H.: Effects of bodily exercise on menstruation, J.A.M.A. **129**:68-72, 1928.
18. Turner, C. E.: Personal and community health, ed. 14, St. Louis, 1971, The C. V. Mosby Co.
19. Wing, J. K.: Early childhood autism, Colorado Springs, Colo., 1966, Maxwell Publishers.
20. Yahraes, H.: Good news about diabetes, Public affairs pamphlet no. 138, New York, 1948, Public Affairs Committee, Inc.
21. Zankle, H. T.: Physical fitness index of diabetic patients, J. Assoc. Phys. Ment. Rehabil. **10**:14-17, 1956.

RECOMMENDED READINGS

Clarke, H. H., and Clarke, D. H.: Developmental and adapted physical education, Englewood Cliffs, N.J., 1963, Prentice-Hall, Inc.

Daniels, A. S., and Davies, E. A.: Adapted physical education, New York, 1975, Harper & Row, Publishers.

Fait, H. F.: Special physical education: adapted, corrective, developmental, ed. 3, Philadelphia, 1975, W. B. Saunders Co.

Muscular dystrophy—the facts, New York, 1959, Muscular Dystrophy Association of America, Inc.

Nolen, J.: Problems of menstruation, J. Health Phys. Educ. Rec. 36:12-65, 1965.

Wallace, H. M.: The muscular dystrophies. In Frampton, M. E., editor: The physically handicapped and special health problems, Boston, 1955, Porter Sargent, Publisher.

PART FOUR

ORGANIZATION AND ADMINISTRATION

Teachers and therapists need to be knowledgeable about plans for district and school programs of adapted physical education. They should know how to plan the curriculum, organize a class, and write daily lesson plans for individuals or for groups. Special facility and equipment needs of the handicapped should be a part of teacher preparation programs. These topics are discussed in Part IV.

18

PROGRAM ORGANIZATION AND ADMINISTRATION

■ No one type of adapted physical education program is suitable for all school levels or for all school districts. Possibly, this is the reason there is a very limited amount of material written about the organization and administration of adapted physical education. Good organization and administration are essential if adapted physical education programs are to be included in increasing numbers in our schools and colleges and if they are to grow and flourish at a time when educational costs are rising and when pressures exist to examine carefully the total curricular offerings at all school levels.

If one believes in the importance of providing worthwhile physical education programs for all students at all school levels, it is then equally important to offer athletic and extramural activities for the gifted student, regular physical education and intramural sports for the large "middle" group, and adapted physical education for those with temporary or permanent physical handicaps. This last group, who probably need physical education and recreation experiences more than either of the other two, have, in the past, been provided with nothing or with inadequate experiences.

A more recent trend, and one that has great promise for the future, is the inclusion of adapted physical education experiences in the *special education* programs of our schools. State and federal legislation, culminating in P.L. 94-142, recently signed into law, should provide quality educational experiences for handicapped persons from the ages of 4 to 21 years. Adapted physical education teachers at all school levels should plan to include special programs for those who are handicapped in their curricular offerings in order to satisfy this mandate. Teacher education institutions must also include information on procedures to be followed for their students specializing in physical education and recreation so that they are prepared to teach classes and offer programs for all types of disabled persons.

Adapted physical education is traditionally offered in one or more ways in districts across the United States. Prior to the signing of P.L. 94-142, many states provided adapted physical education classes for their handicapped students under a state-supported plan. Other plans were supported by the local school district and still others were under the sponsorship of the county. Ideally, these various agencies should offer a cooperative program designed to meet the needs of all disabled persons. One possible solution would be to handle the most severely disabled students in the *special education* program, where the emphasis could be on small classes, assistance from many ancillary specialties (psychiatry, nursing, therapy, speech, and hearing), and the possibility of mainstreaming as the student makes satisfactory progress. Those who are less severely handicapped would be handled in regular schools (special classes when necessary) in the adapted physical education program. This might be a state-supported, federally assisted program. Students with minor handicaps would be handled in district-supported classes and would be mainstreamed whenever possible.

In the final analysis, each state, county, and local district must now face up to the problem of how best to meet their mandated obligation to the disabled student. In any case, the goals, principles, and objectives of such programs are similar.

In 1951, the American Association for Health, Physical Education, and Recreation and the Joint Committee on Health Problems in Education of the American Medical Association and the National Education Association prepared an excellent set of principles that should prove worthwhile to persons interested in organizing, promoting, and evaluating programs of adapted physical education.

GUIDING PRINCIPLES OF ADAPTED PHYSICAL EDUCATION IN ELEMENTARY AND SECONDARY SCHOOLS AND COLLEGES*

It is the responsibility of the school to contribute to the fullest possible development of the potentialities of each individual entrusted to its care. This is a basic tenet of our democratic faith.

1. There is need for common understanding regarding the nature of adapted physical education.

Adapted physical education is a diversified program of developmental activities, games, sports, and rhythms, suited to the interests, capacities and limitations of students with disabilities who may not safely or successfully engage in unrestricted participation in the vigorous activities of the general physical education program.

2. There is need for adapted physical education in schools and colleges. . . .

3. Adapted physical education has much to offer the individual who faces the combined problem of seeking an education and living most effectively with a handicap.

Through adapted physical education the indi-

*Presented by permission of the Committee on Adapted Physical Education, American Association of Health, Physical Education, and Recreation.

vidual can: (a) Be observed and referred when the need for medical or other services is suspected; (b) Be guided in avoidance of situations which would aggravate the condition or subject him to unnecessary risks or injury; (c) Improve neuromuscular skills, general strength and endurance following convalescence from acute illness or injury; (d) Be provided with opportunities for improved psychological adjustment and social development.

4. The direct and related services essential for the proper conduct of adapted physical education should be available to our schools.

These services should include: (a) Adequate and periodic health examination; (b) Classification for physical education based on the health examination and other pertinent tests and observations; (c) Guidance of individuals needing special consideration with respect to physical activity, general health practices, recreational pursuits, vocational planning, psychological adjustment, and social development; (d) Arrangement of appropriate adapted physical education programs; (e) Evaluation and recording of progress through observations, appropriate measurements and consultations; (f) Integrated relationships with other school personnel, medical and its auxiliary services, and the family to assure continuous guidance and supervisory services; (g) Cumulative records for each individual, which should be transferred from school to school.

5. It is essential that adequate medical guidance be available for teachers of adapted physical education.

The possibility of serious pathology requires that programs of adapted physical education should not be attempted without the diagnosis, written recommendation, and supervision of a physician. The planned program of activities must be predicated upon medical findings and accomplished by competent teachers working with medical supervision and guidance. There should be an effective referral service between physicians, physical educators, and parents aimed at proper safeguards and maximum student benefits. School administrators, alert to the special needs of handicapped children, should make every effort to provide adequate staff and facilities necessary for a program of adapted physical education.

6. Teachers of adapted physical education have a great responsibility as well as an unusual opportunity.

Physical educators engaged in teaching adapted physical education should: (a) Have adequate professional education to implement the recommendations provided by medical personnel; (b) Be motivated by the highest ideals with respect to the importance of total student development and satisfactory human relationships; (c) Develop the ability to establish rapport with students who may exhibit social maladjustment as a result of a disability; (d) Be aware of a student's attitude toward his disability; (e) Be objective in relationships with students; (f) Be prepared to give the time and effort necessary to help a student overcome a difficulty; (g) Consider as strictly confidential information related to personal problems of the student; (h) Stress similarities rather than deviations, and abilities instead of disabilities.

7. Adapted physical education is necessary at all school levels.

The student with a disability faces the dual problem of overcoming a handicap and acquiring an education which will enable him to take his place in society as a respected citizen. Failure to assist a student with his problems may retard the growth and development process.

Offering adapted physical education in the elementary grades, and continuing through the secondary school and college, will assist the individual to improve function and make adequate psychological and social adjustments. It will be a factor in his attaining maximum growth and development within the limits of the disability. It will minimize attitudes of defect and fears of insecurity. It will help him face the future with confidence.

The outcomes or objectives of adapted physical education should draw from the objectives of physical education in general, but should be more specific and definitive in terms of the special group of students to be served. The objectives should represent definite behaviors that are attainable by students in the program; however, all students would not be expected to attain all the objectives. An adapted physical education program organized so that all of the objectives are provided for makes it possible for each student to meet those objectives of special importance to their particular needs and interests.

OBJECTIVES OF ADAPTED PHYSICAL EDUCATION

The aim of adapted physical education is to aid students with handicaps to achieve physical, mental, emotional, and social growth commensurate with their potential through a carefully planned program of regular and special physical education and recreation activities.

Specific objectives to help the student accomplish this are as follows:

1. To help students correct conditions that can be improved
2. To help students protect themselves and any conditions that would be aggravated through certain physical activities
3. To provide students with an opportunity to learn and to participate in a number of appropriate recreational and leisure-time sports and activities
4. To improve physical fitness through the maximal development of organic and neuromuscular systems
5. To help each student develop a knowledge and an appreciation of his physical and mental limitations
6. To help students make social adjustments and develop a feeling of self-worth and value
7. To aid each student in developing knowledge and appreciation relative to good body mechanics
8. To help students understand and appreciate a variety of sports that they can enjoy as nonparticipants or spectators

Many government programs and state laws currently require that program administrators and teachers state their program goals and objectives in behavioral or performance terms. This provides for more accurate assessment and accountability of programs, teachers, and students. A meaningfully stated objective is one that succeeds exactly in communicating to the reader the writer's instructional intent. Performance objectives must include the following:

1. A statement of who is going to demonstrate (the performer)
2. A statement of what exactly is included (knowledge, skills, and/or behavior)
3. A statement of the conditions under which the performance will be done
4. A statement identifying the standard of achievement (how *well* and/or how *much*)
5. A statement indicating how the performance will be measured (with what instruments, used by whom)

Chapter 4 of this text includes a more complete discussion of this topic with nu-

merous examples given. Examples are also given in Chapter 5. Three examples are given here to help clarify the technique of writing performance objectives.

EXAMPLE 1: For an obese girl assigned to an adapted physical education class to lose weight: "Jill Jones will lose ½ pound of body weight each week during the 15-week fall semester."

EXAMPLE 2: For a boy with cerebral palsy who wishes to improve his ability and skill in swimming: "Mike Moon will demonstrate his ability to swim a distance of 50 yards using each of two different swimming strokes (with no time limit) by the end of the spring semester."

EXAMPLE 3: For trainable mentally retarded (T.M.R.) persons with severe perceptual-motor problems: "Alex Brooks will demonstrate his ability to roll over from a prone to a supine position and to crawl and creep one body length on a mat by the end of the fall quarter."

In addition to its aims, objectives, and principles, an adapted physical education program is influenced by a number of practical factors that vary from district to district and even between schools located in the same district. These include the following:

1. Community and administrative support
2. Adequacy of the budget
3. Available facilities and equipment
4. Availability of qualified supervisory and teaching personnel
5. Student interest and support

Thus based on sound aims, objectives, and principles and conditioned by practical factors that may influence the curricular offerings of a school, an adapted physical education program must be planned so that it operates most effectively for the students, teachers, and administrators of the particular school or district. Subsequent sections of this chapter should provide helpful suggestions toward this end.

ORGANIZATION OF THE PROGRAM

There should be a long-range plan of organization, whether a new program is being formulated or a well-established one is being evaluated and change suggested for it. The responsibility for the program should be delegated to one person, usually a supervisor at the district level or a well-qualified teacher if one school is being considered. In either case, this person should be aided by an advisory committee or council. This committee helps in such matters as establishment of policy, formation of long-range plans, selection and release of students (at the school level), and interpretation and promotion of the program.

The supervisor and the teacher

The person in charge of the program, together with the teachers, constitutes the program's most important single aspect. For this reason, the supervisor or teacher should be selected because of outstanding qualifications, including personality, experience, training, and knowledge of local, state, and federal regulations.

Personality

Personality, a most important quality of a teacher, is doubly important for the supervisor-teacher of adapted physical education. The very nature of the position, involving as it does both teaching and administration, requires close contact with administrators, counselors, medical personnel, teachers, and students. Students with special needs require a superior teacher, one who can establish close rapport with students; can teach effectively; and can work diplomatically with physicians, nurses, administrators, and other teachers. These qualities are necessary to ensure success in an adapted physical education program.

Experience

Prior teaching experience with adapted classes is a necessary prerequisite for the person who assumes the leadership of an adapted physical education program. Techniques used in teaching disabled persons vary somewhat from those used in teaching regular physical education classes. Generally, more individual teaching and counseling are done in an adapted class and a closer bond is established between teacher and pupil. Special skills and knowledge also are necessary to deal effectively with physicians, nurses, and other medical personnel.

Training

It is desirable that the person heading the adapted physical education program have, as minimum requirements, special training in life and physical sciences, psychology, applied anatomy and physiology, and adapted physical education. Graduate training in adapted or corrective physical education, corrective therapy, or physical therapy would strengthen this background so that expert leadership can be given to members of the adapted physical education teaching faculty and to students in the program.

Recent federal and state legislation has allowed for the expansion of educational programs for the handicapped. To provide better instructional programs for these persons, teacher education institutions have had to expand their training programs to meet this need. Special credentials, certificates, and degrees are granted to those who complete advanced specialized programs in preparation for their work with "inconvenienced" individuals. Extensive fieldwork, internship, and/or student teaching assignments should be parts of such advanced training.

The American Association for Health, Physical Education, and Recreation in cooperation with the Bureau of Education for the Handicapped, United States Department of Health, Education, and Welfare published *Guidelines for Professional Preparation Programs for Personnel Involved in Physical Education and Recreation for the Handicapped*[1] *and included the following recommendations*:

*From Guidelines for professional preparation programs for personnel involved in physical education and recreation for the handicapped, Washington, D.C., 1973, American Association for Health, Physical Education and Recreation and Bureau of Education for the Handicapped, U.S. Department of Health, Education, and Welfare.

Every student needs opportunities for field experiences under the guidance of qualified personnel. Field experience must be an integral part of every [graduate] program in adapted physical education.

1. Careful consideration should be given to providing students with maximum exposure to field experiences commensurate with specialized needs.
2. Course work and theory should be integrated and related to practical situations through appropriate observation and participatory experiences.
3. Formal internships or similar arrangements should be structured to provide increasing opportunities for each student to execute and evaluate learning experiences related to his specialization.
4. Field experiences should be available in a variety of situations within a reasonable geographical area. Field experiences will vary depending on the focus of [graduate] programs, handicapping conditions, and settings in which experiences occur.
5. Supervision of field experiences should be a joint responsibility of faculty and field personnel. Roles of field personnel should be expanded to include participation in developing and modifying [graduate] programs.
6. Specific sites for field experiences may be judged according to such pertinent characteristics as:
   a. Appropriateness to emphases in [graduate] programs
   b. Accessibility to college or university
   c. Availability and adequacy of supervision by faculty and field personnel
   d. Opportunities for interaction and communication with field personnel

The guidelines further elaborate on the preparation necessary for persons to enter programs of training to work with the handicapped and outline the qualifications that teachers and therapists should possess on completion of their training. This information is briefly summarized as follows:

The minimum prerequisite for enrollment in any program preparing a specialist in physical education for impaired, disabled, and handicapped persons should be an undergraduate degree and/or certification in physical education. Individuals with preparation in related professions or disciplines should be considered for graduate specialist programs only if their previous training and experience are supplemented with *essential* professional competencies of the physical education teacher. Ideally every adapted physical education specialist should possess and be able to teach skills and knowledges in a variety of physical activities, to promote a love of activity and participation in a given age group, and to understand and appreciate why such participation is important and vital to all, including impaired, disabled, and handicapped persons.

The specialist in adapted physical education should be able to perform these functions:

1. Assess and evaluate the physical and motor status of individuals with a variety of handicapping conditions.
2. Develop (design, plan), implement (conduct), and evaluate diversified programs of physical education for individuals and groups with any of a variety of handicapping conditions.
3. Participate in interprofessional situations providing special programs or services for individuals or groups, including coordination of such services for a program.

The advisory committee

The advisory committee may be district-wide or may be set up to advise relative to the program at one particular school.

An advisory committee at the district level might consist of the school district physician, a key administrator at the district level, a district or school nurse, the supervisor of adapted physical education, and, possibly, a representative from each of the following groups:

1. The regular physical education teachers
2. The teachers who do not teach physical education
3. The Parent-Teacher Association or other parents' group
4. Representatives of other community groups that are closely associated with physically handicapped children

This committee is advisory in nature and aids the supervisor in the establishment and interpretation of policy; in fostering good public relations; in dealing with physicians', nurses', and parents' groups in the community; and in procuring funds for the program.

An advisory committee at the school level has responsibilities similar to the district committee. It should advise and support the teachers of adapted physical education. It is concerned with interpretation of the program and with public relations at the school level. It also aids in the selection of, and in the release of, students considered for the program. Members of this committee usually include the school physician, the school nurse, an administrator, teachers of adapted physical education for girls and/or for boys, and, often, one or more of the following persons: a teacher from an area other than physical education, a parent or Parent-Teacher Association member, a counselor, a student, the health coordinator, or a representative of the health teachers.

The supervisor and the teachers of adapted physical education will find that the adapted physical education committee can give them invaluable aid in planning for and interpreting this specialized type of program. The members of these committees must therefore be selected with great care.

Interpreting the program

Promoting an adapted physical education program in either a school or a school district requires the ability to demonstrate a real need for the program. It also requires excellence in program planning and teaching, demonstrating that positive results can be obtained through the conduct of a *quality* program.

The need for an adapted program can be demonstrated in a number of different ways: (1) through surveys of the school itself, of schools in the district, or of schools in other nearby districts; (2) by presentation of data obtained from city, county, state, and national bodies showing the need for such programs; and (3) by presentation of published materials by prominent authorities who advocate such classes in the schools. These materials can be presented to school boards, administrators, parents' and teachers' groups, and students to inform them of the need for and value of adapted physical education.

The survey

A survey of a school or district for the purpose of showing a need for adapted physical education should include information about the following factors:
1. The availability of teachers and their background of education and experience
2. The time allotment necessary for the program
3. The cost of the program
4. Existing facilities and equipment and amount of additional space and supplies needed
5. Special problems related to the medical and nursing services
6. Special problems involved in counseling these students and scheduling them for classes at special hours during the day

The caliber of the adapted physical education teacher is the single most important factor of those listed. Money, equipment, support of the physician, nurse, and other teachers all are important, but an enthusiastic, well-qualified teacher is a necessity. The teacher of children who have a physical, mental, or emotional handicap must not only be a good instructor, but must also have the understanding and the ability to establish rapport with students who are seeking an education despite a disability.

Because the adapted physical education program involves special classes for only a portion of the total student enrollment of a school and because class size should be limited to allow for considerable individual instruction, scheduling problems sometimes result. School administrators and counselors must be convinced that this group of students, who have a special need, should be scheduled or programmed into the adapted physical education class early in the selection of their class schedule. In a small school with only 4% to 10% of the students in need of an adapted physical education class, only one class for boys and one for girls may be offered and this may create schedule problems for the students. Some specialists in the field have suggested that these classes be made coeducational to facilitate scheduling the students. This provides twice as many class choices and thus allows for more flexible scheduling procedures.

An adapted physical education program does cost a school or school district additional money. Small classes, special equipment, a special room, and additional medical guidance increase costs over what is spent on regular physical education classes. These costs need not be exorbitant, however. An excellent program can be provided with a minimum of special equipment and even without a special room if one is not available. To help meet the excess expenses, district, state, and federal funds should be made available for classes for handicapped students who have need for special attention in physical education.

Adequate equipment and a well-planned adapted physical education room facilitate the teacher's job and add enjoyment to the program for the student. The teacher who has adequate facilities and equipment can do a better job of meeting the needs of the special student.

The school physician and the nurse play an important role in the adapted physical education program. The support and active backing of these persons are essential if a top quality program is to be presented. The initial screening and assignment of the pupils to adapted physical education should be done by the physician. He should also make the final judgment on when the student returns to the regular physical education class. In between these two times, he may be called on to do further tests on students or he may refer them to another medical specialist for examination. These referrals may result in recommending a change in the student's exercise or activity program.

Considerable data are available to substantiate the importance of providing physical education classes for all students enrolled in school, extending from kindergarten through college or university. Local districts; the American Medical Association; the California Association for Health, Physical Education, and Recreation; the American Alliance for Health, Physical Education, and Recreation; and the President's Council on Physical Fitness have gathered valuable data to substantiate the need for physical education at all school levels. Published materials recommending special programs of adapted physical education in our schools are numerous[2-12] Ample evidence is available to present a strong case for the inclusion of a good adapted physical education program at all school levels. Three such examples are that (1) the Pennsylvania Department of Public Instruction requires all public schools to have adapted physical education programs, (2) the California Education Code provides additional funds to support physical education programs for those who are physically handicapped, and (3) P.L. 94-142, discussed in Chapters 1, 4, and 19, mandates the inclusion of equal educational programs for handicapped persons to commence in 1978.

Teacher and student schedules

Because the adapted physical education class requires a teacher with special training, certain problems may develop in scheduling the classes of that teacher. In a small school, classes may be offered only one or two periods during the day. If more than one class is offered, it is advantageous to have them scheduled consecutively. This will facilitate opening the special adapted physical education room, providing the special equipment necessary, and obtaining the medical records and the exercise and activity cards. It will also give the teacher time between the two periods to counsel students in need of special help. These same advantages prevail for a single class if it is scheduled the first period in the morning, before or after lunch, or the last period in the afternoon.

Some important factors in student scheduling were discussed earlier in this chapter; however, there are some additional matters that also should be considered.

If the special exercise room, the pool, or the special game areas used by the adapted physical education classes are available only during certain periods of the day, the schedule should be arranged so that the adapted classes can use as many of these areas as possible during the course of the year. Often, adapted classes will use the gymnasium; gymnastic, weight-training, or wrestling room; or the dance studio, when vacant. When this is done, it should be a part of the master schedule of this particular facility. Any of these rooms may be used in lieu of a special adapted room or they may be used as a facility for one of the activities offered in the adapted sports and activity program.

The adapted sports and activity program can usually be quite flexible and can be so organized that facilities are used when they are not needed by the other physical education classes that meet during the same period. It is important, however, that a block of time be provided for the adapted class for each activity area, including the pool, so that students in this program have a rich and varied experience in a wide range of physical education activities.

If possible, adapted physical education classes for the boys and for the girls should be secheduled at the same time of day. Thus coeducational classes can be offered or coeducational activities can be arranged for the students in this program when the time and the activities permit.

RELATIONSHIP WITH ADMINISTRATORS, PHYSICIANS, AND PARENTS

The support of five persons or groups of persons is essential if a school or school district is to have a quality program in adapted physical education. They are the administrator, the teacher, the physician, the parent, and the student. The teacher has already been discussed and the student's role will vary with the particular handicap involved.

The administrator

The support of the administration is a necessity if the program is to receive its share of district and school resources. The administrator can help in the following ways:

1. Give enthusiastic support to the total program
2. Provide adequate budget
3. Require adequately trained teachers
4. Support necessary student schedule changes
5. Provide auxiliary services such as medical, nursing, transportation, and maintenance

The physician

The school or district physician plays a very important role in relation to the adapted physical education program. In addition to serving on the advisory committee, where he has the ultimate responsibility for admitting and releasing students, the physician can enhance the program in the following ways:

1. Interpret the program to private physicians in the district, to parents, and to the total school population (Fig. 18-1)
2. Handle or make referrals of students with special problems
3. Fully inform the adapted physical education instructors of the students' conditions and recommend exercises and activities for each student (Figs. 18-2 and 18-3)

The parent

Parents need to be informed about adapted physical education in the school. If possible, they should know, in general, about the adapted program before their child is assigned. This can be done in several different ways. In many schools, an information sheet or brochure is sent to the parents of each new student. This gives an overview of the general rules and regulations of the physical education departments. It may also include information about the adapted program, its aims, its objectives, its activity offerings, and its admission and dismissal procedures. It should be described as an extension and an integral part of the total physical education program, open to any student in the school during a time of special need. The scope of the program can be described to the parent

Text continued on p. 423.

YOURNAME HIGH SCHOOL
LONG BEACH, CALIFORNIA

Alan Walter, M.D.

Dear *Dr. Walter,*

     In order that we may better serve the health needs of our
students, the Yourname High School wishes to acquaint the medical
profession with the service it is prepared to render through its
Physical Education Departments.

     As you know, Physical Education is required, by law, for
all students attending high school in California. As many students
are not physically able to participate in the regular Physical
Education classes, special classes are provided for selected students to engage in corrective work of various kinds, for limited
activity, or for complete rest.

     Classes for girls/boys are conducted by specially trained
teachers and include special programs as follows:

Posture and Body   Preventive and corrective exercise programs
  Mechanics: for feet, ankles, knees, spinal curvatures
                    and other postural problems.

Weak Musculature: Developmental exercises and activities for
                    the sub-fit student.

Restricted Activities: Adapted sports and activities for those
                    students in need of a limited activity
                    program (Cardiac, Asthma, etc.).

Pre and Post   Special exercise programs as prescribed
  Operative: by the physician.

Dysmennorrhea: Counseling and exercise and activity pro-
  (Girls)   grams as advised by the physician.

Rest: Quiet games and activities, relaxation
                    techniques, or rest as prescribed.

     Classes are small and individual attention is given each
student. Your suggestions and your interest in this program are
solicited.

                    Sincerely yours,

                    Marie Carol, M.D.
                    School Physician

Approved: J. Officer
         Principal

A

Fig. 18-1. A, Letter to the private physician from the school doctor.

```
                              Date_____

     To:_____.
              School physician

     _____ High School

     From:_____, M.D.

     Subject:  Recommendations re:  Physical Education for my patient,

             _____

           Based on my examination of _____, his/her physical

     education assignment should be as follows:

     Diagnosis_____

     Permanent_____Temporary_____(How long)_____

     Regular physical education_____

     Adapted physical education_____

     All activities except (please list)_____

     _____

     Only the following activities (please list)_____

     _____

     Special exercises for (please list)_____

     _____

     Complete rest during physical education_____

     The student should be excused from physical education until_____

     _____(date).



     Date_____            Signed_____,M.D.
                                               Personal physician
```

B

Fig. 18-1, cont'd. B, Letter from the private physician to the school.

Continued.

C

YOURNAME HIGH SCHOOL

PHYSICAL EDUCATION DEPARTMENTS

Date *Jan. 15th.*

Dear *Mr. Hunter.*

Your ~~daughter~~/son *Michael*, by recommendation
of *Alan Walter, M.D.* has been assigned to the Adapted
Physical Education program because *of cardiac*
problems and poor posture .

Yourname High School's Adapted Physical Education program
offers each student in the class an opportunity to either correct,
improve, or compensate for physical or organic problems he might
have. Each student is given individual attention in accordance
with the recommendations of a family doctor or a school physician.
Every effort is made to make the time spent in this class safe,
and profitable for your child.

Sincerely yours,

Approved:
Chris Steffy, M.D.
School Physician

David Walter Daniels
Adapted Physical Education Instructor

I would like to have a conference with the Adapted Physical
Education Teacher. Day _____ Time _____. (You
may call for an appointment if you would prefer.)

Signed

_____
Parent or Guardian

Telephone number: 437-0007
437-0707

Fig. 18-1, cont'd. C, Letter to parents from the physical education instructor.

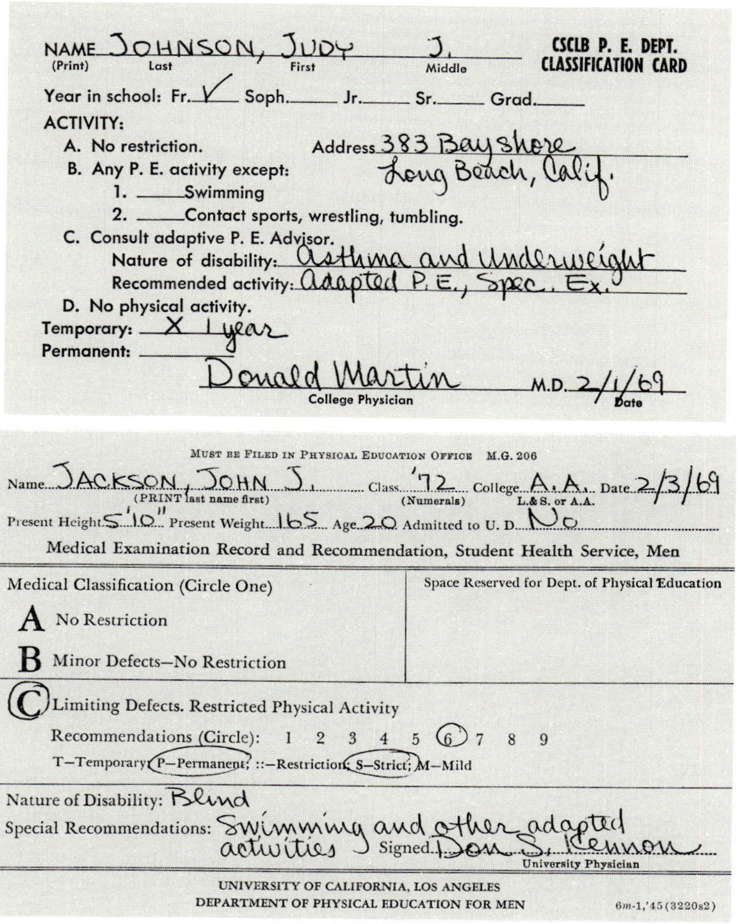

NAME (Print) JOHNSON, JUDY J. — Last First Middle

CSCLB P. E. DEPT. CLASSIFICATION CARD

Year in school: Fr. ✓ Soph.____ Jr.____ Sr.____ Grad.____

ACTIVITY:

A. No restriction. Address 383 Bayshore Long Beach, Calif.

B. Any P. E. activity except:

1. ____Swimming
2. ____Contact sports, wrestling, tumbling.

C. Consult adaptive P. E. Advisor.

Nature of disability: Asthma and underweight

Recommended activity: Adapted P.E., Spec. Ex.

D. No physical activity.

Temporary: X 1 year

Permanent: ____

Donald Martin M.D. 2/1/69

College Physician Date

MUST BE FILED IN PHYSICAL EDUCATION OFFICE M.G. 206

Name JACKSON, JOHN J. (PRINT last name first) Class '72 (Numerals) College A.A. (L.&S. or A.A.) Date 2/3/69

Present Height 5'10" Present Weight 165 Age 20 Admitted to U. D. No

Medical Examination Record and Recommendation, Student Health Service, Men

Medical Classification (Circle One) | Space Reserved for Dept. of Physical Education

A No Restriction

B Minor Defects—No Restriction

C Limiting Defects. Restricted Physical Activity

Recommendations (Circle): 1 2 3 4 5 6 7 8 9

T—Temporary; P—Permanent; ::—Restriction; S—Strict; M—Mild

Nature of Disability: Blind

Special Recommendations: Swimming and other adapted activities Signed Don S. Kennon

University Physician

UNIVERSITY OF CALIFORNIA, LOS ANGELES

DEPARTMENT OF PHYSICAL EDUCATION FOR MEN

6m-1,'45(3220s2)

Fig. 18-2. Sample medical classification cards from the school physician to the physical education department. (See Fig. 18-3 for explanation of code markings and recommendations appearing on these cards.)

LONG BEACH STATE COLLEGE

Division of Health, Physical Education and Recreation

A PLAN OF COORDINATION BETWEEN THE DEPARTMENT OF PHYSICAL EDUCATION AND THE
STUDENT HEALTH SERVICE

Every entering or re-entering student will be given a medical examination by the
student health service. At the conclusion of this examination, the student will be
classified by the examining physician for physical education activities according to
the classifications listed below.

Class A - No restrictions

Class B - Minor restrictions in activity where a student might be excused from
one or two hazardous types of sports but would be cleared for all others.

Class C - Limited (adapted) physical education. The physician should state reason
and briefly describe the types of exercises or activities which would
benefit the student. Assignment to a special class might be necessary.
Use code below where possible and indicate approximate length of time
for restriction.

CODE

1) Output of energy to be reduced: Not to exercise severely enough to become much
out of breath, nor long enough to become much fatigued. This class will include
persons with heart disease, diabetes, severe asthma, hyperthyroidism, neuro-
circulatory asthenia, etc., or convalescing from recent illness.
2) Protect from physical trauma: Should be used for cases too severe or complicated
to be safely handled under a simple "B" classification. Atrophied limbs,
recurrent dislocations, damaged brains, and progressive high myopia are examples.
3) Avoid close contact with other students or with mats: Cases in which there is
mildly infectious or a repulsive skin condition, such as severe acne or exzema.
Infectious cases should be excluded from physical education entirely, until
cured. Persons who have a C-3 classification should also be placed in a "B - no
swimming" class.
4) Not to use legs more than necessary: For persons otherwise OK who have foot
strain, varicose veins, old leg injuries, healed thrombophlebitis, and similar
conditions, which are severe enough to cause them some trouble.
5) Epileptic: MUST BE KEPT OUT OF POOL AND OFF OF HIGH PLACES.
6) Adapt activity to some deformity: Students who are blind or deaf or who have
amputated limbs are often not especially fragile, and do very well in many
activities if given proper assistance.
7) Hernia: Avoid anything that causes increased intra-abdominal pressure, such as
heavy lifting or straining, and anything else that causes pain at the site of
the hernia.
8) Recommended for certain activity only. Specify.
9) Has some physical condition which, while not disabling, may be benefited by
special corrective physical exercises. Examples are spinal curvatures, foot
strain, certain recurrent dislocations, and general muscular underdevelopment.
10) No physical education: If College requirement in Physical Education will be
unfulfilled, this requires also the approval of the Director of the Health
Service on the proper exemption form.

ACCIDENT OR ILLNESS REQUIRING A CHANGE OF CLASSIFICATION

A student who becomes ill or is injured may require a change in his medical
classification. These students should report to the Student Health Service upon their
return to school for a check-up by the attending physician who may or may not change
the student's classification. If a change is necessary, the doctor should fill out
form #HPER 20 which will be attached to the student's permanent record card in the
Department of Physical Education. If no change is necessary, a re-admittance slip
should be filled out to clear the student for full activity in physical education
classes.

Physical Education instructors must not admit a student to an activity class
unless the student has a medical classification card on file in the Physical Education
office, nor should he admit a student to re-enter class if he has been ill, without
either a "readmittance slip" or a "change of medical classification card."

The health and safety of each student at Long Beach State College can best be
guaranteed by close cooperation between the Health Service and the Division of Health,
Physical Education and Recreation. Close observance of these procedures will make
this possible.

Fig. 18-3. Explanation of the code used on the medical report cards from the physician
to the physical education department.

as including provisions for the following:
1. A physically or mentally handicapped person
2. A person who has been injured recently
3. The preoperative or postoperative patient
4. Persons who are convalescing from serious illness
5. Persons in need of special instruction to improve their physical fitness or to ameliorate a postural problem
6. Those individuals having emotional problems related to some physical disability

All of these matters can also be covered if the school provides an orientation day for parents or offers a special program during the year to inform the parents about the curricular offerings of each of the departments in the school. Another way to inform parents about the adapted program is through a form letter from the adapted physical education teacher (Fig. 18-1, C).

SELECTION AND ASSIGNMENT OF STUDENTS

The selection of students for adapted physical education and their assignment to the proper type of activity are two very important phases of the program. Students can be identified (1) through a physical examination, (2) by teachers through their observation of students in classroom or activity situations, and (3) through special testing procedures administered by members of the physical education department.

The physical examination

There are several purposes of giving each student in the school a physical examination. Ideally, the physical examination should identify pupils who need treatment, provide teachers with information concerning students' growth and health status, and identify students whose school and physical education programs need to be modified. The examination must be sufficiently personalized to form a desirable constructive educative experience for the students and their parents and provide the examin-

ing physician with an opportunity to engage in a worthwhile physician-student relationship.

It is more important that the examination be comprehensive and painstaking than that it be given annually. The examination should be given to each pupil at least every third year. The usual pattern is to require an examination in the first grade and then every 3 years through the elementary, secondary school, and college years. Parents should be informed of any disabilities discovered, at the discretion of the examining physician. Many school districts have found that it facilitates scheduling of students for physical education, and especially for adapted physical education in the junior and senior high schools, if the physical examination is given during the last half of the year when the student is enrolled in the sixth and ninth grades. The records of these examinations can then be forwarded to the counseling office of the junior or senior high school where the student will be in attendance the next year, thus facilitating program planning. If, on the other hand, the examination is not given until the student arrives at his new school in the fall of the year, he must either participate in physical education activity without having had a physical examination, which is not recommended, or he must wait for this examination before engaging in activity. Neither of these procedures is recommended, as they either present a danger to the student (and also to the school administration in terms of legal suits) or are wasteful of valuable time of the student and of the teacher.

Some school districts are unable or unwilling to provide physical examinations. In this event, each student should be required to present evidence to the school of an adequate examination from his own physician, stating his clearance for regular physical education or a recommendation for assignment to adapted physical education. There is considerable support for requiring an examination from the private physician rather than from the school phy-

PHYSICAL EDUCATION DIVISION

Physical Education Medical Referral Form
ASAW #1313-1975

Dear Dr. _____ :

(This space can be used for information about state/local physical education requirements, rationale of adapted physical education, objectives and benefits of local programs, organization and administration of local classes, purposes and uses of this form and related areas to improve understanding and communication among physicians, physical educators, parents, and others concerned with and involved in the education, health, and welfare of the student. Procedures for returning the form can be included in this section or at the end of the form.)

John J. Jones, M.D.   George T. Smith, Supervisor
Director, School Health Department   Division of Health, Physical
                                              Education and Athletics

Student information

Name: _____ School: _____
Home address: _____ City _____ State _____ Zip _____
Home telephone: (____) _____ Grade and section _____

Condition

Brief description of condition:

Condition is ☐ permanent   ☐ temporary
Comments: _____

If appropriate, comments about student's medication and its effects on participation in physical activities:

_____

Student may return to unrestricted activity _____ , 19____
Student should return for reexamination _____ , 19____

Functional capacity

☐ *Unrestricted:* No restrictions are placed relative to vigorousness or type of activities.
☐ *Restricted:* Condition is such that intensity and type of activities need to be limited. *(Check one category below.)*
   ☐ *Mild:* Ordinary physical activities need not be restricted, but usually vigorous efforts need to be avoided.
   ☐ *Moderate:* Ordinary physical activities need to be moderately restricted and sustained strenuous efforts avoided.
   ☐ *Limited:* Ordinary physical activities need to be markedly restricted.

Fig. 18-4. Physical education medical referral form approved and endorsed by the Committee on the Medical Aspects of Sports of the American Medical Association, 1975.

Activity recommendations

Indicate body areas for which physical activities should be minimized, eliminated, or maximized.

	Maximized	Minimized	Eliminated	Both	Left	Right	Comments, including any medical contraindications to physical activities
Neck							
Shoulder girdle							
Arms							
Elbows							
Hands and wrists							
Abdomen							
Back							
Pelvic girdle							
Legs							
Knees							
Feet and ankles							
Toes							
Fingers							
Other (specify)							

Remedial

☐ Condition is such that defects or deviations can be improved or prevented from becoming worse through use of carefully selected exercise and/or activities. The following are remedial exercises and/or activities recommended for this student: (Please be specific.)

_____

_____

_____

_____

_____

_____

_____

_____

Signed _____ M.D.

Address _____

_____ Zip _____

Telephone No. (   ) _____

Date _____ 19____

Fig. 18-4, cont'd. For legend see opposite page.

sician, since the private physician should have a better longitudinal picture of the health or health problems of the student.

In no case should students be permitted to engage in physical education activities without proper clearance from a physician.

Type of examination

The physical examination should consist of the following as a minimum:
1. Information obtained by the school nurse should include the student's health history, a vision and hearing test, a record of height and weight, information about the general nutritional status of the student, and a general posture and foot examination.
2. The physician's examination should include heart (before and after exercise), lungs, blood pressure, abdomen, eye, ear, nose, throat, skin, glands, and major posture faults.
3. The student should be referred to his family physician; to a specialist provided by the school district; or to the city, county, state, or other public agencies for additional examinations by specialists when needed and not provided by the district. These special examinations could include psychological examinations, checkups for tuberculosis, or services of other medical specialties such as cardiologists and orthopedists. The service agencies concerned with crippled children, cerebral palsy, neuromuscular disorders, asthma, heart disorders, diabetes, mental retardation, and the like may be consulted as needed.

Medical and physical examination records

An accumulative record card or folder should be prepared during the initial examination and it should follow the student throughout his school years. Many school districts will not forward to a new school district the medical records of the student when he transfers or graduates from that school or district. Since the health record is of such vital importance, provisions

should be made to make inexpensive photostatic copies of the record to forward to the new school along with the academic records that are usually sent. Basic information found on the accumulative record card includes a record of all previous physical examinations, a record of illnesses, immunizations, tests, injuries, referrals and the findings of them, a growth record, defects and their correction, the health history, and information relative to the assignment of students to special classes and activities in physical education (Fig. 18-5).

It is essential that the physical education department receive a written recommendation from the health office, which provides the following information: student's full name, year in school, date of examination, classification for physical education activity, a brief diagnosis and recommendations for the type of exercise and activity approved for those students who should enter adapted physical education classes, length of time a student should remain in the special program, and the signature of the examining physician or of the nurse who transposes the information from the permanent medical record (Fig. 18-2).

This card is filed in the physical education department office. It is then the responsibility of each instructor to check to be sure that all students have had a physical examination and that they are enrolled in the proper type of activity relative to their medical classification for physical education before they engage in any physical activity.

CLASSIFICATION FOR PHYSICAL EDUCATION

Students should be classified by the physician for physical education according to a classification system developed cooperatively by and mutually understood by the medical staff, the school administration, and the instructors in the physical education department. A system frequently used in schools and colleges, which combines simplicity with accuracy and thus facilitates the transfer of important information from the physician to the faculty, is presented in Fig. 18-3.

When the physician, the nurse, and the members of the physical education departments are all familiar with the information presented in the plan just described, "a plan of coordination between the Department of Physical Education and the Student Health Service," rather detailed information can be forwarded by the examining physician to the physical education department by means of the code described. Busy physicians with a large physician-student load can therefore furnish more complete information to the physical education department and, specifically, to the adapted physical education instructor than would be possible if they had to write out a complete description of the student's condition and to make complete recommendations for activity programs for each student.

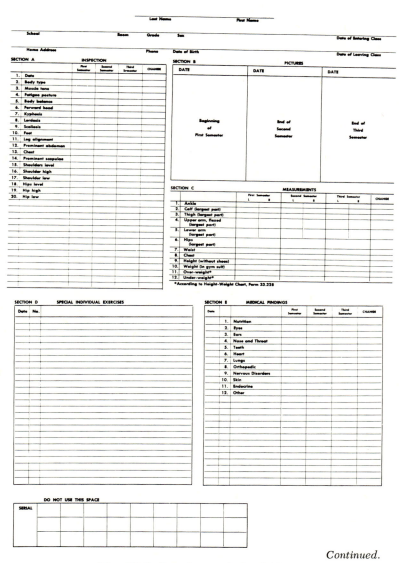

Continued.

Fig. 18-5. Sample cumulative folder.

SECTION F	CORRECTIVE TEACHER'S NOTES	
Date		Signature

SECTION G	DOCTOR'S RECOMMENDATIONS	
Date		Signature

SECTION H   PROGRAM EVALUATION

SECTION J   DISPENSATION OF CASE

	First Semester	Sig.	Second Semester	Sig.	Third Semester	Sig.
Case closed (date)						
Pupil to regular P.E.						
Recommended for further exercise						

LOS ANGELES CITY SCHOOL DISTRICTS
Auxiliary Services Division — Health Education and Health Services Branch
CORRECTIVE PHYSICAL EDUCATION HISTORY FOLDER
INFORMATION AND DIRECTIONS FOR USE OF THIS FOLDER

1. **WHAT IS THE PURPOSE OF THIS INSTRUMENT?** This folder has been prepared for the corrective physical education teacher to use during three semesters as a history record of pupil progress in corrective physical education.

2. **WHO IS TO FILL IT OUT?** This folder is to be filled out by the corrective physical education teacher in whose class the pupil is enrolled.

3. **WHEN IS THE FOLDER TO BE FILLED OUT?** The folder is to be filled out when the pupil first enters the class and each semester period during the time the pupil is enrolled in corrective physical education. Use additional folders when necessary.

4. **TO WHOM IS THE FOLDER TO BE SENT?** The folder is to be sent to the Corrective Physical Education Section of the Health Education and Health Services Branch.

5. **WHEN IS THIS FOLDER DUE?** Upon request. However, if the pupil transfers, the folder should be sent immediately to the Corrective Physical Education Section of the Health Education and Health Services Branch, with pupil's new address or school.

6. **DIRECTIONS FOR SECTION A.** Record date in appropriate column. Record body type as L (lithe), M (medium), S (stout). Record muscle tone as good or poor. Record items 4 to 9 inclusive according to degree using a 1 to 4 scale with 1 (little) and 4 (much). Record feet as N (normal), P (pronated), S (supinated), F (flat). Record leg alignment as N (normal), B (bowed), K (knock-knee). Record prominent abdomen as "yes" or "no." Record chest as N (normal), F (flat), P (pigeon). Record items 14 and 15 as "yes" or "no." Record items 16 through 20 as "yes" or "no"; if "yes," indicate whether left or right.

7. **DIRECTIONS FOR SECTION B.** Place in the appropriate space the photographs taken at the beginning of the first semester and at the end of the second and third semesters.

8. **DIRECTIONS FOR SECTION C.** Using a cloth or steel tape, record measurements in inches to the nearest quarter, and weight (including over or under) to the nearest pound.

9. **DIRECTIONS FOR SECTION D.** Describe all exercises planned by the corrective teacher for the pupil and list these according to the following code numbers, putting the appropriate number in the column for numbers:
   1. Specific individual exercises
   2. Relaxation exercises
   3. Coordination exercises
   4. Head and neck exercises
   5. General trunk exercises
   6. Lateral trunk exercises
   7. Foot and leg alignment exercises

10. **DIRECTIONS FOR SECTION E.** The information for this section should be obtained from the pupil's health record card after conferring with the health coordinator and school nurse if a secondary school, or with the school nurse and principal if an elementary school.

11. **DIRECTIONS FOR SECTION F.** This space is for the corrective teacher to use in recording pupil progress and significant information from home or other sources relative to the child's general health problems, including his feelings regarding his defects.

12. **DIRECTIONS FOR SECTION G.** Information for this section should be obtained also from the pupil's health record card or from the school doctor or private physician.

13. **DIRECTIONS FOR SECTION H.** This space is to be used by the corrective teacher to evaluate the corrective program of the pupil. Record significant developments that have been accomplished for the pupil within the corrective class.

14. **DIRECTIONS FOR SECTION J.** This space is for the corrective teacher to use to record the dispensation of the case, that is, when the pupil leaves the class, when the pupil is returned to regular physical education, or in case the pupil is recommended for more than the three semesters of corrective physical education.

CORRECTIVE TEACHER'S SIGNATURE	DATE
1.	
2.	
3.	

Fig. 18-5, cont'd. Sample cumulative folder.

When physical examinations are conducted at the school, the adapted physical education teacher is often expected to be present during the physical examination. Although this is a time-consuming procedure, it provides an excellent opportunity for the examining physician and the teacher of adapted physical education to communicate. The doctor can ask specific questions regarding the program offerings and can then recommend exercises and activities more adequately. The physical education teacher has the opportunity of seeking detailed information from the physician about the nature and cause of the various disabilities discovered and can obtain specific information about the exercise and activity programs recommended by the physician.

Understanding and free communication between the examining physician and the teacher are essential if the special needs of the child are to be adequately met.

Use of a classification code

In addition to indicating which students should be assigned to adapted physical education classes, the classification code has several other functions (Fig. 18-3). Students who are classified "A" are permitted to enroll in any physical education activity. This often clears them for all intramural sports and the extramural playday type of program for girls. Boys and girls who participate in the interscholastic athletic program are usually given an additional yearly examination to clear them for competition in one or more of the sports activities.

A "B" classification indicates that the student has a disability that limits his participation in one or two specific activities. Using the "B" classification to indicate that a student can participate in all physical education activities except one or two reduces the problem of his assignment to the proper physical education class to one of clerically checking on his enrollment in physical education. Thus the time of the physician and the physical educator can be used on other more important matters. An example would be "Class B, no swimming." The counseling department and the physical education department should be informed to eliminate swimming from the student's schedule.

A limited number of students may need to be restricted from all participation in physical education. They are often classified "D" by the examining physician. The number of students involved should diminish as the quality of the adapted physical education program improves. A good adapted physical education program should be able to provide some type of activity for any student who is well enough to attend regular classes in the school. Students in need of such specialized programs are classified "C" by the doctor and are

assigned to an adapted physical education class. Their exercise and activity assignments are then planned by a physical education teacher with special training. The adapted physical education class offerings are described in detail in other portions of this text. If an adapted physical education program is not offered in a school, students with rather severe limitations can often be used in the capacity of an official, a scorekeeper, a statician, or the like and can then accrue the benefits of socializing with their fellow students and of becoming a participating spectator in the world of sports.

Program adaptations in regular physical education

Students with minor disabilities or posture problems that are functional in nature may receive valuable assistance with their problems if the regular physical education instructor is notified of these conditions and a recommendation is made for a *preventive* program of exercises and activities. Special exercise programs can be given to these students during the regular warm-up period. Possibly, a student would do two regular warm-up exercises with the class; then he might do two or three exercises that are specific for his own problem. Students who need a special sports skill or activity may be allowed to participate in the desired activity alongside the regular class. As an example, a student may need special kicking drills in the swimming pool on a kickboard to strengthen a knee or may need to swim the elementary backstroke for a shoulder or upper back condition. With a little special help and planning, the regular instructor can make a substantial contribution to the physical well-being of students who have minor physical deviations and who must remain in a regular physical education class.

Transfer of students

One of the important features of a quality program of adapted physical education is to provide for the easy transfer of students to and from the special adapted physical education class. Although some students are assigned to an adapted class permanently and some for a year or a semester, there are many students in the school who need to be in the class only for a short period of time to recover from an injury or illness or to complete a program of rehabilitation that will prepare them for their return to a regular physical education section. Often, athletes who are injured during or between seasons can hasten their recovery with a special program of exercises and activities in an adapted class.

In addition to the advantage of meeting the needs of all the students in the school more adequately, the provision of a system of easy transfer of students to and from the adapted class does much to erase the stigma sometimes attached to a class for students who have a disability. When any student in the school may be assigned to this program for rehabilitation, the highly gifted as well as the disabled, there should be no stigma attached to such a transfer.

IDENTIFICATION OF STUDENTS
Identification through activities

There are a number of ways for classroom teachers in the school, and specifically for the teachers of regular physical education classes, to help identify students who are in need of adapted physical education.

Observation of the students in the classroom or on the athletic field will often disclose a physical deviation overlooked by the physician and, often, one of which the students are unaware. Those with posture deviations, the slow learners in physical education activities, the students with poor coordination or balance, and those with limited strength and endurance may be in need of a specially graded program of exercise and activity to bring them up to a level where they can keep up successfully with their peers in a regular physical education class. Such students should be referred to the school physician as possible

candidates for an adapted class or should be scheduled for a special class in developmental physical education.

Teachers, counselors, and the school nurse should also watch for the student who has a change of status because of illness or injury and thus should be transferred to an adapted class until the condition is corrected or fitness level is raised sufficiently to return to a regular class.

Identification through physical education testing

There are a number of different tests that can be administered by the physical education department to aid in the identification of students with some form of physical disability. These tests, combined with the judgment of a qualified instructor, help screen the students who have special needs for a class in adapted physical education.

The method of testing selected would depend on such factors as the specialized training of the instructors, the number of qualified teachers in the physical education department, the space available, the number of students to be tested, when the examinations are to be given, the amount of time available, and the availability of specialized testing and recording equipment.

Individual examinations by one instructor and by several instructors (station-to-station)

There are two types of individual examinations that are commonly used in schools and colleges. In one type, one instructor examines each student individually, covering all of the tests in the battery. In the other method, several stations are set up with a different instructor at each station, each responsible for administering one or more tests.

Individual examination by one instructor is usually very thorough and used to evaluate carefully the individual problems of the student. It would involve the procedures described in more detail in other sections of this text. The instructor usually

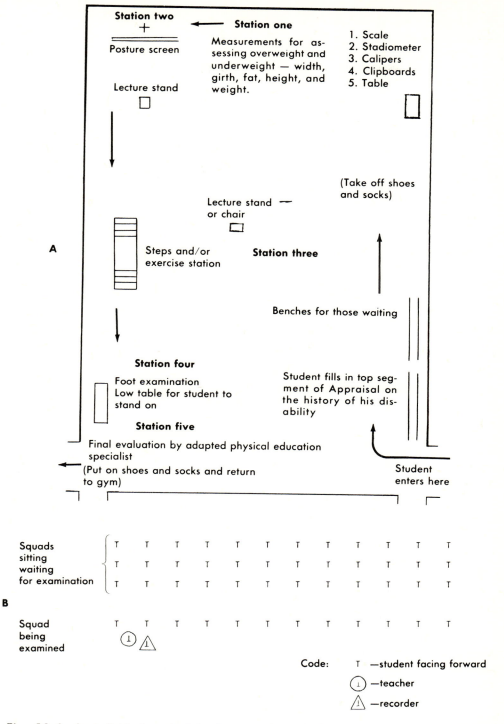

Fig. 18-6. A, Individual method (station-to-station) of conducting a posture and body mechanics examination. **B,** Group method of conducting a posture and body mechanics examination.   *Continued.*

ADAPTED PHYSICAL EDUCATION
GROUP POSTURE EXAMINATION CHECK SHEET

NOTE: Fold up bottom of page
for explanation of symbols

SAMPLE FORM

		BODY		FEET			KNEES		PELVIS			ABD.	CHEST		SHOULDERS			SPINE			HEAD		
Check for dev. from Ant.,Pos.,or Side view																							
	A	S	A&P	A	A	P	A	S	S	A&P	S	S	S	S	S	S	P	A	P	S	S	S	S	A&P
	BB	L	T	L	M	Pro	TT	Hy	Bt	T	FT	BT	Pt	P	F	F	ScW	T	Sc	Lo	Ky	B	F	T
Name of Student																								
Able, Judy																								
Baker, Suzi																								

C

Examine total class from anterior, side and posterior views. Record your eval. of all conditions for each view as you check each student, i.e. check all students from front view and record the major deviations in appropriate columns, then side, then posterior views. (1°=slight, 2°=moderate, 3°=severe)

BODY		FEET		PELVIS		ABDOMEN		SHOULDERS		SPINE	
BB	Body build	L	Long arch	T	Tilt	Pt	Ptosis	F	Forward	Sc	Scoliosis
l	Lithe	M	Meta. arch	FT	Forward tilt			ScW	Winged scap.	Lo	Lordosis
m	Medium	Pro	Pronation	BT	Backward tilt			T	Tilt	Ky	Kyphosis
h	Heavy										
L	Body lean										
T	Body tilt	HEAD		KNEES		CHEST					
		B	Back	TT	Tibial torsion	P	Pigeon				
		F	Forward	Hy	Hyper-extended	F	Flat				
		T	Tilt (side)	B	Bent						

Fig. 18-6, cont'd. C, Form used to record findings of the group type examination. (The information on the bottom half of the illustration is on the back of the form and is used to indicate the meaning of the code letters on the front of the form.)

allows 6 to 10 minutes for each student's examination.

Individual examination by several instructors (station-to-station) can be very thorough or can be used to identify the most pronounced cases. These will later be reexamined with more care by the adapted physical education specialist. As many as six to eight stations are set up, either in a large room like the gymnasium or in a series of small rooms, if they are available. Each instructor must be skillful in the administration of one or more tests and the students move from one room to another to receive the complete examination. A typical station-to-station examination plan is shown in Fig. 18-6, A. Students come to the gymnasium properly dressed for the examination. They fill out the appropriate sections of their appraisal sheet, remove shoes and socks, and proceed to station one for anthropometric measurements and evaluation of nutritional status. Age, height, weight, body width, depth, fat measurements, and girth measurements may be taken. The student then proceeds to station two for an examination with the posture screen or plumb line. Station three is a moving (functional) body mechanics examination. The student walks, performs exercises, climbs steps, sits down in a chair, and the like while the instructor evaluates these movement patterns. The student next proceeds to station four, the foot examination. Here evaluation can be made with the podiascope, pedograph, plumb line, foot tracer, and other devices needed. Stations five to eight may be used for physical fitness, range of motion, relaxation, or perceptual-motor tests, as described in the appropriate chapters of the text. The adapted physical education specialist then reviews the total examination results and prepares the final summary evaluation, which will later be used to determine which students will be placed in special classes and which are in need of special attention and counseling in regular physical education classes.

Group examinations

Lowman and Young[9] and others have suggested procedures for conducting group examinations. A modification of these examinations is presented in Fig. 18-6, *B*. Each instructor may examine his own class using this method, the adapted physical education specialist may conduct the examinations for all classes, or the two instructors may work together to evaluate each class using the group method described.

The entire class is examined by having the students line up in regular (or a predetermined) squad formation. The students are then positioned so that the examiners will have room to pass along each squad and assess each student. The students' names will have been entered previously on a group examination form (Fig. 18-6, *C*) in the same order as they are arranged in squads. The examiner then places all, except one squad, at ease (or has them sit down) while testing this one squad. He, or a recorder, fills out the form as each student is observed. (This is usually conducted as a gross type of screening to identify students who need special programs to improve fitness, body mechanics, coordination, and the like. These students can be examined more carefully at a later date.) Each student is then checked, using the same procedure, from the side and posterior views, if needed, using different tests and activities. The deviations most easily seen from each view are noted. The postural problems most easily identified from each view are so indicated on the group examination form illustrated. The "key" to the abbreviations on the form is found on the back; thus the examiner folds the bottom of the form up to refer to this key (Fig. 18-6, *C*). Records for tests of fitness and coordination can be similarly recorded.

A group examination similar to the one just described can be conducted using a circle formation with the instructor either in the center or on the outside. Recording can be accomplished as described for the other examination. If a moving examination is desired, it can be administered easily in the circle formation. Students can walk, run, skip, exercise, or stand, facing in any direction, to make this a more functional evaluation.

A number of different posture evaluations have been developed using photographic techniques. Still photographs with or without a plumb line or posture screen, motion pictures, and silhouetteographs provide a permanent record to show to a student and to be used for later comparison (Figs. 9-35 and 20-23, *E*). When certain body landmarks are located on these pictures, various semiobjective measurements can be made to assess static posture.

Many other types of tests can be used to aid in the selection of students for the adapted physical education class. These will not be discussed in detail in this section, since they are described in other parts of this text or in most standard texts on physical education tests and measurements. Some of the types of tests and evaluations that should be included in the procedures previously described are the following:

1. Range of motion (goniometry, tracings) (Chapter 20)
2. Perceptual-motor tests (Chapters 3 and 20)
3. Relaxation (Jacobson, Rathbone, Benson) (Chapter 6)
4. Physical fitness (American Association for Health, Physical Education, and Recreation; Canadian Association for Health, Physical Education, and Recreation; Clarke; President's Council on Physical Fitness) (Chapters 7 and 12)
5. Health or personal history of student (health, sleep, rest, relaxation, recreation, etc.) (Fig. 5-47)

THE ADAPTED PHYSICAL EDUCATOR AS COUNSELOR

In general, the function of a counselor is to provide a counselee the opportunity to increase self-understanding.[5] Although counseling and guidance in the school or clinical setting are normally carried out by specially trained personnel, there are many instances in which the adapted physical educator must assume this role. Some of the more common of these counseling situations can be categorized under five distinct headings, namely, (1) modulating energy output, (2) reasonable goal setting, (3) daily living practices, (4) family adjustment, and (5) social adjustment.

Modulating energy output

Persons who have problems of low vitality or who must limit energy expenditure must learn to carefully monitor their activity. Examples of conditions that demand careful monitoring are those affecting respiratory and cardiovascular systems. The adapted physical educator plays an integral part in helping these individuals stay within exercise and activity tolerances. Students who tend to rationalize their problem must be guided and assisted in fully understanding the nature of their problem and in accepting the limitations that it imposes.

Reasonable goal setting

One of the most important areas of assistance that the adapted physical educator can offer handicapped students is to help them set reasonable short- and long-term goals. Very often, handicapped persons either underestimate or overestimate their abilities. Perhaps because of many past failures and physical as well as emotional pain, the disabled person may say covertly, if not overtly, "I don't believe I can succeed, but prove me wrong." Therefore goals may be set either too low or too high. By setting goals that are too low, the individual protects himself; on the other hand, goals that are set too high indicate wishful thinking and fantasizing. This unrealistic attitude may be carried over to everyday living and to the selection of career or occupational goals. By understanding and accepting handicapped persons as worthwhile and helping them establish realistic goals, the adapted physical educator provides a climate that assists disabled persons in gaining a more accurate picture of their assets and liabilities.

Daily living practices

Those who are handicapped often need to develop habits that will enrich their daily lives. The adapted physical educator is often in a position to counsel the student on important aspects of hygienic living, means of coping with and/or avoiding emotional stresses, ways to make life a little easier, and, most importantly, the selection of rewarding leisure-time activities.[3]

Family adjustment

Counseling and guidance in the adapted physical education setting very often include teacher involvement with the student's family. It is of the utmost importance that the adapted physical educator know the families of his students and make himself available to them as a source of information and advice; the lines of communication must always be open between family and teacher.

An interview should take place between the family and teacher at the earliest possible time after the student is admitted to the program. It is highly desirable that the student and both parents be present when the interview takes place. The initial interview gives the teacher an opportunity to describe the program and at the same time discover the expectations of the parents. Moreover, it provides an opportunity for the teacher to determine the parent-child-sibling relationship, besides revealing possible home environmental factors that may enhance or deter the adapted physical education program.

Following the initial interview, periodic contacts with the family should be made as a means of providing feedback as to their child's progress. Such contacts give a continuous opportunity for exchanging ideas, clarifying procedures, and counseling as various problems arise. In essence, there should be a spirit of cooperation between the family and teacher for the betterment of the child.

Of major importance to the guidance of both the family and their handicapped child is the right of parents to know what is being done for their child and why.

Too often, professionals in the helping sciences keep parents in the dark about what services are being rendered to the young client. This attitude is unfortunate and usually stems from the fact that professionals think parents will not fully understand the procedures being employed. Careful communication with parents can help them to become two of the teacher's greatest allies.

To further enhance the counseling and guidance process of parents, several procedures might be tried. The first might be the planning of parent observation periods during the program, after which the teacher should be readily available to answer questions. A second possibility could be the use of parents as aides, assisting children other than their own. A third possibility, requiring highly controlled conditions, could be the utilization of parents as home therapists carrying out the directions of the teacher in helping the child to perform some prescribed activity.

Social adjustment

One of the most important, and sometimes most difficult, areas to deal with is the social adjustment of the handicapped person. Adapted physical education experiences provide major opportunities for helping those who are handicapped develop effective social skills.[12]

It is obvious that social acceptance or rejection cannot be entirely controlled by the handicapped person. For example, the public may be repulsed by the prospect of an epileptic having an unsightly seizure or the drooling individual with cerebral palsy may not be considered aesthetically desirable. The blind person's dependency and the deaf person's communicative problems may often make rewarding relationships difficult. The slowness of those who are mentally limited and the uncommon speech quality of the individual with cleft palate may be factors that disallow typical social adjustment.

The adapted physical educator's role in the social growth of the handicapped student is many faceted. One of the major

factors is for the teacher to help the disabled individual in understanding his own feelings and the reactions of others toward him, while at the same time being able to modify his own feelings. The handicapped student must be counseled into making the most of his social assets, for example, improving his appearance, his manners, his posture, and his personal hygiene. The handicapped individual, although desiring to withdraw from a potentially painful social situation, should be encouraged to take part in group activities whenever possible. Also, it is particularly important that the handicapped student learn many specific game and exercise skills as well as the joy of winning and the ability to lose gracefully.

Adapted physical education offers excellent opportunities for assisting the handicapped student in self-understanding and in acquiring a more rewarding life-style. To be most effective, the adapted physical educator must assume the role of concerned friend and confidant and extend this role into all aspects of the student's life.

ADAPTED PHYSICAL EDUCATION RECORDS

Since all the work of the adapted physical education teacher is directly related to the health and medical well-being of the student, it is essential that accurate, complete, confidential records be maintained. These records should be filed in an orderly manner so that they can be located quickly and used efficiently. All records should be dated, for example, letters sent and received, examination information received or examination performed, photographs taken, and student or parent conferences held. Some of the types of records that should be retained are listed below:

1. Medical examination card
2. Physical education testing cards
3. Posture and body mechanics examinations
4. Letters to and from physicians, the nurse, parents, and administrators
5. Photographic records

STUDENT MOTIVATION

Adapted physical education programs are most successful when they have the support of administrators, physicians, teachers, parents, and students and when the teachers are well qualified, dedicated, and able to highly motivate their students. We have observed programs in adjacent districts and schools having basically the same resources available, with the exception of the qualifications of the adapted physical education teacher: one program proved to be excellent; the other, extremely poor. A good teacher is the single most important factor to be considered in providing for a quality program.

The superior teacher is able to motivate students in many ways. Some of the motivation techniques and devices that work especially well in adapted physical education are the following:

1. Keeping students well informed about:
   a. Their medical diagnosis and the recommendations of the physician (Fig. 9-36, A)
   b. The results of any posture, body mechanics, physical fitness, flexibility, or relaxation tests administered (Fig. 9-36)
   c. Class rules, regulations, and policies, including grading procedures
2. Maintaining teacher enthusiasm and interest in students
3. Using charts and graphs to record student progress (posture examination cards, weight charts; Fig. 5-44)
4. Utilizing photography, that is, photographs of students with posture or disability problems to show them their present problem and to indicate any improvement made (Figs. 20-23, E, and 20-25, B)
5. Using exercise cards to show day-by-day improvements (Fig. 5-2)
6. Employing resistive types of exercises for boys, together with anthropometric measurements (Fig. 20-20)
7. Employing esthetic considerations for girls (nice figure, good posture, proper weight, etc.) and appropriate anthropometric measurements
8. Exercising to music
9. Using good equipment for exercises and testing (Chapters 9 and 20)
10. Maintaining interesting informative bulletin boards[2]
11. Maintaining direct participation of the teacher with the students in games and sports activities
12. Employing interesting adapted sports and games

Each teacher must select the type of motivational techniques that prove successful in the particular situation.[2,9]

Since organization and administration cut across the total adapted physical education program, topics relating to these areas are included in other chapters in this text. Parts of Chapters 3 to 5, 7 to 9, 15, 16, and 19 include detailed information about organizing students for adapted physical education, assignment of exercise routines, and organizational procedures for teaching exercise and adapted sports programs.

REFERENCES

1. Clarke, H. H., and Clarke, D. H.: Developmental and adapted physical education, Englewood Cliffs, N.J., 1963, Prentice-Hall, Inc.
2. Crowe, W. C.: The use of audio-visual materials in developmental (corrective) physical education. Unpublished master's thesis, University of California, Los Angeles, Los Angeles, 1950.
3. Daniels, A. S., and Davies, E. A.: Adaptive physical education, ed. 3, New York, 1975, Harper & Row, Publishers.
4. Guidelines for professional preparation programs for personnel involved in physical education and recreation for the handicapped, Washington, D.C., 1973, American Association for Health, Physical Education, and Recreation and Bureau of Education for the Handicapped, U.S. Department of Health, Education, and Welfare.
5. Hamilton, K. W.: Counseling the handicapped in the rehabilitation process, New York, 1950, The Ronald Press Co.
6. Karpinos, B. D.: Fitness of American youth for military service, Milbank Memorial Fund Q. 38:213, 1960.
7. Karpinos, B. D.: Health of children of school age, Washington, D.C., 1964, U.S. Department of Health, Education, and Welfare.
8. Kelly, E. D.: Adapted and corrective physical

education, New York, 1965, The Ronald Press Co.

9. Lowman, C. L., and Young, C. H.: Postural fitness significance and variations, Philadelphia, 1960, Lea & Febiger.

10. Mathews, D. K., Kurse, R., and Shaw, V.: The science of physical education for handicapped children, New York, 1962, Harper & Row, Publishers.

11. Schiffer, C. G., and Hunt, E. O.: Illness among children, Washington, D.C., 1963, U.S. Department of Health, Education, and Welfare.

12. Vodola, T. M.: Individualized physical education program for the handicapped child, Englewood Cliffs, N.J., 1973, Prentice-Hall, Inc.

RECOMMENDED READINGS

Dexter, G.: Instruction of physically handicapped pupils, remedial physical education, Sacramento, Calif., 1973, California State Department of Education.

Drowatzky, J. N.: Physical education for the mentally retarded, Philadelphia, 1971, Lea & Febiger.

Fait, H. F.: Special physical education, Philadelphia, 1972, W. B. Saunders Co.

Geddes, D.: Physical activities for individuals with handicapping conditions, St. Louis, 1974, The C. V. Mosby Co.

Guide for programs in recreation and physical education for the mentally retarded, Washington, D.C., 1968, American Association for Health, Physical Education, and Recreation and the National Education Association.

Guidelines for adapted physical education, Harrisburg, Pa., 1966, Department of Public Instruction, Commonwealth of Pennsylvania.

Moore, C. A.: The handicapped can succeed, Phys. Educ. 24:163-164, 1967.

Mosston, M.: Teaching physical education, Columbus, Ohio, 1966, Charles E. Merrill Publishing Co.

Physical activity programs and practices for the exceptional individual, third national conference, Long Beach, Calif., 1974, The Alliance.

Physical activity programs and practices for the exceptional individual, fourth national conference, Los Angeles, 1975, The Alliance.

Roice, G. R., and Stoner, W.: Administrative aspects of starting a remedial physical education program. Unpublished data, Los Angeles, 1975.

Slader, C. V.: A workable adaptive program, J. Health Phys. Educ. Rec. 39:71-72, 1968.

Stein, J.: Sense and nonsense about mainstreaming, J. Phys. Educ. Rec. 47:43, 1976.

Techniques and methods for handicapped youth, first national conference, Los Angeles, 1973, The Office of the Los Angeles County Superintendent of Schools, Division of Special Education.

19

CLASS ORGANIZATION

■ Adapted physical education classes can be organized for instruction in several different ways. Conditions vary widely throughout the United States in relation to such factors as whether or not physical education is a required subject, the number of days it is offered each week, the time allowed for the activity phase of the program, whether or not adapted physical education is integrated with the regular physical education program, the availability of specially trained teachers, and special facilities and equipment.

Depending on these factors, the class may be organized formally or informally; may be taught in a group or individually; or may consist of special exercises only, of games and adapted sports only, or of some combination of these types of activities. The special abilities and the preferences of the supervisor and the teachers may also influence the type of instructional program offered. In any event, the major factor to consider is to choose the type of class organization that will enable students in an adapted class to progress to the best of their abilities in physical education activities.

THE SPECIAL EXERCISE AND ACTIVITY PHASE OF THE PROGRAM

Many students in adapted physical education need special exercises to help them correct or prevent a disability or to improve their physical fitness or their perceptual-motor abilities. Exercise and activity programs can be conducted formally, informally, in a group, or by using a combination of these methods of instruction.

Informal (individual) class organization

Adapted classes can be organized for instruction so that each student has an individual exercise and/or activity program. This method is used most frequently at the college and upper grade levels of the secondary school, but it can be used successfully with mature boys and girls of junior high school age. Its major advantage is that students have a program specifically planned to meet their needs and interests. The exercises, the number of repetitions and the resistance used, the rest periods, and the special equipment needed are all assigned to enable students to meet their predetermined objectives. Students can be strongly motivated to work toward correction or improvement of their disabilities in this type of class. The major disadvantages of the informal or individual plan of organization are the lack of teacher control of the class and the time necessary for the teacher to prepare the individual activity programs. Some teachers may find that class control of a group of 20 to 25 students, each working on an individual program, is more difficult than having all the students do the same program simultaneously and under direct teacher control. However, the advantages of having each student engage in an individual program of activities would seem to outweigh such problems. Preparation of individual programs is time-consuming, but certain shortcuts can be used to enable the teacher to prepare these individual programs in a minimum amount of time. A complete plan for the choice and assignment of individual exercise programs is presented in Chapter 5.

Formal class organization

A class organized formally for exercises and other selected activities would be one in which all students performed the same activity at the same time, usually under the direction of the teacher or a student leader. This type of program lends itself well to the instruction of younger children in elementary and junior high school or to the instruction of boys and girls who cannot accept the responsibility of an individual program in the secondary school. The advantages of this type of organization are that it gives teachers good control of the class and

allows them to observe the performance of all the students more adequately than if they were watching 20 students, each doing something different. A disadvantage of this system is the lack of opportunity to give individually assigned activities to students with special needs. Another disadvantage is that some exercises and activities are performed by students who have no need for them and, in some cases, they might even be detrimental in nature. The use of special types of equipment is also more difficult, since each student must have his own piece of apparatus in the formal plan. Real motivation (not just teacher authority) may be lacking in this type of program, since the activities given are assigned to the whole group and not to each individual, based on his interests and his needs.

Group organization

The group organization method of class teaching involves the organization of an adapted physical education class into homogeneous groups based on similarities in the type of disability present or the type of exercise and activity program needed. Students in need of anteroposterior posture correction might be grouped together to perform the same exercises, another group might work on foot exercises, and another group might do special adapted activities and exercises for perceptual-motor growth. These groups of students may remain the same throughout the class period or they may change to allow for more flexibility in their programs. This method combines the advantage of group work with that of individuality of assignment. Dependable students can be used to lead and motivate those with less interest and drive. The teacher can also take advantage of assigning some individual types of programs and still have adequate supervision because of the several homogeneous groups that perform their programs together.

Combined method

Many teachers prefer to use a combination of the preceding types of class organization in an attempt to meet the individual needs of the students, to provide for some small group activity, and also to include formal exercise and activity sessions during which the teacher more directly controls the amount of work done and still maintains discipline and control of the class.

This combination plan might be organized as follows:

5 minutes Formal warm-up consists of all students doing the same exercises under the leadership and direction of the teacher or a student leader.

5 minutes Students are divided into homogeneous groups according to their needs and perform three activities or exercises with the members of their group under direction of a student leader.

10 minutes Each student performs five exercises or activities specifically assigned to him, doing the number of repetitions assigned and recording his progress on his exercise card. (Activities using special equipment can be assigned here, since students are able to take turns in the use of special pieces of apparatus.)

5-10 minutes Games, relays, and contests are organized and led by the teacher, finishing with formal dismissal of the class, if desired.

Additional plans for the organization of the class and of exercise and activity routines are presented in Chapters 3 to 5, 7, 14, 15, and 16.

Activities for daily living and instructional aides

Whether teachers use the individual or the group method of class organization, additional help is always needed, especially as more severely handicapped persons are included in school programs. P.L. 94-142 provides for physical education programs for all; thus there is a need for a change in emphasis in program content and in class organization. A recent trend in working with those who are handicapped is the increased use of aides. Because of the severe nature of the disabilities of those now being handled in special schools and clinics or in spe-

cial classes in regular schools, more direct help and supervision is necessary to meet the activities for daily living (ADL) and the instructionally related needs of those who are handicapped. Both paid and volunteer help are needed to provide this important function. Standards have been developed for the certification of paid aides and many junior colleges have training programs for these important members of the rehabilitation team. Parents, high school and college students in training to become teachers, and members of the PTA and other service groups often serve as volunteers in schools and hospitals. These aides and volunteers allow for an enriched, individualized program of instruction to be given, based on goals and objectives selected for each student. ADL activites such as transfers to and from a wheelchair and getting in and out of bed are examples of activities that might be included or for which special exercise programs would be developed.

THE ADAPTED SPORTS PHASE OF THE PROGRAM

The game and sports phase of an adapted physical education class can be organized in several different ways, depending on the general plan for adapted physical education in the school, how it is coordinated with the regular physical education program, the availability of regular and special facilities and equipment, and the background and skill of the teacher in charge.

Often, the special class in adapted physical education has, as a part of its yearly program, a certain amount of time scheduled for adapted sports and games. This can be organized in one of the three following ways:

1. A part of each period is devoted to a sports program.
2. From 1 to 3 days of each week are set aside for these activities.
3. A period of 1, 2, or more consecutive weeks is blocked out for an activity. There can be as many of these blocks of

time for sports activities during the semester as are deemed desirable.

Some teachers have found that the first method, in which 10 to 15 minutes of each class period are devoted to games and sports (usually after the exercise portion of the class is finished), serves as a good motivation device, keeping interest at a high level in both the exercise and sports parts of the program. Often, the game and sports activities are given in the adapted room and consist of games of low organization, relays, contests, and the like. Time, of course, is a limiting factor in this type of organization, tending to rule out sports and games that require extensive preparations, equipment checkout, instruction, or travel to a specialized location for the activity. This method is often used in elementary school classes and, to some extent, in junior high classes.

Where 1 to 3 days a week are set aside for the adapted sports program, activities that require more time, organization, and instruction can be included. Almost any game or sport can be modified so that it can be participated in by students in the adapted physical education class. Junior and senior high school classes are often organized in this fashion. This type of schedule enables the teacher to keep interest high in both the exercise and sports programs throughout the year. It also gives the student an opportunity to work on a special exercise program continuously throughout the semester or year rather than stopping his exercise routine for an extended period of time while he participates in various types of sports and games.

Some teachers prefer to organize the adapted sports portion of the class into blocks of time for instruction and activity. This type of program might consist of 4 weeks of swimming, 4 weeks of a team sport, 4 weeks of exercise, and 4 weeks of an individual sport. The advantage of this type of organization is that student and instructor attention and interest can be focused on one activity at a time. If the regular physical education classes are scheduled on the block system, it is usually easier to obtain facilities and equipment for the adapted physical education classes if they, too, are scheduled for a single activity for a block of time.

Special students in regular classes

Some teachers prefer to have the students in adapted physical education join a regular physical education class for their work in sports and games in cases in which this will be beneficial or, at least, not detrimental. This is in keeping with the concept of mainstreaming, in which handicapped students are included in regular class activities whenever feasible. The advantage of joining this regular group for various types of activities during the year is that it helps remove any stigma attached to the student's enrollment in a special class for his physical education activity. A free interchange of students between adapted and regular physical education classes, as their needs change, can do much to eliminate any such feelings on the part of the student who is placed in a special class. However, if students in adapted classes are to be assigned to regular classes, they must be screened carefully for each activity by the adapted physical education teacher so that the recommendations of the physician are closely adhered to. The adapted physical education teacher must also provide a special adapted sports program for the students who are left in his class and who cannot participate in the various activities with a regular class.

Some major disadvantages of this system include (1) the interruption of the procedures and organization of both the adapted physical education teacher and the teacher of the regular class and (2) the necessity of closely checking each student in the adapted class for each activity offered. If teachers of regular classes are willing to make the necessary adjustments in their teaching procedures, there is merit in this plan for all the students involved. The adapted sports program is more fully discussed in Chapter 8.

Coeducational classes

Some schools have attempted to offer adapted physical education classes to their students on a coeducational basis with varying degrees of success. In the experimental stage, these programs might have their best chance for success at the elementary school and college level. At the secondary school level, at which time students are especially peer conscious and are sometimes apprehensive about coeducational physical education, even in the regular classes, it would take a strong teacher with excellent backing from the other teachers and the administration to break down some of the traditional feelings associated with a coeducational type of program.

If feasible, there are several advantages to be found in the conduct of a coeducational adapted physical education program; they include the following:

1. The best teacher, male or female, can be used to administer and teach in the program.
2. In small schools, this would increase the flexibility in student scheduling and it also would aid in this problem in schools of all sizes and types, since much more flexibility would be permitted.
3. For the most part, the physical handicaps of boys and girls are similar in nature and the division of the class because of the sex of the individual student is an arbitrary one.
4. The majority of teachers are trained in corrective or adapted physical education in coeducation classes and thus the male and female teachers have a similar educational background for this type of teaching.

The major problems associated with the coeducational class occur in the examination and the exercise phases of the program. Having a male and a female teacher present during the initial posture and other examinations, even though one of them does not have special training in adaptives, and the use of appropriate apparel during both the examination and the exercise phases of the program should minimize these two problems. The traditional pattern of having completely separate classes for boys and for girls in both regular and adapted physical education is gradually being replaced by more coeducational classes. Young, open-minded teachers who are starting new programs have a rare opportunity to show that this coeducational type of program is not only feasible, but also that it may be the most advantageous way to handle classes in physical education for the special student.

GRADING (MARKING) IN ADAPTED PHYSICAL EDUCATION

A grade in any subject should promote educational outcomes and should reflect educational aims and objectives. In order to teach effectively, established objectives must indicate the desired outcomes of instruction so that they may become the criteria on which grades are based. If they are valid criteria, successful measurement will result in valid evaluation.

The complexity of grading physical education classes is magnified when the attempt is made to evaluate the performance of students in an adapted class. The one common denominator among all the students would seem to be their mastery of individual performance objectives. If students are graded on the basis of how well they meet their objectives, a posture student, a cardiac student, an obese student, and a postoperative student can all be properly evaluated for their grade in the course.

A part of the first week of orientation in the adapted physical education class should be used to discuss grading procedures in general. In addition to this, the instructor should sit down with students individually and help them work out their own personal list of objectives. The activity and exercise program is then based on needs and interests as expressed in performance objectives, with the grade (mark) reflecting how well these criteria have been met.

The following criteria might be applied to students to determine how well they have meet objectives in the adapted physical education class:

1. *Performance:* Standard of performance in reference to individual limitations, that is, vigorous work on specific activities and exercises for the posture and obese students, control of the amount and intensity of work for the cardiac and postoperative students, etc.

2. *Persistence:* Accomplishment of individual performance objectives, determined in conference with the instructor and stated in specific terms regarding what is expected.

Suggestions for recording and computing the grade are as follows:

1. Since the grade may involve some subjective judgments on the part of the instructor, the student should be observed and graded many times throughout the semester (weekly, if possible).

2. Either a letter grade or a numerical rating can be given to students evaluated (recorded on the exercise card and in the roll book); in this way, the student and the instructor are always aware of the student's progress toward stated behavior objectives.

3. These letter or numerical grades can be averaged and then should be considered, along with other factors that may influence the final grade (knowledge examinations and health factors, if they are considered), to determine the final mark for the semester.

4. Objective measurements should be used to test skill and knowledge whenever such tests are available.

CURRICULUM PLANNING

Federal and state legislation, administrative codes, and rules and regulations from boards of education provide direction and guidelines for curricular planning at the county and district level. Counties and large cities also furnish curricular direction and materials to local school districts. The curriculum for programs for those who are handicapped may be drawn from all these resources. Currently, legislators and educators in all 50 states are in the process of establishing programs for the handicapped to meet the new "right to education" legislation signed into law in 1975.

The Los Angeles County Schools, Division of Special Education, has also developed extensive curricular materials designed to meet the individual needs of handicapped persons in anticipation of and, ultimately, based on state and federal legislative mandates. These mandates relate to teacher accountability and a special education curriculum that would document pupil movement through measurable objectives, complete with criterion-referenced test measures. The result was the production of "Curriculum including Assessment, Resources, and Evaluation" (CARE). An example of this excellent ongoing program, as it is presently being field-tested, is shown in Fig. 19-1, *A* and *B*. These two illustrations show only one small facet of the psychomotor development area of this generic curriculum for individuals with exceptional needs. This portion of the curriculum is supervised and staffed by specialists in adapted physical education, with particular competencies in special education.

PLANNING FOR TEACHING AND LEARNING

Teaching and learning are facilitated by careful preplanning, whether this takes the form of a skillfully designed curriculum, a plan for a unit of study within the curricular offerings, or a well-organized daily lesson plan.[3, 4, 6, 7] Unit plans and daily lesson plans are discussed briefly in this chapter.

Unit plans

Unit plans usually consist of a systematic program of action for organizing and integrating the learning experiences of pupils around some central theme and, usually, for a given grade level. Adapted physical education classes might have unit plans in physical fitness; therapeutic exercise; per-

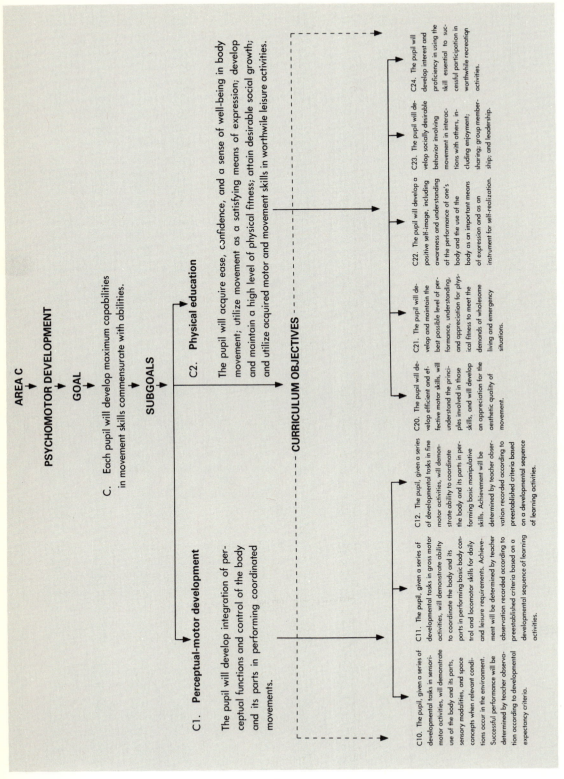

Fig. 19-1. For legend see opposite page.

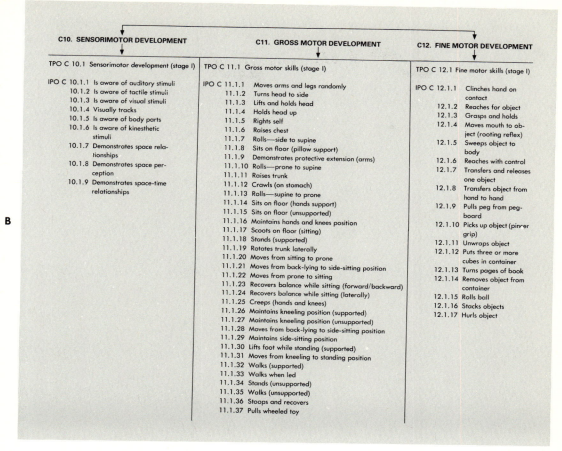

Fig. 19-1. A, Part of the organization plan for the education of handicapped persons in the special education programs of the Los Angeles County Schools. **B,** Sensorimotor, gross motor, and fine motor skills showing terminal performance objectives (TPO) and intermediate performance objectives (IPO) for each. (See part C1 in **A.**) (**A** and **B** by permission of the Office of the Los Angeles County Superintendent of Schools, Los Angeles.)

ceptual-motor activities; or in the more traditional areas of swimming, archery, or bowling; in addition units can be planned to meet the needs of persons with a particular disability.

The values of planning for units of instruction include the following[2, 7]:

1. Making learning more meaningful by avoiding the fragmentation inherent in the daily lesson plans
2. Increasing the retention of learning as a result of the unitary nature of a unit plan

3. Providing flexibility to serve individual differences
4. Helping students develop a stronger feeling of accomplishment as each unit is completed
5. Helping both teacher and learner organize their thinking toward specific ends
6. Permitting more satisfactory means for evaluating or appraising the achievement of objectives

A unit plan is usually composed of several basic elements that allow teachers to better organize guidelines for learning and consists of the following divisions:

1. *Title:* This identifies the area of study.

2. *Introduction:* This provides a general overall view of the content, emphasizes the potential values to participants, and indicates the importance in the total curricular offerings.

3. *Goals and objectives:* Objectives should have meaning to teacher and student alike. They should be clearly stated in terms of student behavior; they should provide an outline of the desired outcomes to be achieved; and the performance level should be clearly indi-

CALIFORNIA STATE UNIVERSITY, LONG BEACH

DAILY LESSON PLAN

Student Teacher_____ Date of Lesson_____ Grade_____

Master Teacher_____ Activity_____ Period_____

Primary Behavioral Objective:

Secondary Objectives:

Equipment and Supplies:

Field or Floor Markings:

TEACHER PROCEDURES AND TIME ALLOTMENT	STUDENT PROCEDURES AND CLASS ORGANIZATION	TEACHING CUES
INTRODUCTION:		
EXPLANATION:		
DEMONSTRATION:		
CLASS PARTICIPATION:		
EVALUATION OR CRITERION REFERENCE TEST:		
CONCLUSION AND TRANSITION TO NEXT LESSON:		

Fig. 19-2. Daily lesson plan form.

cated.[1, 5, 6] Objectives are usually developed in several major categories such as skills, knowledge and understanding, attitudes, and physical fitness.

4. *Development of the unit:* This involves procedures for achieving goals by organization of content, methods, and materials related to the unit. Factors to be included in planning are (1) time; (2) equipment and supplies; (3) grouping for instruction; (4) space and facilities available; (5) teacher resources, including student leaders; (6) sequence of instruction (weekly and daily plans); and (7) teaching aids such as audio visual materials.[2, 4, 6]

5. *Culmination of the unit:* This includes plans for a logical and fitting culmina-

CONSTRUCTIVE STUDENT TEACHER'S SELF-EVALUATION	MASTER TEACHER'S SUGGESTIONS Concerning Lesson Plan and Lesson:
1. Realization of Personal and Professional Objectives	
2. Weakest Part of Lesson	
3. Strongest Part of Lesson	

Fig. 19-2, cont'd. Daily lesson plan form.

tion of the activities that have been engaged in by pupils. It can take the form of skill or knowledge tests, demonstration, play-offs, meets, or individual or group evaluations.

6. *Evaluation:* This should involve the appraisal of the outcomes of learning as related to accomplishment of stated objectives in skill, knowledge, appreciation, and fitness. Objectivity should be sought in all forms of evaluation and the process should involve both the student and the teacher. Evaluation standards should be written, specific, and available to students and teachers from the inception of the unit.

Daily lesson plans

The daily lesson plan is taken from the unit plan so that proper sequences are followed and all of the essential topics and plans are included in the time scheduled for a given unit. Unit plans should not be rigidly followed, however. As student and/or class needs are discovered or more time is found to be necessary for a student in a teaching area, the curricular offerings should be modified to meet such special conditions.

A daily lesson plan, in a similar way, should help teachers and students plan ahead for desired learning experiences. A typical lesson plan should include the following major areas:

1. Name (title of unit)
2. Subunit
3. Topic of the day
4. School level or grade
5. Date
6. Major objective(s)
7. Specific performance objectives (stated in behavioral terms)[1, 5, 7]
8. Procedures
9. Facilities and equipment necessary
10. Evaluation after completion of lesson (Fig. 19-2)

Some adaptations in planning may be necessary in working with impaired and disabled persons. The suggested topics can be modified and the order changed if this will facilitate learning.

REFERENCES

1. Bloom, B. S., editor: Taxonomy of educational objectives, the classification of educational goals, handbook I: the cognitive domain, New York, 1956, David McKay Co., Inc.
2. Cowell, C. C., and Schwehn, H. M.: Modern principles and methods in high school physical education, Boston, 1958, Allyn & Bacon, Inc.
3. Creamer, J. J., and Gilmore, J. T.: Design for competency based education in special education, New York, 1974, Teacher Education Division of Special Education and Rehabilitation, School of Education, Syracuse University.
4. Kemp, J. E.: Instructional design, Belmont, Calif., 1971, Fearon Publishers.
5. Mager, R. F.: Preparing instructional objectives, Palo Alto, Calif., 1962, Pearson Press.
6. Popham, W. J.: Objectives and instruction, AERA monograph series on curriculum evaluation, No. 3, instructional objectives, Chicago, 1969, Rand McNally & Co.
7. Project Curriculum Objectives for Physical Education: Curriculum objectives for physical education, Chipley, Fla., 1974, Panhandle Area Educational Cooperative.

RECOMMENDED READINGS

Anderson, M. H., Elliot, M. E., and LaBerge, J.: Play with a purpose, New York, 1966, Harper & Row, Publishers.

Carr, D. B., et al.: Sequenced instructional programs in physical education for the handicapped, P.L. 88-164, Title III, Dec. 1970, Los Angeles City Schools Special Education Branch, Physical Education Project.

Crowe, W. C., Arnheim, D. D., and Auxter, D.: Laboratory manual in adapted physical education and recreation, St. Louis, 1977, The C. V. Mosby Co.

Daniels, A. S., and Davies, E. A.: Adapted physical education, ed. 3, New York, 1975, Harper & Row, Publishers.

Dauer, V. P.: Essential movement experiences for preschool and primary children, Minneapolis, 1972, Burgess Publishing Co.

Davis, E. C., and Wallis, E.: Toward better teaching in physical education, Englewood Cliffs, N.J., 1961, Prentice-Hall, Inc.

Dexter, G.: Instruction of physically handicapped pupils, remedial physical education, Sacramento, Calif., 1973, California State Department of Education.

Drowatzky, J. N.: Physical education for the

mentally retarded, Philadelphia, 1971, Lea & Febiger.

Educational Research Council of America: Physical education program guide, Columbus, Ohio, 1969, Charles E. Merrill Publishing Co.

Fait, H. F.: Special physical education, Philadelphia, 1975, W. B. Saunders Co.

Geddes, D.: Physical activities for individuals with handicapping conditions, St. Louis, 1974, The C. V. Mosby Company.

Guidelines for adapted physical education, Harrisburg, Pa., 1966, Department of Public Instruction, Commonwealth of Pennsylvania.

Kirchner, G.: Physical education for elementary school children, Dubuque, Iowa, 1970, William C. Brown Co., Publishers.

Nixon, J. E., and Jewett, A. E.: Physical education curriculum, New York, 1971, The Ronald Press Co.

Physical activities for the mentally retarded (ideas for instruction), Washington, D.C., 1968, American Association for Health, Physical Education, and Recreation.

20

FACILITIES AND EQUIPMENT

■ Proper facilities and equipment are as important for classes in adapted physical education as they are for classes in regular physical education. Proper facilities and equipment will help the teacher of adapted physical education make the proper adjustment in the student's program to meet his special needs, whether it is a program of special exercises, of adapted sports and activities, or of rest and relaxation. The lack of such equipment, however, should never be an excuse for the failure to provide an adapted physical education program or for offering a poor program of exercises and activities for the handicapped student. A good teacher of adapted physical education can provide a quality program for students with minimum facilities and equipment if some imagination is used and the instructor is willing to improvise. However, good facilities and equipment make the job of the teacher easier, make the program more meaningful, and provide motivation for the handicapped student.

The facility and equipment needs for adapted physical education programs may vary somewhat, according to the type of student served. Such factors as whether the class consists of all boys or all girls or is coeducational, age and maturity levels of class members, and whether they dress for activity all have an influence on facility and equipment needs. This chapter includes information about the kinds of facilities and equipment that should be provided for adapted physical education classes at the elementary, junior and senior high school, and college levels.

FACILITIES FOR ELEMENTARY SCHOOLS

Facilities for adapted physical education at the elementary school level vary extensively from district to district and from state to state. They may consist of nothing more than using the regular classroom for physical education or, under more desirable conditions, they may include such other areas as the cafeteria, the cafetorium, grass or blacktop areas, or, in a few instances, a gymnasium or a swimming pool. Since many school districts do not hire special physical education teachers for the elementary school level, both the regular program and the adapted physical education program are often severely limited for students enrolled in these schools. Elementary school classroom teachers may, under the best of conditions, have had only one or two courses designed to prepare them for all types of physical education instruction, including adapted physical education. It can readily be seen that an adapted program conducted under these conditions is severely restricted. However, it is possible that some instruction for the handicapped student may be provided under the guidance of a traveling specialist or school district physical education supervisor.

Some school districts have attempted to meet the needs of the handicapped child at the elementary school level by providing special centers, located strategically in the district, where the elementary school student can be taken for this important part of his educational experience. Students from a number of schools in the district are transported to the center where a specialist in adapted physical education, with a properly equipped facility, is able to offer them expert instruction under the guidance of the medical director for the school district or from prescriptions furnished by the student's own family physician. Parents are often encouraged to at-

tend these sessions so that the student will be able to engage in a special program of activities at home, in addition to the work done at the center. Some additional supervised work on these special exercises learned at the center may also be a part of the regular physical education program of the student's home school. The Los Angeles city and Anaheim, California, schools have used visiting teachers and adapted physical education centers to meet the special needs of the children in their district. Hazleton, Pennsylvania, has provided a mobile unit especially designed for adapted physical education. It travels with two special teachers from school to school.

Another possible arrangement that can be used to provide better facilities and equipment for the elementary school child is to schedule children for a class at a nearby junior or senior high school where the adapted room and equipment may be available. Using this arrangement, classroom teachers of several elementary schools can bring their children to the nearby secondary school for an exercise program conducted by a district specialist. Some modifications may be necessary in providing equipment for such a program, but the room and much of the equipment can be adapted for this type of class.

The minimum equipment needs for adapted physical education in an elementary school program would consist of one plumb line or window pole (to be used as a measuring device for anterior, posterior, and lateral posture examinations) and towels. A towel can be substituted for an exercise mat and can be used by the student to perform a large number of special exercises for posture and for general rehabilitation. Sports and game testing and equipment can be the same as that used for the regular classes. Individual exercise mats would be preferred to the towel, since they are more comfortable, can be kept clean, and allow the student to use his towel for his exercise program while he is in the recumbent position on the mat. However, with some ingenuity, the teacher can provide an excellent adapted physical education program for students at the elementary school with minimum equipment.

Special exercises can be performed in the classroom, if sufficient space is provided, or on a blacktop or grass area outdoors. More extensive equipment for an elementary school program is desirable and may consist of many of the items that are described in greater detail in later portions of this chapter in connection with the secondary school and college level programs. Sports and game equipment for adapted physical education students at the elementary school level ordinarily can be borrowed from the regular program. Any adaptations to modify the activities in terms of size of the equipment, size of the court, length of the playing time, and the like could be worked out by the classroom teacher with the help of a district specialist. For added information about the adapted sports program, see Chapter 8. Information on special equipment for perceptual-motor activities is presented in a later part of this chapter.

FACILITIES FOR SECONDARY SCHOOLS AND COLLEGES

Facilities and equipment for adapted physical education in secondary schools and colleges are usually far more extensive than those found in the typical elementary school.

Special exercise room

At least one special room for adapted physical education should be provided for each school at the junior high school, senior high school, and college levels. If the school is large or if the number of students to be accommodated is greater than the number that can be handled in one room, separate facilities for girls and boys are usually provided. Adapted classes can be coeducational, with boys and girls being scheduled into the most convenient class hour.

The size of the adapted room and related facilities adjacent to it are dependent on the philosophy of adapted physical education in each school and in each school district. The adapted room is usually designed to handle a limited number of students. Since students in this program may have individualized programs, whether they are exercise or sports activities, fewer students can be handled satisfactorily than in the regular physical education class. However, it must be remembered that this room must accommodate specialized equipment that occupies a considerable amount of floor, wall, and ceiling space. A clear area must also be provided for exercises and activities that do not involve the use of special equipment. The room therefore must be of sufficient size to meet these special needs comfortably. The minimum size of an adapted physical education room for a junior or senior high school would be 40 feet by 60 feet if the room is limited to the use of adapted classes.[8, 23] If the room is used as a multipurpose facility accommodating regular physical education classes for such specialized kinds of activities as gymnastics or wrestling, additional space is necessary. This multipurpose arrangement has a number of limitations, however, since much of the adapted room equipment must be permanently installed on the floor, ceiling, and walls. The recommended 15-foot ceiling height is not sufficient if this room is also used for gymnastics or activities in which ball games are played, in which case the minimum height should be 20 to 25 feet.

A regular spring construction hardwood floor is preferred for this room, although parquet flooring has been used successfully in some installations. The walls, at least to door height, should be of material that will withstand hard use. The material used should be resistant to scarring and marking and should provide for the mountings of specialized equipment. The ceiling may be of acoustical tile if ball games are not played in the room. High windows

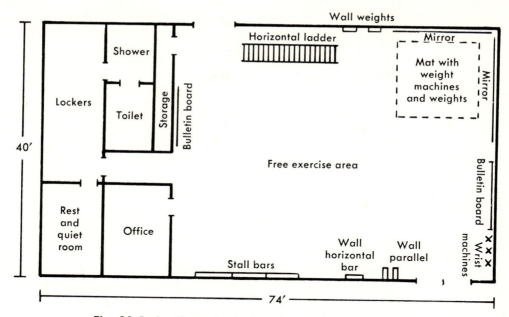

Fig. 20-1. A self-contained adapted physical education room.

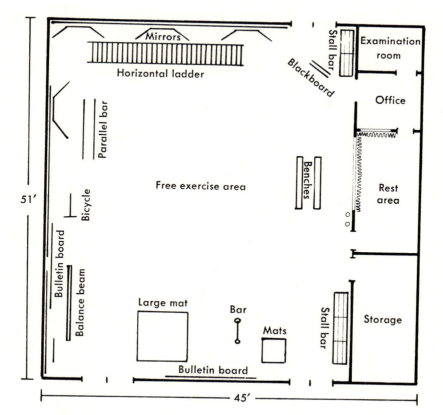

Fig. 20-2. A secondary school girls' adapted physical education room.

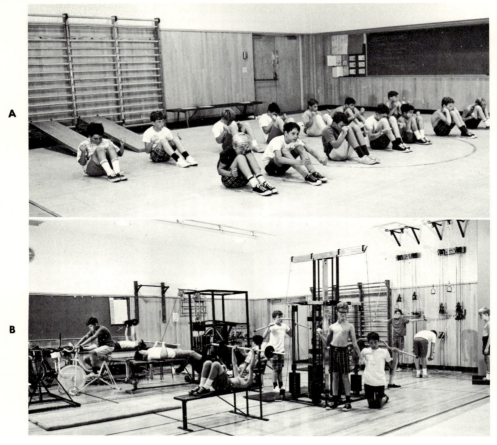

Fig. 20-3. A, Use of the open space area in an adapted physical education room to conduct formal group exercises. **B,** An elementary school class uses a college facility. Each student performs an individual exercise on a piece of equipment.

are needed on two sides of the room to allow for ample light and fresh air and to provide space for installation of equipment on all four walls. Proper lighting and ventilation are important for a special exercise room. Doorways leading to this room from the locker area, hallways, and fields should be extra wide, with ramps leading to them. This arrangement will allow for the easy movement of equipment and for the passing of students who are in wheelchairs or on crutches. Bulletin boards and blackboards should be mounted on the walls to conserve floor space (Figs. 20-1 and 20-2).

Considerable planning is required prior to the time that the equipment is located in the adapted room. It is important that efficient use be made of the space available so that students who are using specialized types of apparatus and equipment are able to use it effectively and so that hazards are not created while students use any special equipment such as barbells, the horizontal ladder, pulleys, and jump ropes (Fig. 20-3). Suitable equipment for such a facility is discussed in a later section of this chapter.

Instructor's office and student rest area

The instructor's office and a room suitable for a rest area and for quiet games should be located immediately adjacent to the adapted room. Observation windows on two sides of the instructor's office will allow him to work at his desk and still supervise both the adapted room and the rest area. Blinds on these windows provide privacy when needed. It is desirable that a lavatory be located adjacent to these facilities. Usually, the room planned for a rest area and quiet games is larger for the girls' program than for the boys' and more cot space is provided for girls in this facility.[7]

Adapted sports area

An adapted sports area may be located immediately adjacent to the adapted room. A doorway connects these facilities. This area should consist of blacktop and grass for multipurpose use and space for specialized games. Activities that can be conducted on the blacktop would include volleyball, paddle tennis, goal-hi, badminton, and deck tennis. A smooth concrete area provides space for shuffleboard, quoits, table tennis, and other adapted activities. A grass or dirt area provides activity space for horseshoes and croquet. The horseshoe-pitching area must be carefully laid out so that student safety is considered.

Other adapted sports activities can often be conducted between or adjacent to the regular physical education classes that are using a facility. They can also be conducted when an activity area such as archery, tennis, or swimming is not being scheduled by other classes. Students in the adapted program should have as many opportunities as possible to participate in activities that are similar to those engaged in by students in the regular physical education program. This can be accomplished easily by making minor adaptations in the games, sports, and activities that are being conducted in the regular physical education curriculum.

There is a recent trend toward the use of community and private facilities by students in adapted physical education. Nearby recreation centers; private pools; bowling alleys; special exercise facilities;

and badminton, racquetball, golf, and archery facilities are often made available and, in some instances, expert instruction is provided for disadvantaged persons by the personnel at the facility.

In most secondary schools and colleges, swimming for students in the adapted classes is conducted during times when others are not using the pool. Sometimes it is possible to conduct an adaptive class in swimming at the same time a small regular class is in session. Since swimming is such an important activity for the handicapped child, every effort must be made to provide pool experiences for as many of the students as possible. A small, warm, therapeutic pool would be an ideal facility for adapted physical education students, but, in the majority of schools, both hydrotherapy activities and special swimming classes for handicapped students must be conducted in the regular pool. Some schools have successfully used portable pools (Fig. 20-4), set up on a blacktop or grass area and then moved from school to school every 2 or 3 weeks, so that all of the handicapped students in a district can participate in a short swimming unit. This works especially well at the elementary school level, where a swimming pool is seldom included in the physical education facilities. One new practice that can be used in either a school or therapy unit for any age level is the portable pool that is built on a trailer. This type of pool can be drained and easily transported to a different facility for use without the extensive labor and time required to take down, move, and set up a portable pool at each new locality.

Chapters 5 and 8 present a more complete discussion of aquatic exercises and activities.

SPECIAL EQUIPMENT

The equipment needs of each of the special facilities just described are somewhat unique, depending on such factors as the number of students using each facility; whether the area is used for boys or girls or is coeducational; whether it is for

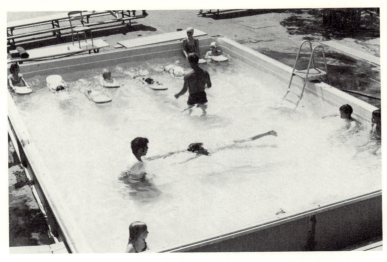

Fig. 20-4. Portable swimming pool. (Courtesy Lyonel Avance, Los Angeles City Unified School District, Special Education Division.)

elementary school, junior or senior high school, or college; and whether minimal or ideal equipment is to be furnished.

Minimum equipment

The minimum equipment needs in an adapted room in a secondary school or college level facility consist of the following: sufficient individual 1-inch thick plastic-covered body mats to accommodate the peak class load, plus five or six more; 2-inch thick mats of sufficient size to cover the floor under hazardous types of equipment such as the horizontal ladder or the horizontal bar; a platform or firm rubber mats to cover the floor where weight-lifting activities will take place; towels for use in the exercise program; a plumb line or posture screen for posture examinations; and miscellaneous, inexpensive pieces of testing equipment such as measuring tapes and skin pencils. Ropes for skipping and school benches can usually be obtained from the maintenance department of the school. Since resistance exercises are desired in most programs, homemade weights can be constructed by the instructor or by the students. Thus with a minimum of expenditure, sufficient equipment

can be obtained to start a good adapted program. Special equipment for perceptual-motor training can be purchased or it can be improvised until funds are made available. Equipment for most adapted sports can be borrowed from the regular physical education program.

Standard equipment

Standard equipment for a remedial or adapted room consists of the minimum equipment already described plus the following items:

1. A posture screen with a built-in conformator on its side (or a separate conformator)
2. A podiascope
3. Manufactured adjustable barbells and dumbbells, together with racks for their storage
4. Stall bars
5. Pulley or chest weights (triplex preferred)
6. Iron boots or special knee exercise apparatus
7. A horizontal ladder
8. An incline board
9. A balance beam
10. Three-way mirrors

11. Special benches
12. Plinths
13. Stall bar stools
14. A wall parallel bar
15. A wall horizontal bar

In addition, the following testing equipment will be standard:
1. Breadth, depth, and skin fold calipers
2. A physician's scale
3. A stadiometer
4. A goniometer
5. Joint-tracing equipment

Equipment for special adapted sports includes that used for the following activities:
1. Shuffleboard
2. Horseshoes
3. Table tennis
4. Paddle tennis
5. Badminton
6. Goal hi
7. Medicine ball
8. Jumping rope

Elaborate equipment

More elaborate equipment consists of some of the following:
1. A multistation heavy resistance machine on which students can exercise a number of different areas of the body (this provides six to eight stations)
2. A rowing machine
3. A stationary bicycle
4. Special wrist and forearm exercise machines
5. Shoulder wheels
6. Sound equipment for rhythmical training
7. Dynamometers
8. Tensiometers

In addition, other specialized exercise and testing equipment, plus additional equipment for the adapted sports and games area, may be desired. Elaborate specialized equipment can be purchased for perceptual-motor activities if this constitutes a substantial part of the program.

Equipment for the other specialized rooms described previously includes, in the instructor's office, desks and work tables,

filing equipment, and sufficient space for the instructor to do small-group counseling. The rest and quiet game area should have bunks or cots to accommodate 2% of the boys and from 2% to 5% of the girls at the peak period of enrollment.[7] Tables and chairs must be provided for quiet game activities. Mattresses, pillows, sheets, and pillowcases must be provided for this facility. A storeroom must be provided in which the quiet game equipment and the adapted sports equipment, plus the testing equipment used in the adapted room, can be stored.

Equipment for perceptual-motor activities

Special equipment for perceptual-motor activities should enhance the offerings of the adapted physical education program. Much of the equipment can be made by the teacher, the maintenance or industrial arts department at the school, or, in some cases, by the students themselves.

Inexpensive equipment

1. Pieces of rope and string of various diameters, composition, and length can be used for many types of activities and for testing purposes, including such activities as rope skipping, making shapes and forms, identifying size and texture, jumping over or climbing under, and tying knots (Fig. 20-5, A).
2. Cardboard boxes of various sizes and shapes can be used as targets, to sit in, to climb through, to walk in, to catch with, and even as a place to store other pieces of equipment.
3. Masking tape has innumerable uses, including to lay out test areas on the floor or walls, to mark boundaries of courts and play areas, to make symbols to identify (numbers, letters, triangles, squares, etc.), to mark special equipment, to mark a right arm or leg (to help a person identify right from left), and to tape things together.
4. Chalk of different colors may be used to do much of the marking of items

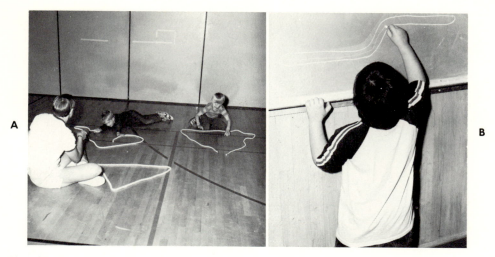

Fig. 20-5. Inexpensive equipment for perceptual-motor activities. **A,** Rope or string. **B,** Chalk. (Courtesy California State University, Audio Visual Center, Long Beach, Calif.)

included in the previous lists to identify color, to draw on the blackboard or on paper (for all types of symbol and color identification), and for "draw-a-man" tests (Fig. 20-5).

5. Plastic bottles or milk cartons can be filled with sand or other materials to serve as weights; different sizes, shapes, and colors can be used for identification; they can be used for games (to run around, to knock over, to catch and throw, to float or sink in the swimming pool) (Fig. 4-13), to hang from strings, to be swung, to be hit, to be avoided, or to be blown.

Low-cost equipment

Since these items can be used for types of activities similar to those discussed in the previous section, the low-cost equipment will merely be listed here, as follows, unless there is some special feature to be discussed:

1. Hula hoops
2. Traffic cones
3. Beads and strings
4. Blocks
5. Balance boards for skill development and testing
6. Yardsticks for testing
7. Balloons

8. Beanbags
9. Plastic and Styrofoam balls
10. Stands to hold crossbars, strings, etc.
11. Wooden boxes to stand on or jump from

More elaborate and/or expensive equipment

Equipment on which to bounce may include any of the following:
1. Trampoline
2. Mini-trampoline
3. Truck tires or inner tubes (or smaller sizes if desired) with canvas laced across the opening on one side to serve as a trampoline
4. Spring-O-Line bounce boards
5. Spring boards, jumping boards, and inner tubes

Protective and padded equipment (Fig. 8-1) may include the following:
1. Mats of various sizes, thicknesses, and consistencies for individual use and to protect under and around the equipment
2. Bolsters to sit on, jump from, or roll on
3. Bataccas to wrestle with, to hit with, and to be hit
4. Large padded boxing gloves and head guards
5. Boxers' heavy bag to hit, tackle, etc.

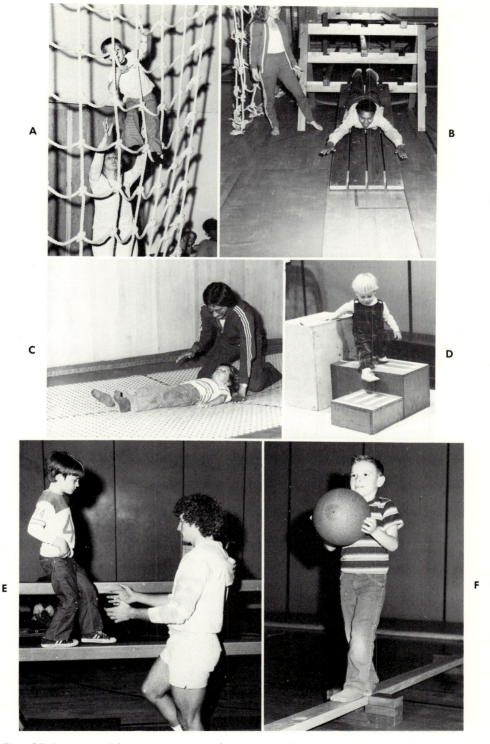

Fig. 20-6. More elaborate equipment for perceptual-motor activities. **A,** Cargo net. **B,** Scooter on incline. **C,** Trampoline. **D,** Wooden boxes. **E,** Stegel. **F,** Balance beam. (Courtesy California State University, Audio Visual Center, Long Beach, Calif.)

6. King-of-the-mountain pad
7. Jousting clubs
8. Specially shaped mats (inclined, round, square, cylindrical, and cone-shaped)
9. Large rubber balls with plastic covers

Special game equipment may include almost every item of equipment used in the *regular* physical education program, as almost all can be adapted for some use with selected students in the perceptual-motor program. Included would be the following:

1. All types of balls (large, small, light, and heavy; of different textures and air pressures; and special balls like the Whiffle ball, the Fleece ball, the Nerf ball, and knitted balls)
2. Things with which to strike the balls, such as bats, rackets, paddles, and clubs
3. Nets of various sizes
4. Bases and goals
5. Standards to hold up nets, goals, and games (tetherball, basketball, volleyball, and goal high)

Specialized types of equipment

Some more specialized types of equipment include children's games, especially those requiring manipulation and allowing for identity of color, shape, texture, number, and letter concepts. These may include the following:

1. Balance beams of various widths and heights
2. A Stegel for balancing and climbing activities
3. Stall bars
4. Incline boards
5. A horizontal ladder
6. Wall parallel and horizontal bars
7. Climbing ropes
8. Ladders
9. A cargo net
10. Pulley weights
11. Rocker boards
12. Scooter boards
13. Wheel toys
14. Stilts
15. Bongo boards
16. T stools

17. Wands
18. Three-way mirrors
19. Pitchbacks
20. Parachutes

Rhythms can provide an opportunity to meet motor development needs, but their use also involves creativity linked to a better self-concept and a broadened self-image (Fig. 20-18). Rhythm equipment might include:

1. Lummi sticks
2. Poi-poi balls
3. A metronome
4. A recorder with tapes or records
5. Tamborines
6. Percussion instruments
7. Song books or song sheets

Aquatic equipment and activities are included in Chapters 5 and 8 (Figs. 5-48 through 5-51, 8-6, and 20-4).

Outdoor play equipment such as slides, swings, teeter-totters, rings, sandboxes, tires, and jungle gyms provides opportunity for a variety of perceptual-motor activities in the fresh air and sunshine.

Tests and testing equipment include markings on mats or the floor, stopwatches, yardsticks and metric tapes or sticks, targets, traffic cones, mats, ropes, hoops, beads, tapping board test equipment, and blocks can be used for *general testing* (Fig. 20-7, *A* to *C*). Some standard tests and test kits that might be used include that following:

1. Roach and Kephart[19]: Purdue Perceptual-Motor Survey
2. Oseretsky[18]: Lincoln Motor Development Scale
3. Stott[21]: Stott Motor Impairment Test
4. Arnheim and Sinclair[2]: Individual Motor Behavior Survey; Diagnostic Motor Ability Test
5. Orpet[17]: Frostig Movement Skills Test
6. Goodenough[12]: Draw-a-Man Test
7. Frostig[11]: Visual Perception Test
8. Fiorentino[10]: Fiorentino Reflex Tests
9. Ayres[3-6]: The Ayres Space Test; Figure-Ground Visual Perception Test; Kinesthesia and Tactual Perception Tests; Motor Accuracy Tests

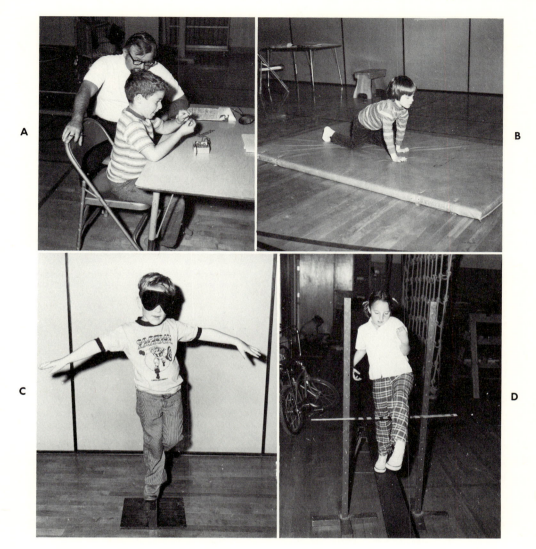

Fig. 20-7. Activities using perceptual-motor testing equipment. **A,** Bead stringing. **B,** Creeping. **C,** Static balance. **D,** Dynamic balance. (Courtesy California State University, Audio Visual Center, Long Beach, Calif.)

10. American Association for Health, Physical Education, and Recreation[23]: Physical fitness tests

Proper use of the room and its equipment

Orientation during the first week of school should include information on the rules and regulations that relate to the use of the adapted physical education room and its equipment. These rules include the following:

1. The room should be used only when proper supervision is present.
2. It is necessary to be instructed in the use of any specialized equipment before using it.
3. Exercises should be performed only when they have been assigned or when

they have been approved for use by the instructor; careful instruction in the execution of each exercise must precede its use, as state previously.

4. It is necessary to be instructed in the proper use and care of barbells, dumbbells, and other resistance equipment prior to the time a progressive resistance program is begun. Students should increase the number of repetitions and the amount of resistance used only when they are capable of executing an exercise properly with the previous amount of weight and the assigned number of repetitions.

5. All equipment must be returned to its proper place immediately after its use.

6. Information about any faulty equipment must be reported immediately to an instructor.

7. Hazardous types of equipment (weights, horizontal ladders, Stegel, trampoline, ropes, cargo ladder, etc.) must be tested by the instructor before student use.

8. A student must stop his exercise or activity program and report to an instructor immediately if he experiences undue pain, dyspnea, or general systemic discomfort.

9. Breath holding is discouraged during lifting activities and abdominal exercises, since this may cause an increase in intra-abdominal pressure and thus possible strain. This also causes the Valsalva effect that constricts the carotid artery.

Construction of equipment

Much of the equipment used in an adapted physical education program can be constructed by the instructor or by the maintenance or industrial arts department in a school. Homemade equipment will often suffice for a number of years until an adequate budget can be obtained to buy the more expensive manufactured equipment. Some items that can be constructed are the following: a three-way mirror, which can be mounted on the wall or placed on a rack or on wheels and moved around the room, with the wings on the sides of the mirror being held in place with piano hinges; posture screens; a podiascope; heel cord stretch boards; foot supinator boards; homemade barbells and dumbbells; pulleys for specialized types of exercises; balance beams; exercise benches; calipers; stadiometers; goniometers; conformators; racks for weights; joint- and foot-tracing devices; bicycle exercisers; and many items for the adapted sports and perceptual-motor programs.[3, 9, 14-17, 23]

Description of equipment and uses for it

This section includes illustrations of a number of different pieces of apparatus that can be used in the corrective room, together with a short description and hints about proper use.

Body mats

Body mats are very useful in an adapted program. They are relatively small and light (usually 3 feet wide, 6 feet long, and 1 inch thick). They are plastic covered and therefore easy to clean and some can be folded in the middle and stacked in a small space. They provide safety and comfort for the student while he is exercising on the floor of the room. These mats are quite durable and will serve their purpose well if they are stacked when not in use. If they are always folded or stacked with the clean sides together, a clean surface is available for each student to use. If they are kept off the floor when not in actual use so that they are not walked on and are not used as crash pads underneath weight lifting and similar types of equipment, they will prove to be quite durable.

Towels

A good, sturdy towel has many uses in the adapted program. Where equipment is limited, the towel can be used instead of the exercise mat or if mats are old and soiled, it can be used as a cover for the mat while the student exercises on it. Many exercises can be performed using a towel. Almost every part of the body can

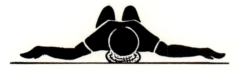

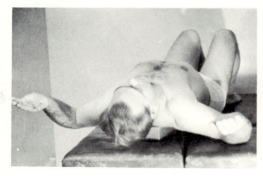

Fig. 20-8. Towel and wood block used to stretch anterior shoulder muscles.

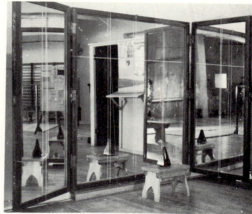

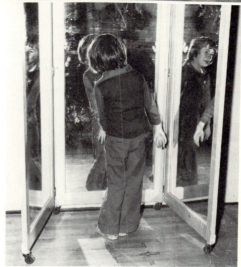

Fig. 20-9. Three-way mirror. Note use of vertical and horizontal lines to aid student with alignment problems. (Lower illustration courtesy California State University, Audio Visual Center, Long Beach, Calif.)

be stretched or resistance can be applied by employing the towel in various ways. The towel can be folded three times lengthwise, then rolled into a tight cylinder and placed directly between the shoulder blades while the individual is resting on the back and can be used thus to stretch the anterior muscles of the chest and shoulder girdle. A folded towel can also be used instead of a headboard and rolled or folded towels can be used for support in certain relaxation exercises (Fig. 20-8 and Chapter 6).

Three-way mirror

Some type of mirror is useful for adapted classes at all grade levels. A mirror with two side wings is preferable, since it allows the student to see three views of his body and thus he understands his posture deviation problems better and can see when he has placed his body in proper alignment. It also allows the student to watch his movements during exercise and therefore to be more accurate in the execution of his exercise program. The instructor can use the mirror to point out to students the kinds of deviations in body mechanics observed while using the plumb line, the posture screen, and various other types of

measuring devices. Students can check their body positions in relation to a gravity line if a plumb line is hung so that it drops straight in front of a section of the mirror. Mirrors can be mounted permanently on the wall in one section of the room or it has been found quite satisfactory to have the three-way or one-way mirror mounted on wheels or on slides so that it can be moved to various areas of the adapted physical education room, thus increasing the flexibility of its use (Fig. 20-9). Besides the upright mirror, overhead mirrors have been found beneficial to students performing in the reclined position.

Resistance equipment

Each year, there are many new types of resistance equipment developed for use in adapted physical education and allied fields. Many of these devices are useful for equipping an adapted physical education room. In addition to the barbells, dumbbells, iron boots, and pulley weights that have been standard equipment for many years, there are a number of other kinds of special resistance equipment that have been developed, consisting of springs, rubber tubing, and many other types of tension-producing or resistance-producing materials. Special exercise equipment has been designed to be used for specific body parts such as the ankles, knees, arms, shoulders, and abdomen. Recently, a number of very large and complex exercise machines have been developed for class use. These exercise machines provide 4 to 10 different exercise stations, each of which allows a student to exercise a certain part of his body and all of which allow him to apply the principle of progressive resistance in his exercise program. The Universal Gym, the Nautilus, and several new types of isokinetic exercise equipment are examples of this type of machine. The instructor actually has a wide choice of resistance-producing devices, ranging from noncommercial equipment made of bags filled with sand and barbells and dumbbells made from tin cans, cement, and pipe to rather highly sophisticated types of manufactured resistance equipment. It is actually a matter of preference regarding the types of resistance equipment selected by the instructor and the influence of budget limitations will guide him in his choice of special pieces of apparatus.

Stall bars

At least one set (three sections) of stall bars should be included in the equipment

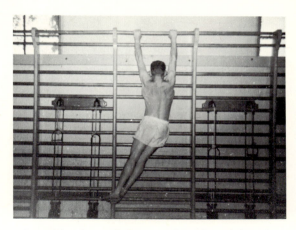

Fig. 20-10. Stall bars and wall weights. Installation of wall weights can be made behind stall bars if space is limited. Note asymmetrical scoliosis exercise.

of the adapted room. The stall bar is a rather flexible piece of apparatus allowing students to perform many types of stretching and developmental exercises. One set of stall bars provides space for three students to exercise at one time and also can be used as a ladder for incline boards where space is at a premium. When wall space is severely limited, a set of pulley weights can be placed behind one section of the stall bars by the removal of one bar and thus two pieces of apparatus can be placed in the space ordinarily occupied by one (Fig. 20-10). A set of exercises for the stall bars is included in Appendix II.

Horizontal ladder

The horizontal ladder should be placed so that one end is higher than the other. This provides additional resistance for students who climb from one end to the other and also allows for certain kinds of asymmetrical hanging exercises to be done by students who have deviations in shoulder height and problems with lateral curvatures of the spine. The horizontal ladder has many uses, ranging from general conditioning kinds of exercises for the arms, shoulder girdle, and trunk to very specific

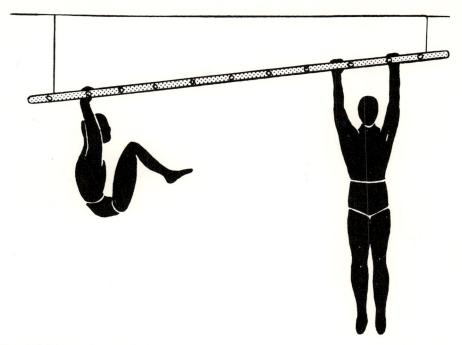

Fig. 20-11. Horizontal ladder. Note abdominal exercise and asymmetrical hanging for scoliosis or low shoulder.

types of stretching and developmental activities for posture and rehabilitation of other types of deviations (Fig. 20-11). (See also exercise No. 21, Chapter 5.)

Pulley weights

Pulley weights have been a standard piece of apparatus in the adapted room for many years. There are several types, ranging from those with handles that are placed at the foot level, the chest level, or overhead to various combinations of these positions. The triplex pulley weight, which is a combination of the three just mentioned, provides for a good deal of flexibility in the assignment of exercises and takes a relatively small amount of space in the adapted room. It is also possible to purchase head straps, foot straps, and hand straps so that specific exercises can be provided for special areas of the body that cannot be exercised with the standard pulley weight machine (Figs. 20-10 and 20-12). A set of

exercises for the pulley weights is included in Appendix III.

Balance beam

The balance beam serves several purposes in the adapted room. It helps students improve their balance and coordination; it helps strengthen and develop the feet and legs; and, when the balance beam is constructed so that it acts as a supinator board, it can also help in the correction of certain foot, ankle, and knee deviations (Figs. 20-6, *F*, and 20-13).

Hand and wrist machines; shoulder and wrestling wheels

There are a number of wall-mounted commercial machines designed to help students develop the musculature in the hands, wrists, forearms, and upper arms. Most of these machines operate on a friction principle, with the amount of resistance adjustable. Musculature of the shoul-

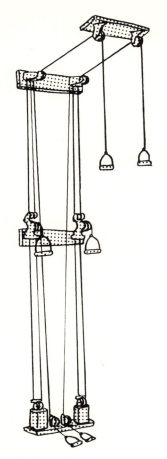

Fig. 20-12. Triplex pulley weight.

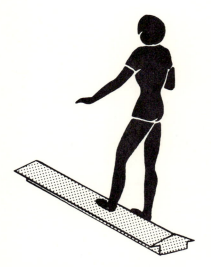

Fig. 20-13. Supinator balance beam.

der girdle, shoulder, elbow, wrist, and hand can be developed or stretched with properly assigned exercises on these pieces of apparatus (Fig. 20-14 and Chapter 5).

Massage plinths

A massage plinth is a very useful piece of apparatus in the adapted room. It can be used for special corrective exercises by the students and for taking special measurements by the instructor. The adaptability of many plinths is increased, since it is possible to adjust the length of their legs and therefore the total slant of the top surface of the plinth. It is further possible to adjust portions of the top surface of the plinth to various angles, affording the student a large number of possible exercise positions.

Benches

Benches, similar to regular playground benches, can be very useful in the adapted room. They provide sitting stations for execution of foot and ankle exercises and because of their long, narrow construction, they are particularly useful for exercises requiring the prone and supine positions (Fig. 20-15).

Rowing machine

The rowing machine is an excellent piece of apparatus for general conditioning exercises. Specific exercises can also be assigned for various posture and disability problems. Many rowing machines are adjustable so that exercise programs can be graded from easy to difficult. A portable treadmill can also be used to develop cardiovascular fitness (Fig. 20-16).

Ropes

Rope skipping is an excellent activity for many students in the adapted physical education class. Since many exercise programs involve, primarily, flexibility and strength development, an endurance activity is often needed. Ropes can be purchased that have special handles and spe-

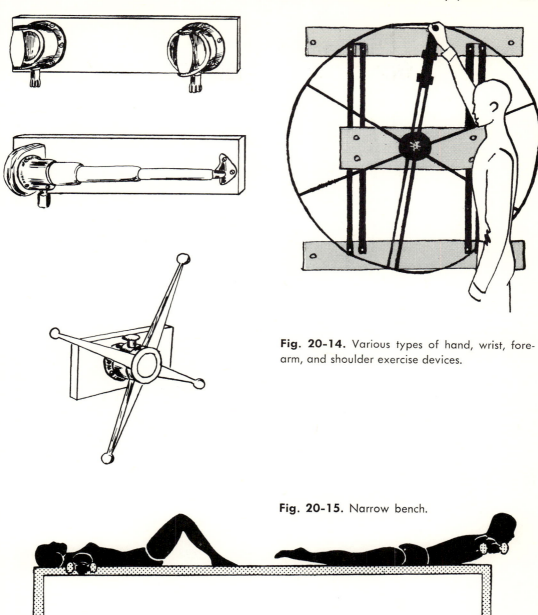

Fig. 20-14. Various types of hand, wrist, forearm, and shoulder exercise devices.

Fig. 20-15. Narrow bench.

cial features or they can be made by the instructor from clothesline rope that can be purchased at a local hardware store. Rope ¼ inch or ⅜ inch in diameter makes a jump rope that is quite satisfactory for the adapted class. (Chapter 8 provides additional information.) Long and short ropes can also be used for many types of perceptual-motor activities and tests, including making letters and geometric shapes and for jumping tests and skills.

Heel cord stretch apparatus

A number of devices can be used to stretch the heel cord, a desirable activity for certain deviations of the foot and ankle. The heel cord can be stretched while standing on one of the lower rungs of the

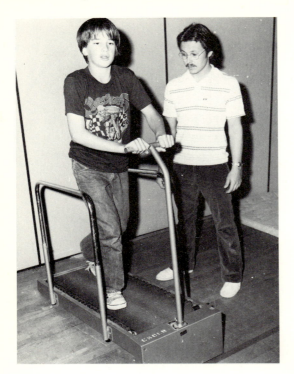

Fig. 20-16. Portable treadmill is used for development of cardiovascular fitness. (Courtesy California State University, Audio Visual Center, Long Beach, Calif.)

stall bar. It can be stretched while the student is standing with the forepart of the foot on a block 1½ or 2 inches thick, lowering the heel down over the edge of the block. Various pieces of apparatus can be constructed to provide a straight stretch in dorsiflexion of the ankle or a stretch of the heel cord can be combined with a stretch of the foot everters by employing a supinator board tilted up at one end to provide for a stretch of the heel cord as well. (The supinator board can be leaned up against one of the lower rungs of the stall bar.)

Bulletin boards and blackboards

Ample bulletin board and blackboard space is needed in the well-planned adapted physical education room. This space can be used for posting announce-

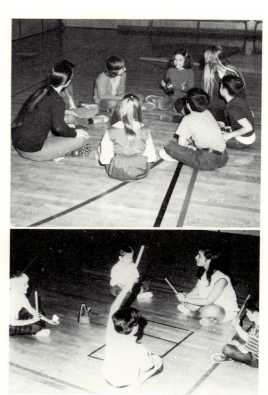

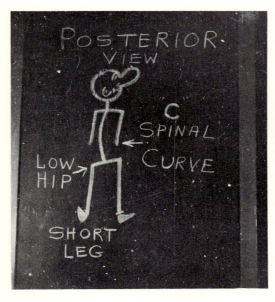

Fig. 20-17. Use of a blackboard as an instructional device.

Fig. 20-18. Rhythmic activities. **A,** Using a tamborine. **B,** Using a metronome and sticks. (Courtesy California State University, Audio Visual Center, Long Beach, Calif.)

ments, pictures, posters, bulletins of interest, exercise cards, instructional information, and all types of motivational devices to interest students in the program. To make the best use of these areas, they should be attractive, material should be interesting and current, and students should be encouraged to contribute materials of interest (Fig. 20-17).

Rhythmic equipment

Many handicapped persons can profit from a variety of rhythmic activities. Some of these include music from tapes or records, which can be used for exercise programs, relaxation, rhythmic training, and dance activities; percussion instruments; lummi sticks; a metronome; or various musical instruments to help establish a rhythm or beat. If special equipment is not available, rhythmic programs can be lead by a teacher or student, using such techniques as clapping, snapping fingers, marching, walking, running, and exercising to rhythmic patterns. The learners capture these beats and rhythms with the eyes and ears, through feeling the beat, or by various combinations of these senses (Fig. 20-18).

ANTHROPOMETRIC TESTS AND TESTING EQUIPMENT

Tests and measurements are important parts of adapted physical education. Consequently, there are a large number of testing devices available that have a number of uses for the instructor and the student. They can be used to show students what their deviations are and to compare tests made at the beginning of the semester with those made at the end. They can be used to identify how much deviation is present in connection with certain kinds of disabilities and therefore to motivate the student in an activity program. A few of the devices having special value for the adapted program are described in this section.

Stadiometer

The stadiometer is used to measure the height of the student. Stadiometers at-

tached to the physician's scale are not always satisfactory, since it is difficult to obtain accurate measurements with these devices. A very satisfactory stadiometer can be constructed by the instructor or by the maintenance or industrial arts department in the school, or one can be improvised on the wall or the door of the room by installing a yardstick or a steel tape (with its distance from the floor measured accurately). Then, by using either a square piece of wood or a right triangle, the height of the student can be measured quickly by sliding the angle firmly down on the top of the student's head and reading his correct height from the measuring device mounted on the wall. This method is quick, accurate, and easy and the equipment is inexpensive to construct (Fig. 20-19).

Instructions for use

The technique for measuring the height of the student must be standardized so that successive measurements will be as meaningful as possible. The following procedures are suggested for the use of a stadiometer:

1. The student is instructed to stand tall, with his heels placed against the wall and with his inner ankle bones touching, if they will do so without discomfort.
2. The student's head should be pressed back against the wall and his chin should be tucked.
3. The examiner should then slide the right triangle firmly down on the student's head.

The reading for the correct height of the individual is made to the nearest centimeter or ¼ inch. Successive measurements should be taken at about the same time each day.

Measuring tapes

A metal or plastic measuring tape can be used by the adapted physical education teacher to perform a number of different tests. Girth measurements can be taken to

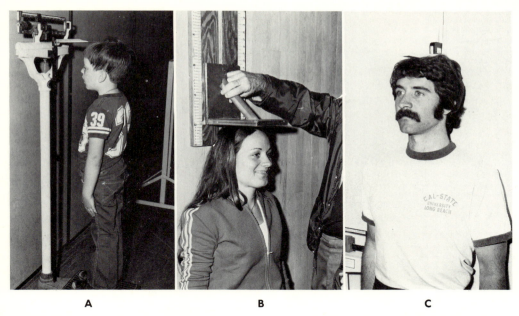

Fig. 20-19. Stadiometers. **A,** Attached to balance scale. **B,** Mounted on wall. **C,** Attached to tape measure. (Courtesy California State University, Audio Visual Center, Long Beach, Calif.)

identify a change in body proportions, particularly those of weight distribution and muscle size. The tape can also be used to measure height, as previously described, and to measure the length of various segments of the body, that is, leg length, the height of various parts of the pelvis from the floor, and the like.

Girth measurements

Description. Girth (circumference) measurements can be taken of many body parts. Tapes with a spring scale attachment at one end can be purchased so that the amount of tension applied during measurement can be standardized. Measurements can be taken of the body and the limbs.

Uses and limitations. Girth measurements, taken as a part of the adapted physical education program, are only as good as the accuracy of the teacher. For this reason, it is important that all techniques be standardized and that systems of recording be developed that are simple and

that can be compared with the measurements made on successive tests. The tests will be most useful if the following procedures are closely followed each time that measurements are made:

1. The same identical area must be measured each time.
2. Measurement is taken under the same conditions, for example, with the arm completely extended and relaxed, with the arm flexed and the muscles at work, or with the chest fully inflated or the air completely expired.
3. The tape is pulled snug, but not tight enough to indent the skin. There are no twists in the tape and it passes in a straight line around the body or body part.
4. The individual is measured at the same time in relation to his workout program so that only permanent changes in the individual's girth would be noted. (He would not be measured before a vigorous workout at one time and after a vigorous workout at another.)

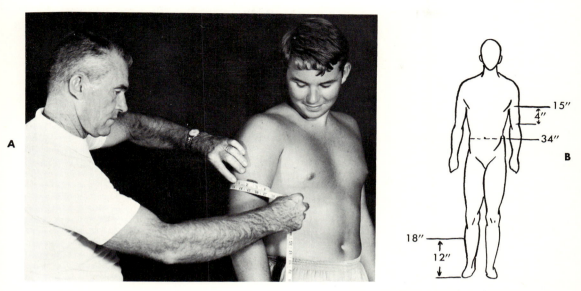

Fig. 20-20. Girth measurements. **A,** Instructor measuring arm girth of student. **B,** System for recording girth measurements by key body landmarks as reference points.

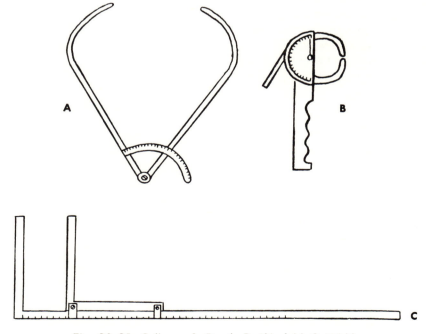

Fig. 20-21. Calipers. **A,** Depth. **B,** Skin fold. **C,** Width.

5. The distance from the reference point of the part measured and the exact girth measurements are carefully recorded (Fig. 20-20).

These tests are used to measure increases or decreases in body size for students engaged in programs of weight gain or loss and where the size of body parts is being increased or decreased.

Calipers

Various types of calipers can be used for anthropometric measurements in the adapted program. Three types are in general use: the width caliper, the skin fold caliper, and the depth caliper. The width caliper is used to measure the width of various segments of the body such as the shoulder (biacromial), chest, and the hip (bi-iliac). These widths are sometimes used in determining the breadth of the skeleton in relation to the nutritional status of the student. The depth caliper is most frequently used to measure the anteroposte-

rior depth of the chest. The skin fold caliper is used to measure the amount of subcutaneous fat as part of an evaluation of the nutritional status of the student (Fig. 20-21). Techniques for the use of these calipers are discussed in Chapter 7.

Joint angle measurements

Joint angle measurements are made to determine whether the individual has a normal range of motion (flexibility) in his joints and to measure the amount of improvement in joint flexibility following various types of illnesses and injuries.

Three types of devices are commonly used to measure the maximum amount of movement possible in a joint. They include a goniometer, a tracer, and the Leighton flexometer.

Goniometer

Instructions for use. The goniometer that is most frequently used in the adapted physical education program is a 180- or

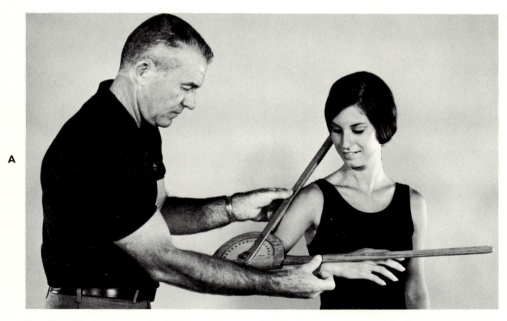

Fig. 20-22. Methods of joint measurement. **A,** Goniometer. **B,** Tracing the arm for elbow flexibility. **C,** Elbow tracing. **D,** Flexometer. (**B** and **C** courtesy California State University, Audio Visual Center, Long Beach, Calif.)

360-degree protractor with two extended arms. One of these arms is stationary and the other is movable around the center of the protractor. The measurements are made by placing one of the arms parallel to one part or limb of the joint to be measured, the axis of the protractor directly over the center of the joint, and the other arm of the goniometer parallel to the other limb of the joint to be measured. The individual moves one body segment as far in one direction as possible and a reading is made on the goniometer. The individual then moves the body segment in the opposite direction to the full range of motion and a second reading is made. Thus the examiner knows the number of degrees of motion in one direction, that is, flexion, and the number of degrees of motion in the other direction, that is, extension. The number of degrees of motion that exist between the two measurements indicates the range of motion possible in that particular joint.

Uses and limitations. The goniometer is only as accurate as the skill of the examiner. Techniques must be standardized so that the protractor is placed on the body

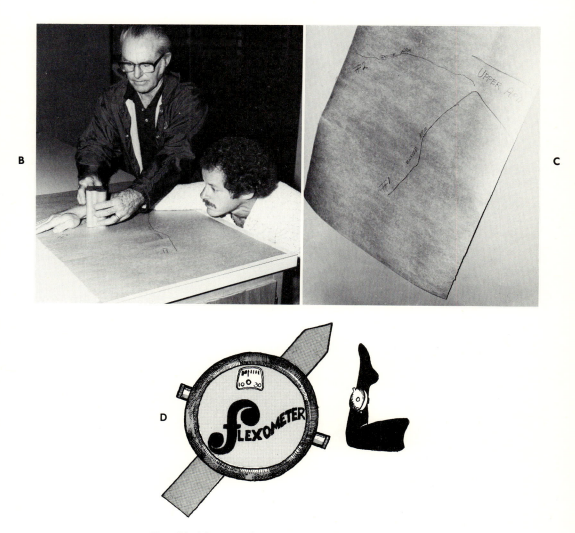

Fig. 20-22, cont'd. For legend see opposite page.

parts to be measured in the same way each time. This necessitates the use of rather exact landmarks so that the readings obtained will be as accurate as possible. Many of the commercial goniometers have very short arms and therefore are quite difficult to use when measuring body parts that are more than 12 to 15 inches in length. It is therefore preferable to use a goniometer with arms that are sufficiently long to reach the total length of the arm or leg. It is possible to construct a goniometer similar to the manufactured types and, in this case, sufficiently long arms can be built into the device (Fig. 20-22, *A*).

Tracer

Instructions for use. The tracing device shown in Fig. 20-22 can be used to measure the flexibility of many of the joints of the human body. This is done by tracing the parts above and below the joint on a large piece of paper spread out on a table or the floor to accommodate the appropriate body part.

To make such a tracing, the individual is seated comfortably in front of a table or a shoulder-high flat surface. A large paper is laid out on the table in front of him and his arm is rested on this paper. The instructor then has the individual extend the elbow as far as possible and, using the tracer, traces both sides of the upper arm to provide a point of reference for future measurements. Then a tracing is made of either the inside or the outside surface of the lower arm. The subject is instructed to flex the elbow as far as possible, keeping the upper arm in the same position. The same surface of the lower arm as was measured previously is then traced in this new position for comparison.

This test gives a reading of the flexibility of the joint in extension and in flexion and the number of degrees of difference between the two gives the range of motion for that joint at that particular time. The tracing should be labeled properly, indicating the method of testing, that is, lateral surface traced; the student's name; and the

date of the examination. By using pencils of different colors in the same tracing device, successive examinations can be made on the same paper and comparisons can be made between the amount of flexibility that the individual had on successive dates after his injury (Fig. 20-22, *B* and *C*).

Uses and limitations. The tracer can best be used on the ankle, knee, wrist, and elbow joints, although, with certain modifications, it can be used to measure actions of the hip and shoulder, including rotation at these joints.

Leighton flexometer

Clark[8] described another device that can be used to measure the range of motion in several joints of the body: the flexometer, developed by Leighton (Fig. 20-22, *D*).

POSTURE AND BODY MECHANICS TEST EQUIPMENT
Posture screen

The posture screen can be used by the instructor to help objectify posture examinations of his students in the standing position. The screen helps the instructor make a more accurate evaluation of the degree of deviation present in a student and assists in making a more meaningful follow-up examination. More information is presented on the use of the posture screen in Chapter 9. The screen should have an adjustable base so that it can be level, proper tension in the strings so that there is no sagging, and a center or gravity line of a different color so that it is easily identified. It should be light enough to be moved easily around the room and may even be so constructed that it can be folded and carried in a car by a traveling teacher. The posture screen may have a conformator built into one side that will permit the same apparatus to be used for measuring the anteroposterior posture deviations with some objectivity (Fig. 20-23, *A*) and will allow the instructor then to record the results of the conformator examination either on a life-size piece of paper or in graph form on his posture ex-

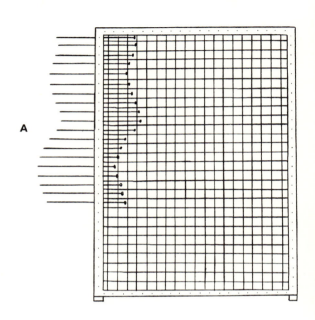
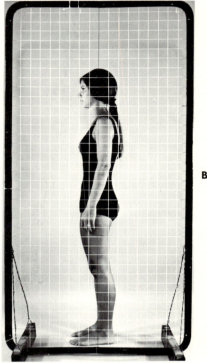

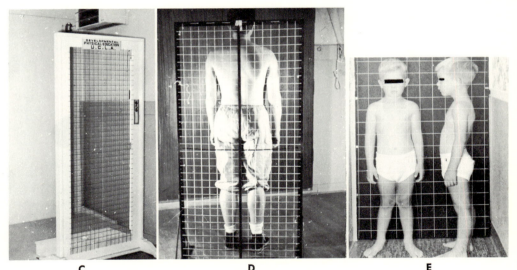

Fig. 20-23. Types of posture screens. **A,** With built-in conformator. **B,** Built from a metal bed frame. **C,** Wood frame with built-in fluorescent lights and platform. **D,** Metal frame that can be folded. **E,** Posture screening through a photographic technique used by Milo Brooks, M.D. It consists of a posture screen painted on the wall. The subject stands in the two positions indicated; a double-exposure photograph is taken, thereby superimposing the screen over the subject.

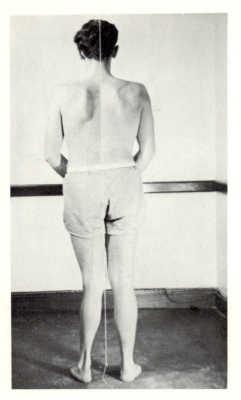

Fig. 20-24. Posture screening with a plumb line. Note knock-knee, atrophy of leg, and winged scapula.

amination sheet. The horizontal and vertical strings form a 2-inch grid on most screens, although some instructors prefer a 4-inch or even a 6-inch grid.*

Plumb line

A plumb line can be purchased from a hardware store or can be constructed easily by the adapted physical education instructor by tying any weight such as a lead fishing sinker to the end of a piece of string. A plumb line is a very useful piece of equipment in the adapted program. It can be used as a gravity line against which both anteroposterior and lateral posture ex-

*Exact specifications of such a posture screen are discussed in Crowe, W. C., Arnheim, D. D., and Auxter, D.: Laboratory manual in adapted physical education and recreation, St. Louis, 1977, The C. V. Mosby Co.

aminations can be taken; it can be used to check the alignment of the leg from the anterior, posterior, and lateral views; and it can be used to check the alignment of the spinal column, all in connection with various posture and body mechanics examinations. It also can be used to align such pieces of equipment as the posture screen and the conformator before they are used to examine students (Fig. 20-24). Chapter 9 describes the use of the posture screen.

Conformator

The conformator is used to identify the amount of anteroposterior curvature in the spinal column. A conformator consists of a number of freely sliding pegs placed in a perpendicular upright frame. The pegs, when placed against the spinal column, conform to the curvature of the skin covering the spinal processes of the spine. If all the sliding pegs are exactly the same length and are sliding freely and if the upright is perpendicular to the floor, a fairly accurate measurement can be taken of the anteroposterior curves. Information can be recorded for future reference in several different ways. A photograph can be taken of the student with the conformator adjusted to his back. The photograph in Fig. 20-25 shows the curvatures of the spine of the student as the examiner would see them from the lateral view and also shows the *actual* curvature of the spine as identified by the conformator. (This eliminates the problem of estimating where the spinal column actually is when the ribs or protruding muscles obstruct the actual curves from the view of the examiner.) Some conformators have a piece of wood hinged in the upright position that swings around so that it lies flat against the pegs of the conformator. After the student's spinal curve has been measured, a long piece of paper is mounted on this piece of wood and it is swung around against the pegs to allow the instructor to record graphically the position of the pegs. Using a skin pencil or ball-point pen, a permanent life-size record

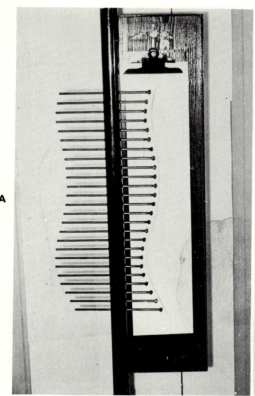

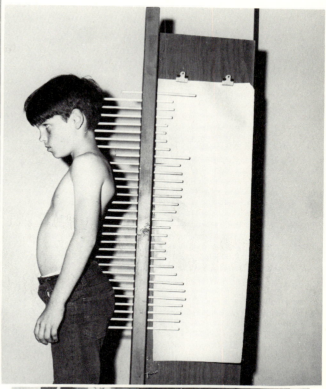

A

B

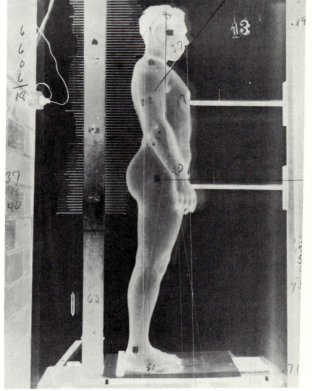

Fig. 20-25. Conformators. **A,** Conformator with attachment to record life-size spinal tracings. **B,** Photography used to record results of a conformator examination. **C,** Silhouetteograph used to record results of a conformator examination. (**B** courtesy California State University, Audio Visual Center, Long Beach, Calif.)

C

of the spinal curve is then traced. So that future tests can be performed and comparisons made, at least one landmark should be identified on this record sheet. Usually, this is the seventh cervical vertebra and the nearest rod to the seventh cervical vertebra is pulled out to show this position. This procedure allows the instructor to make successive examinations on this or a different paper and to place them side by side for comparison of the amount of curve in each segment of the spine (Fig. 20-25, A to C).

Podiascope

The podiascope is used to observe the sole of the foot during weight-bearing conditions. This device allows the instructor to objectify his opinion relative to the mechanics of the foot when the individual has his full weight superimposed on the glass top. To use the podiascope, the student stands on the top glass for approximately 1 minute so that the weight-bearing surfaces of the foot will become readily apparent. The instructor takes a position in front of the podiascope, looking into the slanting mirror so that he can actually observe the bottom of the foot under weight-bearing conditions. The instructor looks for the areas of greatest stress on the bottom of the foot. A towel draped around and over the student's feet helps to reduce the glare and improve the view of the examiner. Good lighting is necessary to use this equipment effectively. Photographs of the bottom of the foot can be taken through the podiascope (Figs. 9-28 and 20-26).

Foot and ankle tracings

Lowman, Colestock, and Cooper[14] described a technique of making a tracing around the foot to identify the amount of pronation that exists in the foot and ankle. They suggested that it is necessary, in order to standardize techniques in this test, to provide some kind of device that will enable the instructor to hold the marking instrument in a perpendicular position in order that lateral deviations of the foot and

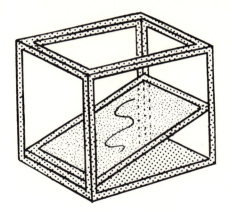

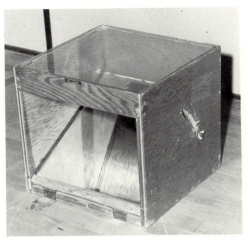

Fig. 20-26. The podiascope. (Lower illustration courtesy California State University, Audio Visual Center, Long Beach, Calif.)

ankle are reflected in the tracing of the foot. This can be accomplished by fastening some type of marking instrument to an object that will hold it in a constant position or by utilizing a tracing device similar to the one shown in Fig. 20-27. Chapter 9 presents instructions on the use of the tracing device (Fig. 9-30).

Pedograph

An inked impression of the print of the sole of the foot under weight-bearing conditions is known as a pedograph print. The device used to make this print consists of a piece of rubber sheeting that is inked on the underside and is mounted on a

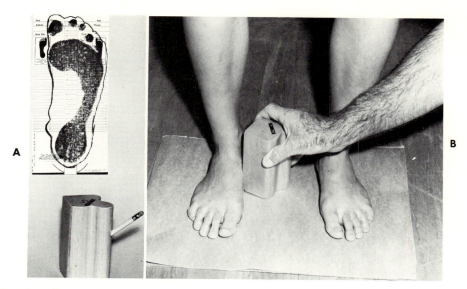

Fig. 20-27. Foot and joint tracer. **A,** Tracing made of foot and ankle and the tracer used. **B,** Making a foot and ankle tracing. (See also Fig. 9-30.) (**B** courtesy California State University, Audio Visual Center, Long Beach, Calif.)

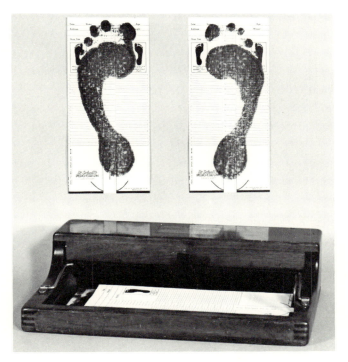

Fig. 20-28. Pedograph machine and pedograph footprints. The pedograph machine and the special paper shown are distributed by the William Scholl Co., Chicago.

frame so that when the student steps on it, an imprint of the foot will be transferred to a piece of paper placed beneath the sheeting. This provides a permanent print of the sole of the foot and supplies information similar to that obtained during an examination of the foot with the podiascope. Information observed during the podiascope examination can be transferred to this sheet to be used for future reference and for comparison with examinations made at a later time. After the ink has dried, the student can step on his pedograph print and a foot tracing can be made to record pronation and other malalignments of the foot and ankle. Thus three types of information can be recorded on this print and it can be used as a permanent record for future use and comparison (Fig. 20-28).

REFERENCES

1. Apgar, V.: A proposal for a new method of evaluation of the newborn infant, Curr. Res. Anesth. **32**:260, 1953.
2. Arnheim, D. D., and Sinclair, W. A.: The clumsy child: a program of motor therapy, St. Louis, 1975, The C. V. Mosby Co.
3. Ayres, A. J.: Manual: Ayres Space Test, Los Angeles, 1962, Western Psychological Services.
4. Ayres, A. J.: Manual: Southern California Figure-ground Visual Perception Test, Los Angeles, 1966, Western Psychological Services.
5. Ayres, A. J.: Manual: Southern California Kinesthesia and Tactile Perception Tests, Los Angeles, 1966, Western Psychological Services.
6. Ayres, A. J.: Manual: Southern California Motor Accuracy Test, Los Angeles, 1964, Western Psychological Services.
7. California Fitness Project, Committee on Evaluative Criteria for facilities: Evaluative criteria for facilities for health, physical education and recreation, Sacramento, Calif., 1958, California State Department of Education.
8. Clarke, H. H.: Application of measurement to health and physical education, Englewood Cliffs, N.J., 1967, Prentice-Hall, Inc.
9. Crowe, W. C.: The use of audio-visual materials in developmental (corrective) physical education. Unpublished master's thesis, University of California at Los Angeles, Los Angeles, 1950.
10. Fiorentino, M. R.: Reflex testing methods for evaluating C.N.S. development, Springfield, Ill., 1963, Charles C Thomas, Publisher.
11. Frostig, M., et al.: Marianne Frostig Developmental Test of Visual Perception, Palo Alto, Calif., 1964, Consulting Psychologists Press.
12. Goodenough, R. L., and Harris, D. B.: Goodenough-Harris Drawing Test, New York, 1963, Harcourt Brace Jovanovich, Inc.
13. Lowman, C. L.: Technique of underwater gymnastics, Los Angeles, 1937, American Publications, Inc.
14. Lowman, C. L., Colestock, C., and Cooper, H.: Corrective physical education for groups, New York, 1928, A. S. Barnes & Co., Inc.
15. Mathews, D. K.: Measurement in physical education, Philadelphia, 1968, W. B. Saunders Co.
16. Mueller, G. W., and Christaldi, J.: A practical program of remedial physical education, Philadelphia, 1966, Lea & Febiger.
17. Orpet, R. E.: Frostig movement skills tests battery, Los Angeles, 1972, Marianne Frostig Center of Educational Therapy.
18. Oseretsky, N. A.: Metric scale for studying the motor capacity of children. In Lassner, R.: Annotated bibliography of the Oseretsky Test of Motor Proficiency: J. Consult. Clin. Psychol. **12**:37-47, 1948.
19. Roach, E. G., and Kephart, N. C.: The Purdue Perceptual-Motor Survey, Columbus, Ohio, 1966, Charles E. Merrill Publishing Co.
20. Stone, E. B., and Deyton, J. W.: Corrective therapy for the handicapped child, Englewood Cliffs, N.J., 1951, Prentice-Hall, Inc.
21. Stott, D. H.: A general test of motor impairment for children, Dev. Med. Child Neurol. **8**:523-531, 1966.
22. Swisher, I.: Facilities and equipment in adapted physical education. Unpublished data, Santa Monica, Calif., 1952.
23. Youth fitness test manual, rev., Washington, D.C., 1961, The American Association for Health, Physical Education, and Recreation.

RECOMMENDED READINGS

Adams, R. C., Daniel, A., and Rullman, L.: Games, sports and exercises for the physically handicapped, Philadephia, 1972, Lea & Febiger.

Anderson, M. H., Elliot, M. E., and LaVerge, J.: Play with a purpose, New York, 1966, Harper & Row, Publishers.

Arnheim, D. D., and Pestolesi, R. A.: Developing motor behavior in children—a balanced approach to elementary physical education, St. Louis, 1973, The C. V. Mosby Co.

Cowart, J., and Dressel, M.: Sport adaptions for a student without fingers, J. Phys. Educ. Rec. **47**:46, 1976.

Dauer, V. P.: Dynamic physical education for

elementary school children, Minneapolis, 1972, Burgess Publishing Co.

Dexter, G.: Instruction of physically handicapped pupils, remedial physical education, Sacramento, Calif., 1973, California State Department of Education.

Frederick, A. B.: 212 ideas for making low-cost physical education equipment, Englewood Cliffs, N.J., 1963, Prentice-Hall, Inc.

Huber, J. H., and Vercollone, J.: Using aquatic mats with exceptional children, J. Phys. Educ. Rec. 47:44, 1976.

Jorris, T. R.: The relationship between abdominal muscle shortening and anterior-posterior pelvis tilt. Unpublished doctoral dissertation, University of California at Los Angeles, Los Angeles, 1960.

Leighton, J. R.: A simple objective and reliable measure of flexibility, Res. Q. 13:205, 1942.

Lowman, C. L., and Young, C. H.: Postural fitness significance and variances, Philadelphia, 1960, Lea & Febiger.

Mathews, D. K.: Measurement in physical education, ed. 3, Philadelphia, 1968, W. B. Saunders Co.

Planning areas and facilities for health, physical education and recreation, Chicago, 1970, The Athletic Institute.

Rarick, L. G., Montoye, H. J., and Seefeldt, V.: An introduction to measurement in physical education, vol. 2, Indianapolis, 1970, Phi Epsilon Kappa Fraternity.

Sloan, W.: The Lincoln-Oseretsky motor development scale, Gen. Psychol. Monogr. 51:183-252, 1955.

Souter, E. B.: Skinfold measurements of fat in college men, Master's thesis, California State University, Long Beach, Calif., 1968.

Werner, P., and Rini, L.: Perceptual-motor development equipment, New York, 1976, John Wiley & Sons, Inc.

GLOSSARY

abduction Moving away from the midline of the body.

accountability Acquisition of short-term instructional objectives of pupils over a specified time frame.

acute Condition having a quick onset and a short duration.

Adam's position Position to determine the extent to which a scoliosis is structural. The subject bends over from the waist with arms relaxed in a hanging position.

adaptive behavior Refers to the effectiveness of adapting to natural and social demands on one's environment.

adduction Moving toward the midline of the body.

aggression Offensive action or procedure.

agonist Muscle that is directly engaged in action.

allergy Hypersensitive reaction to certain foreign substances that are harmless in similar amounts to nonsensitive individuals.

anemia Condition of the blood in which there is a deficiency of hemoglobin.

angina pectoris Sense of suffocating contraction within the chest, usually associated with organic change in the heart.

ankle and foot pronation Abnormal turning of the ankle downward and medially (eversion and abduction).

ankle and foot supination Refers to the foot turned inward and in adduction (inversion and adduction).

ankylosis Abnormal immobility of a joint (fusion).

antagonist Muscle that opposes the action of another muscle.

antigravity muscles Muscles that serve to keep the body in an upright posture.

anxiety Uneasiness that is difficult to describe.

aphasia Impairment in use of words as symbols of ideas.

arteriosclerosis Hardening, thickening, and loss of elasticity of the walls of blood vessels.

arthritis Inflammation of a joint.

arthrodesis Fixation of a joint by surgery.

asthma Labored breathing association with a sense of constriction in the chest.

astigmatism Refractive error caused by an irregularity in the curvature of the cornea of the lens; vision may become blurred.

ataxia Clinical type of cerebral palsy that is characterized by a disturbance of equilibrium.

athetoid Clinical type of cerebral palsy that is characterized by uncoordinated movements of the voluntary muscles, often accompanied by impaired muscle control of the hand and impaired speech and swallowing.

atonia Clinical type of cerebral palsy that is characterized by a lack of muscle tone.

atrophy Wasting away of muscular tissue.

atypical That which is not usual; abnormal.

aura Warning preceding a seizure.

autonomic seizure Seizure that consists of periods of flushing, sweating, fast heartheat, gagging, and heightened blood pressure, in which unconsciousness is absent.

Babinski reflex Elicited by stroking the plantar aspect of the foot and resulting in a dorsal extension of the great toe and spreading of other toes.

barrel chest Abnormally rounded chest.

behavior modification Changing of behavioral characteristics through application of learning principles.

behavior training Anxiety reduction of problem situations for particular individuals.

behavioral objectives Objectives that contain an

action, conditions, and criteria and have not been mastered by the learner.

bilateral Pertaining to two sides.

blind Lacking the sense of sight.

"blue baby" Lack of oxygen transportation to the brain, which may occur during birth.

BMR Basal metabolism rate, expenditure of energy of the body in a resting state.

body image System of ideas and feelings that a person has about his structure.

borderline retarded Mentally retarded persons who are usually capable of competing with most children in activities other than academic ones.

breech extraction Delivery at birth in which the child presents itself feet first.

bronchial asthma Condition that affects the respiratory system and usually results from allergic states in which there is an obstruction of the bronchial tubes or lungs or a combination of both.

cardiovascular disease Inclusive term that describes all diseases of the heart and blood vessels throughout the body.

central deafness Condition in which the receiving mechanism of hearing functions properly, but an abnormality in the central nervous system prevents one from hearing.

cephalocaudal Used to describe development of the individual that proceeds from the head to the feet.

cerebral palsy Conditions in which damage is inflicted to the brain and is accompanied by motor involvement.

chondromalacia Softening of cartilage.

chronic Condition having a gradual onset and a long duration.

circumduction Moving a part in a manner that describes a cone.

competencies Predetermined standards of behavior.

component building Pairing of a positive and a neutral event, then fading the positive in such a manner that there is transfer from the positive to the neutral to make the neutral positive.

condition shifting program Program in which several conditions of behavioral objectives are altered to produce activities that are sequenced from lesser to greater difficulty.

conditions Stipulation of the precise behaviors that are to be displayed when performing an instructional objective; task specifications of the instructional objective.

conductive hearing loss Condition in which the intensity of sound is reduced before reaching the inner ear, where the auditory nerve begins.

congenital Present at birth.

congenital heart disease Condition of the heart at birth.

contracture (muscle) Abnormal contraction of a muscle.

coronary heart disease Condition in which the coronary arteries become sclerotic or hardened and narrowed.

corrective therapy System of therapy utilizing physical activities for the rehabilitation of a disability.

coxa plana Also known as Legg-Calvé-Perthes disease; avascular, necrotic flattening of the head of the femur.

coxa valga Increase in the angle of the neck of the head of the femur to more than 120 degrees.

coxa vara Decrease in the angle of the neck of the head of the femur to less than 120 degrees.

criterion Standard on which judgments may be made for task mastery.

cross education Transfer of a skill from one contralateral body part to another.

cultural-familial mental retardation Mental retardation attributed to child-rearing practices in subcultures, placing children in a disadvantageous position in taking culturally biased intelligence tests.

curriculum Predetermined course of instructional events.

deaf Nonfunctional hearing for the ordinary purposes of life.

decubitus ulcer Bedsore caused by a prolonged pressure.

development To build, to proceed from lower to higher, progression; process of growing to maturity.

developmental period For practical purposes from birth to approximately age 16 years.

diabetes Chronic metabolic disorder that involves the inability of the cells to use glucose properly.

diagnostic-prescriptive integrity Refers to a direct relationship between the assessment and the programming to remediate the assessed disabilities.

diaphysis The shaft of a long bone.

directionality Perception of direction in space.

disability Physical or mental incapacity.

dislocation Abnormal displacement of a bone in relation to its position in a joint.

displacement Disguising of a particular goal by substituting another in its place.

distal Refers to a point away from an origin, as opposed to proximal.

dorsal Refers to back, back of hand, back of thoracic region, or top of foot.

dorsiflexion Refers to the act of bending the ankle upward (flexion).

dysmenorrhea Painful menstruation.

dysplasia Disharmony between different regions of the body; abnormal development.

dyspnea Difficult breathing.

ecchymosis Black and blue area caused by a hemorrhagic condition of the skin.

ECG Refers to the electrocardiograph test, a record of heart muscle action potential.

edema Extended swelling of organs or parts of organs.

educable mentally retarded Persons who are generally able to succeed in early school-related tasks (IQ, 50 to 84).

electromyogram Recording of the action potential of skeletal muscles.

elevation Moving of a part upward.

encephalitis Acute and inflammatory condition of the brain, often characterized by some manifestation of cerebral dysfunction.

epilepsy Disturbance in electrochemical activity of the brain that causes seizures and convulsions.

epiphysis Ossification center at the end of each developing long bone.

etiology Study of the origin of disease (term often misused for "cause").

eversion Lifting the outer border of the foot upward.

exercise intensity Amount of work load in relationship to the functional capacity of the individual.

extension Movement of a part that increases a joint angle.

external evaluation Refers to situation in which person independent of the project evaluates the extent to which predetermined behaviors are acquired by pupils and the processes employed for achieving objectives.

extrinsic Pertaining to being ouside a part.

fading Sequentially reducing the amount of prompting when a performer is attempting a task.

fibrosis Abnormal amount of fibrous tissue.

flexion Movement of a part that decreases a joint angle.

functional capacity Current level of ability to perform activity.

gait Walking pattern.

GAS Refers to the general adaptation syndrome.

general intellectual functioning Assessment of performance on an IQ test.

genu recurvatum Hyperextension at the knee joint.

genu valgum Knock-knee.

genu varum Bowleg.

geriatrics Study of diseases of old age.

gerontology Science of old age.

grand mal seizure Seizure that involves severe convulsions accompanied by stiffening, twisting, alternating contractions and relaxations, and unconsciousness.

growth Development of, or increased size of, a living organism.

hallux valgus (pl. *halluces*) Displacement of the great toe toward the other toes as occurring with a bunion.

handicap Any hinderance or difficulty imposed by a physical, mental, or emotional problem.

hard-of-hearing Those who have hearing impairments, but can function with or without a hearing aid.

heart murmurs Sounds that can be detected by a stethoscope as a result of the blood flowing past the valves of the heart.

Helbing's sign Medial curving of the Achilles tendon occurring in a pronated foot and ankle.

hemarthrosis Blood in a joint cavity.

hemiplegia Neurological affliction of one half of the body or the limbs on one side of the body.

hernia Protrusion through an abnormal opening.

hierarchy Arrangement of activities in which one is prerequisite to a higher, more complex task.

hyperopia Farsightedness; inability to see objects close; the light rays focus behind the retina and cause an unclear image of objects closer than 20 feet from the eye.

hypertensive heart Commonly known as high blood pressure, which places a prolonged stress on the heart and major arteries.

idiopathic Refers to disease of unknown cause.

inflammation Reaction of the tissue to trauma, heat and cold, chemicals, electricity, or microorganisms.

instruction Organized principles with established technical procedure involving action and practice.

interference method Application of operant conditioning in an educational setting.

intrinsic Pertaining to being within a part.

inversion Turning upward of the medial border of the foot.

ischemia Local anemia caused by an obstruction of blood vessels to a part.

isometric muscle contraction Muscle contraction without any appreciable change in its length.

isotonic muscle contraction Muscle contraction whereby origin and insertion move toward one another.

Jacksonian seizure Seizure characterized by local movements of some part of the body spreading to other parts of the body.

kinesthesis Perception of body in space, including rate and extent of movement.

kypholordosis Exaggerated thoracic and lumbar spinal curves (round swayback).

kyphosis Exaggerated thoracic spinal curve (humpback).

laterality Internal awareness of right and left.

learning ability Refers to the facility with which knowledge is acquired as a function of experience.

local edema Excess of tissue fluid in an area.

lordosis Exaggerated lumbar vertebral curve (swayback).

luxation Complete dislocation of articular surfaces at a joint.

main task Of less difficulty than a skill and pre-requisite to skills.

manualism Means by which the deaf communicate by use of hand signals (signing).

maturation Refers to the rate of sequential development of self-help skills of infancy, development of locomotor skills, and interaction with peers, which would occur irrespective of instructional intervention.

menarche Onset of menstruation.

meningitis Acute contagious disease characterized by inflammation of the meninges of the spinal cord.

menstrual cycle Complex process that involves the endocrine glands, uterus, and ovaries and is manifested by the passing of blood from the uterus on an average cycle of 28 days.

mental retardation Subaverage intellectual functioning that originates during the developmental period and is associated with impairment in adaptive behavior.

met Work metabolic rate divided by resting metabolic rate of a subject.

metaphysis Epiphyseal plate, that portion of the developing long bone that lies between the shaft and the epiphysis.

metatarsalgia Also known as Morton's toe; severe pain or cramp in metatarsus in the region of the fourth toe.

mononucleosis Disease of low virulence that affects the lymphocytes.

monoplegia Neurological affliction of one extremity of the body.

morbidity Number of disease cases in a calendar year per 100,000 population.

Moro reflex Startle reflex elicited by noise or by jarring or removing the supporting surface.

mortality Death rate.

motor skill Reasonably complex motor performance.

muscle setting Statically tensing a muscle without moving a part.

muscular dystrophy Chronic, progressive, degenerative, noncontagious disease of the muscular system, characterized by weakness and atrophy of muscles of the body.

myocardial infarcts Limited function of the heart.

myopia Nearsightedness; inability to see objects far away; the rays of light focus in front of the retina when viewing objects 20 feet or more from the person.

neuromotor disorders Conditions in which damage is inflicted to the brain and is accompanied by motor involvement.

nystagmus Impaired muscle function of the eye.

obesity Pathological overweight in which a person is 20% or more above the normal weight (compare *overweight*).

objective Acceptance of events without distortion or prejudice, action toward which effort is directed for a purpose, to achieve outcomes that can be evaluated without prejudice.

ontogeny Historical development of an organism.

ophthalmologist Licensed physician who specializes in the treatment of eye disease and optical defects.

optician Technician who grinds lenses and makes up glasses.

optometrist Person who provides examination of the eye for defects and faults of refraction and the prescription of correctional lenses and exercises.

oralism Method of teaching the deaf by means of lip reading.

organic brain injury Condition in which damage to the central nervous system exists.

orientation Obtaining the response and reinforcing the response.

orthopedics Branch of surgery primarily concerned with treatment of disorders of the musculoskeletal system.

orthoptist Person who provides eye exercises and orthoptic training as prescribed by medical personnel.

orthotics Construction of self-help devices to aid the patient in rehabilitation (braces, etc.).

Oseretsky motor development scale A battery of tests that assesses the level of motor development of a child.

Osgood-Schlatter disease Epiphysitis of the tibial tubercle.

osteoarthritis Chronic and degenerative disease of joints.

osteochondritis Inflammation of cartilage and bone.

osteoporosis Increased porosity of bone by the absorption of calcareous material.

overweight Any deviation of 10% or more above the ideal weight for a person (compare *obese*).

paralysis Permanent or temporary suspension of a motor function because of the loss of integrity of a motor nerve.

paraplegia Neurological affliction of both legs.

paresis Local paralysis.

pathology Study of disease (term often misused for diseased or "pathological conditions").

pattern analysis Study of sequential arrangement of movement behaviors to achieve a purpose.

pelvic tilt Increase or decrease of pelvic inclination.

perceptive deafness Inability to hear caused by a defect of the inner ear or of the auditory nerve in transmitting the impulse to the brain.

pes Refers to the foot.

pes cavus Exaggerated height of the longitudinal arch of the foot (hollow arch).

pes planus Extreme flatness of the longitudinal arch of the foot.

petit mal seizure Nonconvulsive seizure in which consciousness is lost for a few seconds.

phagocytosis Process of ingestion of injurious cells or particles by a phagocyte (white blood cell).

phenylketonuria (PKU) Physiological disturbance caused by an imbalance in the amino acids and resulting in mental limitations.

phylogeny Development of a race or group of animals.

physiatrist Physician in physical medicine.

physical medicine Phase of medicine that utilizes the various therapies to bring about a healing response.

pigeon chest Abnormal prominence of the sternum.

plantar flexion Moving the foot toward its plantar surface at the ankle joint (extension).

pneumonia Disease affecting respiration that is caused by the infection of the air spaces of the lungs.

prescription Specification of action based on diagnosis prior to program implementation.

process Steps that lead to objectives in a particular manner; a progressive series of operations to be followed in a definite order that directs action toward achievement of objectives.

profoundly retarded Mentally retarded persons who require complete custodial care.

prognosis Prediction of the course of a disease.

program Sequential order of behavioral objectives that go from lesser to greater difficulty.

programmed instruction Prearranged behavioral objectives in which technical procedures are applied to cope with individual learning differences.

progressive muscular dystrophy Progressive wasting and atrophy of muscles.

projection Disguising a conflict by excluding one's motives; blaming someone else.

prompting Sensory or physical aid to engage the participant in successful activity.

prone position Lying in a face-down position.

prosthesis Artificial limb or appliance.

protraction Forward movement of a part, for example, shoulder girdle.

proximal Refers to a point nearest to the origin of an organ or body part, as opposed to distal.

proximodistal Used to describe development of the individual that proceeds from the midline of the body outward.

psychogenic deafness Condition in which receptive organs are not impaired, but for emotional reasons, the person does not respond to sound.

psychomotor seizure Seizure in which one may lose contact with reality and manifest bizarre psychogenic behavior.

ptosis Weakness and prolapse of an organ, that is, prominent abdomen.

quadriplegia Neurological affliction of all four extremities.

rationalization Resolution of a conflict by hiding a real motive and substituting another reasonable one.

reaction formation Disguised feeling in which a person acts opposite to the response toward which he may be motivated.

recreation therapy System of therapy utilizing recreation as a means to rehabilitation.

regular class Public school class in which typical children are educated.

regurgitation Imperfect closure of valves to the heart, which permits backflow of blood.

rehabilitation Restoration of a disabled person to greater efficiency and health.

reinforcer Any consequence that follows an action and strengthens that act.

relaxation Lessening of anxiety and muscle tension.

repression Submerging distressing thoughts into the unconscious mind.

retraction Backward movement of a part, for example, shoulder girdle.

rheumatic heart disease Condition caused by rheumatic fever, which damages the heart, its valves, and blood vessels by scar tissue.

rigidity Clinical classification of cerebral palsy characterized by rigid functional uncoordination of reciprocal muscle groups.

risk Used to describe persons who have a majority of factors pointing toward the potential development of coronary heart disease.

round shoulders Postural condition whereby the scapulae are abducted and the shoulders are forward.

salicylates Salt of salicylic acid used to reduce pain and temperature.

scoliosis Lateral and rotation deviation of the vertebral column.

self-concept How persons view themselves.

self-evaluation Accurate interpretation of the consequences of instructional performance without the aid of outside information.

self-instruction To engage in procedures to achieve one's objectives without personal and direct input from the instructor.

senility State of being old.

severely retarded Mentally retarded persons who can be trained to care for some of their bodily needs and develop language, but have great difficulty in social and occupational areas.

shaping Phase of conditioning in which one becomes accustomed to routine of environment and tasks required for performance.

skill Utilization of abilities to perform complex tasks competently as a result of reinforced practice.

social adjustment Degree to which the individual is able to maintain himself independently in the community, achieve gainful employment, and conform to other personal and social responsibilities and standards set by the community.

somatotype Certain body type (endomorphy, mesomorphy, or ectomorphy).

spasm Involuntary muscle contraction.

spastic Clinical type of cerebral palsy characterized by muscle contractures and jerky, uncertain movements of the muscles.

special class Class designed to give special educational help to mentally retarded, emotionally disturbed, deaf, or blind students or children with other handicaps.

spina bifida Congenital separation or lack of union of the vertebral arches.

stenosis Incomplete opening of a valve that restricts blood from flowing.

strabismus Crossed eyes resulting from inability of the eye muscles to coordinate.

stress Condition that causes the inability of an organism to maintain its constant internal environment.

sublimation Substitution of one activity for another, more accessible activity.

subluxation Incomplete dislocation of articular surface of a joint.

submaximal intensity Below the functional level of maximum performance.

subtask Subdivision of a task; several subtasks compose the main task.

supination Rotation of the palm of the hand upward or adduction and inversion of the foot.

supine position Lying on the back and facing upward.

system Interdependent items that relate to a whole operation and function as a unit.

talipes (pl. *talipedes*) Generic term for a foot deformity.

talipes equinovalgus Combination of talipes equinus and talipes valgus; person walks on the border of the big toes (plantar flexion and pronation).

talipes equinovarus Walking on the toes and the outside and anterior portions of the foot (plantar flexion and supination).

talipes equinus Walking on the toes or the anterior portion of the foot.

talipes valgus Walking on the inside of the foot (pronated).

talipes varus Walking on the outside of the foot (supinated).

target level Desired performance level of an individual while participating in activity.

task analysis Separation of tasks of objectives into components and lower order objectives.

tenotomy Surgical operation on the tendons.

tension State of being strained.

terminal objective Synthesis of all subobjectives that enable mastery of the main or general objective.

tetralogy of Fallot "Blue babies"; abnormalities of the opening of the septum between ventricles or positioning of the aorta to the right in such a manner that it lies over the defect of the septum of the left ventricle.

therapeutic modality Device designed to bring about a therapeutic response, for example, heat, cold, light, electrostimulation.

therapy Treatment of a disease or disability.

tibial torsion Refers to the medial twisting of the lower leg on its long axis.

torticollis Also known as wryneck; contraction of neck muscles resulting in drawing the head to one side.

trainable mentally retarded Persons who are characterized by the general inability to succeed in problem-solving tasks and do not have discernible, usable academic skills. They are frequently impaired in both maturation and social adjustment.

tranquilizer Drug that quiets emotionally disturbed patients.

trauma Injury or wound.

tremor Clinical type of cerebral palsy evidenced by a rhythmic movement caused by alternating contractions between flexor and extensor muscles.

Trendelenburg sign Dropping of the pelvis on the unsupported side because of weakness or paralysis of hip abductor muscles.

valgus (valgum) Angling of a part in the direction of the midline of the body (turned out).

varus (varum) Angling of a part in the direction away from the midline of the body (turned in).

vestibular sense Responsible for balance; located in nonauditory portion of the ear.

whiplash injury Deep-tissue neck injury resulting from the head being forcefully snapped forward and backward.

winged scapula Vertebral border of the scapula wings outward because of weakness of the serratus anterior or the middle and lower trapezius muscles.

Wolff's law of bone growth Bone alters its internal architecture and external form according to the manner in which it is used.

APPENDIX I

A RECIPROCAL (PARTNER SYSTEM) EXERCISE SERIES

A system using the principles of isotonic and isometric muscle contraction has been found to be a valuable adjunct to the adapted exercise program. The benefits are as follows: (1) no equipment is needed, (2) maximum workout takes place in minimum time, (3) each student works at his own level, and (4) it is highly motivating for participants.

Operational techniques for resistance

Operational techniques for resistance are as follows:

1. When resistance is applied to a part, it should first be allowed to go through a full range of movement.
2. Isometric resistance should be applied to selected points along the full range of movement.
3. Isometric contractions should be held at least 6 seconds.
4. Three bouts of resistance should be given each individual exercise.
5. Resistance should be discontinued when fatigue occurs.
6. Participants should express their straining with noise and loud verbal encouragement.

Resistance exercises

1. Neck extension and flexion (Fig. I-1)
   a. Purpose: To strengthen the flexors and extensors of the neck
   b. Starting position: Subject takes a four-point position. Operator stands in front of subject, with hands placed on the back of the head of the subject to resist extension and grasping chin for flexion.
   c. Movement: Subject moves up and down against the resistance of the operator. CAUTION!! Start very slowly; neck develops spasms easily.
2. Neck side flexion (Fig. I-2)
   a. Purpose: To strengthen lateral flexors of the neck
   b. Starting position: Subject takes a four-point position. Operator stands in front of subject, with one leg placed against side of subject's face.
   c. Movement: Subject pushes face against knee of operator, attempting to move side of head toward shoulder. As subject applies force, operator gives way to resistance slowly.
3. Hip extension and flexion (Fig. I-3)
   a. Purpose: To strengthen hip flexors and extensors

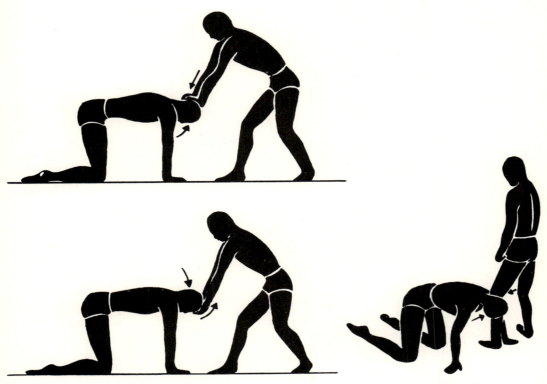

Fig. I-1

Fig. I-2

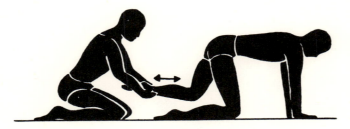

Fig. I-3

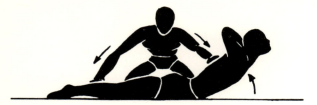

Fig. I-4

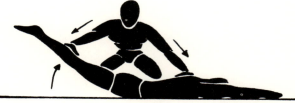

Fig. I-5

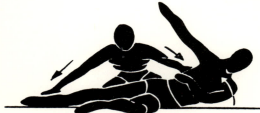

Fig. I-6

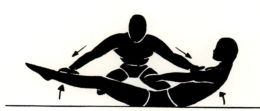

Fig. I-7

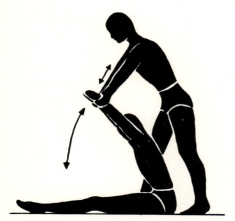

Fig. I-8

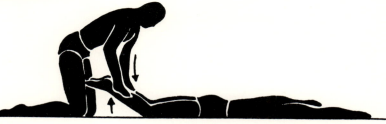

Fig. I-9

b. Starting position: Subject takes a four-point position. Operator kneels to rear of subject, grasping one foot.

c. Movement: As operator resists, subject pulls knee to chest and then pushes thigh backward to full extension.

4. Back extension (Fig. I-4)

   a. Purpose: To strengthen upper back extensors

   b. Starting position: Subject takes a prone position, with hands clasped behind head. Operator addresses himself to the side of subject, placing one hand on his ankles and one hand between scapulae.

   c. Movement: Subject attempts to arch upper back against resistance of operator's upper hand.

5. Low back and hip extension (Fig. I-5)

   a. Purpose: To strengthen low back and hip extensors

   b. Starting position: Subject takes a prone position with arms extended over head. Operator kneels at one side of subject, with lower hand pressing on subject's ankles and upper hand placed between scapulae.

   c. Movement: Subject maintains upper trunk against mat and arches lower back against operator's resistance.

6. Side sit-up (Fig. I-6)

   a. Purpose: To strengthen lateral abdominal muscles

   b. Starting position: Subject takes a side-lying position. Lower arm is placed across chest, whereas upper arm is stretched outward along body line. Lower leg is bent 90 degrees for support, whereas upper leg is kept straight. Operator kneels facing subject's waist and places one hand on subject's ankle or upper leg and the other hand on the side of the trunk.

   c. Movement: While operator stabilizes lower body by pressing down on subject's ankle, subject executes a side sit-up against the resistance of the operator's upper hand.

7. Jackknife (Fig. I-7)

   a. Purpose: To strengthen abdominal muscles and hip flexors

   b. Starting position: Subject lies on his back, lifting legs and trunk off floor, thereby balancing on buttocks. Operator kneels at side of subject, facing hips. Operator places one hand on subject's ankles and the other on subject's chest.

   c. Movement: Subject attempts to maintain jackknife position. Operator forces the subject's legs and trunk back to the floor.

8. Woodchopper (Fig. I-8)

   a. Purpose: To strengthen abdominal muscles

   b. Starting position: Subject takes a long sitting position, with hands clasped and arms extended over head. The operator stands behind subject, bracing knees against subject's back, and grasps subject's clasped hands.

   c. Movement: Against operator's resistance, subject pulls both arms down across body to the floor in a chopping motion. The movement alternates first to the left side and then to the right side of subject.

9. Leg curl (Fig. I-9)

   a. Purpose: To strengthen hamstring muscle group

   b. Starting position: Subject takes a prone position, with arms extended over head. Operator kneels at the foot of subject.

   c. Movement: As subject curls leg toward buttocks, operator resists by holding down against subject's ankles.

10. Knee extension (Fig. I-10)

    a. Purpose: To strengthen quadriceps muscle group

    b. Starting position: Subject takes a prone position, with arms extended overhead. Operator sits on subject's buttocks, facing footward. With

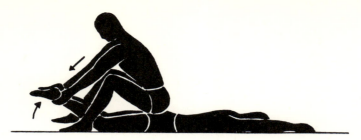

Fig. I-10

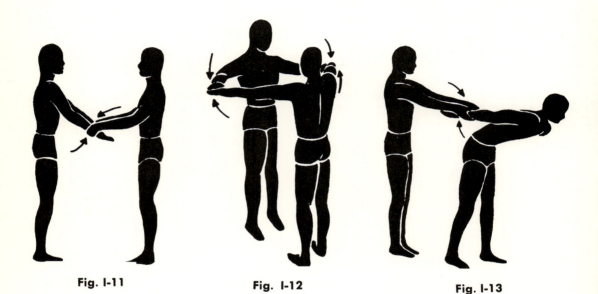

Fig. I-11   **Fig. I-12**   **Fig. I-13**

subject's leg in a flexed position, operator grasps subject's ankle.

c. Movement: Subject extends his leg by kicking downward against the operator's resistance.

11. Front arm raise (Fig. I-11)

a. Purpose: To strengthen shoulder flexors

b. Starting position: Subject stands with arms at side. Operator stands facing subject and grasps both wrists of the subject.

c. Movement: Subject flexes shoulders to 90 degrees while operator resists movement.

12. Side arm raise (Fig. I-12)

a. Purpose: To strengthen shoulder abductors

b. Starting position: Subject stands with arms at side. Operator stands facing subject and grasps both wrists of the subject.

c. Movement: Subject abducts both arms to 90 degrees while operator applies resistance.

13. Back arm push (Fig. I-13)

a. Purpose: To strengthen shoulder extensors

b. Starting position: Subject stands with arms at side. Operator stands behind subject and grasps both subject's wrists.

c. Movement: Subject forces both arms backward through a 50 degree range while operator resists movement.

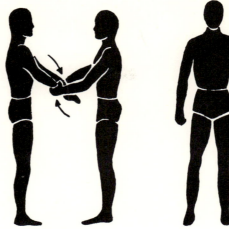

Fig. I-14

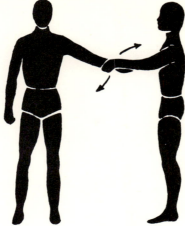

Fig. I-15

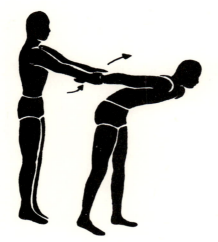

Fig. I-16

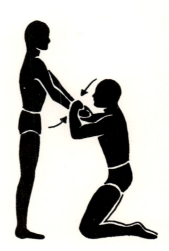

Fig. I-17

14. Front arm pull down (Fig. I-14)
    a. Purpose: To strengthen shoulder extensors and chest
    b. Starting position: Subject stands with arms raised 90 degrees to the front. Operator stands facing subject and grasps subject's wrists.
    c. Movement: Subject attempts to pull both arms straight down to his thighs while operator resists movement.
15. Side arm pull down (Fig. I-15)
    a. Purpose: To strengthen shoulder adductors

    b. Starting position: Subject stands with arms raised to 90 degrees at the side. Operator stands facing subject and grasps both wrists. NOTE! If subject is too strong, one arm may have to be exercised at a time, as illustrated.
    c. Movement: Subject pulls arms downward to his side while operator resists movement.
16. Arm back pull (Fig. I-16)
    a. Purpose: To strengthen shoulder flexors and adductors
    b. Starting position: Operator stands

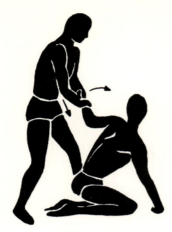

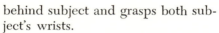

Fig. I-18

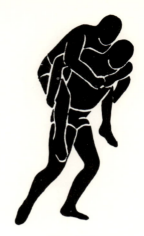

Fig. I-19

behind subject and grasps both subject's wrists.

c. Movement: As subject pulls both
arms forward to the side of his
body, operator resists movement.

17. Arm curl (Fig. I-17)
   a. Purpose: To strengthen arm flexors
   b. Starting position: Subject stands
      with arms raised 45 degrees to the
      front, with one hand over the other.
      Kneeling in front of subject, oper-
      ator places both his forearms over
      the hands of the subject.
   c. Movement: Subject curls both arms
      upward while operator pulls down-
      ward.

18. Arm extension (Fig. I-18)
   a. Purpose: To strengthen arm exten-
      sors

b. Starting position: Subject kneels
   with the arm to be exercised raised
   over head and bent backward at
   the elbow. Operator stands behind
   subject and grasps wrist of arm to
   be exercised.

c. Movement: Subject straightens arm
   over head as operator resists movement.

19. Piggyback exercise for leg (Fig. I-19)
   a. Purpose: To strengthen calves and
      knee, hip, and spine extensors
   b. Starting position: Operator rides
      subject in a piggyback fashion.
   c. Movement: With the resistance
      from the operator's added weight,
      the subject can do toe raises, half
      squats, straddle hops, or short runs.

APPENDIX II

STALL BAR EXERCISES

The stall bar is a traditional piece of equipment in the adapted gymnasium. Figs. II-1 to II-10 provide the reader with a select number of stall bar exercises that may be used by the student, as pictured, or modified, depending on the student's individual needs (see also Chapter 5).

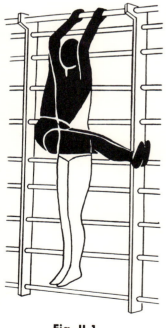

Fig. II-1

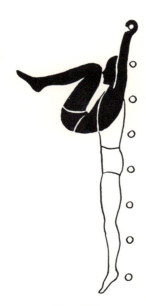

Fig. II-2

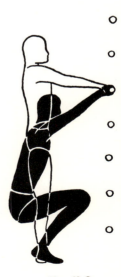

Fig. II-3

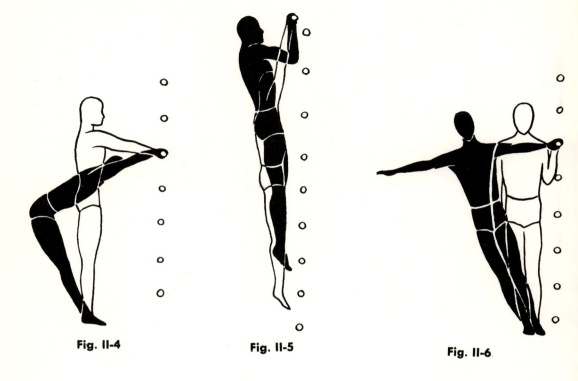

Fig. II-4

Fig. II-5

Fig. II-6

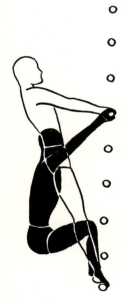

Fig. II-7

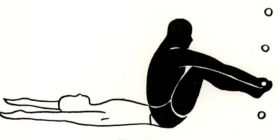

Fig. II-8

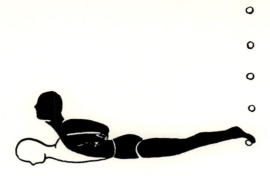

Fig. II-9

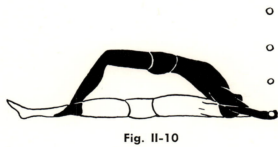

Fig. II-10

APPENDIX III

PULLEY WEIGHT EXERCISES

Pulley weights allow for a variety of progressive resistance exercises. Figs. III-1 to III-10 illustrate suggested routines for various parts of the body. (See also Chapter 5.)

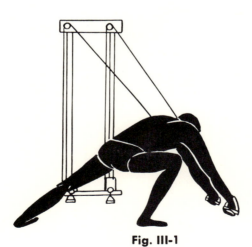

Fig. III-1

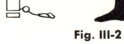

Fig. III-2

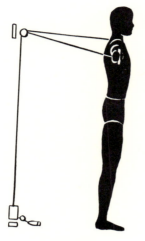

Fig. III-3

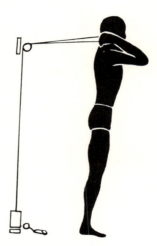

Fig. III-4

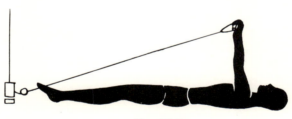

Fig. III-5

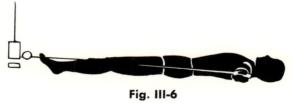

Fig. III-6

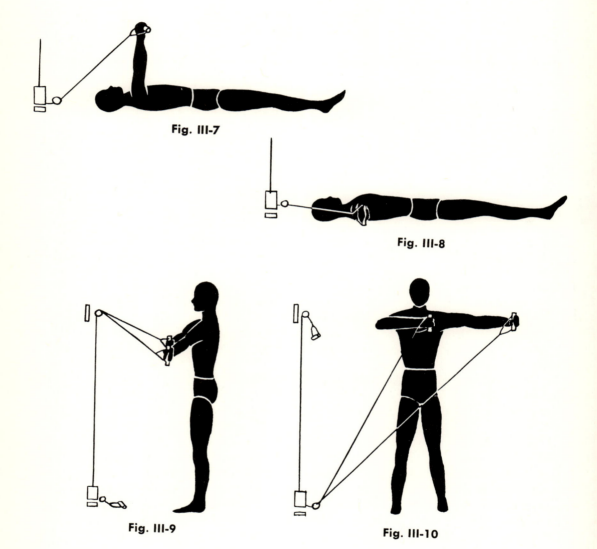

Fig. III-7

Fig. III-8

Fig. III-9

Fig. III-10

APPENDIX IV

CRUTCH AND CANE WALKING

It is desirable that the adapted physical educator understand the intricacies of crutch and cane management. Many students, on entering the adapted program, will incorrectly use the crutch or cane. Improper use of these aids can greatly deter the balance and maneuverability of these students. Individuals who require the use of the crutch or cane are many and varied, ranging from amputees or paraplegics to those who are temporarily incapacitated with some traumatic condition such as a sprained ankle. Whatever the reason for using the crutch or cane, it is imperative that basic principles be practiced by the users.

There are many types of crutches today. The most common, however, are made of hardwood and constructed with a top crosspiece that fits under the armpit and a handgrip that supports the weight of the body. The wood crutch can be made non-adjustable, fitted to the particular requirements of the individual, or, more commonly, as an adjustable type with an extension rod at its support tip and an adjustable handgrip. Metal or leather axillary devices can be added to any crutch in order to better stabilize the arm or wrist. A great number of modifications can be made to provide the user better support and greater

freedom of movement. Recently, the aluminum crutch has come to the fore on account of its light weight and adaptability to individual requirements. Aluminum crutches frequently include an arm piece, adjustable handgrips, and a telescopic rod tip; a variation of this type comes with a forearm cup made of spring steel rather than an axillary piece. Like the crutch, the canes used for medical purposes are often made of hardwood or aluminum.

The fitting of the crutch depends on the individual requirements. However, the most prevalent type of fitting is one in which the measurement is taken from 1 inch below the axillary fold to the bottom of the shoe heel. At all times, accessory rubber arm pieces and tips must be taken into account in the measurement. The hand grip is fixed at a point whereby the elbow is flexed in about a 30-degree angle, the wrist is dorsiflexed fully, and the hand is gripped into a fist. The cane, on the other hand, is measured from the top of the greater trochanter to the floor. In this position, the elbow is flexed about 30 to 40 degrees, according to the patient's particular requirements.

Crutch and cane ambulation are motor skills that require a great deal of physical fitness, along with body control and balance. As in any other motor skill, some individuals have a greater potential than others. It has been suggested that individuals using the crutch or cane to any extent should learn as many different gaits as possible in order to be able to adapt to a variety of situations. In the hospital setting, the patient who needs to learn to walk on crutches will go through a progression of developmental activities, all designed to provide him with strength, balance, and control. Each learned skill is designed to progress to a higher level until ambulation is attained. The progression, in many instances, moves from bed exercises to mat exercises and then continues to standing exercises that provide balance and confidence.

Crutch walking includes two basic types of gait, namely, the point gaits and the swing-through gait. The point gaits are divided into three types: the two point, the three point, and the four point. The two-point gait uses the crutch by moving either the crutch and foot on the same side together or the crutch and the foot on the opposite side (Fig. IV-1). The three-point gait is used by crutch walkers who have the use of one leg that can fully support their weight. While balancing on the nonaffected leg, he moves the crutches forward together. The nonaffected leg then steps through ahead of the planted crutches (Fig. IV-2). In the four-point gait, the right crutch moves forward, then the left foot; then the left crutch advances, followed by the right foot (Fig. IV-3). The swing-through gait, on the other hand, requires greater strength and balance. In the swing-through gait, both crutches are placed ahead of the patient's feet and then the body is swung through to a point ahead of the crutches (Fig. IV-4). The crutches are then recovered and returned to a position ahead of the patient's feet.

In temporary disabilities of the lower limbs, the three-point gait is often used. The patient can either swing to the crutches or swing through, depending on the nature of the disability and his particular requirements. From crutch ambulation, patients may progress to two canes and then to single-cane walking when they are able to engage in limited weight bearing. The most stable technique for the single cane is when it is held in the hand opposite the affected side. However, this rule can be varied according to the nature of the patient's disability.

Once the basis of a gait has been learned, the patient may strive to overcome a variety of obstacles such as hill or ramp walking and ascending or descending curbs and stairs. The principles and methods of these skills can be found in a number of articles and books on the subject.

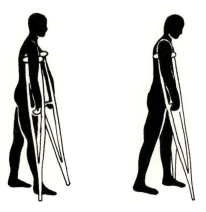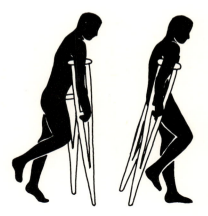

Fig. IV-1. Two-point gait.   **Fig. IV-2.** Three-point gait.

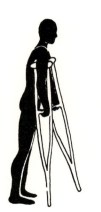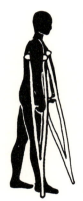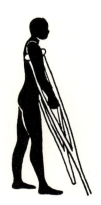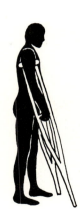

Fig. IV-3. Four-point gait.

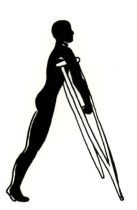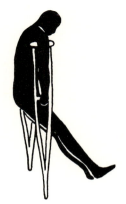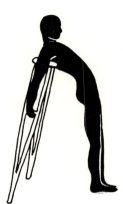

Fig. IV-4. Swing-through gait.

INDEX